TEMPORAL INFORMATION PROCESSING IN THE NERVOUS SYSTEM
SPECIAL REFERENCE TO DYSLEXIA AND DYSPHASIA

ANNALS OF THE NEW YORK ACADEMY OF SCIENCES
Volume 682

TEMPORAL INFORMATION PROCESSING IN THE NERVOUS SYSTEM
SPECIAL REFERENCE TO DYSLEXIA AND DYSPHASIA

Edited by Paula Tallal, Albert M. Galaburda, Rodolfo R. Llinás, and Curt von Euler

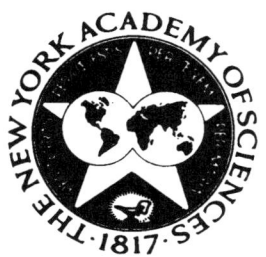

The New York Academy of Sciences
New York, New York
1993

Copyright © 1993 by the New York Academy of Sciences. All rights reserved. Under the provisions of the United States Copyright Act of 1976, individual readers of the Annals are permitted to make fair use of the material in them for teaching or research. Permission is granted to quote from the Annals provided that the customary acknowledgment is made of the source. Material in the Annals may be republished only by permission of the Academy. Address inquiries to the Executive Editor at the New York Academy of Sciences.

Copying fees: *For each copy of an article made beyond the free copying permitted under Section 107 or 108 of the 1976 Copyright Act, a fee should be paid through the Copyright Clearance Center, Inc., 27 Congress Street, Salem, MA 01970. For articles of more than 3 pages, the copying fee is $1.75.*

∞ *The paper used in this publication meets the minimum requirements of American National Standard for Information Sciences—Permanence of Paper for Printed Library Materials, ANSI Z39.48-1984.*

Library of Congress Cataloging-in-Publication Data

Temporal information processing in the nervous system : special
  reference to dyslexia and dysphasia / edited by Paula Tallal, Albert
  M. Galaburda, Rodolfo R. Llinás, and Curt von Euler.
    p. cm. — (Annals of the New York Academy of Sciences, ISSN
  00778923 ; v. 682).
    Includes bibliographical references and index.
    ISBN 0-89766-785-9 (cloth : alk. paper). — ISBN 0-89766-786-7
  (paper : alk. paper)
    1. Language disorders—Pathophysiology—Congresses. 2. Temporal
  lobes—Pathophysiology—Congresses. I. Tallal, Paula, 1947-
  II. Galaburda, Albert M., 1948- . III. Llinás, Rodolfo R., 1934- . IV. Euler, Curt von,
  1918- . V. Series.
    [DNLM: 1. Aphasia—physiopathology—congresses. 2. Dyslexia—
  physiopathology—congresses. 3. Temporal Lobe—physiopathology—
  congresses. W1 AN626YL v.682 1993 / WL 340.5 T288 1992]
  Q11.N5 vol. 682
  [RC423]
  500 s—dc20
  [616.85'5]
  DNLM/DLC
  for Library of Congress   93-17625
                                                                                             CIP

A & PCP
Printed in the United States of America
ISBN 0-89766-785-9 (cloth)
ISBN 0-89766-786-7 (paper)
ISSN 0077-8923

ANNALS OF THE NEW YORK ACADEMY OF SCIENCES

Volume 682
June 14, 1993

TEMPORAL INFORMATION PROCESSING IN THE NERVOUS SYSTEM: SPECIAL REFERENCE TO DYSLEXIA AND DYSPHASIA[a]

Editors
PAULA TALLAL, ALBERT M. GALABURDA, RODOLFO R. LLINÁS, AND CURT VON EULER

Conference Organizers
CURT VON EULER, PER UDDÉN, PAULA TALLAL, RODOLFO R. LLINÁS, ALBERT M. GALABURDA

CONTENTS

Preface. By PAULA TALLAL ix

Keynotes

Neural Mechanisms Underlying Temporal Intregration, Segmentation, and Input Sequence Representation: Some Implications for the Origin of Learning Disabilities. By MICHAEL M. MERZENICH, CHRISTOPH SCHREINER, WILLIAM JENKINS, AND XIAOQIN WANG... 1

A Neurologist's Overview of Developmental Dyslexia. By MARTHA BRIDGE DENCKLA... 23

Part I. The Case for a Basic Temporal Processing Disorder in Dysphasia and Dyslexia

Neurobiological Basis of Speech: A Case for the Preeminence of Temporal Processing. By PAULA TALLAL, STEVE MILLER, AND ROSLYN HOLLY FITCH..................... 27

Is Dyslexia a Dyschronia? By RODOLFO LLINÁS 48

Weakness in the Transient Visual System: A Causal Factor in Dyslexia? By WILLIAM LOVEGROVE 57

Evidence for a Magnocellular Defect in Developmental Dyslexia. By ALBERT GALABURDA AND MARGARET LIVINGSTONE 70

Dyslexia—Impaired Temporal Information Processing? By JOHN STEIN 83

Impaired Temporal Resolution in Developmental Dyslexia. By PETER H. WOLFF 87

[a]This volume is the result of a conference entitled Temporal Information Processing in the Nervous System: Special Reference to Dyslexia and Dysphasia, held in New York City from September 12 to 15, 1992, cosponsored by the Rodin Remediation Academy and the New York Academy of Sciences.

Part II. Temporal Processing in the Auditory System

Neural Representation of Stimulus Times in the Primary Auditory Cortex. *By* DENNIS P. PHILLIPS 104

Temporal Analysis in Normal and Impaired Hearing. *By* BRIAN C. J. MOORE 119

Temporal Auditory Processing in Infancy. *By* SANDRA E. TREHUB 137

Part III. Temporal Processing in Visual and Somatosensory Systems

Temporal Order Determinants in a Somesthetic Frequency Discrimination: Sequential Order Coding. *By* VERNON B. MOUNTCASTLE 150

Temporal Processing in the Visual Brain. *By* RALPH M. SIEGEL AND HEATHER L. READ .. 171

Part IV. Temporal Processing in Motor Systems

Spatiotemporal Motor Processing. *By* JAMES ASHE AND APOSTOLOS P. GEORGOPOULOS ... 179

Neural Disorders of the Linguistic Use of Space and Movement. *By* HOWARD POIZNER AND JUDY KEGL 192

Cerebellar Involvement in the Explicit Representation of Temporal Information. *By* RICHARD IVRY 214

Control of Binocular Eye Movements in Normals and Dyslexics. *By* GUNNAR LENNERSTRAND, JAN YGGE, AND CHRISTER JACOBSSON 231

Part V. Language

Language Functions Related to Prefrontal Cortical Activity: Neurolinguistic Implications. *By* DAVID H. INGVAR 240

Developmental Speech Perception: Implications for Models of Language Impairment. *By* PATRICIA K. KUHL 248

In Speech Perception, Time Is Not What It Seems. *By* ALVIN M. LIBERMAN 264

Understanding Compressed Sentences: The Role of Rhythm and Meaning. *By* JACQUES MEHLER, NURIA SEBASTIAN, GERRY ALTMANN, EMMANUEL DUPOUX, ANNE CHRISTOPHE, AND CHRISTOPHE PALLIER 272

Timing in Speech Production with Special Reference to Word Form Encoding. *By* WILLEM J. M. LEVELT 283

Award Lecture

Phonological Skills and Learning to Read. *By* USHA GOSWAMI 296

Poster Papers

An Operant Conditioning Paradigm for Assessing Auditory Temporal Processing in 6- to 9-Month-Old Infants. *By* APRIL ANN BENASICH AND PAULA TALLAL 312

Successive Information Processing Strategies: WISC-R Sequential Scores and Reading. *By* HADASSAH WEITZMAN BENNETT 315

Effects of Naming Speed Differences on Fluency of Reading after Practice. *By* PATRICIA GREIG BOWERS AND ALLISON KENNEDY 318

Short-circuiting Phonological Limitations in Dyslexia: The Beneficial Effect of Accelerated Reading Pace. *By* ZVIA BREZNITZ 321

Language and Memory in Children with Combined Complex-Partial Epilepsy and Reading Disorder. *By* MELINDA BROMAN 323

Magnocellular Visual Deficits Affect Temporal Processing of Dyslexics. *By* CHRIS CHASE AND ANNETTE R. JENNER 326

Flicker Contrast Sensitivity and the Dunlop Test in Reading-disabled Children. *By* PIERS CORNELISSEN, ALEXANDRA MASON, SUE FOWLER, AND JOHN STEIN............ 330

Alertness: Vigilance and Wakefulness in Developmental Disorders of Reading and Attention. *By* DRAKE D. DUANE.. 333

Dyslexia: A Study of Preserved and Impaired Visuospatial and Phonological Functions. *By* G. F. EDEN, J. F. STEIN, M. H. WOOD, AND F. B. WOOD 335

Auditory and Visual Temporal Processing in Dyslexic and Normal Readers. *By* MARY E. FARMER AND RAYMOND KLEIN 339

Event-related Potentials and Dyslexia. *By* A. J. FAWCETT, A. K. CHATTOPADHYAY, R. H. KANDLER, J. A. JARRATT, R. I. NICOLSON, AND M. PROCTOR 342

Left Hemisphere Specialization for Auditory Temporal Processing in Rats. *By* ROSLYN HOLLY FITCH, CHRISTINE P. BROWN, AND PAULA TALLAL 346

Differential Diagnosis between Learning-disabled and Dysphasic Children. *By* J. FORTIN, J. G. DUDLEY, AND Y. JOANETTE 348

Do Adult Dyslexics Show Low-level Visual Processing Deficits? *By* S. HAYDUK, M. BRUCK, AND P. CAVANAGH 351

Visual Word Recognition in Developmental Dysgraphia: One Lexicon or Two? *By* JAMES M. HODGSON AND GRETCHEN JOHNSON 354

Automaticity and Reading in Learning-disabled College Students. *By* TERESA ANN HUTCHENS 357

Naming and Gesture by Normal and Language-impaired Children: Evidence from a Modified Rapid Automatized Naming Test. *By* WILLIAM F. KATZ, SUSAN CURTISS, AND PAULA TALLAL 359

An Investigation of Frontal Executive Dysfunction in Attention Deficit Disorder Subgroups. *By* SARAH L. KEMP AND URSULA KIRK 363

Deficits in Auditory Sequential Processing found for Both Gifted and Average IQ Reading-impaired Boys. *By* R. HARTER KRAFT..................................... 366

Toward Objective Measurements of Physical versus Mental Overload or Subjective Fatigue when Performing Sequential Eye Scanning and Reading Tasks. *By* E. CHRISTINE KRIS... 369

Auditory–Brainstem Synchronicity in Dyslexia Measured Using the REPs/ABR Protocol. *By* JUDITH L. LAUTER AND SUZANNE B. WOOD........................ 377

Assessing Reading Skills with a Computer-aided Set of Tests Based on the Dual-route Theory of Reading. *By* H. LYYTINEN, S. HAVU, S. LEINONEN, E. HOLOPAINEN, M. ARO, AND T. AHONEN 380

Visible Persistence in Developmental Dyslexia *By* FRANCISCO J. MARTOS AND ANTONIO MARMOLEJO... 383

Children with Dyslexia Classify Pure Tones Slowly. *By* RODERICK I. NICOLSON AND ANGELA J. FAWCETT 387

Children with Dyslexia Automatize Temporal Skills More Slowly. *By* RODERICK I. NICOLSON AND ANGELA J. FAWCETT 390

Innovative Visual–Spatial Powers in Dyslexics: A New Perspective? *By* S. E. PARKINSON AND J. H. EDWARDS 393

Ophthalmologic Aspects of Dyslexia: The Influence of Full Prismatic Correction of Heterophoria on Dyslexic Symptoms. *By* D. PESTALOZZI 397

Dyslexia, Schizotypy, and Visual Direction Sense. *By* A. J. RICHARDSON AND J. F. STEIN 400

Associations of Dyslexia with Epilepsy, Handedness, and Gender. *By* STEVEN C. SCHACHTER, ALBERT M. GALABURDA, AND BERNARD J. RANSIL 402

Correlation of Ocular Motor Reading Strategies to the Status of Adaptation in Patients with Hemianopic Visual Field Defects. *By* DIETER SCHOEPF AND WOLFGANG H. ZANGEMEISTER 404

The Performance of Good and Poor Readers on Simultaneous and Temporal–Sequential Memory Tasks. *By* ANN M. STAUNTON 409

Frequency Modulation Analysis in Children with Landau-Kleffner Syndrome. *By* GERRY A. STEFANATOS 412

Temporal Encoding of Phonetic Features in Auditory Cortex. *By* M. STEINSCHNEIDER, C. E. SCHROEDER, J. C. AREZZO, AND H. G. VAUGHAN, JR. 415

Auditory Temporal Processing in Relation to Reading and Math Disabilities. *By* BETTY U. WATSON AND CHARLES S. WATSON 418

Auditory Perception, Phonological Processing, and Reading Ability/Disability. *By* BETTY U. WATSON AND CHARLES S. WATSON 421

Temporal Information Processing in Adults with Reading Difficulties. *By* JEAN WHYTE . . 424

Long-term Effects of Rehabilitative Interventions for Dyslexic Children. *By* EVELIN WITRUK 426

Memory Deficits of Dyslexic Children. *By* EVELIN WITRUK 430

The Directional Motor Link in Reading Disabilities. *By* ROWE A. YOUNG AND BENSON E. GINSBURG 436

Index of Contributors 441

Financial assistance was received from:

Supporters
- National Institute for Child Health and Development
- National Institutes on Deafness and Other Communication Disorders
- National Institute of Neurological Disorders and Stroke
- The Rodin Remediation Academy

Contributors
- Hoechst-Roussel Pharmaceutical
- Rita Rudel Foundation

The New York Academy of Sciences believes it has a responsibility to provide an open forum for discussion of scientific questions. The positions taken by the participants in the reported conferences are their own and not necessarily those of the Academy. The Academy has no intent to influence legislation by providing such forums.

Preface

PAULA TALLAL
Center for Molecular and Behavioral Neuroscience
Rutgers University
Newark, New Jersey 07102

Traditionally, developmental disorders of language (dysphasia) and reading (dyslexia) have been viewed as distinct clinical syndromes. But, more recent research findings have suggested a close link between these developmental learning disabilities. First, longitudinal studies have demonstrated that children with developmental language disorders are at very high risk to develop reading disabilities. Second, the neuropsychological profiles, specifically focused in the areas of phonological disorders and specific temporal processing deficits, appear to be quite similar for children with developmental language and reading disorders.

Language and reading disorders have been studied from both a linguistic and neuropsychological perspective. Results of linguistic studies have shown that deficits tend to aggregate at the phonological level, with specific problems in phonological processing and awareness. Neuropyschological and neurophysiological studies have revealed a seeming potpourri of disorders in these children that range from auditory and visual processing deficits to fine motor problems. However, recently it has been suggested that language-impaired children have a specific temporal processing disorder that may underlie both their phonological as well as their neuropyschological deficits, and would be parsimonious with their complex sequalea of behavioral symptomatology.

Temporal mechanisms in the nervous system play a central role in fundamental aspects of information processing and production, and may be especially critical for the normal development and maintenance of sensory motor integration systems as well as phonological systems. The goal of this conference was to integrate research findings pertaining to temporal information processing in the nervous system from divergent areas by bringing together scientists whose research focuses on the neural mechanisms underlying temporal integration, mechanisms underlying phonological processes, and studies with language- and reading-impaired children. It is hoped that these proceedings will serve to integrate the relevant anatomical, physiological, and behavioral data pertaining to temporal information processing in the nervous system, with special reference to temporal dysfunctions in children with developmental language and reading disorders.

Neural Mechanisms Underlying Temporal Integration, Segmentation, and Input Sequence Representation: Some Implications for the Origin of Learning Disabilities[a]

MICHAEL M. MERZENICH,[b] CHRISTOPH SCHREINER,
WILLIAM JENKINS, AND XIAOQIN WANG

*W. M. Keck Center for Integrative Neurosciences
and Coleman Laboratory
University of California at San Francisco
San Francisco, California 94143-0732*

INTRODUCTION

The human brain is a powerful, self-organizing machine that facilely generates and manipulates representations of complex input sequences. There has been little study of the physiological mechanisms accounting for several key temporal aspects of perception and behavior, despite their central relevance to our understanding of the neural bases of human cognition and their probable contributions to abnormal operations in special human populations with learning disabilities. Thus, for example, the basic neural mechanisms underlying temporal "integration" and temporal "chunking" or "segmentation" have been incompletely studied. There have been relatively few studies of the representations of temporally sequenced inputs in the brain, and those have been largely limited to piecemeal, single-unit response sampling experiments, or to evoked potential or electroencephalogram (EEG) studies. There have been only a few physiological studies examining the specific conditions under which qualitatively different, temporally simultaneous, and temporally separated stimuli are integrated or are represented categorically, respectively. There has been little specific examination of the nature of distributed neuronal changes accounting for learned, temporally sequenced behaviors underlying the remarkable self-organization of brain function operating throughout a lifetime, but most powerfully in childhood. Finally, there has been little consideration of how what is known about these aspects of dynamic brain function and its ontogeny might account for or relate to the ontogenetic origins of learning disabilities, or to functional brain illnesses.

In this review, we briefly consider our current state of understanding of these important issues of integrative neuroscience from the admittedly limited perspective of our own experiments conducted principally in the somatosensory, auditory, and

---

[a]This research was supported by National Institutes of Health Grant NS-10414, Office of Naval Research Grant 00014-91-J-1317, the Coleman Fund, the Kleberg Foundation, and Hearing Research, Inc.
[b]To whom correspondence should be addressed.

motor cortices. We outline specific hypotheses about the neural origins of psychophysically measured temporal integration, temporal segmentation, and their plasticity. We shall consider basic rules underlying behaviorally and cortically manifested experience-dependent refinement of stimulus representations, and outline some of the principles underlying dynamic cortical contributions to learning. With this background, we then state two testable hypotheses about the causes of abnormal temporal forebrain operations in learning-disabled and other special human populations.

SOME PSYCHOLOGICAL AND NEUROPSYCHOLOGICAL PREMISES

Psychophysical Measures of Temporal Integration and Segmentation

Psychophysicists have measured temporal integration periods for detection of a wide variety of inputs, in all sensory systems. In one psychophysical perspective, the temporal integration period is defined by the minimal duration of a specific, detected stimulus. In another perspective, the temporal integration period is the time epoch over which new inputs can add information to a perceived stimulus event. These basic nervous system processing times have been measured many times in many specific experiments in vision, hearing, and somatosensation.[1-5]

One alternative measure that has been used extensively to measure the basic central nervous system "minimal processing time" or "temporal segmentation time" is the time separation of a stimulus and a following masker requisite for its detection or recognition (called the *stimulus-to-masker asynchrony,* or SOA). In that measure, a briefly applied stimulus is detected only if it is not backward-masked after a liminal post-onset time or post-stimulus-offset no-masker period. The fact that a time period must pass before the arrival of an interfering masker for a signal to be reliably detected or recognized has been interpreted to manifest a requisite time for forebrain "processing" of inputs that commonly extends from tens to hundreds of milliseconds after a brief stimulus.[6,9]

A third, related psychophysical strategy for measuring the brain's processing of temporal chunks has employed tests of the identification of the temporal order of—or the identification of separate elements of—two- to many-component input series (e.g., see P. Tallal[10] and B. Moore,[11] this volume). In highly trained subjects operating in audition[10,11] or somatosensation,[12,13] for example, the spectral identity of sequenced input "segments" or "chunks" can be identified if they are about 20 ms or longer in duration. Much longer stimuli must be applied for correct identification of stimulus order, as a rule, in untrained individuals. In vision, equivalent estimations of temporal segmentation times have come from measures of the persistences of brief stimuli, usually estimated by the use of periodically flashed stimuli.[14,15] Similar stimulus persistence experiments conducted in hearing have measured the temporal conditions under which periodic stimuli are perceived as continuous,[16] or otherwise modify temporally neighboring percepts.[17,18]

Some Features of Perceptual Integration Times

1. *This base integration period reflects cerebral cortex processing times. It does not vary with stimulus complexity. On the other hand, stimulus recognition times differ for tasks of different cognitive complexity.* Studies conducted in vision and in

somesthesis indicate that stimulus persistences and backward masking periods are equivalent for spatially simple and spatially complex stimuli.[19,20] That finding has been interpreted as indicating that the basic temporal smoothing represented by stimulus persistence and perturbed by backward masking occurs relatively early in sensory system processing, in the domain of "primitive" or "preattentive" vision or somesthesis.[21–23] From a number of arguments considering stimulus feature representation at different sensory system levels, preattentive vision and somestheses are believed to arise from primary sensory cortical fields (e.g., see Julesz;[22] Karni and Sagi[24]). At the same time, complex-stimulus recognition requires longer processing times. Prolonged times are attributable in part to the accumulated base integration times that apply to the multiple levels of sensory systems that must be engaged to account for complex image or sound recognition. Thus, for example, the orientation, color, and basic geometrical features of visual "primitives" are recognized separately as integrated features for stimuli flashed in the visual field for a few tens of milliseconds. By contrast, the recognition of transparent motion stimuli believed to require the engagement of a second-level visual cortical field requires several hundreds of milliseconds; while recognition of shape from motion, a task that requires processing of visual information at three or four hierarchical levels, requires many hundreds of milliseconds of processing to emerge.[25] In this example, direct physiological evidence indicates that the overall time required to make progressively more complicated distinctions about these moving visual stimuli partly reflect requirements for successive input sampling for feature extraction, and reflect the base integration periods of the two or three or four essentially engaged cortical fields. At the same time, when the searching of a complex visual image is required for its recognition,[21] the time to recognition must reflect the sums of base integration periods of the preattentive visual process that makes up the search.

2. *Integration "channels."* Within the limits of a base integration or segmentation time, parallel-channel inputs can be added perceptually without substantial interferences. Thus, for example, while color, form, and stereopsis are represented by different neuronal populations that are extracted in parallel with one another, such feature combinations are simultaneously attributable to objects presented to vision within a base time period. Outside of that base time, they are separately perceived and referred.[26] Integration and time chunking are also achieved by input location-specific channels. Thus, to cite one of many examples, successive binaural clicks with shared spectral properties contribute to an improvement of their localization following a square root of 2 integration rule.[27] However, they do not affect the localization of clicks that fall spectrally more than one critical band away in frequency, even when those alternate stimuli are presented in a temporally interleaved stimulus sequence.

3. *Interruption of integration by novel stimuli.* As previously noted, one way to halt integration is by the application of appropriate novel sensory inputs. Backward maskers represent one class of interrupting stimuli. In the auditory realm, that interruption has been demonstrated to apply to the ongoing integration process. Thus, for example, the binaural localization of a train of clicks improves continuously following a square root of 2 rule over a roughly 200–250-ms-long integration time period. If integration is interrupted by introducing a distractor—for example, a tone or noise—at an earlier time, the precision in perceptual location is determined by the number of clicks that preceded the distractor.[28] Such studies (also see Darwin and Ciocca[29]) indicate that the integration process is begun with the introduction of any new input, but can be reset by appropriate, novel subsequent stimuli.

4. *Plasticity of integration time and stimulus onset asynchronies.* One of the most surprising features of base perceptual integration and segmentation periods are their apparent plasticity. Thus, for example, stimulus onset asynchronies (SOAs) representing visual primitives in a limited part of the visual field can be reduced to a fraction of their pretraining durations over a 1- to 2-week practice period.[24,30] Consistent with their relatively "early" representation in the cortex, those severalfold changes in measured integration periods do not apply to other parts of the visual field or to the representation of other visual primitives, that is, they are specific to the submodal and retinal location "channels" that have been trained. Evidence for location-specific shortening of temporal segmentation times has also been recorded in studies of training-dependent changes in the durations of stimuli whose orientations are correctly identified.[31] In a related classical study, the durations of displaced letters required for their recognition were found to be subject to significant learning effects.[32] It might be noted that such perceptual plasticity of temporal integration or chunking phenomena apparently applies to many other aspects of visual acuity, stereopsis, and recognition (e.g., see Gibson;[33] Bruce and Low;[34] Poggio *et al.*;[35] among many others).

In hearing, durations of detected tones and noises can be shortened 3- to 4-fold by practice.[36] Detection of the order of sequenced acoustic inputs are subject to similar training effects.[11] In both behaviors, shortened integration times do not apply to other, untrained frequency domains. In somestheses, we have recently recorded dramatic changes in behaviorally estimated integration times for vibratory stimuli applied to surfaces of the hands of New World owl monkeys[37] (also see Zwislocki *et al.*[38]), again consistent with a capacity for severalfold improvement in integration time with practice in this modality. As in the visual case, that improvement is limited to a spatial channel, that is, to the behaviorally engaged skin and a limited surrounding skin domain. Recorded training-dependent improvements in a variety of other tasks involving detection or discrimination of the most fundamental level have also been documented in somestheses and hearing.[32,39–42]

5. *Ontogenetic shortening of time chunking.* Measures of visual persistence shorten substantially through the course of ontogenetic development.[42] Similarly, basic measures of integration periods, temporal perturbation effects, and segmentation in audition shorten progressively through infancy and early childhood.[43–45] The progressive improvements of many other response distinctions have now been tracked in early childhood. Not surprisingly, nearly *all* have been found to undergo progressive improvement or refinement over tested infancy/early childhood periods (e.g., see Kuhl;[46] Aslin and Smith;[47] Chandna[48]).

Such studies have lead to the general conclusion that subnormal performance in temporal order judgment tasks and in other measures of temporal integration or segmentation times in dysphasic or dyslexic children might reflect a failure in the developmental refinement of temporal processing capabilities. Consistent with that general view, temporal response characteristics for primary visual cortical neurons are substantially degraded in young environmentally deprived animal models, consistent with their having a poor ability to represent rapidly temporally sequenced inputs.[49] However, the effects of such sensory deprivation are not selective for temporal discrimination effects, but appear to apply to *all* aspects of sensation and perception that are subject to performance gains with experience (see Beaulieu and Cynader,[49,50] for review). Thus, while the overall recorded neurological consequences of severe early deprivation include degradation of temporal integration and segmentation capabilities, they extend nonselectively to include virtually every other measured aspects of fundamental stimulus feature representation.

Abnormal Integration Periods and Temporal Segmentation in "Learning-disabled" Human Populations

Previously cited studies indicate that there is a base short integration period and temporal segmentation for identifying stimulus primitives that are: (a) at least roughly equivalent in all sensory systems; (b) progressively shortens in early child development; (c) can be altered throughout life by a period of experience that engages any part of any sensory system; and (d) can be massively degraded along with other basic sensory capabilities by a prolonged early period of experiential deprivation.

The capacity for behavioral plasticity of integration and segmentation periods is important for consideration here because measures of integration times and temporal chunking are found to be abnormal in a number of clinically important human populations. In general, integration times and stimulus persistence measures are significantly longer than normal in several well-studied populations of learning-impaired individuals including dyslexics.[51-55] Integration and segmentation times also appear to be abnormal in at least some hyperlexic, autistic, and schizophrenic individuals.[56,57] An understanding of the origins of cortical integration periods and of possible mechanisms accounting for their plasticity may obviously be important for understanding the origins of these dysfunctional conditions. In this review, we ask: (a) What is the fundamental basis for the nervous system's generation of detectable and recognizable input time chunks? (b) What controls the time duration of the basic detectable and recognizable input chunk? (c) What mechanisms might underlie the experience-dependent shortening of this basic forebrain process? (d) Could relatively poor temporal segmentation of inputs be learned in ontogenetic brain self-organization? (e) How could a practiced behavioral strategy arising in early childhood plausibly underlie the widespread functional manifestations of abnormal temporal processing recorded in dyslexic and auditory language-disabled individuals? (f) Could a defect in the learning machinery account for the panoply of functional signs that mark a language-disabled individual? (g) What single defect might plausibly explain these signs?

SOME RELEVANT NEUROPHYSIOLOGICAL STUDIES

A Methodological Problem: Adaptive Changes in the Brain Underlying Learning Are Distributed

Why have we not made more progress in understanding how representations of behaviors like reading or speech reception are generated by, and altered in the learning brain? Certainly progress in understanding the neural origins of speech reception have been restrained by the arguments that speech and language reception are not specifically sensory and are uniquely human enterprises, and can therefore not be directly studied in animal models (see Lieberman,[58] this volume). While these issues cannot be reviewed in detail in this context, our perspective is that other mammals have the ability to make equivalent distinctions about complex acoustic stimuli including speech features, if they are trained to do so. There is almost certainly nothing fundamentally unique about speech nor about the basic mechanisms that operate in the cortex that represents it. But while many aspects of its ontogenetic origins can be powerfully studied in animal models, in fact very few have been conducted, and those have been of a limited nature and have primarily involved the study of anesthetized experimental preparations.

A fundamental technical problem that has also limited progress is that these brain operations are distributed widely in the forebrain, in two respects. First, even the simplest of learned behaviors generate changes in several to many of the 60–80 human cortical areas. Second, in a cortical zone engaged by inputs important to learning in any one of these areas, neurons are directly interconnected to thousands or tens of thousands of other neurons, and indirectly to millions or tens or hundreds of millions of others. Therefore, (a) stimuli are represented by *distributed* neuronal populations; (b) to reconstruct the very complex representations of multiple-component and time-varying signals like speech elements, speech strings, or scanned orthographic word strings, we must "map" engaged cortical areas completely, and in fine detail; and (c) because the effectiveness of specific, complex interconnections between neurons in the cortical mantle and the thalamus are altered by their behavioral engagement, documentation of learning-induced changes must include a reconstruction of this altered internal functional rewiring.

Thus, one important technical challenge faced by cortical physiologists is the task of reconstruction of distributed cortical representations as they change in learning, on the appropriate spatial scale of the dynamic processes of the neocortex. In practice, neuronal responses must be sampled over a narrow time window in relatively fine grain over a relatively large cortical zone in order to reconstruct changes generated by learning involving even the simplest of stimuli—in even a single cortical area. Most of our own experiments have been conducted in the "primary" somatosensory cortex, specifically because the anatomical projection system delivering inputs into this zone is relatively simple and because extrinsic inputs into that zone are anatomically limited in their spreads, permitting easier reconstruction of the distributed representations of relatively simple stimuli. Other studies conducted in the more complexly organized primary auditory and motor cortices confirm and extend basic findings derived in somatosensory cortex.

Cortical Representational Plasticity: Some Implications for The Ontogeny of Human Behavior

Studies conducted over the past decade have revealed that cortical representations of even the simplest features of sensory stimuli *including the spatiotemporal representations of sequenced inputs* are continuously shaped in detail, by our experiences. Those modifications of the details of sensory representations involve input time-dependent modification of synaptic effectivenesses, both for the afferent inputs delivered into a particular cortical field, and for the intrinsic connections within the cortex (see Merzenich *et al.*,[59-61] for review). Considered in detail, topographic cortical representations of the ear or skin (and presumably, of the retina) are actually time-based constructs, and can be modified at any point in life by changing the weights and sources of temporally correlated inputs. This capacity for modification by experience is limited by the sources and spreads of inputs delivered into any given cortical location, and by competitive influences from inputs delivered into neighboring cortical zones. Representational remodeling also requires that the input be attended; the rate at which it occurs appears to relate to the strength of the cognitive weighting of its significance or correctness. In any event, the time course of changes relate directly to the time course of learning in any given behavioral paradigm. These adaptive changes in distributed cortical responses and cortical cell assemblies must collectively constitute *the* cortical contribution to learning and nondeclarative memory.

To illustrate some aspects of the nature of these changes by a single example, consider the representation of the cochlea or of represented sound frequency in a monkey trained to discriminate differences in frequency.[62] In the example illustrated in FIGURE 1, an adult owl monkey was trained to distinguish frequencies above a 2500-Hz reference frequency in a go/no-go behavioral task. Early in training but after the training was under control, with the animal making few false-positive responses, this monkey could not detect frequency differences of less than about 170 Hz (see FIG. 1A). The animal learned to make progressively finer distinctions as training progressed, so that by the ninety-fifth training session, approximately 20-Hz differences could be detected. At that point, a detailed map reconstruction of the neural representation of sound frequencies within cortical field A1 was recorded. In that reconstruction, the zone of representation of the range of frequencies over which the animal was trained (FIG. 1B) was enlarged severalfold, when compared with control monkeys (FIG. 1C). When we reconstructed sequences of frequency representation within these enlarged zones, very fine shifts in represented frequency were now recorded as a function of cortical location across them (FIG. 1D). In a series of these monkeys, the changes in the territories of representation of the frequencies applied in training were directly correlated with the achieved discriminable differences. Data were consistent with the hypothesis that this finer grained representation resulted in a spatially distinct population being engaged by now-smaller frequency differences.

Note that this experiment reconstructed changes driven within only a single cortical field, the primary auditory cortex, A1. This representation of sound frequency is probably the least mutable of auditory zones, as indicated by its relatively topographically restricted spreads of anatomical inputs, by its relatively predictable representational topography in untrained animals, and by classical conditioning auditory experiments that reveal that far larger and faster changes are induced in several other "secondary" cortical fields in that behavioral context.[63] In any event, behavioral training in even simple forms like this drives representational changes in most if not every cortical field that we study in the given modality. Thus, these changes in A1 almost certainly represent only a fraction of the forebrain zone that is driven to change by this behavior.

Similar representational modeling experiments have been conducted in adult monkeys in which always-innervated islands of skin have been moved to new locations across the hand;[59-61] in both sensory and motor cortical areas in monkeys trained in a pellet retrieval task;[60,64] in monkeys trained in a tactile frequency discrimination task;[65,66] in monkeys trained in a skin pressure regulation task;[67] in monkeys performing limb withdrawals signaled by a tactile cue;[68] in monkeys with restricted profound peripheral input deprivation;[69,70] among many other input manipulations and behaviors (see Merzenich et al.[59]). In these various studies (a) substantial cortical representational remodeling was generated in every case; (b) representational changes were related specifically to stimuli, movements, and responses that applied for the behavior; (c) changes were governed by input timing, that is, were generated by differences in the schedules of temporally nearly simultaneous inputs; (d) when inputs were separated with regard to source and time, changes appeared to involve powerful competitive processes that could divide cortical territory between those competitors; and (e) in several specific series in which appropriate measures have been derived, recorded changes in given cortical fields account for measured behavioral gains that result from the training.

Thus, a few minutes of behavior a day for a few days or weeks can generate changes on a major scale in many cortical areas in the somatosensory or auditory or

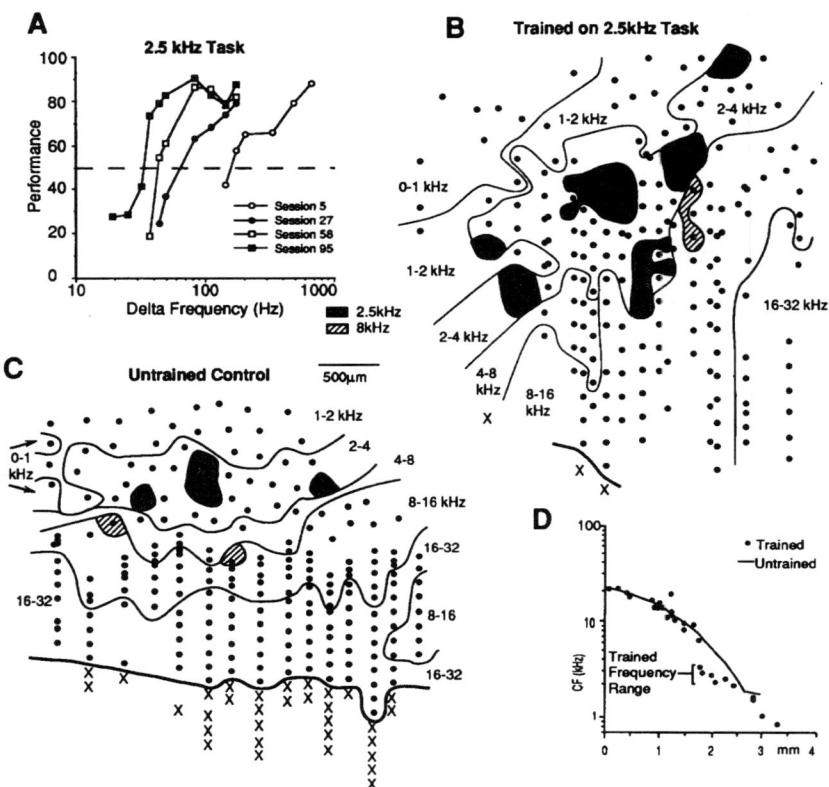

FIGURE 1. A representative primate brain plasticity experiment. An adult owl monkey was trained to discriminate differences in sound frequency around a 2.5-kHz standard (**A**). Once the monkey learned the task and performed it with few false positives, psychometric functions (% correct vs. frequency difference) were recorded over 95 subsequent training sessions. The monkey's discriminative abilites improved progressively with practice, with a roughly 8X finer distinction between frequencies made by the ninety-fifth training session. Neuronal responses in the primary auditory cortical field (A1) were subsequently mapped in detail (**B**). There, *dots* represent neuronal sample sites within A1; *X*'s are sampled sites outside A1. The territory of representation of the trained frequencies (*shaded*), here understated in a unit "best frequency" map, was found to be greatly enlarged in the trained monkey's cortex, as compared with a second, controlled frequency range centered around 8 kHz (*hatching*) or as compared with a normal control (**C**). As a consequence of this expansion of the territory of representation of the trained frequencies, this specific frequency domain came to be represented in finer grain, as is indicated by a purturbation of the function describing the rate of change of represented frequency as a function of position across the frequency representational dimension of A1 (**D**). From the study of a series of these trained monkeys, it was concluded that this emergent, finer grained representation likely accounted for the training-induced gains in frequency discrimination. Every simple behavior that we have assessed by this experimental approach has revealed brain plasticity origins of training-induced behavioral gains. (Figure adapted from Recanzone *et al.*[62])

motor cortical areas in an adult nervous system. What must be the power of the rapidly growing numbers of repetitions of phonemes or detailed spatial visual scenes or motoric rehearsals that apply to the developing forebrains of young children? By the time they begin school, most children have had hundreds of thousands or millions of repetitions of behaviorally important stimuli that might be expected to generate temporally integrated representational constructs and competitive categorical representational constructs in their nervous systems.

Integration Time Periods and Distributed Temporal Response Plasticity in the Neocortex

When repetitive stimuli are delivered into a small sector of the cortical network in a monkey trained to discriminate differences in stimulus rate or frequency, several important changes in the distributed cortical representation of those stimuli occur. Among them, *the cortical network generates a progressively more temporally coherent distributed representation of the stimulus elements of the sequence.*[66,71] In the top panels of FIGURE 2A, the combined responses of *all* the cortical sites representing stimuli delivered at two different frequencies differing (20 and 26 Hz) for a trained finger location are shown from one monkey experiment. In the bottom panels of FIGURE 2A, the responses of all of the sites representing stimuli delivered at the same two frequencies for an adjacent, untrained digit site are shown. In the task in which this monkey was trained, the brain's job was to determine whether the second frequency was higher than the first. Not surprisingly, performance was better for the trained than for the untrained site. The crucial difference lay with the distributed response coherence, which was progressively strengthened by the behavioral training. That difference in population coherence was strongly correlated with the behavioral threshold (FIG. 2B), and almost certainly accounted for the improvements in these animals' behavioral frequency discrimination abilities with practice.[66,71] Other possible contributors, like the sharpness of the temporal responses of individual neurons, the cortical area of representation of these stimuli, the tuning of individual neurons, or the response rates of different neurons, do not change very significantly over this learning period, or were not consistently related to discrimination performance gains.

Consider the implications of this simple result for the representation of input sequences. In a naive individual, the distributed responses generated by a novel input are relatively temporally dispersed. They quickly align temporally with training, to generate a progressively more coherent distributed population neuronal response. As a consequence, a salient signal is generated progressively earlier in time; as coherence grows, the representation of this input becomes progressively less confusable with a following stimulus, and can be distinguished from it if it is presented for a progressively shorter segmentation chunk time. Therefore, with training, temporally finer and finer distinctions between successively presented stimuli can be made.

Formation of Coupled Neuronal Cell Assemblies: Neuronal "Group" Competition

What changes in the cortex likely account for this change in distributed response coherence? Initial studies indicate that it is at least partly due to an increase in

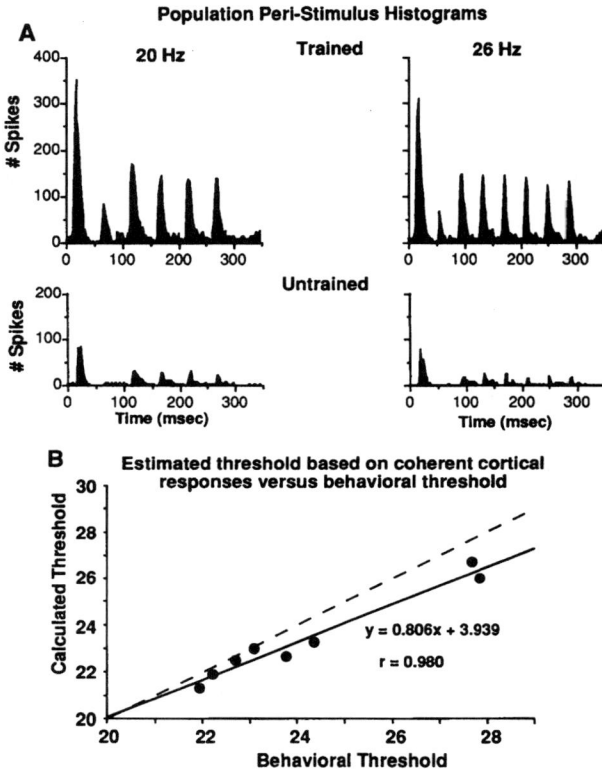

FIGURE 2. Population poststimulus time histograms for neurons sampled all across a primary somatosensory cortical field representing 20-Hz and 26-Hz stimuli, in a monkey trained to distinguish flutter-vibration frequency difference. The responses in the *top panels* are the sum of all responses from a densely sampled map of the hand evoked by vibratory stimuli identical to those used in training, and with the stimulation applied to a *trained* skin site. The reponses in the *bottom panels* in (**A**) are the sum of all distributed responses with identical stimulation at an *untrained* site at the corresponding location on an adjacent finger. The monkey's task was to determine whether or not the frequency represented neurally by the distributed responses shown in the *right column* was higher than (or the same as) the frequency represented in the *left column*. Extensive analyses reveal that *the crucial difference accounting for severalfold performance gains with training was the sharper coherence of representation of individual stimulus events* (**B**).[66] In this series of monkeys, measures of distributed response coherence were correlated with performance gains (**B**) with a correlation coefficient of 0.98. (Figure redrawn from Recanzone *et al.*[66])

positive coupling of neurons that is a probable result of the strengthening of collateral axonal connections between cortical pyramidal cells. That is, when a limited cortical sector is engaged by new inputs, there are plastic changes in the effectivenesses of thalamic inputs delivered into that zone *and* changes in effectivenesses of intracortical connections of those pyramidal cells within a local cortical region.[71–73] When responses from these strongly positively coupled zones are assayed by exciting them with natural stimuli, neurons all across them respond nearly simultaneously to those stimuli. These changes are an instantiation of the classical theorist Donald O. Hebb's two main hypotheses about the changes in cortical synaptic effectivenesses generated in learning to create "representations" of behavior.[74] His first general rule was that inputs that excite neurons when those cells are depolarized will be strengthened. That is another way of saying that two inputs that generate nearly simultaneous volleys into the network will be mutually strengthened; considered in detail, as is now manifested in many experiments,[59] cortical representations are input coincidence-based. His second general rule was that this time-based remodeling of connections will result in the formation, in the cortical network, of newly connected and temporally coherently engaged "cell assemblies" that will specifically represent each newly practiced input combination. These contemporary plasticity experiments reveal that the creation of emergent or remodeled cell assemblies does occur. But further, they reveal that as the synapses between these new cell assemblies progressively strengthen, distributed responses come to be more strongly locked in time, to progressively more coherently and saliently represent the component temporal chunks of the stimulus(i) that induced the network change.

EVIDENCE FOR INTRINSIC (AND EXTRINSIC) CORTICAL "CLOCKS"

1. *Intrinsic oscillators in the cerebral cortex.* One of the more complete studies of temporal response characteristics has come from auditory system investigation of the responses to amplitude modulated stimuli, conducted by Schreiner, Langner and colleagues.[75] Among many other findings, they demonstrated that (a) responses at the level of the auditory nerve to amplitude-modulated (AM) stimuli cannot completely account for the modulation-dependent encoding of the pitches of complex spectra; and (b) an orderly spatial representation of the pitches of complex spectra is generated at the level of the principal midbrain auditory nucleus, the central nucleus of the inferior colliculus. At this subcortical level, neurons representing any given band of sound frequency are distributed across neuronal "isofrequency lamine." Across those functional laminae, predominantly bandpass modulation transfer functions are recorded for the responses of neurons excited by AM stimuli, with neurons at different laminar locations systematically representing "best modulation frequencies" ranging from about 30 Hz to above 1000 Hz.[76] For any given carrier frequency, an orderly representation of best modulation frequency responses spans the normal psychophysical range of periodicity pitch and other complex modulated acoustic signal pitches that apply for that carrier frequency.

Up to and including the thalamic level of the auditory system, some aspects of the spectral and temporal response characteristics of neurons can be *roughly* described by linear spectral–temporal filter relationships.[75] However, a dramatic transformation occurs within the auditory representations in the cerebral cortex. There, neurons have spectral filtering that is similar to that recorded at subcortical levels, and most neurons still have bandpass modulation transfer functions with well-defined "best modulation frequences." However, in the cortex, the best AM frequencies are very low compared with those recorded at subcortical levels. In the primary auditory cortex of cats, for example, they are in the range of about 5 to 25 Hz.[77–79] In one cortical field in the cat, best modulation frequencies (BMFs) can be higher, ranging up to about 100 Hz.[80] However, in most "secondary" auditory cortical fields, BMFs are substantially lower, in the range of 2–5 Hz.[77] Thus, at the level of the auditory cortex, neurons respond strongly to successively presented temporal stimuli only when inputs are "chunked" in time periods (AM cycle lengths) extending from about 50 to 200 ms in cortical field A1, and from about 200 to 500 ms in a series of secondary auditory cortical fields. The shortest of these processing times correspond reasonably well with the minimum durations in which temporal order judgments can be made, and are consistent with the time domains of stimulus persistence or backward masking psychophysical measures recorded in naive human subjects. This A1 temporal chunking is perfectly appropriate for the analysis of inputs at the input rates of speech phonemes. Moreover, the longer best-AM periods of most "secondary" cortical fields blanket the integration time periods appropriate for receiving signals at syllable rates.

During the course of recording these AM response characteristics in auditory cortical fields, Schreiner and Urbas[80] first noted that neurons at many cortical sites had intrinsic oscillations that could be recorded during no-stimulus periods. Moreover, oscillations were often also evoked with application of long unmodulated stimuli, for example, long tonal stimuli. The period of these "intrinsic" oscillations could be determined by autocorrelation. Interestingly, the periods of intrinsic oscillations matched the periods of best-AM stimuli recorded for those same neurons.[78–81] Moreover, corresponding BMFs were also recorded for neurons that exhibited no demonstrable spontaneous oscillations situated above intrinsically oscillating neurons recorded in the same vertical cortical penetrations. *These studies indicate that the time-chunking AM response properties of cortical neurons are influenced by the durations of an intrinsic cortical oscillator.*

Interestingly, with application of novel stimuli, the oscillation phase for the evoked neural responses was reset to zero. This may manifest the neurological basis of the resetting of integration time periods by novel acoustic stimuli reported as a major feature of psychoacoustic studies of temporal integration.[28]

2. *Origins of intrinsic oscillations.* There are several possible sources of these recorded oscillations—and corresponding temporal segmentation stimulus response characteristics—of cortical neurons. First, physiologists have recently discovered a population of neurons in cortical layer 5 with bursting discharge characteristics.[82,83] These large pyramidal cells are coupled to neurons in the layers above, so that with a mild increase in the excitability of a cortical slice, all neurons in a definable cortical "column" have in-phase, periodic bursting discharges. Such studies indicate the presence of an intrinsic cortical "clock" that might bias or control the modulation transfer characteristics of neurons within its particular cortical column. It might be noted that in these models, a number of coupled, bursting neurons probably comprise the "clock" for a given functional column.

There is equally strong evidence that neurons at most cortical locations respond predominantly transiently to new stimuli, with an early excitatory response followed by a period of strong response suppression. In auditory cortex, the timing of excitatory–inhibitory response cycles roughly matches the cycles of intrinsic oscillations or the best modulation frequency for that site.[78,81] It may be that the excitatory modulation contributed by the bursting neurons of layer 5 are strong enough to account for this excitatory–inhibitory cycle, but more likely, intrinsic processes involving sequential excitation-then-inhibition are adapted by mechanisms of plasticity to match—and therefore amplify—the base period contributed by the intrinsic clock.

Other investigators have argued that modulation transfer response characteristics might reflect the operation of intrinsic vertical cortical circuitry. For example, responses in granular and supragranular layers might reverberate through infragranular layers. This and other reverberatory circuitry is certainly in place, and some features of response time in regard to cortical layers recorded in cortical slices and *in vivo* preparations are consistent with this vertical, interlayer cortical reverberation. Again, such circuits may be selected in learning to sharpen temporal representations, and/or may well play a role in amplifying or modulating the base period of an intrinsic cortical clock.

A fourth notion, argued about since the discovery of oscillations of cortical responses in EEG signals many decades ago, is that cortical response oscillations derive from extracortical sources. In classical studies, investigators demonstrated, for example, that cortex could be dominated by oscillatory responses arising in the thalamus during sleep spindle periods. At the same time, it was demonstrated nearly 40 years ago that oscillations can also be recorded in undercut cortex that has no thalamic inputs. These arguments have been resurrected in a modern context by evidence that oscillations in the theta frequency range (25–50 Hz) come from extracortical sources, for example, from the thalamus or hippocampus.[84,85] On the other hand, since the cortex has bursting neurons that can impose temporal chunking response characteristics on the cortical columns they connect with, it has been argued that extrinsic oscillatory inputs may modulate already-present cortical oscillators. This very important issue remains to be clarified.

Are the Base Frequencies of Intrinsic (and Extrinsic) Cortical "Clocks" Plastic?

We have already described one form of temporal sharpening that may relate to the experience-dependent shortening of "temporal chunk" times observed psychophysically. Thus, practice with sequenced inputs results in the generation of more coherent distributed representations of individual stimulus events, which increases their salience and which shortens the time the system requires to identify them, and to separate them from a following masker or distractor or second stimulus. That facet of cortical plasticity may alone account for the plasticity of temporal integration periods, SOAs, pulsation threshold, temporal order judgment, *et alia*. However, the basic temporal segmentation time represented by intrinsic bursting neurons is probably *also* plastic. Thus, for example, Connors and colleagues[83] have shown that a very weak depolarization of these neurons in cortical slices results in significant increases in their burst rates, that is, in a significant shortening of their base clock periods. Changes in input effectivenesses in a cortical column that is differentially engaged by taking up a new behavior would be expected to generate such changes. This important hypothesis is now being tested in animal models, in studies that are ongoing in our laboratories.

Are these two interesting temporal phenomena—that is, best modulation frequency response characteristics probably derived from an intrinsic "clock," and representation of input salience by the distributed response coherence of neurons in the engaged cortical sector—directly linked? In fact, bursting neurons in layer 5 are also coupled by pyramidal cell collaterals, and that coupling is presumably strengthened by any behaviorally important input that selectively engages them. That should result in a positive change in *their* response coherence, and in a progressive increase in the numbers of bursting neurons controlling a given behaviorally exercised column. A second consequence would be that when the behaviorally trained inputs drive the system, these neurons would be more strongly depolarized because of these more coherent connections, which should result in a shortening of their oscillation cycle times. Thus, the same set of plastic changes that generate more coherent—and hence, more easily temporally distinguished—components of temporal sequences hypothetically should also generate changes in the basic "clock" times contributed by intrinsic cortical oscillators. The possible linking of these effects will be resolved in experiments that are now being conducted in our laboratories.

Possible Relationships Between BMF/Intrinsic Oscillation Response Characteristics and Response Bandwidths

In linear systems, there is a direct relationship between input bandwidths and temporal response characteristics. As noted earlier, that condition is roughly maintained in the mammalian auditory system up to the level of the medial geniculate body. In the cortex, there is a highly nonlinear treatment of inputs that are modulated in time. However, it is reasonable to hypothesize that the much slower modulation rates of cortical neurons will still be directly related to spatial bandwidth. In general, the wider the scope of inputs, the more difficult it will be for neurons to generate a strongly coherent representation of incident temporal events, because there should be correspondingly more temporal input dispersion. We have just begun to examine the relationship between input bandwidths and clock periods in cortical field A1. In initial auditory studies, they appear to be related.

Temporal Dispersion of Outputs from First-order Cortical Processing: Implications for Higher Order Processing

Note that the cortical sector representing any given sound frequency in a cortical field like A1 has an orderly representation of neurons with different bandwidths, and a corresponding range of neurons with different best modulation frequencies. That is to say, when a new input is received by A1, its "clocks" are all started roughly in unison; however, the next point at which inputs will be effective will depend upon the unit clock time for each cortical locus, with those times varying in untrained cortex from about 40 ms to about 200 ms. The cortex can provide a strong output representing a second transient input any time over that time period, and it will be fully engaged in representing a second event beyond that time. This constitutes a basis for distributing the representation of a second input in cortical space in a form that permits a selection of inputs for specific temporally sequenced inputs by neurons in higher order cortical areas that have longer chunk times, for example, permitting integration at syllable rates.

Note that this does not mean that cortical neurons cannot selectively represent spectral features that occur in sequence at rates higher than 20–25 events/s. In fact, neurons across the isofrequency representational axis of A1 are *selective* for spectral details like FM sweeps, FM sweep directions, broader spectrum versus narrow-spectrum stimuli, *et alia*,[86] and with training, the cortex can encode and represent them at a level adequate to account for human phonetic discrimination abilities. There is evidence in humans that even the pitches of complex spectra might be represented spatially (not temporally) within the primary auditory cortical field.[87]

The visual cortex also creates an iterative representation of each point on the sensory epithelium in its orderly representation of stimulus bandwidth or "spatial frequency" within primary visual cortex "hypercolumns." This infers that the higher levels of the visual system also treat inputs across a range of "chunk times," again conferring a capacity to create highly selective representations of specific time-varying input sequences.

CONCLUSIONS: HYPOTHESES

From these observations, we proffer two basic testable hypotheses about the origins of speech and language disabilities including dyslexia of central nervous system origin that are marked by longer than normal temporal integration and segmentation period lengths that apply to inputs in all three principal sensory modalities and to the production of fine movements.

HYPOTHESIS 1: *"Deficiencies in Temporal Processing Are Learned.* Could dyslexia and developmental dysphasia arise because some infants adopt more global hearing or looking strategies? Many aspects of eye movement behavior as well as studies of abnormal peripheral masking effects and improved reading with peripheral masking are consistent with the hypothesis that these special children operate in vision with a wider-than-normal field of attention. A consistently wider field of view should result in a degraded ability of the system to generate temporally sharpened representations from always-wide-bandwidth—and hence, temporally noiser—inputs. Heavy experience with such inputs might be expected to alter the base oscillation periods of visual cortical fields downward, because (a) those base periods are plausibly linked to input bandwidth and/or (b) as a rule, the strength of depolarization of clock neurons would depend upon the strengths of their own intrinsic inputs, and the more temporally dispersed those inputs, the lower their states of depolarization, and therefore the lower their base clock rates.

Note that very early visual practice with a wider field of view does not necessarily represent a "deficient" or "negative" or "dysfunctional" behavior. To the contrary, it would probably represent a practice strategy that, from the visual system's point of view, presents advantages for the rapid processing of relatively complex, spatially distributed inputs, especially for a very young brain. Such an alternative learning strategy might be expected to arise with higher probability in preterm infants because their oculomotor and focus control is more primitively developed when visual behavior is initiated.[88]

Once a "bad" looking (or listening) strategy is in place, by this hypothetical scenario, visual scene representation at every cognitive level as well as eye movement representations would be powerfully reinforced by the many tens or hundreds of thousands or millions of input repetitions. When reading was initiated, it would be initiated in a brain that had been powerfully trained and reinforced in countless operations to scan visually with a wide field of view. When the reading lesson stopped, the visual operations of the nervous system continue to work to reinforce and to sustain inappropriate forms of representation. In this scenario, reading practice that did not control for the field of view would only work to further reinforce the enduring problem, and to forestall its ultimate resolution. For example, vergence control for small visual targets would not be expected to have developed normally.[89–91] because this behavior would have been unpracticed. On the other hand, vergence control for larger visual targets would develop more normally. In a childhood reading lesson, thousands of repetitions involving vergence with larger visual targets could occur, further strengthening the dominance of the burned-in strategy. No matter how intensive, training from this and other specific learning perspectives could have substantially negative—not positive—consequences. Moreover, away from the reading class, a child's other lessons, addressed without visual control, could further reinforce "bad" looking, and coupled with the rest of the day's rich visual operations frustrate the small neurological consequences of a reading lesson. In many children, lack of success in reading would result in an attenuation of possibly corrective practice in any event.

How might an "error" in brain self-organization account for a general error in processing of rapidly sequenced inputs that also applies to auditory, somatosensory, and motor operations? Recent studies have revealed that activity is normally temporally coupled over long distances in the cerebral cortex, between modalities, and to some extent between hemispheres.[85,92–94] This cross-modal and cross-region coupling is manifested by recording in-phase oscillations in brain activity, for example, across the somatosensory and motor cortex in a monkey performing a tactually guided motor task, or between area 17 and "higher" visual cortical areas. It is probable, then, that a basic deficiency in timing input sequence would reflect the operations of the weakest cortical link in this chain of temporally coordinated processes: *All must track the slowest participant in their temporally coupled representation.*

Could the timing problem first originate with an "inappropriate listening" or haptic strategy? Hearing, like vision, could very well be the usual source of the inappropriate field of focus, and could well impose its "bad" timing on visual operations. For reasons that are beyond the scope of this brief review, the somatosensory system is less likely to be the original source of time chunking deficiencies.

If these special temporal processing-based learning disabilities arise by a learning scenario, on the basis of what we understand about brain plasticity and learning ontogeny, can they be reversed? That question cannot be answered with clarity, nor can there be any certainty that all cases are alike in this respect. However, the brain of a child and even an adult is capable of remarkable representational remodeling. If a learning-origins hypothesis applies, then what must be overcome in retraining is the massive accumulated weight of experience derived from all earlier life, as well as the potentially daily confounding inputs that occur away from the reading class. Reversal of this situation could be painstakingly slow, but is clearly possible. Several potential manipulative strategies for greatly accelerating the rates of change in learning systems are under investigation. They might be expected to ultimately greatly facilitate the training process in learning-disabled children.

HYPOTHESIS 2: *There Is a Locally or Globally Expressed Physical Defect in the Learning Machine.* We have earlier noted that the temporal integration periods and segment lengths shorten through development, and can be shortened throughout life by practice. The creation of more coherent representations of stimuli in learning and the probable plasticity of basic cortical "clock" times in child development and throughout life are dependent upon the operation of basic mechanisms of synapse strengthening. The list of the molecular elements of the forebrain machinery underlying the modification of synaptic effectivenesses in learning is a very long one; a defect in any one of at least several hundred proteins, for example, could potentially result in some attenuation of rates of learning, and hence, in prolonged temporal integration and segmentation times. It has been established that dyslexic children are of normal intelligence, when evaluated in nonreading tests. That would suggest that (a) reading challenges a mildly deficient system in a way that does not have substantial impacts on other aspects of associative learning; and (b) that the physical defect must apply *selectively* to plastic changes that control aspects of the temporal processing of inputs, or perhaps to strategies for looking or for controlling eye movements (see before). A recent gene-deletion study in mice has argued that the deletion of one key protein kinase believed to be critical for a fundamental learning process can result in a deficit in some aspects of learning in some brain regions, while other behaviors and other brain regions may not be significantly affected.[95,96] Given the almost innumerable possible consequences of genetic mutation, it is very possible that specific genetic defects could produce functional deficits selective for temporal processing in these learning systems. At the same time, a far more common expectation would be the appearance of a general learning deficiency.

With a small established defect, it might be difficult to reduce temporal chunk times down to their usual minima. For example, a defect might result in a dispersion of temporal inputs that limits the achievable levels of response coherence or "clock" times. It might limit the achievable changes in depolarization, and hence, the possible reductions in base "clock" times because of a limitation in the power of presynaptic or postsynaptic contributors to long-term potentiation. Moreover, (a) when the self-organizing mechanisms of the brain operate behaviorally with the defect in place, suboptimal experiential driving of the system would further reinforce and distribute its prolonged minimum temporal chunking, à la the scenario outlined earlier; and (b) lack of effective practice in a learning-disabled child ensures that these *specific* aspects of learning usually remain underexercised, an experiential fact that could be expected to contribute to the stabilization of deficient temporal processing.[49] A defect in the learning machine would not necessarily have to be expressed globally; a disabling defect applying principally to vision or to hearing could presumably impose its timing limitations on other sensory systems.

Concluding Remarks

Functional limitations imposed by "inappropriate" learning strategies adopted by our self-organizing nervous systems early in life must occur—indeed, must account for many aspects of the rich variety of human abilities that stamp us all as individual. We are now entering an era in experimental neuroscience in which we are beginning to understand how experiences generate changes in the nervous system that shape our language, our visual world, our coordinated movements, our cognition. A vision of how our ontogenetic, day-by-day experiences might account for our individual limitations and for the remarkable variability in human performance abilities is gradually emerging from these studies.

In parallel, neuroscientists are defining the organizational details and mechanisms of the learning machinery of the brain. The complex, neuronal circuit, cellular, and molecular processes that account for acquisition of complex "basic" skills like speech reception and reading are subject to many possible inherited deficiencies. Genetic defects partially disabling the learning machinery must occur. We are now entering an era in which the consequences of such mutations and gene dropouts can be assessed.

Both of these growing neuroscience subdisciplines must be tasked with determining whether and how the adoption of specific early learning strategies and/or how specific genetic defects might selectively alter the neural representations of temporal integration and segmentation. Our challenge is to press consideration of these two origins hypotheses along with their alternatives (e.g., Livingstone and Galaburda[97]), from the special perspective of the psychophysical and operational capabilities of these very extraordinary human populations.

ACKNOWLEDGMENTS

The authors thank Dr. Bruno Preilowski for his helpful comments on his manuscript.

REFERENCES

1. GREEN, D. M. 1985. Temporal factors in psychoacoustics. *In* Time Resolution in Auditory Systems, A. Michelsen, Ed.: 122–140. Springer-Verlag. Berlin/New York.
2. DE BOER, E. 1985. Auditory time constants: A paradox? *In* Time Resolution in Auditory Systems, A. Michelsen, Ed.: 141–158. Springer-Verlag. Berlin/New York.
3. GERKEN, G. M., U. K. BHAT & M. HUTCHISON-CLUTTER. 1990 Auditory temporal integration and the power function model. J. Acoust. Soc. Am. **88:** 767–768.
4. DILOLLO, V. 1980. Temporal integration in visual memory. J. Exp. Psychol. **109:** 75–97.
5. VERILLO, R. T. 1965. Temporal summation in vibrotactile sensitivity. J. Acoust. Soc. Am. **37:** 843–846.
6. BREITMEYER, B. G. 1984. Visual Masking. Oxford Univ. Press. New York.
7. CRAIG, J. C. 1989. Interference in localizing tactile stimuli. Percept. Psychophys. **45:** 343–355.
8. HORNER, D. T. & J. C. CRAIG. 1989. A comparison of discrimination and identification of vibrotactile patterns. Percept. Psychophys. **45:** 21–30.
9. SHERRICK, C. 1991. Vibrotactile pattern perception: Some findings. *In:* The Psychology of Touch, M. A. Heller and W. Schiff, Eds.: 189–218. Erlbaum. Hillsdale, N.J.
10. TALLAL, P., S. MILLER & R. H. FITCH. 1993. Neurobiological basis of speech: A case for the preeminence of temporal processing. This issue.
11. MOORE, B. 1993. Temporal analysis in normal and impaired hearing. This issue.
12. HIRSCH, I. J. & C. E. SHERRICK. 1961. Perceived order in different sense modalities. J. Exp. Psychol. **62:** 423–432.
13. CRAIG, J. C. & B. H. XU. 1990. Temporal order and tactile patterns. Percept. Psychophys. **47:** 22–34.
14. COLTHEART, M. 1980. Iconic memory and visible persistence. Percept. Psychophys. **27:** 183–228.
15. LONG, G. M. 1985. The varieties of visual persistence. Percept. Psycholphys. **38:** 381–385.
16. HOUTGAST, T. 1974. Lateral Suppression in Hearing, Ph.D. Thesis, Free University, Amsterdam, the Netherlands.
17. DANNEBRING, G. L. & A. S. BREGMAN. 1978. Streaming vs. fusion of sinusoidal components of complex waves. Percept Psychophys. **24:** 369–376.
18. BREGMAN, A. S. 1990. Auditory Scene Analysis: The Perceptual Organization of Sound. MIT Press. Cambridge, Mass.
19. IRWIN, D. W. & J. M. YEOMANS. 1991. Duration of visible persistence in relation to stimulus complexity. **50:** 475–489.
20. HORNER, D. T. 1991. The effects of complexity on the perception of vibrotactile patterns. Percept. Psychophys. **49:** 551–562.
21. JULESZ, B. 1984. Toward an axiomatic theory of preattentive vision. *In* Dynamic Aspects of Neocortical Function, G. M. Edelman, E. Gall, and M. Cowan, Eds.: Wiley. New York, 585–615.

22. ———. 1990. Early vision is bottom-up, except for focal attention. Cold Spring Harbor Symp. Quant. Biol. **55**: 973–978.
23. TRIESMAN, A., A. VIERA & A. HAYES. 1992. Automaticity and preattentive processing. Am. J. Psychol. **105**: 341–362.
24. KARNI, A. & D. SAGI. 1991. Where practice makes perfect in texture discrimination: Evidence for primary visual cortex plasticity. Proc. Natl. Acad. Sci. **88**: 4966–4970.
25. ANDERSEN, R. A., R. J. SNOWDEN, S. TREUE & M. GRAZIANO. 1990. Hierarchical processing of motion in the visual cortex of monkey. *In* Cold Spring Harbor Symp. Quant. Biol. **55**: 741–748.
26. TREISMAN, A. 1988. Features and objects. Q. J. Exp. Psychol. **40**: 201–237.
27. HAFTER, E. R., T. N. BUELL & V. M. RICHARDS. 1988. Onset-coding in lateralization: Its form, site and function. *In* Auditory Function. Neurobiological Bases of Hearing, G. Edelman, E. Gall, and M. Cowan, Eds.: 647–678. Wiley. New York.
28. HAFTER, E. R. & T. N. BUELL. 1990. Restarting the adapted binaural system. J. Acoust. Soc. Am. **88**: 806–812.
29. DARWIN, C. J. & W. CIOCCA. 1992. Grouping in pitch perception: Effects of onset asynchrony and ear of presentation of a mistuned component. J. Acoust. Soc. Am. **91**: 3381–3390.
30. WOLFORD, G., F. NARCHAK & H. HUGHES. 1988. Practice effects in backward masking. J. Exp. Psychol: Hum. Percept. Perform. **14**: 101–112.
31. BALL, K. & R. SEKULAR. 1987. Direction-specific improvement in motion discrimination. Vision Res. **27**: 953–965.
32. SANFORD, E. C. 1988. The relative legibility of small letters. Am. J. Psychol. **1**: 401–435.
33. GIBSON, E. J. 1969. Principles of Perceptual Learning. Appleton–Century–Crofts. New York.
34. BRUCE, R. H. & F. N. LOW. 1951. The effect of practice with brief exposure techniques upon central and peripheral visual acuity and a search for a brief test of peripheral acuity. J. Exp. Psychol. **41**: 275–280.
35. POGGIO, T., M. FAHLE & S. EDELMAN. 1992. Fast perceptual learning in visual hyperacuity. Science **256**: 1018–1021.
36. FLORENTINE, M. Northeastern University, personal communication.
37. JENKINS, W. & M. MERZENICH, unpublished work in progress.
38. ZWISLOCKI, J., F. MAIRE, A. S. FELDMAN & H. RUBIN. 1957. On the effect of practice and motivation on the threshold of audibility. J. Acoust. Soc. Am. **30**: 254–262.
39. GIBSON, E. J. 1953. Improvement in perceptual judgments as a function of controlled practice or training. Psychol. Bull. **50**: 401–432.
40. ANDERSON, J. R. 1981. Cognitive Skills and Their Acquisition. Erlbaum. Hillsdale, N.J.
41. CRAIG, J. C. 1988. The role of experience in tactual pattern perception: A preliminary report. Int. J. Rehabil. Res. **11**: 167–171.
42. TELLER, D. Y. 1990. The development of visual function in infants. Res. Publ. Assoc. Res. Nerv. Ment. Dis. **65**: 109–118.
43. RUBEN, R. J. 1992. The ontogeny of human hearing. Acta Otolaryngol. **112**: 192–196.
44. WERNER, L. A., G. C. MAREAN, C. F. HALPIN, N. B. SPETNER & J. M. GILLENWATER. 1992. Infant auditory temporal acuity: Gap detection. Child Dev. **63**: 260–272.
45. NOVAK, G. P., D. KURTZBERG, J. A. KREUZER & H. G. VAUGHAN, JR. 1989. Cortical responses to speech sounds and their formants in normal infants. Natural sequences and spatiotemporal analysis. Electroencephalogr. Clin. Neurophys. **75**: 295 and 305.
46. KUHL, P. 1993. Developmental speech perception: Implications for models of language impairment. This issue.
47. ASLIN, R. N. & R. B. SMITH. 1988. Perceptual development. Ann. Rev. Psychol. **39**: 435–473.
48. CHANDNA, A. 1991. Natural history of the development of visual acuity in infants. *Eye* **5**: 20–26.
49. BEAULIEU, C. & M. CYNADER. 1989. Effect of the richness of the environment on neurons in cat visual cortex. II. Spatial and temporal frequency characteristics. Dev. Brain Res. **53**: 82–88.

50. ———. 1989. Effect of the richness of the environment on neurons in cat visual cortex. I. Receptive field properties. Brain Res. (Dev. Brain Res.) **53:** 71–81.
51. TALLAL, P. & M. PIERCY. 1979. Defects of auditory perception in children with developmental dysphasia. *In* Developmental Dysphasia, M. A. Syke, Ed.: 63–84. Academic Press. Orlando, Fla.
52. LOVEGROVE, W. J., R. P. GARZIA & S. R. NICHOLSON. 1990. Experimental evidence for a transient system deficit in specific reading disability. J. Am. Optom. Assoc. **61:** 137–146.
53. LOVEGROVE, W. J. 1993. Weakness in the transient visual system: A causal factor in dyslexia? This issue.
54. WILLIAMS, M. C. & K. LECLUYSE. 1990. Perceptual consequences of a temporal processing deficit in reading disabled children. J. Am. Optom. Assoc. **61:** 111–121.
55. SCHAPIRO, K. L., N. OGDEN & F. LIND-BLAD. 1990. Temporal processing in dyslexia. J. Learn. Disabilities **23:** 99–107.
56. MERRITT, R. D. & D. W. BALOGH. 1990. Backward masking as a function of spatial frequency. A comparison of MMPI-identified schizotypics and control subjects. J. Nerv. Ment. Dis. **178:** 186–193.
57. TALLAL, P. 1992. Rutgers University, personal communication.
58. LIEBERMAN, J. 1993. In speech perception, time is not what it seems. This issue.
59. MERZENICH, M. M., K. A. GRAJSKI, W. M. JENKINS, G. H. RECANZONE & B. PETERSON. 1991. Functional cortical plasticity. Cortical network origins of representational changes. Cold Spring Harbor Symp. Quant. Biol. **55:** 873–887.
60. MERZENICH, M. M., T. ALLARD & W. M. JENKINS. 1990. Neural ontogeny of higher brain function; implications of some recent neurophysiological findings. *In* Information Processing in the Somatosensory System, O. Franzén and P. Westman, Eds.: 293–311. Macmillan. London.
61. MERZENICH, M. M., G. H. RECANZONE & W. M. JENKINS. 1990. How the brain functionally rewires itself. *In* Natural and Artificial Parallel Computations, M. Arbib and J. A. Robinson, Eds.: 177–210. MIT Press. New York.
62. RECANZONE, G. H., C. E. SCHREINER & M. M. MERZENICH. 1993. Plasticity in the frequency representation of primary auditory cortex following descrimination training in adult owl monkeys. J. Neurosci. **13:** 87–104.
63. WEINBERGER, N. M. & D. M. DIAMOND. 1989. Dynamic modulation of the auditory system by associative learning. *In* Auditory Function. Neurobiological Bases of Hearing, G. Edelman, E. Gall, and M. Cowan, Eds.: 485–514. Wiley. New York.
64. MILLIKEN, G. W., R. J. NUDO, R. GRENDA, W. M. JENKINS & M. M. MERZENICH. 1992. Expansion of distal forelimb representations in primary motor cortex of adult squirrel monkeys following motor training. Soc. Neurosci. Abstr. **18:** 506.
65. RECANZONE, G. H., W. M. JENKINS, G. H. HRADEK & M. M. MERZENICH. 1992. Progressive improvement in discriminative abilities in adult owl monkeys performing a tactile frequency discrimination task. J. Neurophysiol. **67:** 1015–1030.
66. RECANZONE G. H., M. M. MERZENICH & C. E. SCHREINER. 1992. Changes in the distributed temporal response properties of SI cortical neurons reflect improvements in performance on a temporally-based tactile discrimination task. J. Neurophysiol. **67:** 1071–1091.
67. JENKINS, W. M., M. M. MERZENICH, T. T. ALLARD & E. GUIC-ROBLES. 1990. Functional reorganization of primary somatosensory cortex in adult owl monkeys after behaviorally controlled tactile stimulation. J. Neurophysiol. **63:** 82–104.
68. RECANZONE, G. H., M. M. MERZENICH & W. M. JENKINS. 1992. Frequency discrimination training engaging a restricted skin surfaces results in an emergence of a cutaneous response zone in cortical area 3a. J. Neurophysiol. **67:** 1057–1070.
69. MERZENICH, M. M., R. J. NELSON, M. P. STRYKER, M. S. CYNADER, A. SCHOPPMANN & J. J. ZOOK. 1984. Somatosensory cortical map changes following digit amputation in adult monkeys. J. Comp. Neurol. **224:** 591–605.
70. PONS, T. P., P. E. GARRAGHTY, A. K. OMMAYA, J. H. KAAS, E. TAUB & M. MISHKIN. 1991. Massive cortical reorganization after sensory deafferentation in adult macaques. Science **252:** 1857–1860.

71. RECANZONE, G. H. & M. M. MERZENICH. 1991. Alterations of the functional organization of primary somatosensory cortex following intracortical microstimulation or behavioral training. In Memory: Organization of Locus of Change, L. Squire, G. Lynch, N. Weinberger, and J. McGaugh, Eds.: 217–238. Oxford Univ. Press. Oxford.
72. RECANZONE, G. H., M. M. MERZENICH & H. R. DINSE. 1992. Expansion of cortical representation of a specific skin field in primary somatosensory cortex by intracortical microstimulation. Cereb. Cortex **2:** 181–196.
73. DINSE, H. R., G. H. RECANZONE & M. M. MERZENICH. 1990. Direct observation of neural assemblies during neocortical representational reorganization. In Parallel Processing in Neural Systems and Computers, R. Eckmiller, G. Hartmann, and G. Hauske, Eds.: 1–21. Elsevier. Amsterdam, the Netherlands.
74. HEBB, D. O. 1949. The Organization of Behavior: A Neuropsychological Theory. Wiley. New York.
75. SCHREINER, C. E. & G. LANGNER. 1988. Coding of temporal patterns in the central auditory nervous system. In Auditory Function. Neurobiological Bases of Hearing, G. Edelman, E. Gall, and M. Cowan, Eds.: 337–362. Wiley. New York.
76. ———. 1988. Periodicity coding in the inferior colliculus of the cat: II. Topographic organization. J. Neurophysiol. **60:** 1823–1840.
77. SCHREINER, C. E. & J. V. URBAS. 1988. Representation of amplitude modulation in the auditory cortex of the cat: II. Comparison between cortical fields. Hear. Res. **32:** 49–64.
78. EGGERMONT, J. J. 1992. Stimulus induced and spontaneous rhythmic firing of single units in cat primary auditory cortex. Hear. Res. **61:** 1–11.
79. PHILLIPS, D. 1993. Neural representation of stimulus times in the primary auditory cortex. This issue.
80. SCHREINER, C. E. & J. V. URBAS. 1986. Representation of amplitude modulation in the auditory cortex of the cat: I. Anterior auditory field. Hear. Res. **21:** 227–241.
81. SCHREINER, C. E. & P. X. JORIS. 1986. Intrinsic oscillations in the primary auditory cortex of cats. In Proceedings, IUPS Satellite Symposium on Hearing: 81. Univ. of California. San Francisco.
82. CONNORS, B. W. & M. J. GUTNICK. 1990. Intrinsic firing patterns of diverse neocortical neurons. Trends Neurosci. **13:** 99–104.
83. SILVA, L. R., Y. AMITAI & B. W. CONNORS. 1991. Intrinsic oscillations of neocortex generated by layer 5 puramidal neurons. Science **251:** 432–435.
84. LLINAS, R. 1993. Is dyslexia a dyschronia? This issue.
85. JAGADEESH, B., C. M. GRAY & D. FERSTER. 1992. Visually evoked oscillations of membrane potential in cells of cat visual cortex. Science **257:** 206–211.
86. SCHREINER, C. E. 1991. Functional topographies in the primary auditory cortex of the cat Acta Otolaryngol. Suppl. **491:** 7–15.
87. PANTEV, C., M. HOKE, B. LUTKEN & K. LEHNERTZ 1989. Tonotopic organization of the auditory cortex: Pitch versus frequency representaion. Science **246:** 486–488.
88. MOLTENO, A. C., I. J. HODGKINSON, C. J. HEWITT & G. F. SANDERSON. 1992. The development of fixing and focusing behaviour in normal human infants as observed with the Otago photoscreener. Aust. N. Z. J. Opthal. **20:** 197–205.
89. STEIN, J. F., P. M. RIDDELL & S. FOWLER. 1988. Disordered vergence control in dyslexic children. Brit J. Opthal. **72:** 162–166.
90. HUNG, G. K. 1989. Reduced vergence reponse velocities in dyslexics: A preliminary report. Opthal. Physiol. Opt. **9:** 420–423.
91. BUZZELLI, A. R. 1991. Stereopsis, accommodative and vergence facility: Do they relate to dyslexia? Opt. Vis. Sci. **68:** 842–846.
92. MURTHY, V. N. & E. E. FETZ. 1992. Coherent 25- to 35-Hz oscillations in the sensorimotor cortex of awake behaving monkeys. Proc. Natl. Acad. Sci. **89:** 5670–5674.
93. ENGEL, A. K., A. K. KREITER, P. KONIG & W. SINGER. 1991. Synchronization of oscillatory neuronal responses between striate and extrastriate visual cortical areas of the cat. Proc. Natl. Acad. Sci. **88:** 6048–6052.
94. RIBARY, U., A. A. IOANNIDES, K. D. SINGH, R. HASSON, J. P. BOLTON, F. LADO, A. MOGILNER & R. LLINAS. 1991. Magnetic field tomography of coherent thalamocortical 40 Hz oscillations in humans. Proc. Natl. Acad. Sci. **88:** 11037–11041.

95. SILVA, A. J., R. PAYLOR, J. M. WEHNER & S. TONEGAWA. 1992. Impaired spatial learning in alpha-calcium-calmodulin kinase II mutant mice. Science **257:** 206–211.
96. SILVA, A. J., C. F. STEVENS, S. TONEGAWA & Y. WANG 1992. Deficient hippocampal long-term potentiation in alpha-calcium-calmodulin kinase II mutant mice. Science **257:** 201–206.
97. GALABURDA, A. & M. LIVINGSTONE. 1993. Evidence for a magnocellular defect in developmental dyslexia. This issue.

heterogeneous if task-analyzed for what specific visual competence each requires). Fractionation of language has not yet been matched in sophistication by fractionation of visual processes, at least in the published research on dyslexic mechanisms. Then there is the confounding of "visual" with "spatial" functions, often eliding the distinction that not all spatial tasks are visual and, even more important, certainly not all visual tasks are spatial. So it is inappropriate to conclude that dyslexia has nothing to do with *any* visual dysfunction, in spite of the fact that a great many visually based tasks have been shown to be areas of strength among dyslexic populations. To reiterate: because some of these visually based strengths may be in the spatial domain irrelevant to reading, and because some others may be so complex that deficient subskills may have been masked with "success," it is premature to dismiss all possibility of some visual deficit contributing to dyslexia. One need not set up a categorical "straw man" called *the visual subtype*. Rather, adhering to the multi-dimensional quantitative view that brains may have mixed weaknesses in various proportions and combinations of modular systems, there may be a discrete visual factor in the equation. A hint that this may be so, in a limited developmental manner, comes from clinical experience of the poor copy-forms scores ("visual–motor integration") of many young (less than eleven year old) dyslexic children, even the "pure" type; in their teens, such children make at least acceptable scores on such tests without any training. My own research on map-walking yielded similar results (poor below eleven years, superior after that). Since these visually presented tasks require organization and production of motor output, however, the locus of deficit (or "outgrowing" the deficit) is still to be determined. Perhaps the oculomotor system plays a mediating role. Perhaps, as is suggested by their anterior brain width on MRI scans, even pure dyslexics are subtly deficient in executive function.[6]

The problem for neurologically oriented research, compounded by the longitudinal aspects of development, is how to compromise between purification and generalization. If we insist on the detailed study of the relatively rare (yet not impossible) pure dyslexic case, we may never see the brain of that exquisitely explored case. Clinical samples are well known to suffer from more co-morbidities than epidemiologic samples (unless, like this writer, you draw referrals from highly sophisticated families who worry about any child not getting straight A grades). Clinical samples, however, do submit to more extensive and intensive study than do epidemiological samples (the "more" about whom we tend to know "less"). For any type of sample there is the problem of longitudinal follow-up, environmental and/or psychosocial instability/stress, and differential therapeutic interventions over time. Correlative anatomic and physiologic neuroimaging is obtained in even tinier samples and by as-yet-unstandardized methods. No wonder studies "do not replicate" or generalize each other.

With all these issues, it is amazing how much consensus exists. Clinical and epidemiological samples have cross-validated; genetics has, while failing to pin down the gene, provided further confirmatory evidence with respect to phonological and executive functional domains. As long as each case study, clinical study, family study, or epidemiological study describes its subjects and its terminology clearly and operationally, avoiding vague descriptors and grandiose constructs, there is a good chance that we will continue to refine a neurologically based profile of the differences underlying developmental dyslexia.[7]

Finally, although this is primarily a clinically based overview of what is meant by the diagnostic label of developmental dyslexia, I would like to add two recently acquired perspectives that have resulted from the research of the Learning Disabilities Research Center of which I am Principal Investigator. The work summarized here comes from the progress report of my esteemed colleague, Dr. Frank Vellutino, who is Principal Investigator of our Project Four (school-based and "in the field"). These two perspectives are on the (1) issues of gender ratios as relevant to the biology of dyslexia, and (2) nature/nurture interactions in the production of the reading disability phenotype.[8]

1. In kindergarten (KG) children tested with an extensive battery of cognitive, linguistic, visuospatial, prereading, and early arithmetic skills, gender differences do emerge. That is, 65 percent of the KG children whose reading readiness skills were in the lowest 10 percent of the distribution were boys, while only 41 percent of those in the top 10 percent were boys. For general verbal ability, gender is evenly distributed in the lowest 10 percent, but girls are somewhat over represented in the top 10 percent. For early arithmetical abilities, there were twice as many boys as girls in both the lowest 10 percent and highest 10 percent of the arithmetic distribution. Thus, at this early age when cultural factors (although not absent) are minimal, gender differences that run in opposite directions for prereading and arithmetic emerge despite no gender disadvantage in verbal ability.
2. Instructional differences: Vellutino and co-investigators have data on first grade classrooms in the same geographic area/system during the past two academic years (1990–1991 and 1991–1992): they find that the proportion of the school day spent on language-arts (reading-related) instruction ranges from 15 to 41 percent, while the type of relative emphasis (code-versus-meaning-oriented) within that time allocation varies from 1 to 45 percent on code and from 16 to 75 percent on meaning.

This difference in reading "nurture" is bound to interact with factors of "nature" to produce, ultimately, the achievement level that enters into the calculation of discrepancy-based reading disability. Without factoring in the instructional variables, equating reading disability with the presumed biologic entity "dyslexia" is doomed to produce confusion.

REFERENCES

1. AMERICAN PSYCHIATRIC ASSOCIATION. 1987. Diagnostic and Statistical Manual of Mental Disorders, 3d ed. (Rev.). American Psychiatric Association. Washington, D.C.
2. HUGHES, J. R. & M. B. DENCKLA. 1978. Outline of a pilot study of electroencephalographic correlates of dyslexia. In Dyslexia: An appraisal of Current Knowledge, A. L. Benton and D. Pearl, Eds.:112–122. University Press. New York.
3. VELLUTINO, F. R., D. M. SCANLON & M. S. TANZMAN. 1991. Bridging the gap between cognitive and neuropsychological conceptualizations of reading disability. Learn. Individ. Differ. **3**:181–203.
4 LYON, G. R. 1992. Research in Learning Disabilities: Research Directions. Report prepared for the National Institute of Child Health and Human Development. National Institutes of Health. Bethesda, Md.
5. DENCKLA, M. B. & J. M. RUMSEY. 1992. Developmental dyslexia. In Diseases of the Nervous System, 3d ed., Vol. 1, Clinical Neurobiology, A. K. Asbury, G. M. McKhann, and W. I. McDonald, Eds.: 636–645.
6. HYND, G. W., et al. 1990. Brain morphology in developmental dyslexia and attention deficit disorder/hyperactivity. Arch. Neurol. **47**:919–926.
7. PENNINGTON, B. F. 1991. Dyslexia and other developmental language disorders. In Diagnosing Learning Disorders, chap. 4:45–81. Guilford Press. New York.
8. VELLUTINO, F. R. & D. M. SCANLON. 1991. Intervention-resistant reading disability. Progr. Rep, Project IV. P50 HD25806 Neurodevelopmental Pathways to Learning Disabilities. M. B. Denckla, PI.

Neurobiological Basis of Speech: A Case for the Preeminence of Temporal Processing

PAULA TALLAL, STEVE MILLER, AND
ROSLYN HOLLY FITCH
Center for Molecular and Behavioral Neuroscience
Rutgers University
197 University Avenue
Newark, New Jersey 07102

INTRODUCTION

Epidemiological surveys have reported that somewhere between 3 and 10 percent of preschool children exhibit some form of developmental speech or language disorder that cannot be attributed to a known cause such as hearing impairment, general mental retardation, or frank neurological disorder (e.g., seizures or an acquired brain lesion).[1] Research is now showing that dysfunction of higher level speech processing, necessary for normal language and reading development, may result from difficulties in the processing of basic sensory information entering the nervous system in rapid succession (within milliseconds). In this paper we present evidence supporting the hypothesis that a basic temporal processing impairment in language-impaired children underlies their inability to integrate sensory information that converges in rapid succession in the central nervous system. We provide data showing that this deficit is pansensory, that is, affects processing in multiple sensory modalities, and also affects motor output within the millisecond time frame. We also provide data that links these basic temporal integration deficits to specific patterns of speech perception and speech production deficits in language-impaired children. We suggest that these basic temporal deficits cause a cascade of effects, starting with disruption of the normal development of an otherwise effective and efficient phonological system. We propose further that these phonological processing deficits result in subsequent failure to learn to speak and to read normally. That is, both the language and reading problems have their basis in deficiently established phonological processing and decoding. Finally, we use data derived from our ongoing behavioral studies with language-impaired children to address some fundamental issues pertaining to the neurobiological basis of speech perception and production (e.g., hemispheric specialization) underlying these processes. We suggest that results from magnetic resonance imaging (MRI) and positron emission tomography (PET) studies, as well as studies of behavioral performance in normal adults and adults with acquired lesions, combined with more recent results from animal studies, all support the view that a left-hemispheric specialization for speech initially developed through evolution as a specialization for processing and producing sensory and motor events that occur in rapid succession.

EXPERIMENTAL STUDIES OF SPECIFICALLY LANGUAGE-IMPAIRED CHILDREN

The term *specific language impairment* (LI) has come to refer to the diagnostic classification which, for research purposes, is based on quantitative exclusionary and inclusionary criteria. For the purposes of the studies reviewed below, LI refers to children who were developing normally in every respect, but failed to develop language at the expected rate. Criteria for inclusion as an LI subject in our research studies began with exclusion of all children with sensory hearing loss, general mental retardation, paralysis or lack of sensation in the oral musculature, or frank neurological or psychiatric disorders (including attention deficit disorder). In addition, potential subjects had to demonstrate a nonverbal performance IQ of 85 or above, and a significant discrepancy between both their chronological and mental age in receptive and/or expressive language development (based on standardized clinical tests). The results of the behavioral experiments reported below have been replicated on three separate samples of LI children meeting these criteria, and control children matched on age, IQ, and socioeconomic status. The sample sizes for these replications included 12 subjects per group, 36 subjects per group, and 100 LI and 60 controls. Details of subject selection, test scores, and demographics for these populations are given by Tallal and Piercy,[2] Stark and Tallal,[3] and Zeigler et al.[4]

Our studies began in 1970 with an interest in understanding the severe deficits in both phonological perception and production that characterized most LI children. We reasoned that before studying speech *per se*, it would be important to assess the integrity of the component acoustic processes that are critical to the analysis of the complex acoustic spectra of speech. Put simply, it is clearly important to determine that a child can hear normally before interpreting deficits in their ability to process or produce speech. Similarly, even where it can be shown that the sensory organ is intact, it is still important to assess other central aspects of auditory processing to ensure that the fundamental components of acoustic analysis throughout the nervous system are intact and functioning normally.

With this premise in mind we began by developing a hierarchical battery of subtests for assessing detection, temporal integration, association, discrimination, sequencing, rate processing, and serial memory for acoustic events. In order to avoid verbal instructions or response requirements, Tallal and Piercy[5] developed an operant conditioning paradigm in which subjects were trained to detect and discriminate varied sequential presentations of two complex steady-state tones with different fundamental frequencies (100 Hz and 305 Hz), and to respond by pressing panels on a response box.

We used two test methods. In the association method subjects were trained to respond to each tone separately by pushing the top panel to Tone 1 and the bottom to Tone 2. Discrimination training continued until criterion was reached. Subjects were then trained to respond to each of the four possible two-tone sequences (1–1, 1–2, 2–1, 2–2) by pushing the panels in the corresponding order. In the first series, the interstimulus interval (ISI) was constant at 428 ms. In the second series, subjects were tested on the same two-tone sequences, but with ISIs ranging from 8 ms to 4062 ms, presented in random order. A similar procedure was used to test serial memory using the same two tones in sequences of three to seven elements (ISI 428 ms).

Because a subject may have been able to perceive the elements of a temporal sequence, but unable to reproduce a corresponding motor pattern, a same–different method was also used. The response panel was turned through 90° to avoid confusion between methods. Subjects were initially presented with the two tones in varied sequences (ISI 428 ms), and were trained to press the right panel if the tones were the same and the left panel if different. Training again continued until criterion was reached. The same series of two-tone sequences, 24 with ISI 428 ms and 48 with ISI varied as earlier, were then presented, and the subject indicated whether the two tones were the same or different. Half of the subjects in each group performed the association task first; half performed the same–different task first.

In the first series of experiments, twelve 6- through 9-year-old LI children and matched controls were tested on these procedures using a fixed duration (75 ms) for tones 1 and 2.[5] In trials in which more than one tone was presented, the ISI was varied between 8 and 4062 ms. Results showed that there were no significant differences between the performance of LI and control children on the detection, association, or sequencing subtest when the ISI was at 428 ms or longer. As can be seen in FIGURE 1, however, the performance of the LI children deteriorated rapidly with shorter ISIs. No LI subject reached a criterion of 75 percent correct at a 150 ms ISI or shorter. In contrast, all controls were able to reach 75 percent correct at ISIs of 8 ms or longer. A similar pattern of results was demonstrated in both the same–different and sequential ordering paradigms. That is, at rapid rates of presentation, LI children were significantly impaired in their ability to both discriminate and sequence auditory stimuli.

Two points should be emphasized regarding the pattern of data presented in FIGURE 1. First, the processing time needed by LI subjects to respond correctly on this basic auditory processing test was *orders of magnitude* greater than that required by matched controls. Second, the perceptual function for the LIs was bimodal rather than linear. That is, at sufficiently slow presentation rates, LI children were unimpaired in their ability to identify, discriminate, and sequence basic acoustic information. But, when the rate of presentation was speeded up by decreasing the interval between stimuli the LIs' performance dropped to chance levels. These data suggest that when given sufficient input time for signal processing, LI children are able to

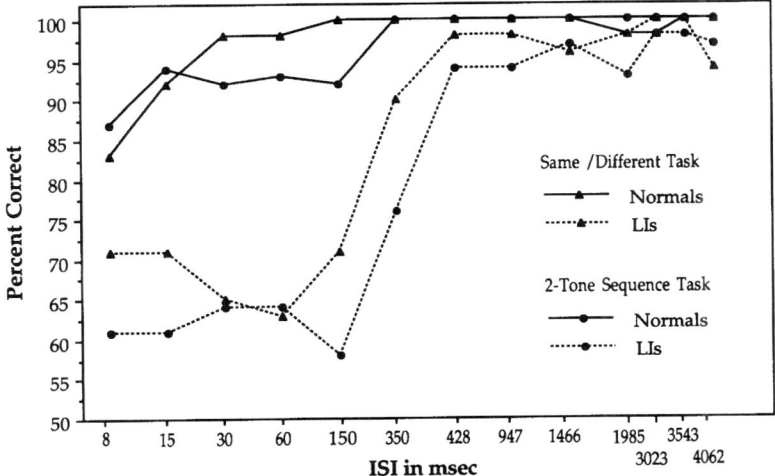

FIGURE 1. Percent correct for normals and LIs with varied ISIs. Duration of complex tones = 75 ms (tone 1 = 100 Hz, tone 2 = 305 Hz). (Adapted from data presented in Tallal and Piercy.[5])

utilize central auditory processes for discrimination and sequencing of sensory information normally. However, they need orders of magnitude more time between the input of basic sensory events in order to access these higher level processes.

In the next set of experiments the role of stimulus duration on auditory perception was examined.[2] The most significant findings were on the serial memory task. Whereas all controls (100 percent) reached criterion on the three-element serial memory task at 75-ms tone durations, only 2 out of 12 LI children (17 percent) reached this same criterion. When the stimulus duration was lengthened to 250 ms, however, 10 out of 12 LIs reached criterion on this same three-element task. It is important to note that control performance did not deteriorate significantly as a function of increasing the number of elements in a sequence (up to five items), even at 75-ms tone durations. However, severe deterioration in the LI subjects' performance was seen at sequence lengths above three elements, even with longer stimulus durations. Thus it is clear from these results that even though increasing the duration of the stimulus improved the serial memory performance of LI children, serial memory remained impaired for LIs in comparison to controls.

In conclusion, the time available for acoustic processing is clearly important for sequential memory performance. However, since increasing stimulus duration did not completely ameliorate deficits in serial memory for tone sequences of greater than three elements for LI children, the impairment of serial memory may be independent of the temporal processing deficit. Conversely, given the developmental nature of language impairment, it is possible that a primary temporal processing deficit may result in a form of auditory deprivation that, in turn, alters neuronal mapping and connections across the auditory system (see Merzenich et al.[6]) with cascading effects on other higher level auditory processes. The effects of this deprivation may result in, among other things, retarded development of complex acoustic processes (e.g., auditory serial memory), as well as deficits in the perception of rapid and sequential transients within speech.

STUDIES OF SPEECH PERCEPTION AND PRODUCTION

The previous nonverbal acoustic studies clearly showed that LI children exhibited a profound deficit in processing rapidly presented acoustic information. How could such a basic temporal integration dysfunction undermine speech and language development? The results of the psychoacoustic studies reviewed pointed to an area of temporal dysfunction within the tens of milliseconds range. This time frame led us, in turn, to focus our attention on the phonemic level of speech processing, as specific temporal elements of the acoustic signal within a phoneme occur within this time frame and are essential for perceptual discrimination of speech. For example, vowels transmit the same acoustic information throughout their spectra and are thus referred to as steady state. Stop consonant syllables (such as /ba/, /da/, /ga/, /pa/, /ta/, and /ka/), on the other hand, have a transitional period during which the frequencies (called *formants*) change very rapidly over time (see FIGURE 2). Information carried within these brief formant transitions are critical for syllable discrimination. We predicted that LI children would be particularly impaired in discriminating brief-duration temporal cues within speech, such as the brief formant transitions within stop-consonant/vowel syllables. However, we predicted that they would be unimpaired in discriminating between speech sounds that were characterized by steady-state acoustic spectra, such as vowels.

FIGURE 2 shows two pairs of computer-synthesized speech stimuli used in these initial studies. The first pair shows the spectra of two steady-state vowels, /ɛ/ and /æ/. Note that the acoustic spectra of these speech stimuli are constant (and differ from each other) throughout their entire 250-ms duration. The second pair represent the acoustic spectra of the syllables /ba/ and /da/. Here we see that these syllables differ only over the initial 40 ms, during which the frequencies change very rapidly in time, followed immediately by the vowel /a/, which is steady-state throughout the remainder of both 250-ms syllables. That is, for most of the 250 ms both syllables are comprised of identical steady-state formant frequencies of the vowel /a/. Consequently, discrimination of these two syllables critically depends on an accurate analysis of the initial 40-ms formant transitions.

Using the same response paradigm described for the nonverbal acoustic studies just reported, we investigated LI children's ability to detect, associate, and sequence these two pairs of speech sounds. The experimental results were clear. The LI children were unimpaired in performing any of these tasks with the steady-state vowel stimuli. However, when the stop consonant–vowel (CV) syllables, incorporating 40-ms formant transitions, were used as stimuli, 10 out of 12 of the LI children were unable even to reach criterion on the association subtest. That is, they were unable even to learn to associate the bottom button on the response panel with the stimulus /ba/ and the top button with the stimulus /da/. The children insisted that they could not hear the difference between the two stimuli being presented.[7]

In a subsequent experiment, we sought to determine whether the poor performance found on tests with CV syllables derived from an impaired ability to process transitional elements of auditory information *per se,* or was due to an inability to resolve other brief-duration cues typically found within phonemes as well.[8] In this experiment the preceding paradigm was modified by using computer-generated speech stimuli whose spectral or temporal characteristics had been systematically

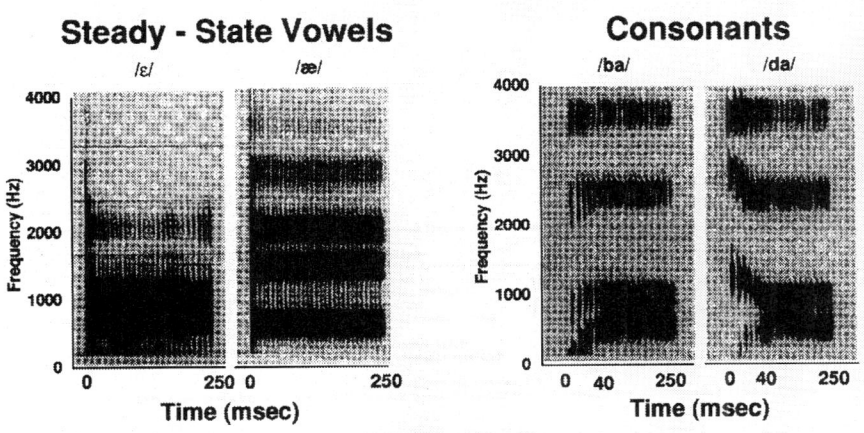

FIGURE 2.

manipulated. The first stimulus pair was a set of computer-generated vowel–vowel syllables based on the temporal characteristics of the CV syllables /ba/ and /da/. In the new pair, however, the initial 40-ms segment of each syllable was steady state rather than transitional, and represented the acoustic spectra for one of the vowels /ɛ/ or /æ/. The remaining portion of the 250 ms in each syllable was comprised of the same steady-state vowel, /I/. A second pair of stimuli based on the original /ba, da/ syllables was also generated. In this stimulus pair, however, the initial 40-ms formant transition within each of the CV syllables /ba/ and /da/ was synthetically extended, to approximately 80 ms.

Again, the LI children were tested using the sequential associative response paradigm described earlier, this time using the two new pairs of stimuli. The results were quite intriguing. This time, the LIs were *impaired* in their ability to discriminate the vowel–vowel stimuli (incorporating a critical 40-ms-duration segment), but *unimpaired* in processing the CV syllables where the duration of the critical formant transition had been extended to 80 ms. Subsequent studies asking subjects to discriminate many different speech sounds based on a variety of temporal and/or spectral cues, confirmed the hypothesis that LI children were impaired in their ability to integrate brief acoustic components of information occurring within tens of milliseconds in the ongoing speech stream, regardless of phonetic classification.[9] Results from other laboratories assessing the perceptual speech abilities of language and/or learning-impaired children, as well as adults with a lifelong history of dyslexia, also support this conclusion.[10–12]

We were interested in determining whether the influence of this temporal integration deficit would extend beyond the domain of speech perception. In a series of studies,[13,14] we undertook detailed spectrographic analyses of speech production data from LI and control children, specifically focusing on the temporal aspects of their speech production. We found a remarkable similarity between the pattern of temporal production impairments and temporal perception impairments at the phonetic level in the LI subjects. That is, we demonstrated that language-impaired children were not only impaired in their ability to process the temporal components of the acoustic spectra that characterize speech syllables, but were also impaired in their ability to control the *production* of these brief temporal events in their motor output. This remarkable mirroring of specific temporal constraints in both sensory and motor systems subserving speech has important implications for theories that pertain to neural mechanisms underlying speech in humans.

We were also interested in whether the degree of deficit in temporal integration would correlate with the degree of language impairment beyond the phoneme level. We hypothesized that the degree of impairment in temporal processing would be highly correlated with the overall degree of receptive language delay in LI children. In order to investigate this hypothesis we rank ordered the LI subjects according to which child showed the greatest impairment and which the least on our temporal processing tests. Next, we rank ordered the same children based on their performance on a battery of standardized clinical receptive language tests. The results were clear-cut. There was a highly significant multiple correlation ($r = 0.85$, $p < 0.001$) between the degree of temporal processing impairment and the degree of receptive language impairment.[15]

On the basis of the multiple studies reviewed here, we conclude that a primary inability to process acoustic information that enters the nervous system in rapid succession (within a time frame of tens of milliseconds) will serve to disrupt or delay the development of phonological processes, and subsequently lead to more global delayed development of receptive language.

MODALITY SPECIFICITY

The previous experiments clearly support the existence of an auditory temporal processing deficit in LI children that affects their performance in both speech perception and production, as well as the degree of their receptive language impairment. In the next set of experiments we addressed whether this temporal processing deficit is specific to the auditory modality. In this series of studies, we used a comprehensive battery of sensory and motor tests designed to assess visual, tactile, and cross-modal sensory integration, as well as rapid sequential motor output. Studies were well-controlled to compare performance in these modalities using verbal and nonverbal stimuli. The hierarchy of processing subtests described earlier for the auditory experiments were employed to assess visual and cross-modal temporal processing. The assessment of tactile processing utilized a modification of these procedures based on discrimination of single, sequential, or simultaneous touches to the fingers, hands, and/or cheeks. Motor tasks included the ability to make rapid sequential nonverbal finger and mouth movements, as well as the ability to rapidly produce single or sequential speech syllables and words.[16-19]

The results of this extensive series of studies can be summarized in the following manner. Language-impaired children were significantly impaired in comparison to matched controls in their ability to discriminate, sequence, or remember any brief stimulus if followed in rapid succession (tens of milliseconds) by another stimulus, regardless of the modality of stimulation. Importantly, LI children were unimpaired on precisely the same tasks when the interval between the offset of one stimulus and the onset of another was extended. A similar pattern was found for the production of rapid, sequential, and fine-grained oral or manual movements. These deficits were found regardless of whether the stimuli were verbal or nonverbal.[19]

The results of these studies demonstrate that LI children have a pervasive pan-sensory/motor deficit that impedes their ability to perceive or produce information within a tightly delineated time frame of tens of milliseconds. Importantly, in a study of 36 LI and well-matched control children, we found a striking bimodal distribution in the performance of these groups on temporal sensory/motor tasks. FIGURE 3 shows the results of a discriminate function analysis that incorporated six variables representing auditory, visual, tactile, and cross-modal temporal integration, as well as rapid sequential motor performance obtained from LI versus control children. As can be seen in this figure we found virtually *no overlap* between the ranges in performance for these two groups.[19]

IMPLICATIONS FOR DYSLEXIA

There appears to be a striking convergence of experimental data obtained from language-impaired and reading-impaired (dyslexic) children. Longitudinal studies have demonstrated that the vast majority of children identified in preschool as developmentally language impaired exhibit inordinant difficulty learning to read when they reach elementary school (see Tallal *et al.*,[20] 1988, for review). A broad body of research now suggests that phonological awareness and decoding deficits may be at the heart of developmental reading disorders.[21] But, what is the physiological basis of disorders in phonological awareness and decoding? We have been struck by the considerable overlap between the performance profiles reported in the literature for developmentally language-impaired and dyslexic children. Both groups

(a) Discriminant Function Analysis Summary

Variable step number	Variable entered	F value to enter	p
1	Rapid speech production	50.5	.001
2	Finger identification (two touches)	14.6	.001
3	Discriminating /ba/ vs. /da/	10.1	.01
4	Sequencing cross-modal nonverbal stimuli presented rapidly	5.6	.05
5	Sequencing letters presented rapidly	7.2	.01
6	Simultaneous tactile stimulation (face/hand)	8.0	.01

(b) Discriminant Function Equation

$Y = -1.684 \text{ (constant)} + 0.049 \text{ (Variable 1)} - 0.401 \text{ (Variable 2)} - 0.148 \text{ (Variable 3)} - 0.467 \text{ (Variable 4)} + 0.242 \text{ (Variable 5)} - 0.570 \text{ (Variable 6)}$

(c) Histogram of Canonical Variables

```
                                                            N
                                                        N   N
                                                        N   N
                                                      N NN  N
                                                      N NNN N
                                    L                 N NNNNNNNN N NNN       N   N
     L     L LLL     L LLL    LLLLL L LL       L  N   N NNNNNNNNNN N NNN     N   N
..+....+....+....+....+....+....+....+....+....+....+....+....+....+....+....+..
-5.0  -4.0  -3.0   -2.0   -1.0    0.0    1.0    2.0    3.0   4.0
```

FIGURE 3. (a) The discriminant analysis summary lists the actual variables entering the discriminant function equation, in the order of their effect on discrimination and the F-test value and appropriate significance level (p) at each step. (b) The discriminant function equation itself is displayed. (c) A discriminant function value is calculated for each subject, based on individual performance on the test variables, and is converted to a probability score as displayed in the histogram of canonical variables. (L = language impaired; N = normal control.) (From Tallal et al.[19] Reprinted with permission.)

show specific deficits at various levels of temporal integration of basic sensory information, although most of the research with language-impaired children focuses on these deficits in the auditory modality, while the research with reading-impaired children focuses on similar deficits in the visual modality.[22] Similarly, both LI and dyslexic children appear to be plagued by deficits in rapid sequential, fine motor performance.[23,24]

In an attempt to investigate the similarities and differences between LI and dyslexic children, the same series of auditory, visual, cross-modal, tactile, and motor tasks described earlier were administered to two groups of dyslexic children. One group showed not only a significant discrepancy from normals on standardized reading tests (an expected finding), but also differed from controls on measures of oral language. The other group of dyslexics was impaired in reading, but fell within normal limits on all tests of oral language. In studying these two groups we were specifically interested in identifying a relationship between deficits in phonological decoding (reading nonsense words) and temporal processing abilities, as well as assessing how the dyslexics compared to LI children on these measures. The results were clear. The dyslexic children *with* concomitant oral language disabilities showed, like the LI children, a significant deficit in both nonsense word reading and nonverbal temporal processing. Furthermore, these deficits were highly correlated ($r = 0.81$; $p < 0.001$) in this subgroup of dyslexics. As can be seen in FIGURE 4, there was a striking correspondence between the degree of deficit in nonverbal auditory temporal processing and the degree of deficit in reading nonsense words (decoding skills). On the other hand, the dyslexics with normal oral language scores had neither phonological decoding nor temporal processing deficits in *any* sensory modality. Their reading difficulties appeared to occur at a higher level of analysis.

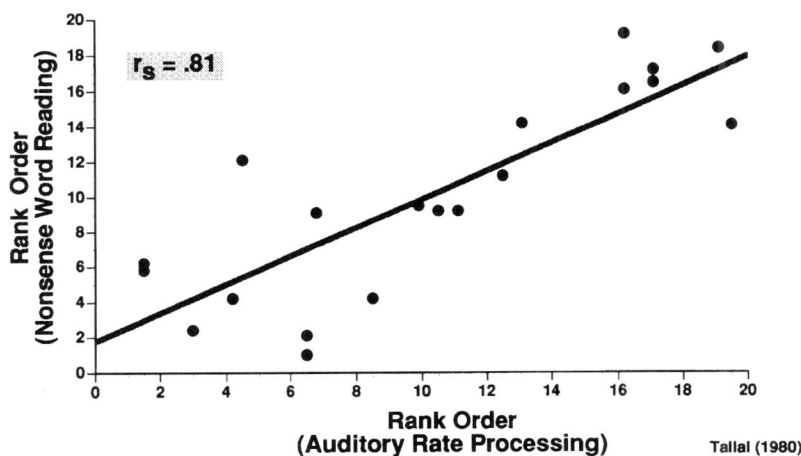

FIGURE 4. Dyslexics—Correlation between nonsense word reading and auditory rate processing. (Adapted from data presented in Tallal.[53])

CONCLUSIONS OF BEHAVIORAL STUDIES WITH LANGUAGE-IMPAIRED AND DYSLEXIC CHILDREN

This large body of data derived over a 20-year period led us to the conclusion that some children have a severe developmental deficit in processing brief components of information that enter the nervous system in rapid succession, and a concomitant motor deficit in organizing rapid sequential motor output. Importantly, this deficit appears to be highly specific, impinging primarily on neural mechanisms underlying the organization of information within the tens of millisecond range. The neurobiological basis of this deficit is, as yet, unknown. However, this deficit appears to account for the pattern of aberrations in the development of several aspects of higher level cognitive processes that are known to characterize children with developmental language and reading impairment.

One hypothesis about the emergence of the processing deficit described here is provided by Merzenich et al.[6] In his keynote address, Merzenich suggested that pansensory temporal/motor deficits could emerge through a lack of "sharpening" of temporal processes in a single modality. He theorized that a lack of critical experience in early development could bias the nervous system, rendering it unable to process rapidly presented information. In addition, because the brain has to assure that it keeps the external world in sync, processing in all modalities would have to adjust to the slowest processing rate of any single modality.

Galaburda and Livingstone[25] offer another plausible hypothesis. Based on neuroanatomical as well as physiological studies of adult developmental dyslexics, they report differences both in the structure and function of thalamocortical magnocellular systems, but intact parvocellular systems. At the physiological level, the magnocellular system appears to respond most strongly to rapid, transient, or moving stimuli presented in peripheral fields, while the parvocellular system responds most strongly to detailed, static stimuli presented foveally. Importantly, Galaburda and Livingstone report that they have found significant cellular differences at the thalamic level in the magnocellular system, but not in the parvocellular system of dyslexic brains. These cellular differences occur not only in the lateral geniculate nucleus (LGN) of the thalamus, which carries visual information, but also in the medial geniculate nucleus (MGN) of the thalamus, which carries auditory information to the cortex (including language areas). These results are very powerful, as they are the first empirical data that provide a potential direct link between anatomical, physiological, and behavioral data in dyslexia. Importantly, they pinpoint a specific neuroanatomical and physiological deficit that is compatible with the behavioral evidence of a pansensory temporal deficit in phonologically language- and reading-impaired children.

Llinas[26] offers still another hypothesis. He suggests that a specific intrinsic "clock" controlling the rate of neuronal firing patterns or oscillations might be impaired in some LI and dyslexic individuals. Interestingly, he reports that an oscillation in neuronal firing rates in the cortex of normal human subjects can be characterized in the 40-Hz range (i.e., 1 cycle every 25 ms). Furthermore, these neuronal oscillations have been hypothesized to be an essential and important component for gating or "binding" sensory information in cortico–thalamo–cortical networks. If these intrinsic oscillation rates of neural firing were "slowed" due to some developmental variation in CNS organization, one of the main functional results would be an inability to process either sensory and/or motor information presented in rapid succession within tens of milliseconds—precisely the deficit we have described for language- and reading-impaired children having concomitant phonological disorders.

The suggestion of deficient cortico–thalamo–cortical networks is intriguing in light of our recent data from magnetic resonance imaging (MRI) studies with LI children. Jernigan et al.[27] report finding significant reduction in gray matter volume in subcortical structures (including striatum and thalamus), as well as in cortical structures known to subserve language. In addition, we reported strikingly aberrant patterns of cerebral lateralization in the brains of LI children as compared to well-matched controls, in both prefrontal and parietal regions. It is compelling to note that highly significant correlations were found between the extent of aberrant hemispheric asymmetry of these cortical regions, and the degree of deficit on our tests of auditory temporal processing for these LI children.[56]

Each of these hypotheses is extremely provocative, and not necessarily mutually exclusive. We are currently investigating several of these hypotheses empirically in studies with language- and reading-impaired individuals.

One last point needs to be addressed before moving away from our studies with LI and dyslexic children. The question has frequently been asked as to how these children function relatively normally if they have such a severe and basic temporal processing deficit. It must be emphasized that the time frame that we have identified for the temporal processing disorder is in the range of tens of milliseconds. Therefore, it would be expected that only processes critically dependent on information presented (or movements produced) within this time frame would be affected.[28] Processing of information presented over longer durations, such as environmental noises, scene analysis, or coordination of gross motor movements, would not be expected to be impaired. However, the phonological processes subserving both speech perception and production *would* be expected to be particularly vulnerable to this type of temporal dysfunction. This would be the case for both oral or written language, although the effect of a temporal processing deficit on written language may be more difficult for the reader to relate to this hypothesis.

While it is true that letters remain static on the page for the reader to observe for any length of time, the visual identification of graphemes is useful only if the visual representation can be associated with a neural representation of the appropriate phoneme. We suggest that language- and reading-impaired children, due to their basic auditory temporal processing deficit, are unable to establish stable and invariant phonemic representations. As suggested by Isabelle Liberman, these children never become proficient at "phonemic awareness."[21] Many studies support such an assumption.[29] These data suggest that auditory temporal phonologic deficits are sufficient to disrupt reading development. Thus it is important to note that although temporal processing deficits are pansensory, the deficits in the other modalities, such as the transient visual system, may not in themselves affect reading directly.

HEMISPHERIC SPECIALIZATION—WHAT IS SPECIALIZED?

Shifting gears, we would like to focus on issues pertaining to hemispheric specialization for speech perception. If there is one tenet in neuropsychology that is consistently supported by numerous and diverse studies, it is that speech is processed and produced preferentially by the left cerebral hemisphere. Support for this important hypothesis derives both from studies of adults who have sustained selective brain damage leading to specific functional disorders, and from studies designed to evaluate differences in information processing within and between the cerebral hemispheres in normal intact subjects. Although there is considerable discussion about the distribution of processing of various components of language between the right and the left hemisphere, there is strong support from craniotomy and split brain studies[35,55] that phonological perception and production is primarily specialized in the left hemisphere. But, what is the neurobiological basis of this specialization? Put simply, how do neural networks or assemblies in the auditory system "know" that certain acoustic events are "speech," leading these acoustic stimuli to be selectively processed and represented in the left hemisphere? And, why did processing of such complex motor and sensory patterns become specialized in a single hemisphere? Finally, are there evolutionary precursors to hemispheric specialization for speech?

Our studies with developmental language and reading-impaired children have led us to focus on mechanisms that could subserve rapid temporal integration of ongoing streams of information within a time frame of tens of milliseconds. These data also led us to hypothesize a critical role for these temporal processes in speech perception and production. Indeed, our studies with LI and dyslexic children demonstrate clearly that major deficits in temporal analysis, in the tens of milliseconds range, may preclude the normal development of perceptual and motor phonological systems.

We turn now to a series of studies in which we addressed whether processes that have been interpreted to be hemispherically specialized for speech may in fact be specialized, more generally, for the analysis of rapidly changing acoustic information. The results from four different studies are reported. The first addresses the interpretation of speech processing studies in adults with acquired brain lesions. The second questions the results derived from speech processing studies using the dichotic listening technique. The third reports very recent data from a PET study with normal adult listeners. The final study questions the notion that hemispheric specialization is specific to humans, by investigating functional hemispheric laterlization for auditory temporal processing in rats.

Adult Acquired Lesion Studies

It is well-established that damage to the left cerebral hemisphere in humans often results in disruption of speech and language processing, a deficit known as *aphasia*. Receptive and expressive phonological processing disorders are a common sequelae of both Broca's aphasia, which results from damage to the anterior quadrant of the left hemisphere, and Wernicke's aphasia, which results from damage to the posterior quadrant of the left hemisphere. While damage to the left hemisphere is usually associated with impaired phonological processing, damage to the right hemisphere has been associated with impairments in speech prosody and other nonverbal aspects of acoustic analysis.[30-32] If this assumed dissociation between verbal and nonverbal processing of acoustic events is valid, and verbal versus nonverbal acoustic processing functions are in fact subserved by different hemispheres, such a dichotomy would raise grave questions regarding common mechanisms postulated to underlie nonverbal rapid tone processing and perceptual speech processing disorders in LI and dyslexic children.

In order to investigate this paradox, we studied a very well-characterized group of men with acquired missile wounds to either the right or left hemisphere of the brain. These subjects had previously been extensively assessed by Dr. Freda Newcombe in Oxford, England. The questions we asked were as follows: (1) Does damage to the left or right cerebral hemisphere disrupt nonverbal rapid temporal processing? (2) Are adult aphasics with acquired left-hemisphere damage impaired in perceiving all speech sound contrasts, or, like language-impaired children, selectively impaired in perceiving only those speech sound contrasts that require them to process very rapid acoustic change? (3) Is there a correlation between the degree of temporal processing impairment and receptive language impairment in adult aphasics? The results, reported in Tallal and Newcombe,[33] can be seen in FIGURE 5. Clearly, selective damage to the left, but not the right, cerebral hemisphere disrupted the ability to respond correctly to two tones with short, but not long, interstimulus intervals (ISI). Importantly, neither left- nor right-hemisphere damaged subjects differed significantly from controls in processing these nonverbal stimuli when the stimuli had longer duration ISIs. Thus, contrary to expectation, processing of rapidly changing *nonverbal* acoustic information was severely disrupted by *left*-hemisphere, not right-hemisphere, brain damage in adults.

A pattern of results that is similar to those reported earlier for LI children regarding impaired speech perception were also found for these adult aphasics. That is, adult aphasics only showed deficits in discriminating between speech sound contrasts that incorporated brief, rapidly changing temporal cues. They were completely unimpaired in the discrimination of other speech sounds that had longer

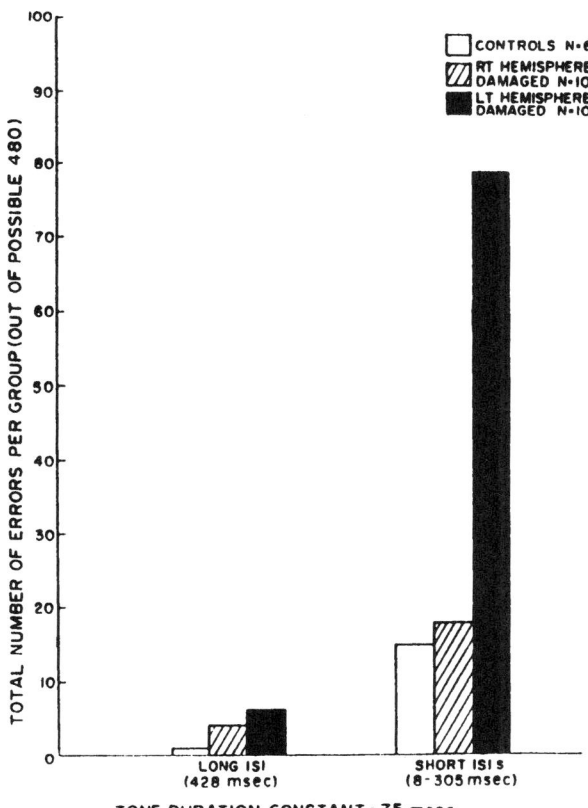

FIGURE 5. Sequencing nonverbal auditory stimuli presented at various rates. (From Tallal and Newcombe.[33] Reproduced by permission.)

duration steady-state, or more slowly changing, acoustic spectra. Finally, as can be seen in FIGURE 6, there was a highly significant correlation between the degree of receptive language impairment and the number of errors made in processing rapidly presented sequential tones for left-hemisphere damaged, adult aphasic patients.

The result of these studies with adult aphasics showed a pattern identical to results obtained from children with developmental language impairments. Furthermore, the current results demonstrate that damage to the left cerebral hemisphere disrupts the processing of rapidly changing acoustic spectra, regardless of whether stimuli are verbal or nonverbal, while leaving intact the mechanisms underlying the processing of steady-state or slowly changing information, again regardless of whether the stimuli are verbal or nonverbal.

These results support the conclusion that what is selectively damaged by left-hemisphere lesions involves mechanisms critical to the processing of information within a time frame of tens of milliseconds. We suggest that it is a disruption of this mechanism that leads to the phonological disorders so commonly seen in aphasia. We would hypothesize that these mechanisms are common to both the perception and production of speech information within this time range, and point to the work of Kimura and Archibald,[34] and Ojemann and Mateer,[35] in support of this hypothesis.

Dichotic Listening Studies

One technique that has been used extensively to study hemispheric specialization in intact, normal subjects is the dichotic listening paradigm[36] (see also Hugdahl[37] for review). This paradigm utilizes the fact that in humans, information from each ear travels primarily via a contralateral (crossed) auditory pathway, and also via an ipsilateral auditory pathway, to respective cerebral hemispheres. Information entering one hemisphere is also transferred across the corpus collosum to the opposite hemisphere. The dichotic listening technique sets up an unusual competition between these pathways by simultaneously presenting different auditory stimuli to the two

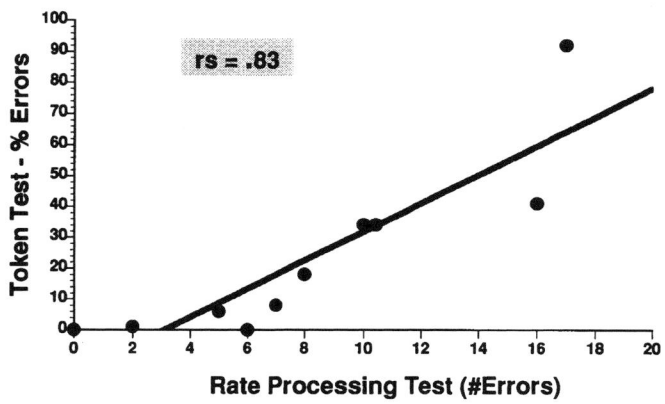

FIGURE 6. Adult aphasics—Correlation between auditory rate processing and language comprehension. (Adapted from data presented in Tallal and Newcombe.[33])

ears. A myriad of studies have shown that when competing *verbal* information is presented to the two ears, subjects more often respond correctly to the information presented to the right, as compared to the left ear. This right ear advantage (REA) has been hypothesized to result from the right ear having primary access, via contralateral pathways, to the left hemisphere. The preferential processing of speech information presented dichotically to the right ear has, historically, been used as strong evidence of left-hemisphere specialization for speech perception.

What is it about speech stimuli that gain them specialized access to left-hemisphere processing? Put a different way, what is it about left-hemisphere processing that results in more accurate perception of speech? We[38] hypothesized that the left hemisphere has specialized mechanisms allowing sensory information in the range of tens of milliseconds to be processed more effectively than in the right hemisphere. Since many components of speech fall within this critical temporal range, our hypothesis would predict that speech sounds should be processed preferentially by the left hemisphere. That is, we hypothesized that the left hemisphere is specifically specialized for the processing of information changing rapidly in the temporal dimension. We suggest that it is the temporal requirement, not the requirement for verbal analysis *per se,* underlying the observed REA for speech.

To address this hypothesis we prepared two sets of computer-generated speech stimuli. Each set derived from the consonant–vowel (CV) syllables /ba/, /da/, /ga/, /pa/, /ta/, /ka/. Recall that each of these syllables is characterized by rapidly changing formant transitions lasting approximately 40 ms. In one set of computer-generated stimuli these CV syllables were synthesized to contain the typical 40-ms-duration formant transitions. For the second set of syllables, however, we extended the duration of the formant transitions to approximately 80 ms. To ensure the "validity" of these computer-generated stimuli, we demonstrated that normal listeners and trained phonetic transcribers were equally proficient at correctly identifying the six CV syllables in both the 40- and 80-ms set. These initial results demonstrated that the temporal manipulation had not distorted phonological perception.

The two sets of CV syllable stimuli were then used to test the ear preference of normal adult listeners in a dichotic listening paradigm. Presentations of all stimuli were counterbalanced across subjects. FIGURE 7 shows the results of the study. As expected, we found a significant REA for the dichotically presented syllables with

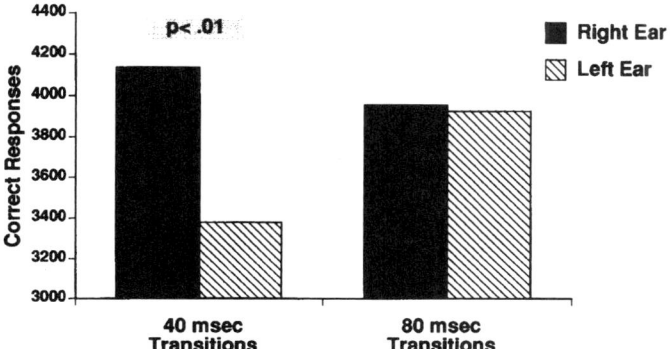

FIGURE 7. Dichotically presented CV syllables 40- vs. 80-ms formant transitions. (Adapted from data presented in Schwartz and Tallal.[38])

40-ms-duration formant transitions, replicating the results of numerous other studies performed with similar stimuli. When the CV syllables with extended-duration formant transitions were presented dichotically to subjects, however, the REA was significantly reduced.[38]

This critical result prompts a reevaluation of hypotheses regarding mechanisms underlying hemispheric specialization for speech. These data demonstrate that the left hemisphere may be specialized for processing rapidly changing temporal information, rather than speech *per se*. Previous studies have shown that speech stimuli that are steady state, or do not incorporate brief or rapidly changing temporal cues, fail to show an REA.[39] It could be argued that category differences, or differences between vowels and consonants, may have contributed to these results. In our studies, however, we used an identical set of speech syllables in each condition; these syllables were equally identifiable with respect to the intended syllable, and differed *only* in the duration of critical temporal cues. Thus, these data provide strong support for the hypothesis that, even in normal listeners, what is specialized in the left hemisphere relates to temporal constraints rather than phonological processes *per se*.

In a recent study, Poizner and Tallal (unpublished data) investigated the modality specificity of this hemispheric specialization for temporal processing. In this study, visual nonsense letters were presented tachistoscopically to either the right or left visual hemifield of normal adults, in the time range of tens of milliseconds. Right-handed adults showed superior performance in responding to the temporal order of two briefly presented visual stimuli when the stimuli were presented to their right visual field (left hemisphere) as compared to when the same stimuli were presented to their left visual field. These data taken in combination with the dichotic listening results support the hypothesis that the left hemisphere is better equipped to process temporal events that converge in the nervous system within tens of milliseconds regardless of sensory modality, and regardless of whether stimuli are verbal or nonverbal.

PET Studies

At the 1992 Annual Meeting of the Society of Neuroscience, Tallal and collaborators at Washington University in St. Louis (Steve Petersen, Julie Fiez, and Marcus Raichle), reported[40] the results of a study using positron emission tomography (PET) scanning to investigate neural aspects of speech and temporal perception in healthy adult volunteers. Subjects listened to four sets of sounds that were designed to determine which areas of the brain were significantly activated during speech and nonspeech acoustic processing. Speech stimuli that either did (syllables, words) or did not (vowels) incorporate rapidly changing acoustic spectra were used. In addition, complex acoustic stimuli that incorporated temporal changes within the range that occur in speech, but did not have verbal meaning, were used. Significant decreases in activity occurred bilaterally for all four sets of stimuli in a number of regions in the parietal lobe. Increases in activity were found in both the left and right temporal and frontal cortex. One area (Brodmann 45) in the left frontal cortex was particularly interesting. This area was near Broca's area, a frontal area that when damaged, is known to lead to aphasia. The left frontal area was significantly activated only by the sets of stimuli that incorporated rapid acoustic change (syllables, words, and brief tone sequences). Importantly, significant distinctions in activation in the left hemisphere did not occur along verbal versus nonverbal lines, as may have been expected. The vowels, which are verbal, but do not incorporate a rapidly changing acoustic spectrum, did not significantly activate the same left frontal brain region as the three sets of stimuli that did incorporate brief temporal cues.[41]

These PET data, derived from imaging metabolic activity in the brains of healthy adults, are consistent with the findings from studies of children who experience developmental language and reading disorders. These children have great difficulty processing stimuli incorporating brief temporal cues (rapidly presented auditory, visual, or tactual sequences, syllables, and words), but have no problem processing steady-state vowels and other verbal and nonverbal stimuli that do not require the integration of sensory information within the tens of milliseconds range. They are also consistent with the results of a magnetic resonance imaging (MRI) study in which Jernigan and Tallal found that language-impaired children failed to show expected cerebral asymmetry in the frontal and parietal regions.[27] The degree of aberrant cerebral asymmetry in these two brain regions was highly correlated with deficits in processing rapidly presented tone sequences.[56]

Animal Studies

The belief has long been held that the ability to perceive and produce human speech represents a unique and special process. Even though the basic mechanisms for encoding speech stimuli are, technically, a form of acoustic information processing, many have held fast to the notion that speech processing is distinct from the discrimination of other complex but nonverbal acoustic sounds. Central to this philosophy is the assumption that key components in speech processing are to be found only in the human brain, and not in any other species.[42] However, accumulated evidence from our behavioral studies with LI children suggest that: (1) a common mechanism underlies the discrimination of verbal *and* nonverbal acoustic stimuli characterized by rapid change in the temporal domain; and (2) disruption of this auditory temporal processing ability impairs *both* the ability to discriminate speech sounds and nonverbal stimuli such as tone pairs. Given these results, one can introduce the evolutionary hypothesis that auditory temporal processing represents a "precursor" to speech processing, and further, that left-hemisphere specialization for this basic process might be expected in other species. To assess this hypothesis, we designed a series of studies to investigate the potential origins of left-hemisphere specialization for speech processing in an animal model.

While other researchers have identified left-hemisphere specialization for the discrimination of species-typical calls in both monkeys and mice,[43-45] these results have typically been interpreted as evidence of left-hemisphere specialization for communicative information processing. Such an interpretation, however, is called into question by findings that monkeys exhibit left-hemisphere specialization for performing complex auditory discriminations of stimuli with *no* communicative relevance,[46,47] and also findings that the key information used by monkeys in discriminating species-typical calls is peak frequency position, a specifically temporal cue.[48] Thus, we would argue that the preceding results may reflect left-hemisphere specialization for auditory temporal processing in other species, and that this mechanism is critical to the discrimination of both coo calls in monkeys and ultrasonic noise bursts in mice.

To further investigate this hypothesis, Fitch *et al.*[49] have trained adult rats in a modified operant conditioning procedure that culminated in a test paradigm similar to a human dichotic listening test. Sequences of two tones separated by an interstimulus interval were presented selectively to the right or left ear, while white noise was presented to the contralateral ear. Rats were trained to use a go/no go strategy to identify one "target" sequence out of three other possible negative sequences. Correct responses resulted in water reinforcement. It is important to note that these tone sequences carried no intrinsic communicative relevance for the rat. Results showed that adult male rats were significantly better at discriminating these tone sequences with the right as compared to the left ear, a finding that has been replicated in two additional studies.[50,54]

Interestingly, human dichotic listening tests and tests of language recovery after left-hemisphere damage have shown a gender difference suggesting stronger left-hemisphere specialization of language function in males (e.g., see Kimura and Harshman[51] and McGlone[52]). We were interested in whether this result might reflect stronger lateralization of auditory temporal processing in males and, if so, whether the same effect might be seen in a nonlingual species. Thus adult male and female rats were simultaneously tested in the paradigm just described. Results showed a highly significant interaction between sex and ear advantage across two separate studies; male rats were, in fact, significantly more lateralized to the left hemisphere than females.[54]

These results are of significant interest for two reasons. First, they support the critical importance of a basic, nonlingual process—auditory temporal processing—to the existence of left-hemisphere specialization for language processing in humans, by suggesting that critical precursors to this function can be found in other species. Thus, in addition to studies with LI children that argue that basic temporal processing abilities are critical to the development of speech processing, we now argue that this function may underlie the very evolution of speech processing mechanisms as well. Second, the identification of neural mechanisms for this critical function in an animal model provides the opportunity for asking questions that cannot be easily addressed in human subjects. Further studies are currently in progress to (1) examine the effects of hormonal manipulations and stress on lateralization for auditory temporal processing; (2) examine the effects of specific neuropathologies that mimic those observed in adult dyslexic brains on auditory temporal discrimination in rats; and (3) to assess the relative organization of this function within the CNS.

The long-term goal of our studies is to shed light not only on key issues underlying the mystery of developmental language and reading disorders, but also on fundamental questions pertaining to the neurobiological basis of phonological systems in humans and the origins of hemispheric specialization for language.

REFERENCES

1. BEITCHMAN, J. H., R. NAIR & P. G. PATEL. 1986. Prevalence of speech and language disorders in 5-year-old kindergarten children in the Ottawa-Carlton region. J. Speech Hear. Disord. **51:** 98–110.
2. TALLAL, P. & M. PIERCY. 1973. Developmental aphasia: Impaired rate of non-verbal processing as a function of sensory modality. Neuropsychologia **11:** 389–398.
3. STARK, R. E. & P. TALLAL. 1981. Selection of children with specific language deficits. J. Speech Hear. Disord. **46:** 114–122.
4. ZEIGLER, M., P. TALLAL & S. CURTISS. 1990. Selecting language impaired children for research studies: Insights from the San Diego Longitudinal Study. Percept. Motor Skills **71:** 1079–1089.

5. TALLAL, P. & M. PIERCY. 1973. Defects of non-verbal auditory perception in children with developmental aphasia. Nature **241**: 468–469.
6. MERZENICH, M. M., C. SCHREINER, W. JENKINS & X. WANG. 1993. Neural mechanisms underlying temporal integration, segmentation, and input sequence representations: Some implications for the origin of learning disabilities. This issue.
7. TALLAL, P. & M. PIERCY. 1974. Developmental aphasia: Rate of auditory processing and selective impairment of consonant perception. Neuropsychologia **12**: 83–93.
8. ———. 1975. Developmental aphasia: The perception of brief vowels and extended stop consonants. Neuropsychologia **13**: 69–74.
9. TALLAL, P. & R. E. STARK. 1981. Speech acoustic-cue discrimination abilities of normally developing and language-impaired children. J. Acoust. Soc. Am. **69**: 568–574.
10. ELLIOT, L. L., M. A. HAMMER & M. E. SCHOLL. 1989. Fine-grained auditory discrimination in normal children and children with language-learning problems. J. Speech Hear. Res. **32**: 112–119.
11. STEFFENS, M. L., R. E. EILERS, K. GROSS-GLENN & B. JALLAD. 1992. Speech perception in adults subjects with familial dyslexia. J. Speech Hear. Res. **35**: 192–200.
12. TOMBLIN, J. B., P. R. FREESE & N. L. RECORDS. 1992. Diagnosing specific language impairment in adults for the purpose of pedigree analysis. J. Speech Hear. Res. **35**: 832–843.
13. R. STARK & P. TALLAL. 1979. Analysis of stop consonant production errors in developmentally dysphasic children. J. Acoust. Soc. Am. **66**: 1703–1712.
14. TALLAL, P., R. E. STARK & S. CURTISS. 1976. Relation between speech perception and speech production impairment in children with developmental dysphasia. Brain Lang. **3**: 305–317.
15. TALLAL, P., R. E. STARK & D. MELLITS. 1985. The relationship between auditory temporal analysis and receptive language development: Evidence from studies of developmental language disorder. Neuropsychologia **23**: 527–534.
16. JOHNSTON, R. B., R. E. STARK, E. D. MELLITS & P. TALLAL. 1981. Neurological status of language-impaired and normal children. Ann. Neurol. **10**: 159–163.
17. KATZ, W. F., S. CURTISS & P. TALLAL. 1992. Rapid automatized naming and gesture by normal and language-impaired children. Brain Lang. **43**: 623–641.
18. TALLAL, P., R. STARK, C. KALLMAN & D. MELLITS. 1981. A reexamination of some nonverbal perceptual abilities of language-impaired and normal children as a function of age and sensory modality. J. Speech Hear. Res. **24**: 351–357.
19. TALLAL, P., R. E. STARK & D. MELLITS. 1985. Identification of language-impaired children on the basis of rapid perception and production skills. Brain Lang. **25**: 314–322.
20. TALLAL, P., S. CURTISS & R. KAPLAN. 1988. The San Diego longitudinal study: Evaluating the outcomes of preschool impairment in language development. *In* International Perspectives on Communication Disorders, S. E. Gerber & G. T. Mencher, Eds.: 86–126. Gallaudet Univ. Press. Washington, D.C.
21. LIBERMAN, I. Y. & D. SHANKWEILER. 1985. Phonology and the problems of learning to read and write. Rem. Spec. Educ. **6**: 8–17.
22. LOVEGROVE, W. 1993. Weakness in the transient visual system: A causal factor in dyslexia? This issue.
23. WOLFF, P. H. 1993. Impaired temporal resolution in developmental dyslexia. This issue.
24. KATZ, W. F., S. CURTISS & P. TALLAL. 1993. Naming and gesture by normal and language-impaired children: Evidence from a modified rapid automatized naming test. This issue.
25. GALABURDA, A. & M. LIVINGSTONE. 1993. Evidence for a magnocellular defect in developmental dyslexia. This issue.
26. LLINAS, R. 1993. Is dyslexia a dischronia? This issue.
27. JERNIGAN, T., J. HESSELINK & P. TALLAL. 1991. Cerebral structure on magnetic resonance imaging in language-learning impaired children. Arch. Neurol. **48**: 539–545.
28. PHILLIPS, D. P. 1993. Neural representation of stimulus times in the primary auditory cortex. This issue.

29. GOSWAMI, U. Phonological skills and learning to read. This issue.
30. BLUMENSTEIN, S. & W. E. COOPER. 1974. Hemispheric processing of intonation contours. Cortex **10:** 146–158.
31. MILNER, B. 1962. Laterality effects in audition. *In* Interhemispheric Relations and Cerebral Dominance, V. Mountcastle, Ed.: 177–195. Johns Hopkins Univ. Press. Baltimore, Md.
32. ZATORRE, R. J., A. C. EVANS, E. MEYER & A. GJEDDE. 1992. Lateralization of phonetic and pitch discrimination in speech processing. Science **256:** 846–849.
33. TALLAL, P. & F. NEWCOMBE. 1978. Impairment of auditory perception and language comprehension in dysphasia. Brain Lang. **5:** 13–24.
34. KIMURA, D. & Y. ARCHIBALD. 1974. Motor function of the left hemisphere. Brain **97:** 337–350.
35. OJEMANN, G. A. & C. MATEER. 1979. Human language cortex: Localization of memory, syntax, and sequential motor-phoneme identification systems. Science **205:** 1401–1403.
36. KIMURA, D. 1961. Cerebral dominance and the perception of verbal stimuli. Can. J. Psychol. **15:** 166–171.
37. HUGDAHL, K., Ed. 1988. Handbook of Dichotic Listening: Theory, Methods and Research. Wiley. New York.
38. SCHWARTZ, J. & P. TALLAL. 1980. Rate of acoustic change may underlie hemispheric specialization for speech perception. Science **207:** 1380–1381.
39. CUTTING, J. E. 1974. Two left hemisphere mechanisms in speech perception. Percept. Psychophys. **16:** 601–612.
40. FIEZ, J. A., P. TALLAL, F. M. MIEZIN, S. DOBMEYER, M. E. RAICHLE & S. E. PETERSEN. 1992. PET studies of auditory processing: Passive presentation and active detection. Soc. Neurosci. Abstr. **18:** 932.
41. FIEZ, J. A. Functional anatomy of lexical processing: Pet activation and performance studies. Washington Univ. St. Louis, Mo.
42. LIBERMAN, A. M. 1993. In speech perception, time is not the enemy. This issue.
43. EHRET, G. 1987. Left hemisphere advantage in the mouse brain for recognizing ultrasonic communication calls. Nature **325:** 249 and 249–251.
44. HEFFNER, H. E. & R. S. HEFFNER. 1986. Effects of unilateral and bilateral auditory cortex lesions on the discrimination of vocalizations by Japanese macaques. J. Neurophysiol. **56:** 683–701.
45. PETERSEN, M. R., M. D. BEECHER, S. R. ZOLOTH, D. B. MOODY & W. C. STEBBINS. 1978. Neural lateralization of species-specific vocalizations by Japanese macaques *(Macaca fuscata)*. Science **202:** 325–327.
46. DEWSON, J. H. III. 1977. Preliminary evidence of hemispheric asymmetry of auditory function in monkeys. *In* Lateralization in the Nervous System, S. Harnad, R. W. Doty, L. Goldstein, J. Jaynes, and G. Krauthamer, Eds.: 63–71. Academic Press. New York.
47. GAFFAN, D. & S. HARRISON. 1991. Auditory-visual associations, hemispheric specialization and temporal-frontal interaction in the rhesus monkey. Brain **114:** 2133–2144.
48. MAY, B., D. B. MOODY & W. C. STEBBINS. 1989. Categorical perception of conspecific communication sounds by Japanese macaques. *Macaca fuscata.* J. Acoust. Soc. Am. **85:** 837–847.
49. FITCH, R. H., C. BROWN & P. TALLAL. 1992. Left hemisphere specialization for auditory discrimination in male and female rats. Soc. Neurosci. Abstr. **18:** 1039.
50. ———. 1993. Left hemisphere specialization for auditory temporal processing in rats. This issue.
51. KIMURA, D. & R. HARSHMAN. 1984. Sex differences in brain organization for verbal and non-verbal functions. *In* Progress in Brain Research, Vol. 61, G. J DeVries *et al.* Eds. Elsevier. Amsterdam, the Netherlands.
52. MCGLONE, J. 1980. Sex differences in human brain asymmetry: A critical review. Behav. Brain Sci. **3:** 215–263.
53. TALLAL, P. 1980. Auditory temporal perception, phonics, and reading disabilities in children. Brain Lang. **9:** 182–198.

54. FITCH, R. H., C. BROWN, K. O'CONNOR & P. TALLAL. 1993. Functional lateralization for auditory temporal processing in male and female rats. Behav. Neurosci. In press.
55. GAZZANIGA, M. S. 1970. The Bissected Brain. Appleton-Century-Crofts. New York.
56. TALLAL, P., R. SAINBURG & T. JERNIGAN. 1991. Neuropathology of developmental dysphasia. Read. Writ. **4:** 65–79.

Is Dyslexia a Dyschronia?

RODOLFO LLINÁS

Department of Physiology and Biophysics
New York University Medical Center
550 First Avenue
New York, New York 10016

INTRODUCTION

This quite unique conference has convened a variety of clinical and basic scientists concerned with language disorders and dyslexia. We seek to enhance through dialogue our mutual understanding of language dysfunctions.

An important step in this direction would be to widen our concept of the dyslexic syndrome to encompass more than the issues that relate to language, writing, and reading skills. Ultimately, dyslexia is a nervous system dysfunction, and as such, must be reducible to problems at a level more basic than that at which it is expressed (behavior), that is, to the realm of neuronal or synaptic malfunction. In addition, the dyschronicity of dyslexia may interfere with rapid processing and could lead to problems with the ability to learn associatively and, therefore, with phonologically learned skills.

Viewing the dyslectic syndrome most broadly, as would a nonspecialist, one salient point seems to be the difficulty that dyslexics have with certain tasks that fall outside the purely linguistic domain. These include at least two global types of dysfunction: (a) the abnormal delay in the ability to discriminate between different sensory stimuli if they are presented nearly simultaneously,[1,2] and (b) a difficulty in generating active movements that require rapid succession.[3] The latter includes speed deficits in lexical tasks[4] and recently discovered processing-speed deficits with visual tasks,[5,6] with choice-reaction tasks to pure tones,[7] and with the ability to compensate sufficiently quickly for slight losses of balance.[8] These two dysfunctions are present in many severe cases of dyslexia[9] and add significantly to other documented problems of dyslexics, concerning memory acquisition and category formation. One may surmise that given the difficulty dyslexics have in dealing with rapid sequence in sensory and motor performance, the issue of timing may be one of the responsible elements in the syndrome just cited.

Timing is essential in the functioning of even the simplest dynamic system. For example, in a combustion engine, the timing between the compression of the gasified gasoline and its ignition by the activation of the spark plug is absolutely essential for the engine to function as an efficient source of kinetic energy. Indeed, an improperly tuned car generates a host of problems that may manifest themselves in a rich repertoire; the car may not start as readily as expected, it may not climb a hill well, acceleration may be sluggish, and it may stall easily. By correcting the *timing* of the engine, all of these problems disappear, since they all derive from a single cause— the dynamics of the system. Indeed, nothing is missing, yet events do not follow each other exactly as they should. It is my feeling that such "dyschronia" may be a significant factor in dyslexia.

It may be concluded at the outset, therefore, that in dyslexics a set of fundamental properties of the central nervous system (CNS) is altered, which in turn disrupts specific aspects of CNS function. Yet, we must keep in mind that those affected function successfully and even thrive in our complex society.

TIMING AND BRAIN FUNCTION

At this point we should consider what we mean by timing in reference to brain function. In this context, timing has to do with three seemingly disparate neuronal properties, those of (i) time intervals (in the sense of duration), themselves deeply embedded in the kinetics of the neuronal electrophysiological processes; (ii) simultaneity, that is, neuronal events happening at the same time, but not necessarily next to each other in the brain; and (iii) the intrinsic rhythmic activity of neurons, from which oscillatory coherence among groups of cell ensembles arises. These three properties are the basis for our view of temporal conjunction or binding,[10,11] in which brain function is conceived as anatomically dispersed over specific sensory and motor maps, but bound together by time, in the sense of being capable of temporal resonance. These two features of neuronal events, specificity of location and resonance generate a particular functional space, the "where-when domain." Such a domain can be considered at the basis for cognitive brain functions. Since this timing component is central to brain function, we must consider the mechanisms by which it is generated. Not surprisingly, rhythmicity—the ability to generate repeated events at fixed time intervals—arises mostly, but not exclusively, from the intrinsic electrical properties of neurons.[11] Synchronicity, the ability of cell groups to generate electrical signals at the same time, depends also on the properties of synaptic transmission and on the conductance properties of the pathways that carry such rhythmic events. Rhythmic entrainment (resonance) may be generated as rhythmic events are locked to each other in time to generate a pacemaker.

A good example of rhythmic resonance generating synchronicity in a neuronal network is the olivocerebellar system, in which rhythmic firing in the inferior olive nucleus reaches all sites of the cerebellar cortex at the same time, regardless of the distance between the various portions of these two brain regions.[12] This synchronicity, which varies less than one millisecond, is accomplished by varying conductance velocities of the olivocerebellar axon such that their conduction time is the same to all parts of the cortex.[12] This means that while the cerebellar cortex is deeply folded, and thus the distance between the most superficial and the deepest regions may vary as much as 50 percent of the length of the olivocortical path, conduction time differences are tuned during development to allow such synchronicity.[12] If we now consider that such a principle is present in areas other than the cerebellum,[12] it becomes evident that if different cell groups having similar intrinsic rhythmicity are interconnected, resonance between these distant sites or neural systems can easily occur. Thus, while such systems may be physically separated in space, they are next to each other in time.

NEURONAL OSCILLATIONS

Before considering what types of neuronal oscillation may be altered in dyslexics, a quick review of the phenomenologies observed in single neurons may be important, since they suggest possible ways to address the problem, especially from a pharmacological point of view. With a few well-known exceptions, neurons are capable of generating action potentials, which for all practical purposes can be considered to be single-wave oscillations. Their propagation down an axon is a bit like the solitons in rivers or the wave that travels to the end of a whip that is cracked. By contrast, subthreshold membrane oscillations are the ionic events that generate the sinusoidal-like membrane potential waves that are present in many neurons of the CNS, most notably the inferior olive and thalamus. Because disruptions of such type of activity may be an important part of dyslexia, I will describe their properties briefly.

Inferior Olivary Neurons: Threshold and Subthreshold Oscillations

In vitro experiments in brain slices have demonstrated that mammalian inferior olivary (I.O.) neurons possess a set of ionic conductances that promote single-cell oscillatory electrical activity.[13-16] That is, I.O. neurons may be considered to be single-cell oscillators. The firing of I.O. cells is characterized by an initial fast-rising action potential—a somatic sodium spike—followed by a 10–15-ms after-depolarization that is generated by a powerful calcium-dependent dendritic spike (FIG. 1A). Subsequently, calcium-dependent potassium conductances are activated, generating a long after-hyperpolarization (AHP) that shunts most synaptic input and silences the spike-generating activity. During this AHP a somatic calcium conductance is deinactivated and, as the membrane potential begins to depolarize, these channels open, an active calcium rebound response brings the membrane to spike threshold and a low-threshold calcium spike is generated[13] (FIG. 1B). Accordingly, if the dendritic-calcium action potential is narrow, the duration of the AHP will be short, the low-threshold calcium conductance deinactivation may be incomplete, the rebound response will have a low amplitude, and spike threshold will not be reached.

The latter point is central to our understanding of the oscillatory properties of I.O. cells. It demonstrates that calcium entry probably determines the cycle time and the robustness of this neuronal oscillator by influencing the strength of the AHP, and therefore the generation of rebound spikes.

In addition to oscillations that reach spike threshold, subthreshold membrane-potential oscillations may also be recorded intracellularly (FIG. 1C). Close to sinusoidal, these spontaneous oscillations represent an emerging property of the I.O. neuronal ensemble. The frequency of these spontaneous oscillations is independent of the electroresponsive state of any individual neuron, but depend on the fact that I.O. cells are linked by gap junctions. Indeed, direct activation of the recorded cell does not alter the oscillation frequency.[15,16] However, the oscillation can be altered substantially via electrical activation of the ensembles of neurons.

The electrical properties previously described enable I.O. neurons to resonate at two distinct frequency ranges: (1) 3 to 6 Hz, or (2) 9 to 12 Hz, depending on whether the dendritic or somatic calcium electroresponsiveness predominates. In a cell slightly depolarized from its resting level the firing frequency will be determined by the calcium entering during the dendritic spike, which in turn governs the size and duration of the AHP (through activation of a calcium-dependent potassium conductance). At more hyperpolarized levels, however, active invasion of the dendrites is decreased and the firing frequency is dominated by the deinactivating rebound somatic-calcium conductance[15] (through the deinactivation and subsequent opening of the somatic calcium conductance).

In vivo experiments have shown that intrinsic properties, such as those generating membrane oscillations, are a prerequisite for the timing required for motor execution, for example, that which characterize the cerebellar control of motor coordination.[17]

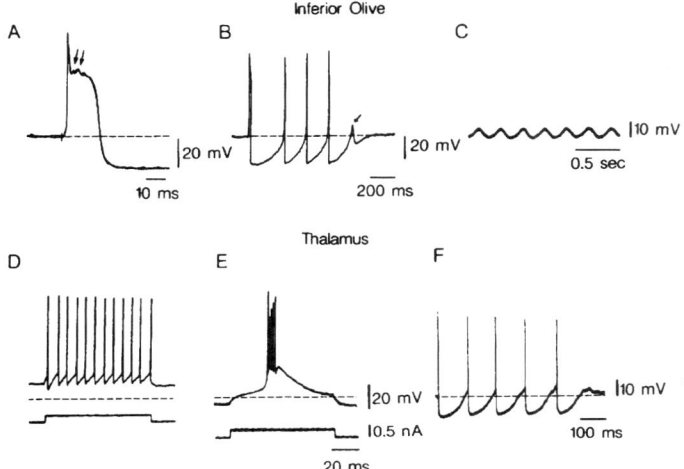

FIGURE 1. Oscillatory properties of CNS nuclear cells. A–C. Oscillatory properties of I.O. neurons recorded *in vitro*. A. Antidromically activated action potentials recorded intracellularly. Initial fast depolarization followed by an after-depolarization and after-hyperpolarization can be seen. *Arrows* mark firing of axon. B. Spontaneous burst of spikes. The initial spike is followed by three action potentials and a subthreshold rebound indicated by an *arrow*. Note that the threshold for the rebound response is negative to the resting membrane potential. C. Spontaneous oscillatory potentials in inferior olivary cells. Oscillatory potentials occurring at close to resting potential, having a peak-to-peak average of approximately 8 mV and a peak-to-peak frequency of approximately 5 Hz *in vitro*. D–F. Oscillatory properties of thalamic cells. D. A depolarizing current pulse produces a train of action potentials if superimposed on a slightly depolarized membrane potential level. E. The cell was directly stimulated while being hyperpolarized by a constant current injection. The outward current pulse, which had the same amplitude as those in **D**, now triggers an all-or-none burst of spikes. F. Depolarization of a thalamic neuron from rest triggered self-maintained oscillation at 9 Hz. (Parts **A, B,** and **C** modified from from Llinás and Yarom;[13,15] parts **D, E,** and **F** modified from from Llinás.[11])

Thalamic Neuron Oscillations: Two Modes of Firing

Because cognition is so closely tied to thalamocortical activity, a review of thalamic neuron physiology may be quite useful in the context of this conference. In contrast to the rather stereotypical membrane oscillations of I.O. cells, thalamic cells may oscillate or may fire tonically. In the latter mode they resemble most other CNS neurons in that their firing frequency is proportional to membrane depolarization.

Thalamic neurons are able to fire at high frequencies because their dendritic calcium conductance is not large, making their Ca-dependent AHP shorter than in the I.O. (FIG. 1D). When thalamic cells are hyperpolarized, however, a low-threshold calcium spike comparable to that in the I.O., triggers a short phasic burst of spikes[18] (FIG. 1E). This burst is activated by a low-threshold calcium spike comparable to that in the I.O.[13] These two types of electrical behavior allow thalamic cells to switch from a tonic to a phasic firing pattern by modulation of the membrane potential.

In addition to the ability to fire in two distinct modes, thalamic cells fire at one of three preferred frequencies: near 6 Hz,[18] near 10 Hz,[18] or near 40 Hz.[19] The ionic mechanisms underlying thalamic neuron oscillatory behavior are in some aspects quite similar to those encountered in I.O. cells. In addition to having rather limited dendritic calcium-dependent excitability, however, thalamic cells display an early potassium conductance ("A" current) similar to that described in invertebrate neurons.[20,21] This particular conductance allows oscillatory single-cell response near 6 Hz at negative membrane potentials. When depolarized, the activation of a persistent sodium conductance, similar to that seen in Purkinje cells,[11] dominates neuronal excitability and triggers fast sodium-dependent spikes at close to 10 Hz (FIG. 1F).

The point of interest here is that the switching of firing modes in thalamic neurons can trigger macroscopic changes in functional states as dramatic as the difference between wakefulness and sleep.[22,23]

Neocortical Interneurons: Two Types of Subthreshold Oscillations

Subthreshold membrane potential oscillations have been recorded from layer IV neocortical interneurons *in vitro*.[24,25] Oscillations were present at the resting membrane potential in about half the neurons recorded and were elicited by depolarization in the other cells. Two types of layer IV interneurons were identified according to the characteristics of their subthreshold oscillations: broad-frequency oscillators and narrow-frequency oscillators.[25]

Broad-frequency Oscillators

In these cells injection of low-amplitude current pluses elicited a burst of action potentials followed by irregular single-spike firing. As in the ECII stellate cells, the oscillations are generated by the sequential activation of voltage-gated sodium and potassium conductances. The oscillatory frequency of these calls was sensitive to membrane potential level within a range of 10–40 Hz.

Narrow-frequency Oscillations

In the second type of interneuron the frequency of the subthreshold oscillations was independent of the membrane potential. Subthreshold oscillations were rarely observed at the resting membrane potential, but were invariably evoked by membrane depolarization. These cells demonstrated a clear persistent sodium-dependent plateau potential upon which subthreshold oscillations were generated. The average frequency at 37°C was 44.7 ± 4.64 Hz. In this type of cell a depolarizing pulse delivered during the subthreshold oscillation increased the likelihood that the oscillation reached spike threshold. The spiking occurred at the peak of the oscillation potentials and, unlike the broad range oscillators, membrane depolarization did not alter their oscillatory frequency.

Intracellular staining has shown that these cells belong to the sparsely spinous group of cortical neurons,[25] and their axonal projection fields are consistent with their classification as cortical inhibitory interneurons.[26]

40-Hz Oscillation in CNS Function

Now, in order to place single-cell properties as previously described into a framework that relates to a more global description of brain function, I would like to address the question of 40-Hz oscillation and its relation on the one hand, to cell function, and on the other hand, to cognition. Indeed, rhythmic oscillatory potentials have been found within a given cortical column in the visual cortex.[27] These oscillations are well correlated with single-unit activity within the column and are thought to serve as an associative mechanism in the temporal domain via synchronized oscillatory rhythmicity.[27] This temporal association or "binding" has been demonstrated using cross correlation between columns.[27,28]

The neuronal source of this high-frequency oscillation has not yet been resolved. It was proposed that the thalamus serves a linking function allowing conjunction by coherent resonance between different cortical regions.[28] This view is supported by the finding that thalamic-projection neurons fire at 30 to 40 Hz, following activation of brainstem cholinergic inputs.[29]

At least two classes of cortical interneurons are capable of subthreshold oscillatory rhythms at frequencies similar to those found in the "activated" cortical column.[27] Of these, the broad-frequency (ECIIsc) oscillators increase their frequency with membrane depolarization. This tendency may allow "coherent resonance" that may facilitate phase locking of the oscillations in these neurons, depending on the excitatory synaptic activity in layer IV of the cortex.

These findings suggest that inhibitory interneurons may play a role in cortical associative processing as outlined previously.[24] According to that hypothesis: (1) the thalamus would activate, in addition to the well-known excitatory input to all cortical layers,[30] layer IV inhibitory interneurons that, when sufficiently depolarized, would oscillate at close to 40 Hz. (2) Superimposed on the specific excitatory activity generated in the cortex by the incoming thalamic activity, the inhibitory interneurons would elicit inhibitory postsynaptic potentials (IPSPs) in other cortical neurons, including the pyramidal cells of layer VI. (3) These IPSPs would shape the rhythmic inhibition of pyramidal-cell activity at 40 Hz, or at a harmonic frequency, producing the rhythmicity observed in the visual cortex.[27]

BINDING BY SPECIFIC AND NONSPECIFIC 40-Hz RESONANT CONJUNCTIONS

Summarizing recent findings on oscillation then, 40-Hz activity is present at many levels in the CNS, to include such sites as the retina[31] and olfactory bulb;[32] the specific[33] and nonspecific[34] thalamus; and the neocortex.[25]

Moreover some 40-Hz activity recorded in the visual cortex is correlated with retinal 40-Hz activity.[31] Thus, such oscillation involves not only cortical but also thalamocortical interactions. In this scheme[33] (FIG. 2, left), 40-Hz oscillation of specific thalamic neurons[34] can establish thalamocortical resonance as reviewed earlier via fourth-layer inputs, which resonates with inhibitory interneurons at that level.[25] Such oscillation can reenter the thalamus via the layer VI pyramidal cells and resonate with both the nucleus reticularis and in the specific thalamic nuclei.[25]

On the other hand, a second system (FIG. 2, right) is represented by the intralaminary cortical input to layer I of the cortex and its return-pathway projection via layers V and VI pyramidal systems to the intralaminary nucleus, directly and indirectly via collaterals to the nucleus reticularis.[35] Since, as stated earlier, these cells have been shown to oscillate in 40-Hz bursts and to be organized in a toroidal nucleus,[36] which could result in recurrent activity that is the ultimate cause of the rostrocaudal cortical activation found in the magnetoencephalographic recordings.[33]

Finally, it is also evident from the literature that neither of these two circuits alone can generate cognition. Indeed, damage of the nonspecific thalamus produces deep disturbances of consciousness, while damage of specific systems produces loss of the particular modality. As such, consciousness may arise by the resonant 40-Hz coactivation of at least these two systems, which would temporarily conjoin cerebral cortical sites specifically activated at or around 40-Hz frequency. In this manner the specific system would provide the content and the nonspecific system that would generate the temporal binding of such content into a single cognitive experience.

One can easily imagine how a slight modification of oscillatory properties could result in a well-defined functional deficiency in behavior. Two frequencies in particular may be considered when considering dysfunction. One would be the 10-Hz oscillation that seems to be the timing signal for movements and which, as in the case

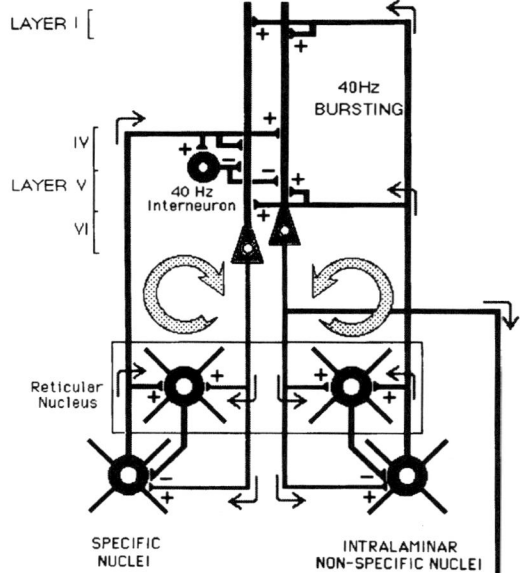

FIGURE 2. Thalamocortical circuits proposed to serve temporal binding. (A) Diagram of two thalamocortical systems. (**Left**) Specific sensory or motor nuclei project to layer IV of the cortex, producing cortical oscillation by direct activation and feed-forward inhibition via 40-Hz inhibitory interneurons. Collaterals of these projections produce thalamic feedback inhibition via the nucleus reticularis. The return pathway *(circular arrow on the right)* reenters this oscillation to specific and reticularis thalamic nuclei via layer VI pyramidal cells. (**Right**) Second loop shows nonspecific intralaminary nuclei projecting to the most superficial layer of the cortex and giving collaterals to the reticular nucleus. Layer V pyramidal cells return oscillation to the reticular and the nonspecific thalamic nuclei, establishing a second resonant loop. The conjunction of the specific and nonspecific loops is proposed to generate temporal binding. (Modified from Llinás and Ribary.[33])

of physiological tremor, can interfere with timing of precise movements or motor coordination. However, a likely possibility for the abnormal behavior of dyslexia may instead be related to the 40-Hz rhythmicity, since such rhythmicity is associated with higher levels of brain function. In particular, if one agrees with the hypothesis that the rostrocaudal scan produced by the 40-Hz organization of thalamocortical pathways represents the functional basis of cognition, then one could easily see how an abnormality in this type of function may be ultimately responsible for the temporal binding that allows cognition to be unified into well-defined temporal sets of sequences. It then would follow that by being altered they could interfere partially or completely with the perception of stimuli presented at short intervals. Such a hypothesis may then be proposed as related to the physiological basis for dyslexia.

THE CONCEPT OF DYSCHRONIA

Thus the proposal advanced here is that in dyslexia, due to cellular dysfunction, the normal properties of neuronal circuits responsible for temporal aspects of cognition are modified in a particular range. It is suggested further that this modification allows the nervous system to function only within particular temporal windows, within which its function is close to normal. However, neuronal abnormalities are such that ensemble oscillations may fall within a particular range (one may consider 25 ms as such a range). We propose that such abnormalities, if present, may generate two significant brain events: (1) the inability to generate sharp enough ensemble oscillations at higher frequencies (i.e., 35–45 Hz), and (2) the inability to reset such rhythmicity following close-interval sensory stimulation.

In fact, one would predict that the absence of the proper triggering, or resetting, of 40-Hz or 10-Hz activity, could give rise to consequences similar to those presented in dyslexia. This is a working hypothesis that is currently being tested experimentally. If such thinking were to be correct, then the implications would be significant and promising, as they would demand a well-focused effort to determine the mechanism by which the intrinsic rhythmicity of the brain is altered. And, given what we know of the origin of oscillatory events, a further question would be whether there are any pharmacological tools that can improve the timing properties in CNS circuits in dyslexia.

While considering dyslexia as a dyschronia may lead to possible pharmacological activation of this syndrome, it must be kept clearly in mind that this is only one aspect of the problem. There is ample evidence that dyslexia is accompanied by modifications of brain-cell numbers and distributions as well as gross morphological problems,[3] so this syndrome must be more than a purely electrophysiological function. Nevertheless, given our stage of knowledge, it seems quite legitimate to forward general hypotheses and to discuss further steps to be taken to clarify and ultimately to alleviate the behavioral difficulties that arise from these subtle and yet disruptive alterations in CNS function.

REFERENCES

1. NICOLSON, R. I. & A. J. FAWCETT. 1992. Q. J. Exp. Psychol. Section A. In press.
2. ———. 1993. Children with dyslexia classify pure tones slowly. This issue.
3. TALLAL, P. 1993. Neurobiological basis of speech: A case for the preeminence of temporal processing. This issue.

4. DENCKLA, M. B. & R. G. RUDEL. 1976. Neuropsychologia **14:** 471–479.
5. LIVINGSTONE, M. S., G. D. ROSEN, F. W. DRISLANE & A. M. GALABURDA. 1991. Proc. Natl. Acad. Sci. U.S.A. **88:** 7943–7947.
6. LOVEGROVE, W. J., R. P. GARZIA & S. B. NICHOLSON. 1990. J. Am. Optometric Assoc. **61:** 137–146.
7. NICOLSON, R. I. & A. J. FAWCETT. 1993. Q. J. Exp. Psychol. In press.
8. ———. 1990. Cognition **30:** 159–182.
9. ———. 1993. Children with dyslexia automatize temporal skills more slowly. This issue.
10. CRICK, F. & C. KOCH. 1990. Cold Springs Harbor Symposium on Quant. Biol. **55:** 953–962.
11. LLINÁS, R. 1988. Science **242:** 1654–1664.
12. SUGIHARA, I., et al. 1993. J. Physiol. In press.
13. LLINÁS, R. & Y. YAROM. 1981. J. Physiol., London. **315:** 549–567.
14. ———. 1981. J. Physiol., London. **315:** 569–584.
15. ———. 1986. J. Physiol., London. **376:** 163–182.
16. BENARDO, L. S. & R. E. FOSTER. 1986. Brain Res. Bull. **17:** 773–784.
17. LLINÁS, R. & K. SASAKI. 1989. Eur. J. Neurosci. **1:** 587–602.
18. JAHNSEN, H. & R. LLINÁS. 1984. J. Physiol. London. **349:** 227–248.
19. STERIADE, M., et al. 1991. Proc. Natl. Acad. Sci. U.S.A.
20. CONNOR, J. A. & C. F. STEVENS. 1971. J. Physiol. **213:** 21–30.
21. HAGIWARA, S., K. KUSANO & N. SAITO. 1961. J. Physiol. **155:** 470–489.
22. STERIADE, M., P. GLOOR, R. LLINÁS, F. LOPESDA SILVA & M. M. MESULAM. 1990. Electroencephalogr. Clin. Neurophysiol. **30**.
23. LLINÁS, R. & D. PARÉ. 1991. Neuroscience **44**(3): 521–535.
24. LLINÁS, R. 1990. Intrinsic electrical properties of mammalian neurons and CNS function. *In* Fidia Research Foundation Neuroscience Award Lectures. Raven Press. New York.
25. LLINÁS, R., A. A. GRACE & Y. YAROM. 1991. Proc. Natl. Acad. Sci. U.S.A. **88:** 897–901.
26. JONES, K. A. & R. W. BAUGHMAN. 1988. J. Neurosci. **8:** 3522–3524.
27. GRAY, C. M., P. KONIG, A. K. ENGEL & W. SINGER. 1989. Nature **338:** 334–337.
28. GRAY, C. M., A. K. ENGEL, P. KONIG & W. SINGER. 1990. Eur. J. Neurosci. **2:** 607–619.
29. STERIADE, M. 1992. Personal communication.
30. COLONNIER, M. 1967. Arch. Neurol. **16:** 651–657.
31. GHOSE, G. M. & R. D. FREEMAN. 1992. J. Neurophys. **68:** 1558–1574.
32. BRESSLER, S. L. & W. J. FREEMAN. 1980. Electroencephalogr. Clin. Neurophysiol. **50:** 19–24.
33. LLINÁS, R. & U. RIBARY. 1993. Proc. Natl. Acad. Sci. U.S.A. **90:** 2078–2081.
34. STERIADE, M., R. CURRÓDOSSI, D. PARÉ & G. OAKSON. 1991. Proc. Natl. Acad. Sci. U.S.A. **88:** 4396–4400.
35. JONES, E. G. 1985. The Thalamus. Plenum. New York.
36. KRIEG, W. J. S. 1966. Functional Neuroanatomy. Brain Books.

Weakness in the Transient Visual System: A Causal Factor in Dyslexia?

WILLIAM LOVEGROVE

Department of Psychology
University of Wollongong
Wollongong, Australia 2500

INTRODUCTION

The research to be described concerns the nature of visual processing in dyslexic and normal-reading children. The central issue for our research for some time was whether these children differ from normal readers in basic visual processes. The major question has now become, what are the implications of the visual processing differences between dyslexics and controls that we and others have now demonstrated? Both questions are considered here.

For some years the commonly accepted view within the reading disability literature has been that reading disability is not attributable to visual deficits and that normal readers and dyslexics do not differ systematically in terms of visual processing.[1,2] Extensive work over the last ten years in a number of laboratories, however, has clearly demonstrated that the two groups do differ in terms of visual processing even though we know less about the possible implications of these findings. Much of this recent research has resulted in part from developments in theoretical vision that have been applied to reading, thus providing a more suitable theoretical framework in which to consider reading and vision. The following section briefly outlines one approach to vision that has been usefully applied. A more detailed discussion of this framework is found in the article by Galaburda and Livingstone in this volume.[3]

THE SUSTAINED AND TRANSIENT SUBSYSTEMS

One approach to vision research[4,5] indicates that information is transmitted from the eye to the brain via a number of separate parallel pathways. The separate pathways are frequently referred to as channels. Each channel is specialized to process information about particular features of visual stimuli. This research has identified a number of channels, each sensitive to a narrow range of spatial frequencies (or stimulus widths) and orientations in cats, monkeys, and humans.

Spatial frequency or size-sensitive channels are relevant to reading because when we read we process both general (low spatial frequency) and detailed (high spatial frequency) information in each fixation. We extract detailed information from an area approximately 5–6 letter spaces to the right of fixation. Beyond this we also extract visual information, but only of a general nature such as word shape.[6] These two types of size information must in some way be combined.

It has also been shown that the different channels transmit their information at different rates and respond differently to different rates of temporal change. Some channels are sensitive to very rapidly changing stimuli and others to stationary or slowly moving stimuli. Similarly some channels primarily respond at stimulus onset and offset, whereas others respond throughout stimulus presentation. Such results have led to the proposal of two subsystems within the visual system. Many of the properties of these two subsystems have been identified and are shown in TABLE 1. An extended discussion of the properties of these systems and how they are identified can be found in Breitmeyer[7] and Galaburda and Livingstone.[3] Breitmeyer also discusses the evidence indicating the physiological basis of these two systems, as have Galaburda and Livingstone.[3] The magnocellular system and the parvocellular systems are often equated with the transient and sustained, respectively.

It has been demonstrated physiologically[8] and psychophysically that the two systems may inhibit each other.[9] In particular if the sustained system is responding when the transient system is stimulated, the transient will terminate the sustained activity. Breitmeyer[9] and Matin[10] have argued that such transient on sustained inhibition is important in metacontrast. Metacontrast, in turn, is important in saccadic suppression. These two subsystems and the interactions between them may serve a number of functions essential to reading.

Since the transient system is predominantly a flicker- or motion-detecting system transmitting information about stimulus change and general shape, it is well suited for transmitting peripheral information in reading. The sustained system, being predominantly a detailed pattern system, should be most important in extracting detailed information during fixations. Below we shall see that the two systems also interact in important ways.

SUSTAINED AND TRANSIENT SUBSYSTEMS AND READING

When reading, the eyes move through a series of rapid eye movements called saccades. These are separated by fixation intervals when the eyes are stationary. The average fixation duration is approximately 200–250 ms for normal readers, and it is during these stationary periods that information from the printed page is seen. The average saccade length is 6–8 characters or about 2 degrees of visual angle.[6] Saccadic eye movements function to bring unidentified regions of text into foveal vision for detailed analysis during fixations. Foveal vision is the area of high acuity in the center of vision extending approximately 2 degrees (6–8 letters) around the fixation point on a line of text. Beyond the fovea acuity drops off rather dramatically.

The role of transient and sustained subsystems in reading has been considered by

TABLE 1. General Properties of the Transient and Sustained Subsystems

Transient System	Sustained System
Highly sensitive to contrast	Low sensitivity to contrast
Most sensitive to low spatial frequencies	Most sensitive to high spatial frequencies
Most sensitive to high temporal frequencies	Most sensitive to low temporal frequencies
Fast transmission times	Slow transmission times
Responds at stimulus onset and offset	Responds throughout stimulus presentation
Predominates in peripheral vision	Predominates in central vision
The transient system may inhibit the sustained system	The sustained system may inhibit the transient system

Breitmeyer.[7,9] Breitmeyer[9] has implicated transient and sustained system interactions in reading via saccadic suppression. He has argued that two forms of transient–sustained interactions are involved in saccadic suppression: metacontrast and the peripheral shift effect. For this reason much of the work to be reported has been carried out within the framework of transient–sustained interactions. The following is a selective review of some recent research carried out in a few laboratories, including ours.

TRANSIENT AND SUSTAINED PROCESSING IN DYSLEXICS AND CONTROLS

Even though we have used a range of measures to identify transient and sustained system processing, I will primarily focus on those involving uniform-field flicker. Some of our earliest studies concentrated on measuring visible persistence. Visible persistence is a measure of temporal processing, and refers to the continued perception of a stimulus after it has been physically removed. This is assumed to reflect ongoing neural activity initiated by the stimulus presentation. In adults, duration of visible persistence increases with increasing spatial frequency.[11] Several studies have compared dyslexics and controls on measures of visible persistence. These have shown that dyslexics have a significantly smaller increase in persistence duration with increasing spatial frequency than do controls[12] (FIG. 1).

In an attempt to understand further the nature of these differences between dyslexics and controls in visible persistence as a function of spatial frequency, Slaghuis and Lovegrove[13] used uniform-field masking to reduce transient system

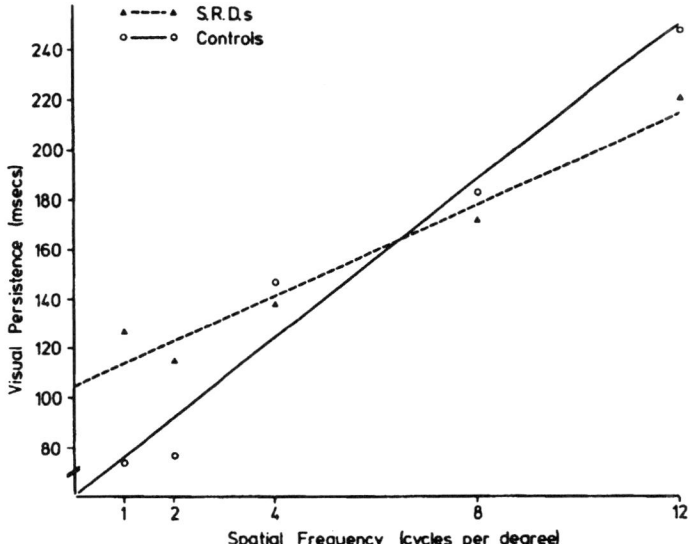

FIGURE 1. Duration of visible persistence as a function of spatial frequency for controls and reading disabled. (From Lovegrove *et al.*[12] Permission to reprint applied for.)

involvement in the persistence task (see Breitmeyer et al.[14] for a full discussion of the rationale of this procedure). In brief, uniform-field masking should reduce transient system involvement without any significant effect on sustained system processing (FIG. 2). When visible persistence is measured in both groups under these conditions, persistence differences between the groups disappear.[13] This is precisely what would be expected if the transient system in dyslexics was already weak.

Further supporting evidence has recently been provided by Lehmkuhle et al.[15] They recorded visual evoked potentials (VEP) from controls and dyslexics with and without uniform-field flicker. Under nonflicker conditions, they showed that the latencies of early VEP components were longer for dyslexics at low but not high spatial frequencies. Uniform-field flicker significantly increased the latency and reduced the amplitude of the early VEP components in normal readers. In dyslexics the uniform-field flicker only reduced the amplitude of the same components. The net outcome was that the results for the two groups did not differ as much under uniform-field flicker masking conditions. This strongly reinforces the visible persistence data, but under conditions where it is essentially impossible to interpret the results in terms of criterion differences between the two groups.

We also attempted to measure transient system functioning more directly by determining flicker thresholds under a range of conditions in dyslexics and controls. In these experiments subjects are shown a sine-wave grating counterphasing. Subjects are required to detect the presence of the flickering grating. In a number of experiments we and others have shown dyslexics to be less sensitive than controls to counterphase flicker, as shown in FIGURE 3.[16-18] The differences between the groups sometimes become larger as the temporal frequency increases,[18] and sometimes do not.[16,17] This more direct measure of transient system processing distinguishes well between individuals in the two groups.[18]

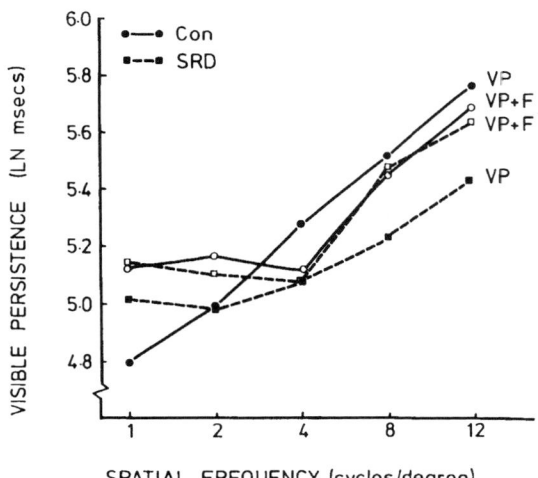

FIGURE 2. Mean in visible persistence, as a function of spatial frequency, for the controls (*circles*) and dyslexics (*squares*) without masking (*solid symbols*) and with 6-Hz flicker masking (*open symbols*). (From Slaghuis and Lovegrove.[13] Permission to reprint applied for.)

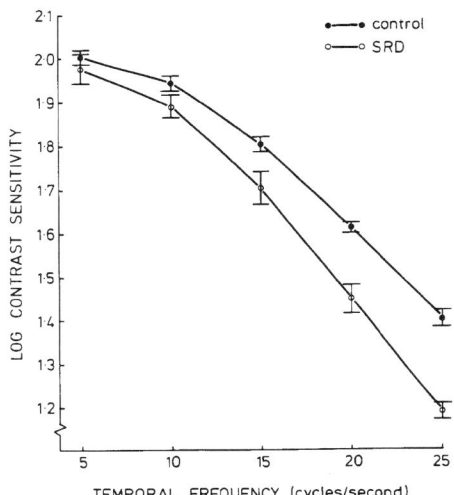

FIGURE 3. Flicker contrast sensitivity for a counterphasing 2 cycles/deg grating as a function of temporal frequency for controls and reading disabled. (From Martin and Lovegrove.[17] Permission to reprint applied for.)

Additional support for differences in transient system activity between the groups has been found in other VEP[19,20] and anatomical studies.[19] The data collected by May et al. is discussed in more detail below.

Lovegrove and associates have also conducted a series of experiments comparing sustained system processing in controls and dyslexics (see reference 21). These studies measured orientation and spatial frequency tuning and the magnitude of the oblique effect.[22] Using similar procedures, equipment, and subjects as the experiments outlined earlier, this series of experiments failed to show any significant differences between the two groups. This implies that either there are no differences between the groups in the functioning of their sustained systems or that such differences are smaller than the transient differences demonstrated.

It should be noted that both Williams and Bologna[23] and Ruddock[24] have demonstrated differences between the two groups on a visual search task. This task should have involved some sustained system activity. Furthermore, Williams et al.[25] have shown some interesting facilitation effects in a metacontrast experiment (this experiment is discussed in more detail below). While the precise interpretation of these data is not clear, the data do suggest some differences between the groups in the sustained system. The exact nature of these differences requires further research, but it is likely that many tasks involving transient–sustained interactions are likely to show differences between the groups.

In summary, a number of measures of low-level visual processing suggest a transient deficit in dyslexics. The differences between the groups are quite large on some measures and discriminate well between individuals in the different groups, with approximately 75 percent of dyslexics showing reduced transient system sensitivity.[26] At the same time evidence to date suggests that the two groups do not differ as clearly in sustained system functioning.

HIGHER LEVEL PERCEPTUAL PROCESSES AND DYSLEXIA

It is known that the transient and sustained systems may be involved in higher level perceptual processes than those discussed previously.[27,28] Williams and colleagues have recently investigated the question of how a transient deficit may manifest itself in a number of such perceptual processes. Their general conclusion is that dyslexics manifest difficulties on a large number of perceptual tasks, most of which are believed to involve the transient system.[29]

In an important study Williams et al.[25] plotted the time course of transient–sustained interactions using a metacontrast masking paradigm. In metacontrast masking a target is briefly presented, followed at various delays by a spatially adjacent masking stimulus. It is normally found that the visibility of the target first decreases, and then increases as the pattern mask follows it by longer and longer delays. Breitmeyer and Ganz[27] and Weisstein et al.[28] have argued that metacontrast masking is due to the inhibition of the sustained response to the target by the transient response to the mask. Maximal masking occurs when the transient response to the mask and the sustained response to the target overlap most in time in the visual system. The point of maximal masking, then, provides an index of the relative processing rates of the target sustained response and the mask transient response. If the difference in rate of transmission is small, the dip in the masking function occurs after a short delay and vice versa. The magnitude of masking provides an index of the strength of transient-on-sustained inhibition. It should be noted that this is one of the mechanisms proposed to be involved in saccadic suppression.

In an experiment using line targets Williams et al.[25] showed that maximal masking occurred at a shorter delay in dyslexics than in controls. This result is direct evidence that dyslexics have a slower transient system, or at least a smaller difference between the rates of processing for their transient and sustained systems than controls. They also found that in peripheral vision, dyslexics experienced almost no metacontrast masking, which further supports this position. The magnitude of masking was also less in central vision, showing that the transient inhibition was also weaker. The visible persistence differences reported earlier suggested visual timing differences between controls and dyslexics. This study provides clearer evidence of timing differences.

RELIABILITY OF MEASURES

Given the conflict on the issue of reading disability and vision in the literature, there are a number of questions that follow from the data outlined previously. The first is how many dyslexics differ from controls on these measures, and the second concerns the reliability of these measures. Each of these questions is considered in turn.

In an attempt to address the first question, Slaghuis and Lovegrove[26] combined data from a number of studies measuring duration of visible persistence as a function of spatial frequency in dyslexics and normal readers. They calculated a regression coefficient for the slope of this function for each subject in each group. To permit combining of the scores from different experiments, all regression coefficients were converted to z scores. A discriminant analysis was then performed on the z scores for 61 dyslexics and 61 controls. The results are shown in TABLE 2. This table shows that 75 percent of the dyslexics differed from the controls on this measure, while 5

TABLE 2. Number of Subjects Classified with and without Visual Deficits[a]

	Visual	No Visual	Total
SRDs	46 (75.4%)	15 (24.6%)	61
Controls	5 (8.0%)	56 (92.0%)	61

Sources: From Slaghuis and Lovegrove.[26] Permission to reprint applied for.
[a]Using discriminant analysis on regression coefficients (converted to z scores) representing the slope of the spatial frequency by visible persistence function. The data are from five studies as discussed in the text.

percent of controls had functions like the majority of the dyslexics. It is not clear why this is so, but it possibly relates to measurement error.

A second approach to this problem has been to use the latency scores from visual evoked potential data.[20] In their study subjects were presented with sine-wave gratings ranging in spatial frequency from 0.5 to 8.0 cycles per degree flickering at a rate of 2 hertz (Hz). Stimulus duration was 200 ms. This allowed analysis of two components of the VEP elicited by both stimulus onset and by stimulus offset. The major findings indicated that poor readers had significantly lower amplitudes and significantly shorter latencies for components produced by stimulus offsets when low spatial frequency stimuli were used.

Factor analyses of these data revealed two factors for both the low and high spatial frequency stimuli.[30] With the low spatial frequency stimulus, Factor II was associated with the latencies on the first onset component and Factor I with the latencies of all components. These scores were subject to a discriminant analysis based on the differential scores on the two factors. This analysis showed that good and poor readers were well differentiated by the factor scores on the low spatial frequency but not the high spatial frequency factor. Thus, this measure also differentiates well between individuals in the two groups.

We have addressed the question of the reliability of the measures within the subjects by measuring the consistency of the regression coefficients for the spatial frequency by the duration of the visible persistence function referred to earlier. Slaghuis measured this function a number of times in the same children in a series of studies separated by three to six months. This issue is important in light of the claim by Georgeson and Georgeson[31] that this is an extremely unreliable measure. Our analyses showed that in the children we tested there were significant correlations on these measures over the three testing occasions.[32] Consequently, our measures appear to be more reliable than those reported by Georgeson and Georgeson.[31]

VISION, DYSLEXIA, AND CAUSALITY?

Hulme[33] has argued that it is most unlikely that there is a causal link between transient system processing and dyslexia. Lovegrove[34] has countered that this question still should be regarded as open. I will consider this issue in two ways. The first will look at possible relationships between visual deficits and phonological processing. The second will take up the question of whether it is possible to make predictions about conditions that may improve reading in dyslexics.

IS THERE ANY LINK BETWEEN TRANSIENT SYSTEM AND PHONOLOGICAL PROCESSING?

Independent Contributions to Dyslexia?

It is well documented that dyslexics experience major difficulties in phonological awareness[35] and phonological recoding.[36] Less is known, however, about possible relationships between transient processing and phonological processing. This issue was considered in a study of approximately 60 dyslexics and 60 controls.[37] These authors took measures of transient system processing (flicker sensitivity), phonological awareness (segment comparison[38]), and phonological recoding (nonsense words and sentence verification[39]) in each child. These measures were subjected to a factor analysis that showed that the phonological recoding measures and the phonological awareness measure loaded on the same factor as the measure of transient processing used. This analysis shows some relation between the two processing areas without revealing the precise nature of that relationship.

Further information on this issue has been provided by Stein and his colleagues. Cornelissen *et al.*[40] measured the number of nonword errors made by groups of dyslexics and controls. They divided the subjects into two groups depending on whether or not they passed the Dunlop test of stability of ocular dominance.[41] Subjects were required to recognize words printed in different sizes. Cornelissen *et al.*[40] argued that nonword errors generally may be attributed to phonological awareness abilities. On the other hand, if errors varied with print size, they are more likely to reflect visual problems of the sort frequently studied by the Stein group. Their results showed that children who passed the Dunlop test made more nonword errors than children who failed the Dunlop test when reading large print, but they made fewer nonword errors with medium and small print. This group by print size interaction indicates a causal role for the visual problems.

Eden *et al.*[42] measured the contribution made by measures of visual processing (a binocular fixation index) and phonological recoding (pig latin completion time) to reading scores in a large groups of dyslexics and controls. Their data showed that chronological age and IQ accounted for 38 percent of the variance. When phonological recoding data were added in, the percentage of the variance accounted for rose to 50 percent. With the addition of the visual measures, the percentage of the variance accounted for rose to 65 percent. This study also showed some evidence of left-field neglect in the dyslexic group.

It should be noted that Stein[43] also argues that the visual anomalies his group have identified in dyslexics reflect transient system processing. In particular his group's work implicates the posterior parietal cortex, which receives primarily magnocellular input.[44] Stein's[43] conclusion is based partly on the evidence of left-field neglect in dyslexics referred to above.

Evidence is also found in work that shows that there are dyslexics who have no phonological recoding problems, but do have visual problems as measured by a visual segmentation task.[45] This suggests that phonological awareness is an important part of the explanation of dyslexia, but not the full explanation in all cases.

Common Underlying Mechanisms?

Another possibility is that both the deficits in vision and phonological processing reflect some common underlying process or processes. Indirect support for this hypothesis comes from a number of sources. For example, it is possible that some of these different deficits are related by virtue of the fact that some dyslexics have a problem in processing rapidly presented stimuli in more than one sensory modality. Tallal,[46] for example, has shown dyslexics to have problems in audition that are similar to those we have measured in vision. She has shown that dyslexics perform as well as control readers on an auditory temporal order judgment task or an auditory fusion task when the two stimuli are separated by an interval of 428 ms. When this interval was reduced to 8–305 ms, dyslexics performed clearly worse than controls. Furthermore, Tallal showed a highly significant positive correlation between her auditory temporal measures and nonsense word performance.

There is evidence, then, showing a relationship between rapid visual processing (as measured by transient system processing) and measures of both phonological awareness and phonological recoding. Similarly, a strong relationship has also been demonstrated between rapid auditory processing and nonsense word performance. It has not been easy to integrate these various findings in previously available theoretical frameworks. Lovegrove et al.[37] suggested the possibility of a general sensory timing problem in dyslexics. More recently this tentative suggestion has received further support. Livingstone et al.[19] have noted that, like the visual system, the auditory and somatosensory systems may also be subdivided into fast and slow components. They speculated further that problems may occur in dyslexics in the fast system of more than one modality. Their speculation was based in part on their finding of smaller magnocellular cells in dyslexics than in controls. Even though this possibility has not yet been directly investigated, it is an exciting prospect that may help to integrate a large amount of apparently discrepant data. It is currently being investigated in our laboratory among others.

WHAT CAN WE PREDICT FROM A TRANSIENT DEFICIT?

The issue of causality may also be considered by predicting conditions that would lead to different levels of performance in normal readers and dyslexics based on transient system deficits. In terms of Breitmeyer's theory outlined earlier[9] a transient deficit should lead to more errors for dyslexics when reading continuous test than when reading isolated words. This is because the reading of continuous text requires integration of peripheral information from one fixation with central information on the next. Breitmeyer has argued that this task would largely involve the transient system. We have recently tested this conclusion by varying the mode of visual presentation when reading. The general aim of this work was to vary the mode of visual presentation while holding semantic context constant.

Three conditions of visual presentation on a computer monitor were used while holding the semantic context constant. This was done by presenting stories in three different ways. In the first condition, one word at a time was presented in the middle of the screen. Thus the subjects never had to move their eyes and never had information presented to the right of fixation. In the second condition, one word was presented at a time, but its position was moved across the screen. Here the subjects were required to move their eyes across the screen, but still were never presented with information to the right of fixation. The final condition was a whole line presentation that most closely approximated normal reading. Rate of word presentation was held constant across the three conditions.

The results in FIGURE 4[47] show that normal readers were most accurate in the two eye movement conditions and made slightly more errors in the one-word-at-a-time

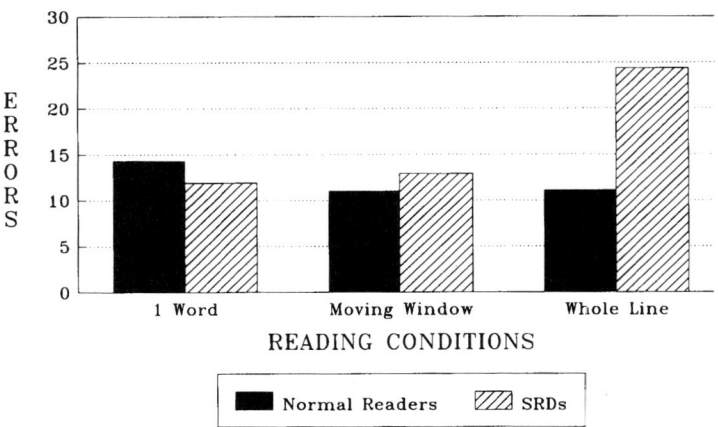

FIGURE 4. Mean number of errors for dyslexics and controls as a function of type of text presentation.

condition. The reverse was true for the dyslexics. They read significantly more accurately in both one-word conditions than in the whole-line condition. The mode of presentation of written material that maximized reading accuracy in controls therefore produced the most errors in dyslexics. These findings have both theoretical and practical implications. Theoretically, they support the prediction based on Breitmeyer's theory that dyslexics with a transient deficit should have difficulties integrating peripheral and central information. Practically, these results offer a means of presenting written text to beginning readers that may facilitate their attempts to learn to read.

CONCLUSIONS

While none of the preceding constitutes conclusive evidence that there is a causal link between transient system processing and dyslexia, the data do show this to be a more open question than has been the case for some time. Some of the data from several types of studies indicate that visual factors make an independent contribution to dyslexia. They also indicate that the issue warrants further investigation that may lead to a fuller understanding of the problem of dyslexia. Finally, the possibility of a general sensory timing deficit shows that the study of visual processing in dyslexics has provided a useful window on nervous system functioning in dyslexics.

REFERENCES

1. BENTON, A. L. 1962. Dyslexia in relation to form perception and directional sense. *In* Reading Disability: Progress and Research Needs in Dyslexia, J. Money, Ed.: 81–102. Johns Hopkins Press. Baltimore, Md.
2. VELLUTINO, F. R. 1979. Dyslexia: Theory and Research. MIT Press. London.
3. GALABURDA, A. & M. LIVINGSTONE. 1993. Evidence for a magnocellular defect in developmental dyslexia. This issue.
4. CAMPBELL, F. W. 1974. The transmission of spatial information through the visual system. *In* The Neurosciences Third Study Program, F. O. Schmidt and F. S. Worden, Eds.: 95–103. MIT Press. Cambridge, Mass.
5. GRAHAM. N. 1980. Spatial frequency channels in human vision. Detecting edges without edges detectors. *In* Visual Coding and Adaptability, C. S. Harris, Ed.: 215–262. Lawrence Erlbaum. Hillsdale, N.J.
6. RAYNER, K. 1975. The perceptual span and peripheral cues in reading. Cogn. Psychol. **7**: 65–81.
7. BREITMEYER, B. G. 1988. Reality and relevance of sustained and transient channels in reading and reading disability. Paper presented to the 24th International Congress of Psychology. Sydney, Australia.
8. SINGER, W. & N. BEDWORTH. 1973. Inhibitory interaction between X and Y units in the cat lateral geniculate nucleus. Brain Res. **49**: 291–307.
9. BREITMEYER, B. G. 1980. Unmasking visual masking: A look at the "why" behind the veil of "how." Psychol. Rev. **87**(1): 52–69.
10. MATIN, E. 1974. Saccadic suppression: A review and an analysis. Psychol. Bull. **81**: 899–915.
11. MEYER, G. E. & W. M. MAGUIRE. 1977. Spatial frequency and the mediation of short-term visual storage. Science **198**: 524–525.
12. LOVEGROVE, W., M. HEDDLE & W. SLAGHUIS. 1980. Reading disability: Spatial frequency specific deficits in visual information store. Neuropsychologia **18**: 111–115.
13. SLAGHUIS, W. & W. J. LOVEGROVE. 1984. Flicker masking of spatial frequency dependent visible persistence and specific reading disability. Perception **13**: 527–534.
14. BREITMEYER, B., D. M. LEVI & R. S. HARWERTH. 1981. Flicker-masking in spatial vision. Vision Res. **21**:1377–1385.
15. LEHMKUHLE, S., R. P. GARZIA, L. TURNER, T. HASH & J. A. BARO. 1992. A defective visual pathway in reading disabled children. New Eng. J. Med. In press.
16. CORNELISSEN, P. 1992. Fixation, contrast sensitivity and childrens reading. Submitted for publication in Stud. Visual Inf. Process.
17. BRANNAN, J. & M. WILLIAMS. 1988. The effects of age and reading ability on flicker threshold. Clin. Visual Sci. **3**: 137–142.
18. MARTIN, F. & W. LOVEGROVE. 1987. Flicker contrast sensitivity in normal and specifically-disabled readers. Perception **16**: 215–221.
19. LIVINGSTONE, M., F. DRISLANE, G. ROSEN & A. GALABURDA. 1991. Physiological evidence for a magnocellular defect in developmental dyslexia. Proc. N.Y. Acad. Sci. **88**: 7943–7947.
20. MAY, J., W. LOVEGROVE, F. MARTIN & W. NELSON. 1991. Pattern-elicited visual evoked potentials in good and poor readers. Clin. Vision Sci. **2**: 131–136.
21. LOVEGROVE, W., F. MARTIN & W. SLAGHUIS. 1986. A theoretical and experimental case for a residual deficit in specific reading disability. Cog. Neuropsychol. **3**: 225–267.
22. LOVEGROVE, W., F. MARTIN A. BOWLING, D. BADCOCK & S. PAXTON. 1982. Contrast sensitivity functions and specific reading disability. Neuropsychologia **20**: 309–315.
23. WILLIAMS, M. & N. BOLOGNA. 1985. Perceptual grouping in good and poor readers. Percept. Psychophys. **38**: 367–374.
24. RUDDOCK, K. 1991. Visual search in dyslexia. *In* Vision and Visual Dyslexia, J. Stein, Ed.: 141–146. Macmillan. London.

25. WILLIAMS, M. K. MOLINET & K. LECLUYSE. 1989. Visual masking as a measure of temporal processing in normal and disabled readers. Clin. Vision Sci. **4:** 137–144.
26. SLAGHUIS, W. & W. J. LOVEGROVE. 1985. Spatial-frequency mediated visible persistence and specific reading disability. Brain Cogn. **4:** 219–240.
27. BREITMEYER, B. & L. GANZ. 1976. Implications of sustained and transient channels for theories of visual pattern masking, saccadic supression, and information processing. Psychol. Rev. **83:**1–36.
28. WEISSTEIN, N., G. OZOZ & R. SZOC. 1975. A comparison and elaboration of two models of metacontrast. Psychol. Rev. **2:** 325–342.
29. WILLIAMS, M. & K. LECLUYSE. 1990. Perceptual consequences of a temporal processing deficit in reading disabled children. J. Am. Optom. Ass. **61:** 111–121.
30. MAY, J., W. DUNLAP & W. LOVEGROVE. 1991. Visual evoked potentials latency factor scores differentiate good and poor readers. Clin. Vision Sci. In press.
31. GEORGESON, M. & J. GEORGESON. 1985. On seeing temporal gaps between gratings: A criterion problem for measurement of visible persistence. Vision Res. **25:** 1729–1733.
32. LOVEGROVE, W. & W. SLAGUIS. 1989. How reliably are visual differences found in dyslexics? Irish J. Psychol. **10:**542–550.
33. HULME, C. 1988. The implausability of low-level visual defects as a cause of children's reading difficulties. Cogn. Neuropsychol. **5:**47–48.
34. LOVEGROVE, W. 1991. The visual deficit hypothesis. *In* Current Perspectives in Learning Disabilities: Nature, Theory and Treatment, N. Singh and I. Beale, Eds. Springer-Verlag. New York.
35. BRADLEY, L. & P. BRYANT. 1983. Categorising sounds and learning to read— A causal connection. Nature **301:** 419–421.
36. SNOWLING, M. 1981. Phonemic deficits in developmental dyslexia. Psychol. Res. **43:**219–234.
37. LOVEGROVE, W., D. MCNICOL, F. MARTIN, B. MACKENZIE & K. PEPPER. 1988. Phonological recoding, memory processing and memory deficits in specific reading disability. *In* Human Information Processing: Measures, Mechanisms and Models, D. Vickers and P. Smith, Eds.: 65–82. North-Holland. Amsterdam, the Netherlands.
38. TRIEMAN, R. & J. BARON. 1978. Segmental analysis ability: Development and relation to reading. *In* Reading Research: Advances in Theory and Practice, Vol. 2, T. G. Waller and G. E. MacKinnon, Eds. Academic Press. New York.
39. BARON, J. 1973. Phonemic stage not necessary for reading. Q. J. Exp. Psychol. **25:** 241–246.
40. CORNELISSEN, P., L. BRADLEY, S. FOWLER & J. F. STEIN. 1991. What children see affects how they read. Developmental Medicine and Child Neurology. In press.
41. DUNLOP, P. 1972. Dyslexia: An orthoptic approach. Aust. J. Orthopt. **12:** 16–20.
42. EDEN, G., J. F. STEIN & F. B. WOOD. 1991. Visuospatial ability and language processing in reading disabled children. Paper presented at the 18th Rodin Conference, Berne, Switzerland. (Submitted for publication in Stud. Visual Inform. Process.)
43. STEIN, J. F. 1991. Visuospatial sense, hemispheric asymmetry and dyslexia. *In* Visual Dyslexia: Vision and Visual Dysfunction, Vol. 13, J. Stein, Ed. Macmillan. New York.
44. LIVINGSTONE, M. & D. HUBEL. 1987. Psychophysical evidence for separate channels for the perception of form, color, and movement, and depth. J. Neurosci. **7:** 3416–3468.
45. JOHNSTONE, R., M. ANDERSON & L. DUNCAN. 1991. Phonological and visual segmentation problems in poor readers. *In* Dyslexia: Integrating Theory and Practice, M. Snowling and M. Thomson, Eds. Whurr. London.
46. TALLAL, P. 1985. Auditory temporal perception, phonics and reading disabilities in children. Brain Lang. **9:** 182–198.
47. HILL, R. & W. LOVEGROVE. 1992. One word at a time: A solution to the visual deficit in SRDs? *In* Visual Aspects of Dyslexia and Its Remediation, S. F. Wright, R. Groner, and R. Kaufmann-Hayoz, Eds. North-Holland. Amsterdam, the Netherlands. In press.
48. LOVEGROVE, W. J., A. BOWLING, D. BADCOCK & M. BLACKWOOD. 1980. Specific reading disability: Differences in contrast sensitivity as a function of spatial frequency. Science **210:** 439–440.

49. MARTIN, F. & W. LOVEGROVE. 1984. The effects of field size and luminance on contrast sensitivity differences between specifically reading disabled and normal children. Neuropsychologia **22:** 73–77.
50. ———. 1988. Uniform and field flicker in control and specifically-disabled readers. Perception **17:** 203–214.
51. WILLIAMS, M., J. BRANNAN & N. BOLOGNA. 1988. Perceptual consequences of a transient subsystem visual deficit in the reading disabled. Paper presented at the 24th International Congress of Psychology, Sydney, Australia.

Evidence for a Magnocellular Defect in Developmental Dyslexia[a]

ALBERT GALABURDA[b-e] AND
MARGARET LIVINGSTONE[d,e]

[c] *Department of Neurology*
Beth Israel Hospital
330 Brookline Avenue
Boston, Massachusetts 02215

[d] *Department of Neurology*
Children's Hospital
Boston, Massachusetts 02115

[e] *Department of Neurobiology*
Harvard Medical School
Boston, Massachusetts 02115

INTRODUCTION

Developmental dyslexia is the selective impairment of reading skills despite normal intelligence, visual acuity, motivation, and instruction. Several lines of evidence suggest that dyslexic subjects process visual information more slowly than normal subjects. The flicker fusion rate, which is the fastest rate at which a contrast reversal of a stimulus can be seen, is abnormally slow in dyslexic children at low spatial frequencies and low contrasts.[1] Moreover, such visual abnormalities were reported to be found in over 75 percent of the reading-disabled children tested.[2] When two visual stimuli are presented in rapid succession, the two images fuse and appear as a single presentation; the temporal separation necessary to distinguish two presentations measures visual persistence, and this is up to 100 ms longer for dyslexic than for normal children.[3-6] In contrast, dyslexics perform normally on tests having prolonged stimulus presentations.[2]

These perceptual studies suggest that dyslexia affects some part of the visual system that is fast and transient and has high contrast sensitivity and low spatial selectivity. Exactly these properties characterize the magnocellular subdivision of the visual pathway. The primate visual system is composed mainly of two major processing pathways that remain largely segregated and independent throughout the visual system. This subdivision begins in the retina but is most apparent in, and was first discovered in, the lateral geniculate nucleus (LGN), where cells in the ventral, or magnocellular, layers are larger than cells in the dorsal, or parvocellular, layers. The magno and parvo subdivisions differ physiologically in four major ways: magno cells are much more sensitive than parvo cells to luminance contrast,[7-9] they respond faster and more transiently than parvo cells,[10-14] parvo cells are color coded and magno cells are not,[10,12,15-17] and magno cells have slightly lower spatial resolu-

---

[a]This work was supported by grants from the National Institutes of Health, the Office of Naval Research, and The Orton Dyslexia Society.

[b]To whom correspondence should be addressed.

tion.[14] This functional segregation, begun in the retina, is largely maintained throughout the visual system, possibly even up through higher cortical association areas. Therefore a problem selective to the magnocellular pathway could arise at any level from the retina to peristriate visual cortical areas, and it would be difficult, using behavioral tests, to localize the perceptual defects described in dyslexia.

PHYSIOLOGICAL EVIDENCE FOR A MAGNOCELLULAR DEFECT IN DEVELOPMENTAL DYSLEXIA

In this study we used physiological rather than perceptual methods to measure the contrast sensitivity and visual temporal resolution of normal and dyslexic adult subjects. The dyslexic subjects (3 males, 2 females; mean age 27.4 ± 3.8 years) all had reading levels well below normal, despite above average intelligence. The control subjects (4 males, 3 females; mean age 25.8 ± 4.5 years) were all normal readers and were matched to the dyslexic subjects in age, intelligence, education, and professional level.

We first recorded averaged visual cortical evoked potentials (VEP) in response to the contrast reversal of a binocularly presented checkerboard pattern at both low and high contrasts (FIG. 1). At 40 percent contrast the VEP looked similar for the two groups. At 4 percent contrast the VEP between 40 and 90 ms differed in the two populations, and, by inspection, this difference could be interpreted as a small broad negative wave being delayed by 20 to 40 ms in the dyslexic sample. In addition, the more distinct large positive wave at around 100 ms was delayed in the dyslexic population. There were differences beyond 150 ms as well, but these were uninterpretable.

Source location studies using multiple electrodes have indicated that the earliest component of the VEP originates in Visual Area 1 (V-1), or in geniculate afferents to V-1, and that the large positive potential peaking around 100 ms (the P100) represents activity in both V-1 and peristriatevisual areas.[18-20] Therefore the earliest abnormalities in the dyslexic VEP suggest that a substantial population of early responding cells in V-1 or geniculate afferents respond abnormally, possibly more slowly, in response to low-contrast stimuli. Since the cellular correlates of the visually evoked potential are poorly understood, we cannot distinguish whether these early differences indicate differences in size or timing of the neuronal responses in the dyslexic population. The slowing of the P100 wave suggests a delay either in an early phase of the peristriate response or a late phase of the V-1 response. We could interpret both the early and the P100 differences as a slowing of the magnocellular response, since the broad negative wave occurring before 50 ms is likely to represent magnocellular activity in V-1, and the P100 is likely to reflect the approximately simultaneous occurrence of parvocellular activity in V-1 and magnocellular activity in subsequent visual areas.

To explore the question of whether the early component of the evoked response in the dyslexics was abnormal in size or simply delayed, we looked at the binocularly evoked response to alternating counterphase contrast reversals of the same checkerboard pattern at several alternation frequencies and contrasts [FIG. 2(a)]. At high contrasts the VEP of all the subjects showed oscillatory responses, phase-locked to the visual stimulus. At lower contrasts the responses of the normal subjects were slightly reduced, but the responses of the dyslexic subjects appeared markedly reduced. We quantified these differences by calculating a Fourier spectrum for each evoked response and measuring the power of the spectrum at twice the stimulating

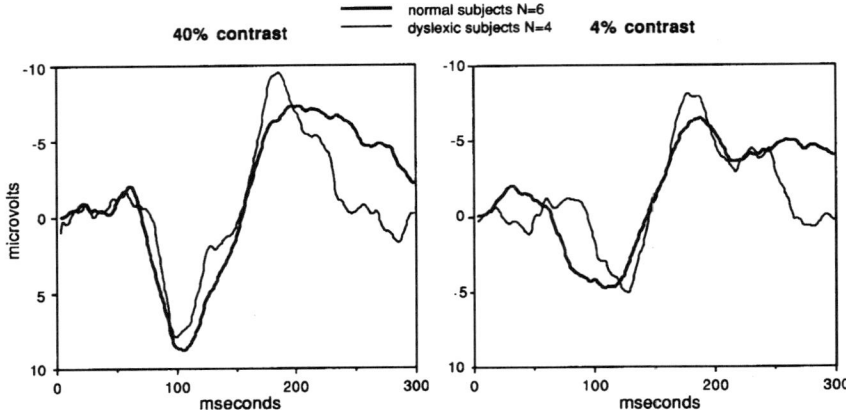

FIGURE 1. Cortical evoked responses were recorded from 4 dyslexic and 6 normal subjects. Copper-cup surface electrodes were placed at OZ and at CZ.[80] Stimuli were generated by a Grass Visual Pattern Generator, model 10VPG, on a Grass model VPGM black-and-white monitor with a 60-Hz refresh rate. The stimulus consisted of a 24-cm × 18.5-cm rectangular checkerboard of 36 rectangles, each 4 × 3 cm, presented at a viewing distance of 60 cm. (The spatial frequency of the stimulus was thus 0.16 cycles/degree vertically and 0.12 cycles/degree horizontally.) The contrast of the checkerboard was reversed in a counterphase square-wave temporal pattern at 0.5 Hz (1 contrast reversal/second). Responses were recorded and averaged with a Grass Bio-response Averager, model BA10CD. The signals were amplified 20,000 times and filtered with a low-frequency cutoff of 1 Hz and a high-frequency cutoff of 100 Hz. The light intensity of the monitor was measured with an SIE photometer, and, for all contrasts tested, the luminance averaged over the entire stimulus was 4.0 cd/m². The different contrasts used produced approximately equal increments and decrements around the average luminance. Contrast is expressed as a percentage—$[(L_{max} - L_{min})/2(L_{max} + L_{min})] \times 100$. For each subject 128 responses, triggered by the stimulus-contrast reversal, were averaged. Then the responses from 6 normal and 4 dyslexic subjects were scanned, digitized, and averaged together. Negative is upward.

frequency (since each cycle of the counterphase reversal pattern consists of two contrast reversals). The results for three contrasts and three stimulating frequencies are shown in FIGURE 2(b) and (c). At both 2 and 4 percent contrast the dyslexic subjects showed significantly (Mann-Whitney U test, $p<0.01$) smaller responses to a 15-Hz stimulus, but their responses to slower stimulation frequencies or to 30 percent contrast at all stimulating frequencies were all within the normal range. This pattern of results is consistent with a selective defect in the magnocellular system.

Cells in the magnocellular system respond well to low-contrast stimuli, and cells in the parvocellular system do not.[7–9,21] Therefore the normal responses of the dyslexic subjects to low-contrast stimuli only at the slower stimulation frequencies suggest that the magnocellular system of dyslexics can respond to low-contrast stimuli, but the response is simply slower than normal. The normal responses of the dyslexic subjects to the 15-Hz stimulus at 30 percent contrast could be accounted for by a speeding up of their magno system at high contrasts or to a high-frequency response of the parvo system. We have no way to distinguish between these two possibilities, since in monkeys the magno system does respond more rapidly at high contrasts than at low contrasts,[15,16] but the parvo system can also respond to frequencies as fast as 15-Hz stimuli at high contrasts.[15,16,22]

From our results we draw conclusions similar to those drawn from perceptual experiments—that dyslexic subjects are less sensitive to low-contrast, fast visual stimulation and that the characteristics of the abnormalities are suggestive of a defect in the transient, or magnocellular, subdivision of the visual pathway. Furthermore, because abnormalities in the VEP are evident as early as 50 ms after a visual stimulation, we can say that a defect exists at a very early stage in the magnocellular pathway, at least as early as the input stage of V-1.

ANATOMICAL EVIDENCE FOR A MAGNOCELLULAR DEFECT

Lateral Geniculate Bodies

In view of the findings from the evoked-potentials experiments, we examined the brains of 5 dyslexic subjects (4 male, 1 female; mean age 34.2 ± 13.7 years) and 5 nondyslexic subjects (all male; mean age 40 ± 11.2 years). The dyslexic brains came from subjects who were diagnosed in life and had been used in previous anatomical studies.[23-25] The control subjects had received sufficient testing during life to permit exclusion of the diagnosis of developmental dyslexia. The tissue processing methods have been described before.[23-26] We used the Yakovlev method for processing whole brains in serial histological sections.[26] Brains are sectioned at 35 μm, usually every twentieth and twenty-first section is stained for Nissl substance with cresylechviolett and for myelin by the Loyez method. The section thickness makes the preparations unsuitable for cell counting, but large numbers of unencumbered neurons are available for measuring cell area. Images representing the medial, middle, and lateral portions of parvocellular and magnocellular layers were digitized (512 × 512 × 8) using a GOULD FD-5000 image analysis system interfaced to a DEC VAX 11/750 computer. For each image, a grey-level threshold was selected such that the Nissl-stained neurons were fully filled. Using this threshold, object borders were drawn using an artificial intelligence-based algorithm, after which the investigator selected for measurement every object that was fully isolated from its neighbors and was identifiable by morphology as a neuron.

On inspection of the lateral geniculate nuclei (LGN) the parvocellular layers appeared similar in the two groups, but the magnocellular layers were more disorganized in the dyslexic brains, and the cell bodies appeared generally smaller and more variable in size and shape (FIG. 3). We measured cell bodies in the magnocellular and parvocellular layers of 6 to 9 fields from each LGN. Three independent observers carried out the entire set of measurements. The second and third observers, but not the first, were blind to the identity of the subjects. An average of 320 magno cells and 740 parvo cells were measured by each observer in each brain. Since there were no systematic regional differences, a single measurement was obtained for each type of neuron, for each brain, for each observer. Across observers both the mean and the median magnocellular areas were significantly smaller in the dyslexic brains [$p < 0.05$ in all cases; FIG. 4]. As compared with the control brains, the mean magno cell area was on average 27 percent smaller in the dyslexic brains. There were no significant differences in the mean parvocellular neuronal areas ($F[1,8] < 1$ in all cases), which also suggests that there are no systematic differences in the degree of tissue shrinkage or staining between the two groups. Two observers found no

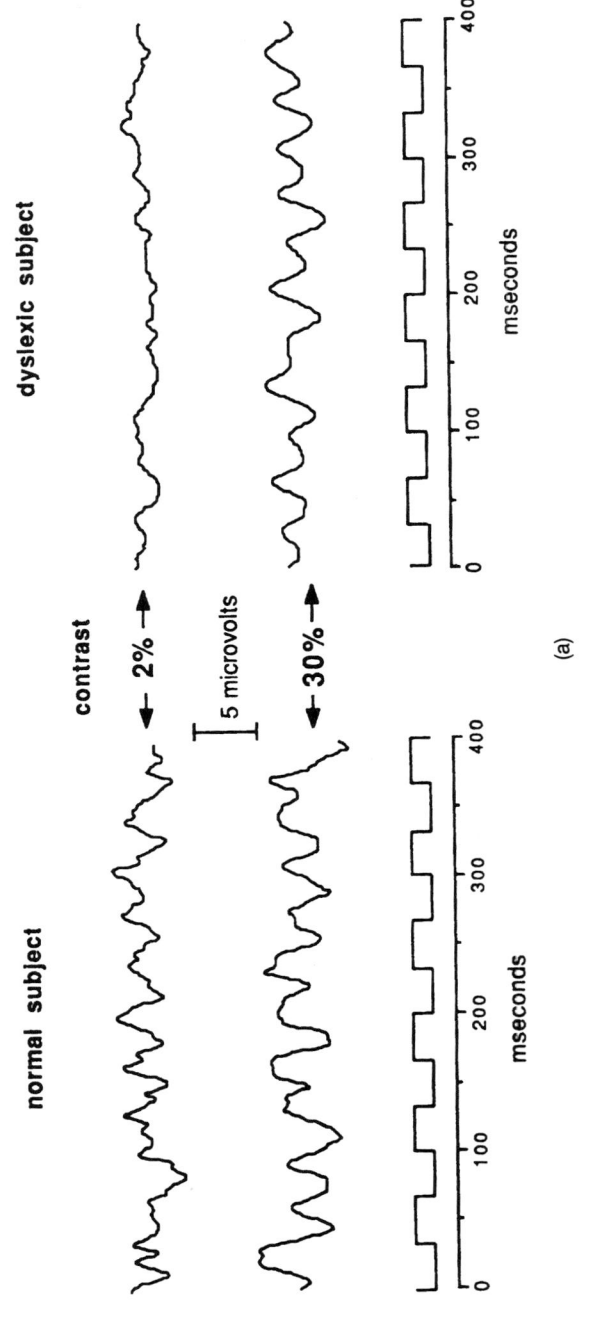

(a)

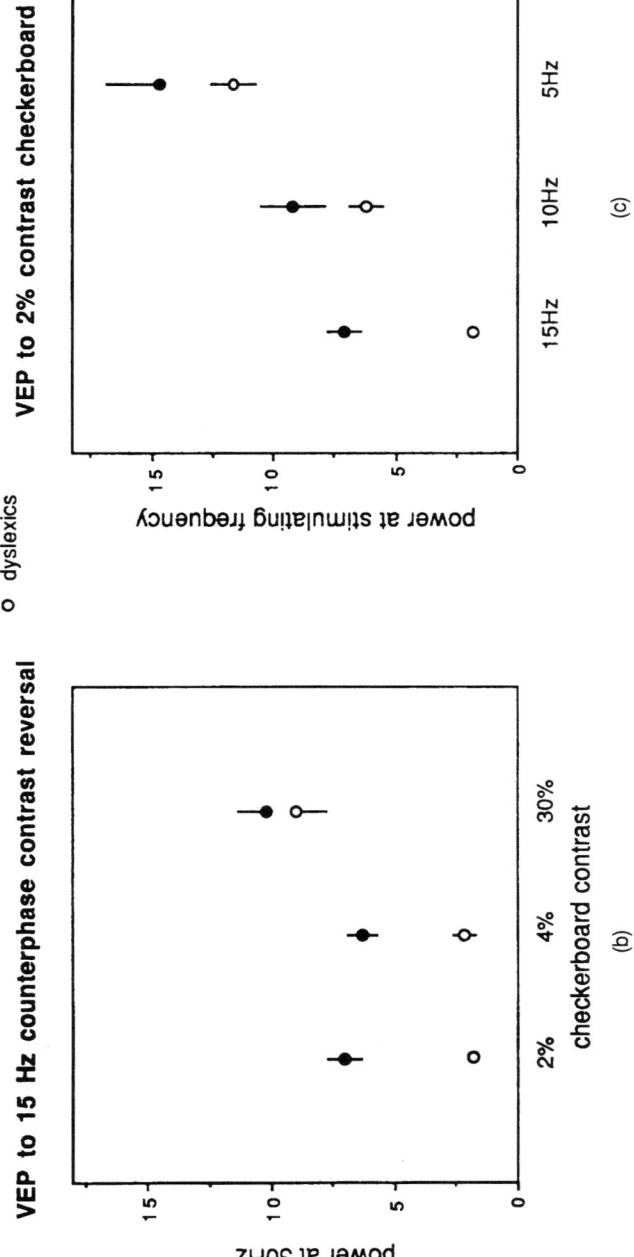

FIGURE 2. (a) Cortical evoked responses in two subjects to 15-Hz contrast reversal at two contrasts (2% and 30%) of the same checkerboard pattern as in FIGURE 1. Negative upward. As indicated at the bottom, the contrast of the checkerboard was reversed in a counterphase square-wave temporal pattern at 15 Hz (30 contrast reversals/second). Each tracing represents the average of 64 sweeps. The *bottom tracings* indicate the luminance of one square in the checkerboard pattern. (b) and (c) Fourier spectrum analyses of evoked potentials, such as those shown in FIGURE 2(a), at different contrasts and stimulation frequencies for 7 normal subjects and 5 dyslexic subjects. For each contrast level and stimulus frequency 64 sweeps were averaged, then each response was scanned, digitized, and a Fourier spectrum was calculated. The ordinate indicates the power in the Fourier spectrum at the same frequency as the contrast reversal rate (twice the counterphase reversal rate) of the visual stimulus. Values indicate mean ± SEM. We used a Mann-Whitney U test to determine that the responses of the dyslexic and normal populations differed significantly for 2% and 4% contrast patterns at 15 Hz ($p<0.01$).

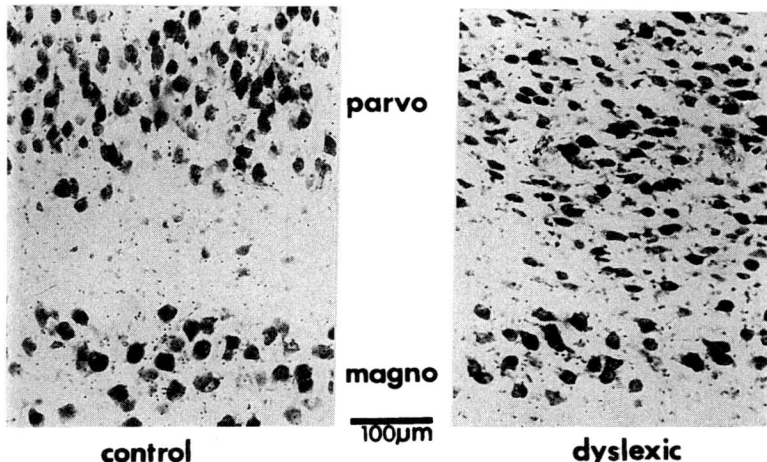

FIGURE 3. Nissl-stained sections of lateral geniculate nuclei from a control and a dyslexic brain. The fields include the ventralmost parvocellular layer and the dorsalmost magnocellular layer. Note that the magnocellular cells in the dyslexic geniculate are generally smaller and more variable in size and shape. Also the lamination is more disorganized in the dyslexic geniculate. (Magnification: 42×.)

difference in the distribution of cell sizes in the parvo layers, while observer 1 found a greater percentage of larger cells in the dyslexic sample ($\chi^2 = 20.0$, $df = 8$, $p < 0.05$).

These results raise the question of whether abnormalities are also present at earlier or later stages in the visual pathway. The magnocellular geniculate layers get their retinal inputs selectively from the large, Type A, retinal ganglion cells, and the parvocellular layers get their inputs from the smaller, Type B, ganglion cells.[27,28] It would therefore be very interesting to compare retinal ganglion cell size distributions in dyslexic and normal subjects, but the retinas of these subjects were unavailable for study. The Type A ganglion cells have larger diameter axons than the Type B cells,[27,29] so an abnormality in the large-cell population in the retina might be manifest as a difference in axon diameter distribution at the level of the optic nerves and optic tracts. Tissue prepared for electron microscopy, which is unavailable to us, is needed to measure axon diameter in these structures reliably (c.f. reference 30). Since magnocellular geniculate cells normally have larger diameter axons than parvocellular cells,[31] we might expect dyslexic brains to show an abnormal axon diameter distribution in the optic radiation, but again, our material did not allow us to make this measurement. The next place we could look for an abnormality in the visual system was V-1. On inspection the overall appearance and lamination of V-1 in the two populations was similar. We wanted to be able to measure some aspect of V-1 that specifically reflected the magnocellular component of the geniculate input. Our first choice would have been to compare the thickness of layer 4Cα, which receives input from the magnocellular geniculate layers, with layer 4Cβ, which receives parvocellular input.[32,33] Unfortunately these two layers are not clearly distinguishable in either Nissl- or myelin-stained sections. But in the myelin-stained sections we could easily distinguish layer 4B, which receives its input almost entirely from layer

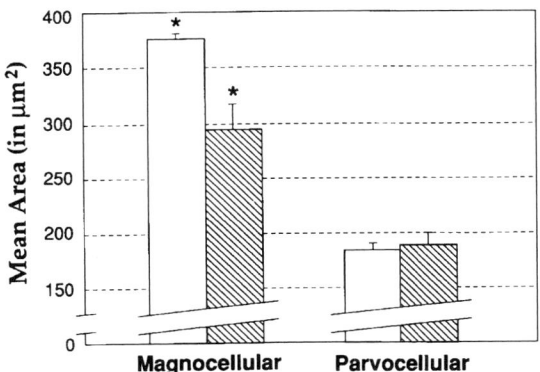

FIGURE 4. Bar graph showing differences in average cell size between dyslexic and control brains in the magno- and parvocellular layers of the lateral geniculate nuclei.

$4C\alpha$,[34–36] and therefore from the magnocellular geniculate layers indirectly. We compared the thickness of layer 4B to the thickness of layers 2 and 3 together, which receive input predominantly from $4C\beta$.[32,33] The ratio of 4B to 2–3 did not differ in the two groups. This particular negative finding does not, of course, rule out other abnormalities in V-1.

The decreased size of the magnocellular geniculate neurons might be expected to have functional consequences and, indeed, the results presented previously suggest that in dyslexic subjects the early stages of the magnocellular subdivision of the visual system process low-contrast information abnormally slowly. Smaller cell bodies would be expected to have thinner axons, and thinner axons would be expected to have slower conduction velocities.[37,38] But slower conduction between geniculate and cortex cannot be the sole difference, because a 30 percent decrease in magnocellular axon diameter would result in only about a millisecond delay in geniculo–cortical conduction time, and even a two- or threefold decrease in diameter would result in only a few milliseconds delay. Despite our inability to find other abnormalities in the visual pathway in our material, it is nevertheless quite possible that the magnocellular division of the visual pathway may be affected in dyslexia at many levels. If so, then the processing abnormalities or delays might be cumulative, resulting in observed 20–50-ms delays in the evoked potential and 100–200-ms delays in tasks that require visual discrimination.

ANATOMICAL EVIDENCE FOR DIFFERENCES IN THE AUDITORY SYSTEM

Several workers have suggested that the analysis of fast temporal auditory transitions, critical for language, is specifically handled by the left hemisphere:[39–41] In dichotic listening studies rapid acoustic stimuli show left hemisphere dominance, but reduction of the rate of acoustic change diminished lateralization.[39] Tallal[42,43] has argued convincingly that children with developmental language deficits may suffer from fundamental disturbances in sound perception. Individuals with developmental reading disorders, too, have been reported to exhibit difficulties with temporal sound processing and sequencing.[44-46] Tallal and colleagues[47-49] have suggested that the development of adequate reading competence depends on normal auditory perception. Zinkus et al.,[50] Webster et al.,[51] and others have reported pervasive language and reading disturbances in children with chronic, severe otitis media. Shucard et al.[52] found amplitude asymmetries of auditory evoked responses that were in opposite directions in dyslexics and controls, and Pinkerton et al.[53] found early and late amplitude and asymmetry differences consistent with a disturbance in both early and late auditory processing in dyslexics, but not all studies have agreed on these findings.[54,55] A high frequency of spelling errors was found to correlate with low auditory evoked potential amplitudes at P50 and P300 by Byring and Jarvilehto,[56] and related findings have been reported by others (reference 57; see review by Obrzut et al.[45]).

We examined the medial geniculate nuclei (MGN) in autopsy specimens from the same subjects described in the abovementioned LGN study prepared in the same fashion. Each MGN was thoroughly sampled without regard to nuclear subdivision and 600–700 neurons per brain were drawn using a camera lucida setup under 500× magnification. Measurements were made with a MOP-3 Zeiss plannimeter. Sections were coded and randomly right–left reversed so that the morphometrist was not aware of group (dyslexic versus non) or side (right versus left). There was no overall difference in mean area between dyslexic and control MGN neurons, but the difference between cell areas of left dyslexic MGN and left control MGN neurons approached significance. When cells were grouped into bins of 50 or 100 μm^2, the distribution of neuronal sizes differed between dyslexics and controls, with the dyslexic sample showing a relative paucity of large neurons and a relative excess of small neurons. This was because the left MGN of dyslexics, as compared to controls, showed more small cells and fewer large cells. There was an asymmetry in the proportion of large cells in the direction of the left MGN in the control sample and in the direction of the right MGN in the dyslexic sample.

DISCUSSION

Despite many gaps, the picture beginning to emerge from anatomical and physiological studies of the visual system is that the segregation apparent at very early stages gives rise to separate and independent parallel pathways. Physiological studies indicate that the magno system carries information about motion and stereopsis, and perceptual studies suggest that it may be largely responsible for motion perception, spatial localization, depth perception from many kinds of depth cues (stereopsis, perspective, shading, and motion), hyperacuity, figural grouping, illusory border perception, and figure/ground segregation (for references, see reference 58). The parvo system seems to be concerned with color perception, object recognition, and high-resolution form perception. The observations that dyslexics often have poor stereoacuity,[59] visual instability, and problems in visual localization[60] are all consistent with a selective deficit in the magnocellular pathway, but as far as we know no one has compared dyslexics and normals for any of the other proposed magno functions.

The role of the magnocellular system in reading is still unknown. Lovegrove et al.[61] have suggested that the transient system rapidly transmits information about spatial organization (for reading this would involve the arrangement and overall shape of words and letters), and then the slower sustained system deciphers the details (syllables and letters). They have also suggested that an even more important role might be that with each saccade the transient system inhibits the sustained system, erasing the otherwise persistent image of the previous fixation, which is consistent with the prolonged afterimages experienced under conditions of impaired magno activity.[58]

If the problem in dyslexia is that a slower magnocellular system does not sufficiently precede the information from the parvo system, then manipulations that slow the parvo system more than the magno system might restore the proper temporal relationship. Indeed, simply reducing the contrast of black letters on a white page by a factor of 2.5, which would be expected to slow processing more in the parvo system than in the magno system,[14–16] has been reported to improve reading performance in reading-disabled children.[62] Since diffuse red light, and not white or shorter wavelength light, produces a sustained inhibition of many magnocellular geniculate cells,[10] the use of colored filters[63,64] may alter the performance of the magno system.

Orton[65] suggested that dyslexia may arise not from high-level cognitive problems, but rather from perceptual deficits. Since then, however, many authors have argued that dyslexia is a specifically linguistic problem arising from a poor understanding of the phonological structure of words.[66–69] There may be a link, however, between perceptual processing and phonological capabilities. Language- and reading-impaired children have trouble distinguishing both consonant–vowel phonemes and nonlinguistic cues if they have rapid (around 40 ms) auditory transitions, but they perform normally with other auditory discriminations, both linguistic and nonlinguistic.[47,70,71] Studies that test the temporal resolution of the visual system find that most reading-disabled children show defects only in rapid visual information processing, and that these same children do poorly on tests of phonological skills.[2,72] Dyslexia and dysphasia (specific developmental language delay) have both been thought to be very high-level, even cognitive, defects, since these children do poorly in some auditory, somatosensory, visual, and motor tasks as well as linguistic tasks. But Tallal et al.[73] found that language-impaired children did poorly in each of these modalities only for tasks that required very rapid information processing. Thus defects in rapid information processing may not be limited to the visual modality, and problems in the ability to discriminate rapid auditory transitions may underlie the linguistic problems. The preliminary findings in the MGN previously described may represent the anatomic substrate of the defect in rapid auditory processing seen in dyslexics. Thus, the relative paucity of large cells in the left MGN of dyslexics may prevent the lateralization of rapid processing to the left hemisphere, which is likely to represent an important factor in language lateralization. Normal acquisition of phonological competence may depend on normal auditory perception at critical developmental times.

The linguistic changes may also relate to anatomical findings described in several earlier studies of these same autopsy specimens—anomalous cerebral asymmetry of a language area known as the planum temporale and developmental cortical abnormalities affecting parts of this and other language areas.[23–25] The relationship between the previous and present anatomic findings is not known. The anatomy of the cortical language areas may be modified by abnormal early sensory input. In that case, the changes in the language areas of dyslexic brains could reflect abnormal early sensory input. On the other hand, the pathologic factors that disturb the visual and auditory thalamic nuclei may also act directly on the development of the language areas and other cortical areas themselves. Indeed, the language areas of the planum temporale, which are characterized by the presence of large pyramidal neurons and rich intracortical myelination,[74] may form part of the fast components of the auditory system and could therefore be affected by a disease process that targets fast subsystems.

Other sensory and motor systems are also functionally subdivided,[75-78] and it is likely that these areas, like the visual system, are segregated into fast and slow subdivisions. This is particularly likely in light of the observations of McGuire *et al.*,[79] who found that an antibody, CAT 301, selectively stains the magnocellular subdivision of the visual pathway, from the geniculate through primary and secondary visual cortices up through higher parietal visual areas; this same antibody stains many other cortical areas, including some, but not all, somatosensory areas, a subset of the motor areas, and many other less well-defined areas. Most of these areas differ from areas that do not stain with CAT 301 in that they are heavily myelinated, suggesting that these areas all have in common the ability to process information rapidly. The neuronal subdivisions involved in fast information processing in each modality thus may share particular molecular entities and might thereby be vulnerable to the same pathogenic factors. We suggest therefore that dyslexics and dysphasics have a specific defect in the rapid subdivisions, the magnocellular homologues, of many forebrain systems.

ACKNOWLEDGMENTS

We thank Rita Burke and Jane McGuiggin for technical help with the evoked potentials. We thank Antis Zalkalns, who processed the human specimens for histology, and William H. Baker, Jr., and The Orton Dyslexia Society, who helped establish access to brain donors for this research project.

REFERENCES

1. MARTIN, F. & W. LOVEGROVE. 1987. Perception **16:** 215.
2. LOVEGROVE, W. R., R. MARTIN & W. SLAGHUIS. 1986. Cogn. Neuropsychol. **3:** 225.
3. STANLEY, G. & R. HALL. 1973. Child Dev. **44:** 841.
4. LOVEGROVE, W. J., G. BILLING & W. SLAGHUIS. 1978. Cortex **14:** 268.
5. LOVEGROVE, W. J., M. HEDDLE & W. L. SLAGHUIS. 1980. Neuropsychologia **18:** 111.
6. DiLOLLO, V., D. HANSON & J. S. McINTYRE. 1983. J. Exp. Psychol. **9:** 923.
7. SHAPLEY, R. M., E. KAPLAN & R. SOODAK. 1981. Nature **292:** 543.
8. KAPLAN, E. & R. M. SHAPLEY. 1982. J. Physiol. (London) **330:** 125.
9. ———. 1986. Proc. Natl. Acad. Sci. U.S.A. **83:** 2755.
10. WIESEL, T. N. & D. H. HUBEL. 1966. J. Neurophysiology **29:** 1115.
11. DREHER, B., Y. FUKADA & R. W. RODIECK. 1976. J. Physiol. (London) **258:** 433.
12. SCHILLER, P. H. & J. G. MALPELI. 1978. J. Neurophysiol. **41:** 788.
13. HICKS, T. P., B. B. LEE & T. R. VIDYASAGAR. 1983. J. Physiol. (London) **337:** 183.
14. DERRINGTON, A. M. & P. LENNIE. 1984. J. Physiol. (London) **357:** 219.
15. DEVALOIS, R. L., E. ABRAMOV & G. H. JACOBS. 1966. J. Opt. Soc. Am. **56:** 966.
16. DEVALOIS, R. L., D. M. SNODDERLY, JR., E. W. YUND & N. K. HEPLER. 1967. Sens. Processes **1:** 244.
17. DERRINGTON, A. M., J. KRAUSKOPF & P. LENNIE. 1984. J. Physiol. (London) **357:** 241.
18. JEFFREYS, D. A. & J. G. AXFORD. 1972. Exp. Brain Res. **16:** 1 and 22.
19. MAIER, J., G. DAGNELIE, H. SPEKREIJSE & B. W. VAN DIJK. 1987. Vision Res. **27:** 165.
20. SREBRO, R. 1987. Vision Res. **27:** 901.
21. HUBEL, D. & M. LIVINGSTONE. 1990. J. Neurosci. **10:** 2223.
22. LEE, B. B., P. R. MARTIN & A. VALBERG. 1989. J. Physiol. **414:** 223.

23. GALABURDA, A. M. & T. L. KEMPER. 1979. Ann. Neurol. **6:** 94.
24. GALABURDA, A. M., G. F. SHERMAN, G. D. ROSEN, F. ABOITIZ & N. GESCHWIND. 1985. Ann. Neurol. **18:** 222.
25. HUMPHREYS, P., W. E. KAUFMANN & A. M. GALABURDA. 1990. Ann. Neurol. **28:** 727.
26. YAKOVLEV, P. I. 1970. *In* Neuropathology: Methods, Diagnosis, C. G. Tedeschi, Ed.: 371–378. Little, Brown. Boston.
27. LEVENTHAL, A. G., R. W. RODIECK & B. DREHER. 1981. Science **213:** 1139.
28. PERRY, V. H., R. OEHLER & A. COWEY. 1984. Neuroscience **12:** 1101.
29. CONLEY, M. & D. FITZPATRICK. 1989. Visual Neurosci. **2:** 287.
30. REESE, B. E. & R. W. GUILLERY. 1987. J. Comp. Neurol. **260:** 453.
31. BLASDEL, G. G. & J. S. LUND. 1983. J. Neurosci. **3:** 1389.
32. HUBEL, D. H. & T. N. WIESEL. 1972. J. Comp. Neurol. **146:** 421.
33. HENDRICKSON, A. E., J. R. WILSON & M. P. OGREN. 1978. J. Comp. Neurol. **182:** 123.
34. LUND, J. S. 1973. J. Comp. Neurol. **147:** 455.
35. LUND, J. S. & R. G. BOOTHE. 1975. J. Comp. Neurol. **159:** 305.
36. FITZPATRICK, D., J. S. LUND & G. G. BLASDEL. 1985. J. Neurosci. **5:** 3329.
37. HURSH, J. B. 1939. Am. J. Physiol. **127:** 131.
38. COPPIN, C. M. L. & J. J. B. JACK. 1972. J. Physiol. (London) **222:** 91P.
39. SCHWARTZ, J. & P. TALLAL. 1980. Science **207:** 1380.
40. HAMMOND, G. R. 1982. Brain Cogn. **1:** 95.
41. EFRON, R. 1963. Brain **36:** 403.
42. TALLAL, P. & M. PIERCY. 1973. Nature **241:** 468.
43. TALLAL, P. 1978. Language Acquisition and Language Breakdown: Parallels and Divergences, A. Caramazza and E. B. Zurif, Eds.: 25–61. Johns Hopkins Press. Baltimore, Md.
44. BAKKER, D. J. 1971. Temporal Order in Disturbed Reading: Developmental and Neuropsychological Aspects in Normal and Reading-Retarded Children. Rotterdam Univ. Press. Rotterdam, the Netherlands.
45. OBRZUT, J. E., G. L. MORRIS, S. L. WILSON, J. M. LORD & L. E. CARAVEO. 1987. Int. J. Neurosci. **32:** 811.
46. WOOD, F., L. FLOWERS, M. BUCHSBAUM & P. TALLAL. 1991. Read Writ. **4:** 81.
47. TALLAL, P. 1980. Brain Lang. **9:** 182–198.
48. ———. 1984. Appl. Psycholing. **5:** 167.
49. ———. 1980. Bull. Orton Soc. **30:** 170.
50. ZINKUS, P. W., M. I. GOTTLIEB & M. SCHAPIRO. 1978. Am. J. Dis. Child. **132:** 1100.
51. WEBSTER, A., J. M. BAMFORD, N. J. THYER & R. AYLES. 1989. J. Child. Psychol. Psychiatry **30:** 529.
52. SHUCARD, D. W., K. R. CUMMINS & M. G. MCGEE. 1984. Brain Lang. **21:** 318.
53. PINKERTON, F., D. R. WATSON & R. J. MCCLELLAND. 1989. Dev. Med. Child. Neurol. **31:** 569.
54. GRONTVED, A., B. WALTER & A. GRONBORG. 1988. Acta Otolaryngol. Suppl. (Stockholm) **449:** 171.
55. POBLANO, A., N. DRUET, Y. PEÑALOZA & R. JIMÉNEZ. 1991. Bol. Med. Hosp. Infant. Mex. **48:** 434.
56. BYRING, R. & T. JARVILEHTO. 1985. Dev. Med. Child. Neurol. **27:** 141.
57. ORTIZ ALONSO, T., M. MAVARRO & E. VILA ABAD. 1990. Funct. Neurol. **5:** 333.
58. LIVINGSTONE, M. & D. HUBEL. 1987. J. Neurosci. **7:** 3416.
59. STEIN, J., P. RIDDELL & S. FOWLER. 1987. *In* Aphasia, C. Rose, Ed. Whurr Wyke. London.
60. ———. 1989. Brain Reading. C. von Euler, I. Lundberg, and G. Lennerstrand, Eds.: 139–157. Stockton Press. New York.
61. LOVEGROVE, W. J., R. P. GARZIA & S. B. NICHOLSON. 1990. J. Am. Optom. Assoc. **61:** 137.
62. GIDDINGS, E. H. & S. L. CARMEAN. 1989. Perceptual and Motor Skills **69:** 383.
63. IRLEN, H. 1980. Paper presented at the 91st Annual Convention of the American Psychological Association, Anaheim, Calif.
64. BREITMEYER, B. G. & M. C. WILLIAMS. 1990. Vision Res. **30:** 1969.
65. ORTON, S. T. 1937. Reading, Writing, and Speech Problems in Children. Chapman & Hall. London.

66. LIBERMAN, I. Y. & D. SHANKWEILER. 1985. Redial Spec. Educ. **6:** 8.
67. LIBERMAN, I. Y. 1989. Brain and Reading, C. von Euler, I. Lundberg, and G. Lennerstrand, Eds.: 207–220. Stockton Press. New York.
68. VELUTINO, F. R. 1977. Dyslexia: Theory and Research. MIT Press. Cambridge, Mass.
69. VELLUTINO, F. R. & D. SCANLON. 1987. Merrill-Palmer Q. **33:** 321.
70. TALLAL, P. & M. PIERCY. 1974. Neuropsychologia **12:** 83.
71. ———. 1975. Neuropsychologia **13:** 69.
72. TALLAL, P., R. STARK, C. KALLMAN & D. MELLITS. 1981. J. Speech Hear. Res. **24:** 351.
73. TALLAL, P., R. E. STARK & E. D. MELLITS. 1985. Brain Lang. **25:** 314.
74. GALABURDA, A. M. & F. SANIDES. 1980. J. Comp. Neurol. **190:** 597.
75. MOUNTCASTLE, V. B. J. 1957. J. Neurophysiol. **20:** 408.
76. ABELES, M. & M. H. GOLDSTEIN, JR. 1970. J. Neurophysiol. **33:** 172.
77. WOOLSEY, T. A. & H. VAN DER LOOS. 1970. Brain Res. **17:** 205.
78. GOLDMAN, P. & W. J. H. NAUTA. 1977. Brain Res. **122:** 393.
79. MCGUIRE, P. K., S. HOCKFIELD & P. S. GOLDMAN-RAKIC. 1989. J. Comp. Neurol. **288:** 280.
80. JASPER, H. H. 1958. Electroencephalogr. Clin. Neurophysiol. **10:** 371.

Dyslexia—Impaired Temporal Information Processing?

JOHN STEIN
*University Laboratory of Physiology
Parks Road
Oxford, OX1 3PT, England*

The question that the New York Academy of Sciences Rodin Conference attempted to answer was, can the problems that children with developmental dyslexia have with learning to read and spell be attributed to a generalized defect in the processing of rapidly changing signals by the central nervous system (CNS)? Accordingly the bulk of the presentations described what is known about temporal information processing in the normal brain in the somaesthetic, auditory, visual, and motor domains. However, no one was brave enough to attempt to educe anatomical or physiological features that are common to all these structures in order to answer whether there can be said to be a specialized system of neurones for dealing with rapid temporal modulations all over the nervous system. Clearly if dyslexics do have a generalized impairment of temporal processing there would need to be, in normals, a generalized system, transcending sensory and motor boundaries, to be impaired in dyslexics.

The magnocellular component of visual processing that probably is impaired in dyslexics, does have anatomical counterparts in the somaesthetic, auditory, and motor systems: the dorsal column, magnocellular medial geniculate, and the gigantocellular motor pathways, respectively. These cells share many common histological and immunohistochemical features. But although it is known in a general way that they can follow rapid temporal modulations accurately, their physiological and psychophysical properties have not yet been worked out in anything like the degree of detail that the visual magnocellular pathway enjoys. Nevertheless, although no one of the conference did so, there is probably enough evidence to speculate that there is indeed a generalized neuronal system transcending sensory and motor boundaries specialized for processing rapidly changing signals, and that since such a system exists it could conceivably be impaired in dyslexics.

The most important question from the point of view of understanding the aetiology of dyslexic symptoms was discussed by only a few of the contributors to the conference, namely, is there evidence that the ability to process rapid temporal modulations is actually impaired in dyslexics? Bill Lovegrove[1] reviewed the evidence that he and others have collected that favors the hypothesis that the transient, magnocellular component of dyslexics' visual processing is mildly impaired. At low spatial frequencies visible persistence is prolonged and flicker contrast sensitivity under mesopic conditions is reduced in many dyslexics, whilst visual evoked potentials in response to stimuli selective for the transient system are reduced. The same visual evoked potential (VEP) result was reported by Margaret Livingstone[2] who also gave us some striking illusions that result from the "color blindness" of the transient system. Piers Cornellisen and colleagues[3] have confirmed Lovegrove's results in children who failed the Dunlop test of binocular stability. Likewise Chris Chase and Annette Jenner[4] showed that the flicker fusion frequency of dyslexics for motion stimuli exciting the transient system was some 30 percent lower than for equiluminent colored stimuli that excite only the sustained system. Thus there is now quite strong evidence that dyslexics probably do suffer a mild impairment of their visual transient, or magnocellular, system.

The question whether this impairment is truly specific to dyslexia was not addressed by anyone. But there is circumstantial evidence that it is not. Alex Richardson[5] presented evidence that many dyslexics score highly on a scale measuring schizotypal personality, and that subjects who score highly on this scale, whether or not they are dyslexic, do badly in a dot localization task that is thought to reflect the functioning of the visual transient system. So it is possible that both dyslexics and high schizotypal personalities have impaired transient systems. The feature common to both these groups may be maldevelopment of the right posterior cortex, which in humans is specialized for visuomotor control.

Paula Tallal[6] presented evidence, mainly from developmental dysphasics rather than dyslexics, demonstrating that impaired temporal processing is not confined to the visual sphere. Learning impairment is associated with defective ability to analyze rapidly changing sounds, so that developmental dysphasics require an interstimulus interval up to 10 times longer than normals to hear two tones as separate. Angela Fawcett and Rod Nicholson's demonstration[7] of a delayed P300 in the auditory evoked potential of dyslexics performing an auditory oddball task suggests that dyslexics share the same impairment of rapid auditory processing as developmental dysphasics.

In the motor sphere analogous timing problems have been found in dyslexics as well. Peter Wolff[8] showed that the variability of dyslexics' tapping at 10 Hz in various bimanual tasks is much greater than normal controls; whilst Fawcett and Nicholson[9] showed that they have longer choice reaction times, and much greater difficulty in balancing on a beam if given mental arithmetic to perform at the same time or even if merely blindfolded. Although the skills required to perform these tasks are not by any means confined to the motor system, one interpretation of the impairments is that they are all caused by defective processing of rapidly changing sensorimotor signals in dyslexics.

How might such a generalized defect of temporal processing cause problems with learning to read? One hypothesis advanced by Breitmeyer and Lovegrove to explain how impairment of the visual transient system may impede reading is that saccadic suppression is reduced. The transient system is thought to be responsible for switching off, during each reading saccade, signals provided by the sustained system that would otherwise persist, so that the images gained during one fixation are erased before the next. If this process does not take place properly, the letters seen in one fixation might blur into the next. However, the reduction in transient system function seen in dyslexics is very slight; and it is difficult to believe that such a small change could give rise to the degree of blurring that many dyslexic children report.

We have put forward an alternative hypothesis that links our findings regarding binocular instability in dyslexics with the transient system defect that we find to be associated with it (Cornelissen *et al.*).[3] The control of eye movements is known to be dominated by the transient system because it provides the motion signals essential for their guidance. It is also known that the magnocellular system is mainly responsible for processing binocular disparity signals; many of Margaret Livingstone's illusions[2] were designed to demonstrate this fact. The main cue that the vergence system employs to lock the two eyes onto objects at different depths is binocular disparity. Thus integrity of the magnocellular system is essential for binocular stability. Slight defects in its operation could well lead to the slightly unsteady fixation that we find in many dyslexic children, and we have shown that this is enough to cause their unstable visual perceptions, poor visual direction sense, visual confusion, and characteristic "visual" reading errors.

One can postulate analogous mechanisms to explain how a "transient" system defect in auditory processing could lead to the kind of phonological processing deficits so frequently found in dyslexics. As Liberman pointed out at the conference, breaking speech down into phonemes is not as simple an operation as it may at first seem, because speech is a continuous series of articulatory gestures that do not map directly onto the arbitrary phonemic description that humans have invented for the purpose of writing. Unlike speech gestures themselves, the phonemes corresponding to them have to be learnt, using rapid changes in acoustic frequency and amplitude as cues to categorize them. If, as a result of an auditory transient system defect, a child could not process these differences properly, then clearly she or he would not be able to categorize them successfully.

A further question that was not much discussed at the conference was how the visual and auditory impairments that result from a magnocellular, transient system defect might relate to the anomalies of cortical organization that are found in dyslexics (Galaburda).[10] The general opinion still appears to be that these anomalies predominate in the left hemisphere, offering the basis of a possible explanation for impairments in phonological processing. But Galaburda and colleagues[10] have clearly shown that cortical microgyriae and ectopias occur on the right side as well; these may well underlie dyslexics' visuospatial deficiencies. There is as yet, however, no detailed explanation of how a defect of the magnocellular system might give rise to these cytological abnormalities.

Nor on a larger scale is there any understanding of how a magnocellular defect might be related to the alterations of cerebral asymmetry that are seen in dyslexics. Whereas the planum temporale is larger on the left in two-thirds of normals, most dyslexics have the same size on both left and right, or the right side is larger. This is probably the result of failure of developmental pruning down of the right side rather than failure of the left side to grow larger. But how a magnocellular defect might lead to this result is again unclear.

Nevertheless, so long as these questions can be answered in the future, the hypothesis that dyslexics suffer an impairment of the magnocellular system of neurones in their CNS does provide the basis for a theory of possible physiological mechanisms underlying reading difficulties. Defective temporal processing in many domains, particularly when this occurs during crucial phases of development, may translate into the great variety of different impairments of perceptual and motor skills that have been discovered in dyslexics.

REFERENCES

1. LOVEGROVE, W. 1993. Weakness in the transient visual system: A causal factor in dyslexia? This issue.
2. LIVINGSTONE, M. 1992. Parallel processing of form, color, motion and depth: Anatomy, physiology, art and illusion. Paper presented at the Rodin Remediation Academy Conference on Temporal Information Processing in the Nervous System: Special Reference to Dyslexia and Dysphasia, New York, Sept. 12–15.
3. CORNELLISEN, P. L. 1993. Flicker contrast sensitivity and the Dunlop test in reading-disabled children. This issue.
4. CHASE, C. & A. R. JENNER. 1993. Magnocellular visual deficits affect temporal processing of dyslexics. This issue.

5. RICHARDSON, A. J. & J. F. STEIN. 1993. Dyslexia, schizotypy, and visual direction sense. This issue.
6. TALLAL, P. 1993. Neural basis of temporal perceptual motor processing: Implications for speech and reading. This issue.
7. NICOLSON, R. I. & A. J. FAWCETT. 1993. Children with dyslexia classify pure tones slowly. This issue.
8. WOLFF, P. H. 1993. Impaired temporal resolution in developmental dyslexia. This issue.
9. NICOLSON, R. I. & A. J. FAWCETT. 1993. Children with dyslexia automatize temporal skills more slowly. This issue.
10. GALABURDA, A. M. 1992. Neuropathological evidence for elective affliction of the magnocellular visual subsystem. Paper presented at the Rodin Remediation Academy Conference on Temporal Information Processing in the Nervous System: Special Reference to Dyslexia and Disphasia, New York, Sept. 12–15.

Impaired Temporal Resolution in Developmental Dyslexia[a]

PETER H. WOLFF

The Children's Hospital
Harvard Medical School
Boston, Massachusetts 02215

INTRODUCTION

Developmental dyslexia (hereafter DD) is widely recognized as etiologically and functionally heterogeneous groups of learning disabilities, whose common denominator is "unexplained" reading and spelling failures in individuals who show little or no impairment in the everyday use of oral language.[1-3] Yet, extensive clinical and experimental studies have neither led to operationally precise definitions for distinguishing DD from other "specific" learning disabilities; nor have they resolved enduring questions about its etiology, pathophysiology, or natural history. For example, investigators still debate whether DD is essentially a biological disorder,[4,5] the result of inappropriate reading instructions, or a normal developmental variation in rates of reading skill acquisition.[6] Similarly, they continue to debate whether language deficits are the necessary and sufficient causes of DD,[1,7,8] or only the surface expression of "deeper" biological dysfunctions that must be made explicit to clarify the basic causes of reading and writing disorders.[4,5]

Although most contemporary dyslexia research assumes that DD is fundamentally a biologically, and in many cases a genetically mediated disorder, humans in large numbers have been reading for at most 300 years. Therefore, it must be concluded that the genetic variations resulting in the dyslexia phenotype have no direct effect on reading and writing but must be mediated through intervening third factors on which selective pressure operates. Furthermore, the condition would almost certainly not be recognized as a disability in preliterate societies, and one might conclude that the invention of the printing press has played as important a causal role in DD as all biological variables combined.

Nevertheless, children or adults who are severely affected by the disorder suffer inordinately from societal demands to adapt to the educational and economic requirements of allegedly literate societies. As such, it merits the attention of investigators from many disciplines, provided they keep in mind that DD does not come in well-defined homogeneous phenotypes, and that its causes are neither linear nor unidirectional—for example, from brain to behavior. By the same token, they must consider the possibility that the prevailing neuropsychological models on human brain–behavior relations are not necessarily the most fruitful for resolving enduring theoretical and clinical issues raised by this complex syndrome.

---

[a]This work was supported by National Institute for Child Health and Development Grant HD-26630.

THEORETICAL MODELS

At least two major directions of contemporary research on dyslexia can be identified for purposes of exposition. One of these starts from the truism that learning to read builds on the child's speech and language processes at many levels, and from extensively documented evidence indicating that nearly all dyslexic children show deficits in one or more components of language perception and production in addition to their primary reading difficulty.[1,2,8] Most investigators informed by this "linguistic–cognitive" orientation focus exclusively on the language performance of dyslexic individuals, and they may consider it theoretically insupportable and clinically uninformative to reduce the complex language phenomena to neuroanatomical substrates or neurophysiological component processes.[7,9]

A very different research strategy assumes that although language deficits may be the most salient clinical features of DD, they are not self-explanatory. Instead, the strategy assumes that the detailed investigation of the language deficits is an important entry point for neuropsychological investigations on the relation between anomalous brain functions and behavior. One of the general findings from experimental studies under this model is that dyslexic children differ from normal readers in the temporal resolution and serial-order perception of linguistically neutral and verbally meaningful auditory and visual events,[10–12] in their ability to impose serial order on sequences of finger or hand movements, and in their ability to impose rhythmic structures on word strings to establish phrase boundaries in the reception and production of connected text.[13]

Such observations have motivated the generic hypothesis that impaired temporal resolution in perception and action is one major physiological source of domain-general dysfunctions, and that the left cerebral hemisphere is the primary anatomical locus.[14,15] The hypothesis has served as a useful theoretical framework for empirical research on the neuropsychology of DD, integrating a wide range of apparently disparate findings and legitimizing specific reading retardation or DD as a real condition with biological causes. However, it has not materially advanced our theoretical understanding of DD, nor has it perceptibly influenced current strategies of clinical interventions. Knowing, for example, that DD is causally related to structural anomalies or dysfunction of the parietal lobe of the left cerebral hemisphere is at best a gratuitous piece of information for those who have to teach dyslexic students how to read and write. Likewise, the finding that sequencing difficulties, dysrhythmic behavior, or impaired temporal information processing are domain-general characteristics of DD will remain relatively uninformative until it has been empirically demonstrated which variables of temporal organization (e.g., frequency, timing precision, and serial ordering) are impaired in DD, how they interact during the performance of temporally complex tasks, and what basic units of behavior are being sequenced.[3]

Several clinical presentations at this symposium have presented evidence supporting the more specific hypothesis that DD is selectively associated with difficulties in processing auditory and visual stimuli in the high-frequency domain, and that this deficit is associated with a neurological impairment of mechanisms dedicated to the processing of high-frequency events. The hypothesis is a fruitful point of departure for focused empirical studies, but it also does not explain how discrete physiological dysfunctions impinge on higher level language processes and "organizational" difficulties in putting isolated components together. Nor does it specify how the presumably autonomous neural mechanisms for processing high- and low-frequency events deal with events in the intermediate frequency range, or interact with other dedicated mechanisms of timing precision and serial ordering, and the like.

TEMPORAL RESOLUTION IN MOTOR COORDINATION

Our studies on DD have focused primarily on coordinated bimanual action, with a particular emphasis on temporal variables of timing precision and serial ordering.[16–18] There is no obvious or direct causal relation between bimanual coordination and learning to read, but a substantial body of experimental studies on humans and other mammals suggests that neural mechanisms for the control of timing precision and serial ordering in speech and language overlap extensively with neuronal processes for the temporal organization of unimanual and bimanual motor skills, at a neuroanatomical, physiological, and behavioral level of description.[19, 20] Assuming that motor coordination and expressive language share common principles of temporal organization, we argued that the analysis of temporal parameters in the coordinated motor action may be particularly instructive for examining temporal resolution deficits in dyslexic individuals because coordinated motor action can be measured objectively and decomposed systematically into relevant component variables of timing control without distorting the phenomenon of interest beyond recognition. We did not assume that impaired motor coordination *causes* reading retardation, but did assume that a third factor of impaired temporal resolution is expressed outwardly in both the manual motor skills and language performance of dyslexic individuals.

The experimental groups on whom I will report comprised more than 230 dyslexic individuals, including children, adolescents, and adults. By detailed clinical history, intelligence and academic achievement tests, and some additional language measures, all of the experimental subjects (including males and females) met generally accepted inclusion and exclusion criteria for DD. Matched control groups of normal readers were included in all studies; additional groups of "pathological controls" or learning-disabled students reading and spelling at or above grade level were included in some studies.

Temporal resolution in bimanual coordination was tested by a modified version of the conventional finger-tapping paradigm. Subjects were instructed to tap two touch-sensitive plates by moving the index fingers on one or both hands vertically at the metacarpo–phalangeal joints while supporting the rest of the hand on a soft pad and lifting each finger after each contact. Finger contact produced voltage signals that measured the actual duration of contact to within 1-ms accuracy were interfaced with a DAC input/output (I/O) interface, and sampled at a rate of 1000/s by an IBM-compatible microprocessor.

The three basic tasks of bimanual coordination were (1) tapping in *synchrony;* (2) tapping in rhythmic *alternations,* each finger tapping at half the prescribed frequency in an alternating pattern; and (3) tapping in *asymmetric* 2:1 patterns so that the "leading" finger responded to *each* metronome signal, the other finger responded to every *other* signal in synchrony with the leading finger, and the two fingers performed in a ratio of 2:0 (leading/nonleading finger). Each condition was tested at several metronome rates, the range of frequencies varying with the nature of the task and the age of subjects.

The outcome variables for the first set of studies were (1) variability of interresponse intervals (IRI) reported as standard deviations for each finger (in milliseconds); (2) mean tapping frequency over a trial relative to metronome rate, as a general measure of the subject's ability to maintain the prescribed response frequency; and (3) the ratio of responses by the left and right fingers over a trial, as a global measure of the subject's ability to preserve the prescribed bimanual pattern throughout a trial. In most of the studies conventional analyses of variance on grouped data were used to test for group differences. Subsequently, more refined qualitative analyses were introduced to examine *how,* as well as *how well,* individual subjects performed the bimanual tasks.

To locate the specific findings in a larger context, I begin with a summary of the results:

1. Dyslexic individuals performed the bimanual tasks with significantly greater variability of IRI than age-matched controls in each of the groups tested ($p<0.01$; 0.001); they also deviated more from the prescribed response frequency.
2. Pathological controls did not differ from controls, but like normal controls they differed significantly from dyslexic subjects.
3. The various tasks were not equally discriminating at each age:
   (a) None of the dyslexic students differed from controls on analogous *unimanual* tapping tasks
   (b) Nine–ten-year-old dyslexic students differed from controls on bimanual *synchronous* tapping tasks that were no longer discriminating at 11–13 years (see FIG. 1)
   (c) Bimanual alternation tasks discriminated dyslexic adolescents and normal or pathological controls until the age of 17–18 years, but were not discriminating in adults (FIG. 2)
   (d) Asymmetric bimanual coordination tasks were discriminating in all age groups (see FIG. 3).
4. The findings just summarized were based on conventional analyses of variance and did not indicate how many dyslexic subjects actually differ from normal controls, or how many normal readers performed like dyslexic individuals. When one standard deviation from the mean performance of normal controls was set as the classifying criterion, more than 50 percent of dyslexic students and less than 10 percent of normal or pathological controls deviated from expected performance on each age-sensitive measure of bimanual coordination. By *post hoc* analyses, there were no differences between dyslexic subjects with and without motor deficits on conventional academic achievement tests of reading and spelling, standardized intelligence tests, or the extended clinical examination for minor neurological signs.

In sum, impaired temporal resolution in bimanual coordination appears to be a developmentally invariant finding in a substantial proportion of all dyslexic subjects. However, the findings are of little theoretical interest unless one can demonstrate a plausible functional relation between impaired bimanual coordination and reading or writing disorders in well-defined subtypes of dyslexia. Given the heterogeneity of DD subtypes, and the complexity of their causal conditions, conventional learning hypotheses that posit a direct linear causal chain *from* motor coordination *to* reading, or conversely *from* reading *to* motor coordination are so implausible that they can probably be rejected at face value. Moreover, our earlier studies had indicated that the motor deficits were already evident in 9-year-old dyslexic children who were still in the early stages of learning to read. On the other hand, there is no convincing

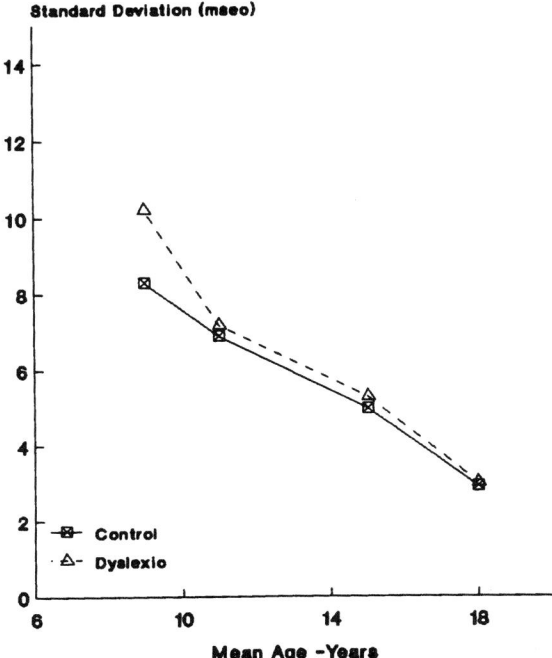

FIGURE 1. Synchronous bimanual tapping as a function of age. Response frequency: 1.5 Hz.

evidence that remedial sensorimotor training has even the slightest effect on the reading skill of dyslexic children.

Neuropsychological models typically identify either neuroanatomical anomalies[14] or deficits of domain-general computational processes in the left cerebral hemisphere[14,15] as third factors that impinge on both language and motor functions, but are not isomorphic with either behavioral domain. The strongest evidence for left hemisphere involvement in DD is observation of adult neurological patients with localized left hemisphere lesions, who frequently exhibit deficits of temporal resolution in language processing and skilled manual motor performance that are remarkably similar to the language and motor deficits of dyslexic children. As a first approximation, one might therefore conclude that our findings on impaired bimanual coordination are simply one more piece of evidence for domain-general left hemisphere involvement in DD.

However, the temporal variable of language and motor performance that is most frequently implicated in adult neurological patients with localized left hemisphere lesions is the processing of serial ordering, or the ability to superimpose a hierarchic pattern on discrete units of behavior in flexible sequences.[21] The temporal variables that clearly discriminated dyslexic subjects from normal readers in our studies were *timing precision, response frequency,* and their interactions. Because, on the other hand, the cerebellar hemispheres have sometimes been identified as a domain-

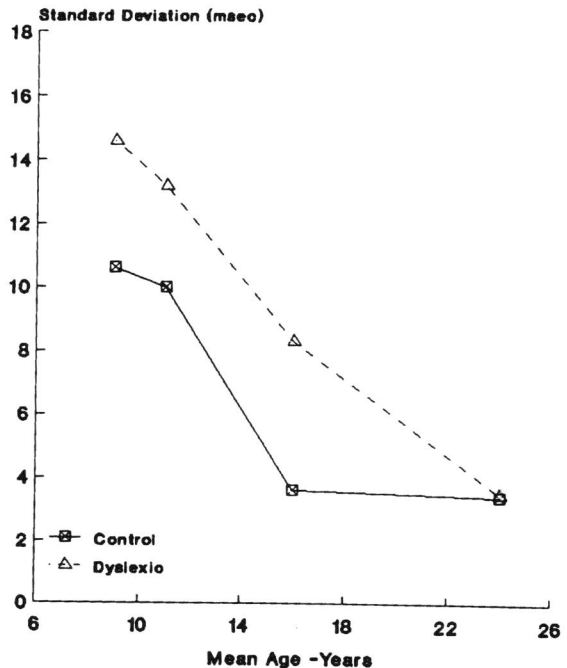

FIGURE 2. Bimanual alternation tapping as a function of age. Response frequency: 3.0 Hz.

general neurological locus for the control of timing precision,[22] we might then conclude instead that the impaired temporal resolution of dyslexic subjects identified a dysfunction of the cerebellar hemispheres. Yet, even 8–9-year-old dyslexic children performed as well as normal controls on tasks of *unimanual* finger tapping, so that our findings do not justify the conclusion of a basic deficit in timing precision in DD.

The motor tasks that most clearly discriminated dyslexic individuals and controls all involved the integration of asymmetric or asynchronously timed movements between the right and left fingers to achieve the target goal. Performance of such bimanual tasks depends on the suppression or inhibition of unintentional bilateral coactivation of homotopic muscles on both sides of the body, or "mirror movements," and therefore presumably on efficient transmission of motor commands between the hemispheres.[23–25]

Callosectomized adults exhibit remarkably few behavioral deficits on familiar tasks, but they find it virtually impossible even after extensive training to perform novel bimanual skills that require the integration of asynchronous or asymmetric movements of the left and right hands to achieve a coordinated bimanual goal, when the task has to be performed under time constraints and without visual feedback.[26] Under such conditions, the adults behave as if the two hands or fingers were constrained to act as a single unit, or as intrinsic spatiotemporal synergies. By

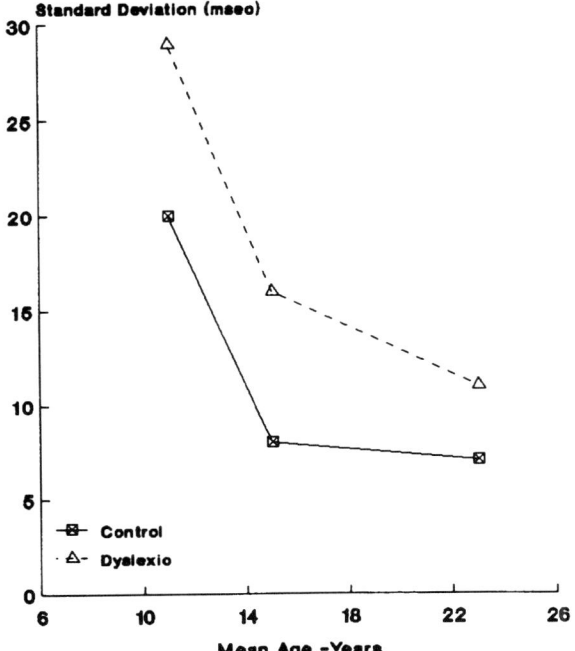

FIGURE 3. A symmetric 2:1 pattern. Tapping as a function of age. Response frequency, leading finger: 3.0 Hz.

contrast, they have no difficulty performing either automatized bimanual tasks, or novel tasks that can presumably be regulated by a single timing command to both hands, such as bimanual tapping in synchrony. The apparent similarities between motor coordination deficits of dyslexic individuals and acallosal patients is still another possible locus for the functional impairment of dyslexic individuals, namely a reduced efficiency of interhemispheric information transfer.[27]

To be sure, most dyslexic individuals probably have a grossly intact corpus callosum, and surgical callosectomy does not render adult neurological patterns dyslexic. Nevertheless, growing up with structurally intact but functionally impaired major cerebral commissures probably has very different consequences for the performance and automatization of complex behavior patterns that involve component processes from both hemispheres than the acute surgical callosectomy in adult patients whose cerebral commissures were presumably normal before surgery. Growing up with grossly intact but dysfunctional cerebral commissures might, for example, be associated with the *adequate* transmission of degraded information (as in the case of left or right hemisphere anomalies), or in a *slow rate* of information transfer for time-distributed functions that require the precise temporal integration between the hemispheres, or in a failure to suppress redundant or conflicting information between the hemispheres.

Our findings on bimanual motor coordination in DD are therefore approximately consistent with at least two, and possibly three, different hierarchic models on human brain behavior relations. Each model assumes that perceptual and motor deficits of temporal resolution for nonverbal events are the outward expression of underlying neuropsychologically mediated dysfunctions. One neuropsychological model assumes anomalous information processing within the left cerebral hemisphere, the second stresses a reduced efficiency of interhemispheric communication, and the third might propose selective dysfunctions of the cerebellar hemispheres as the primary source. Experiments that would persuasively adjudicate among alternative possibilities are difficult to perform in individuals with a grossly intact central nervous system; more often than not, the same behavioral evidence can be adduced to support the alternative models. The pertinent question to be addressed at this time may therefore not be *which* of the competing neuropsychological hypotheses best accounts for the evidence, but *whether* the general hierarchic model on which all of the hypotheses are based is theoretically supportable or clinically useful.

As an alternative approach to the study of DD, we started from the premise that the complex behavior patterns of dyslexic individuals, like the complex behavior of all living things, are not determined by hard-programmed central nervous system prescriptions, but constitute the emergent properties of nonlinear coalitions among very large numbers of potentially independent degrees of freedom in the nervous and motor systems.[25,28]

ALTERNATIVE MODELS OF IMPAIRED TEMPORAL RESOLUTION IN DEVELOPMENTAL DYSLEXIA

The neuropsychological models on DD summarized previously are all based on the *a priori* assumption that humans behave like steady-state systems; and that their behavioral attributes can all eventually be reduced to a few fundamental interactions in terms of linear deterministic laws.[29] From this assumption follows a widely held perspective that the central nervous system operates according to a hierarchy of control centers, each higher center in the tier controlling the behavior of the next lower center in a unidirectional downward flow of information. The clearest exposition of this model is the one proposed by Tinbergen as the basis for studying animal behavior from an ethological perspective.[30] Within neuropsychology proper, the hierarchic model has been elaborated by a number of additional assumptions: (1) each functional control center corresponds to a specific neuroanatomical locus; (2) single degrees of freedom can centrally control many degrees of freedom peripherally; (3) information flow is unidirectional from the center to the periphery; and (4) injuries or developmental anomalies in a given control center will result in one or a set of related behavioral disorders, whose detailed analysis will reveal the brain centers that control the functions of interest.

Although the model has long served as an integrative and explanatory framework for research in the clinical and experimental behavioral sciences, its explanatory power for human behavior in general, and for the behavioral phenotype of DD in particular, is very limited. By positing a linear and hard-programmed causal link from specific centers in the brain to manifest behavior, it forecloses any coherent explanations for the remarkable plasticity of the neuromotor system. It fails to account for the organism's exquisite sensitivity to its initial internal conditions, and for the reciprocal interactions or circular causation between the center and the ecological context.[28,31] Therefore, it also gives no plausible account of how individuals with localized brain lesions or abnormal patterns of neurological development can frequently achieve the same intended goal by alternative pathways when the usual flow of information is blocked or dysfunctional. Most generally the model fails to deal with a fundamental characteristic of all living things, that they invariably induce novel patterns of behavioral coordination during development from antecedent conditions that do not exhibit such novel properties (for a detailed discussion of these issues, see reference 31).

The need for a qualitatively different theoretical perspective on behavioral coordination in dyslexic individuals came to our attention when we examined in greater detail *how*, rather than how badly, dyslexic individuals performed the various bimanual coordination tasks. Experimental investigations by others using rigorous methods of measurement and analysis under a "dynamical systems perspective" have demonstrated that the frequency at which tasks of bimanual coordination are performed is a critical variable or control parameter of spontaneous pattern formation. On the assumption that a more detailed analysis of response frequency as a determinant of timing precision in bimanual coordination might provide potentially important clues about the functional differences between dyslexic individuals and controls on domain-general processes of temporal resolution, we tested subjects on the same tasks but over a wider range of response frequencies, and introduced more exact methods of analysis to display the "natural history" of bimanual coordination over the course of a trial.

Initially, we used conventional methods for analyzing grouped data and plotted the variability of IRI of dyslexic adults and controls on bimanual alternation tasks over a wider range of response frequencies (see FIG. 4). Although dyslexic adults no longer differ from controls when performing at response frequencies up to 3 Hz (see earlier), they differed significantly at higher prescribed metronome rates, and the differences between groups increased as the response was scaled up to 5 or 6.5 Hz (2.5, 3.75 Hz for each finger). The same effect was demonstrated on asymmetric tasks of tapping 2:1 ratios, where dyslexic adults had increasing difficulties relative to controls in maintaining the required asymmetric 2:1 pattern as the response frequency was scaled up.

Whenever dyslexic subjects performed "poorly," in other words, when they showed a rapid increase in variability of IRI, their performance did not simply degenerate. Instead, they frequently began to tap their fingers in new patterns that had not been prescribed by the instructions. These preliminary experiments suggested that response frequency is at least as critical an independent variable (or control parameter) for demonstrating group differences of timing precision as the structure of the bimanual task. However, comparisons based on group statistics for variability of IRI were not sufficient to reveal how subjects actually behaved when they exceeded their critical frequency threshold.

Therefore, we plotted individual IRI over a trial within and between fingers during the performance of various bimanual patterns over a wider range of response frequencies. FIGURE 5 graphs a bimanual alternation trial of a *normal* adult performing at a rate of 6.5 Hz (3.25 Hz for each finger). The top panel plots the IRI *within* each finger and indicates that (1) the subject tapped at the prescribed response frequency; (2) the two fingers responded the same number of times in the course of the trial; (3) the ratio of tapping responses (left/right finger) was, as expected, 1.00; and (4) the IRI were the same for the two fingers. The bottom panel displays the IRI *between* fingers. It indicates that (1) IRI were the same from left to right, and from right to left; and (2) the IRI between fingers was half that within fingers, as the task required.

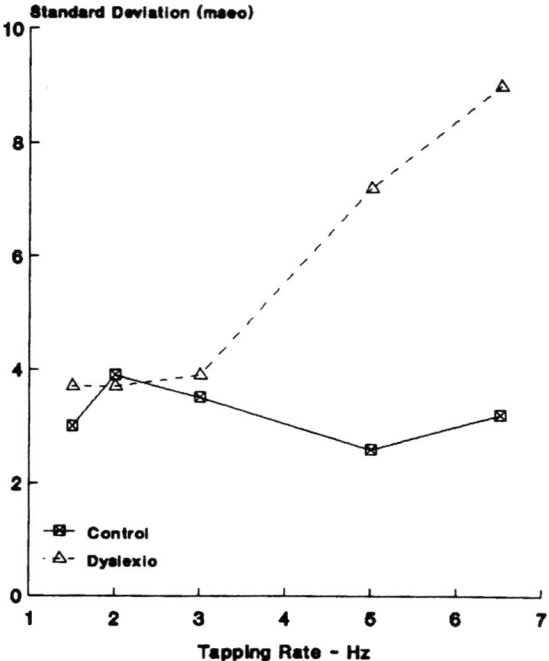

FIGURE 4. Effects of response frequency on stability of bimanual alternation—adults.

FIGURE 6 graphs the performance of a severely dyslexic adult (reading level, below fourth-grade level) on the same bimanual task at the same response frequency. The top panel (IRI within fingers) indicates that (1) the subject tapped with substantially greater variability of IRI than the normal reader; (2) both fingers tapped faster than the metronome specified; and (3) the two fingers tapped at different frequencies so that the interdigit tapping ratio deviated significantly from the expected ratio of 1.00 (faster/slower finger, 1.38). The bottom panel (IRI *between* fingers) in turn indicates that (1) one finger often touched the plate almost immediately after the other (within 1–2 ms) rather than at the appropriate IRI prescribed for the alternation pattern; (2) the IRI between fingers was not the same from left to right as from right to left, and fluctuated constantly throughout the trial; and (3) contrary to what would be predicted by a dynamical systems perspective,[25, 28] the subject did not maintain the new relative phase (tapping in synchrony) once he or she had shifted from the prescribed alternation pattern; instead, the subject switched back and forth between alternation and synchronous patterns.

FIGURES 7 and 8 graph the performance of a dyslexic adult and a normal reader on the same asymmetric 2:1 task, except that the dyslexic subject was being tested at a substantially slower prescribed rate. FIGURE 7, for example, indicates that the normal reader (1) tapped at a low and constant variability of IRI with each finger, and maintained distinct IRI for the leading and nonleading fingers throughout the trial; and (2) tapped in the expected ratio of 2.00 (leading/nonleading finger) at the

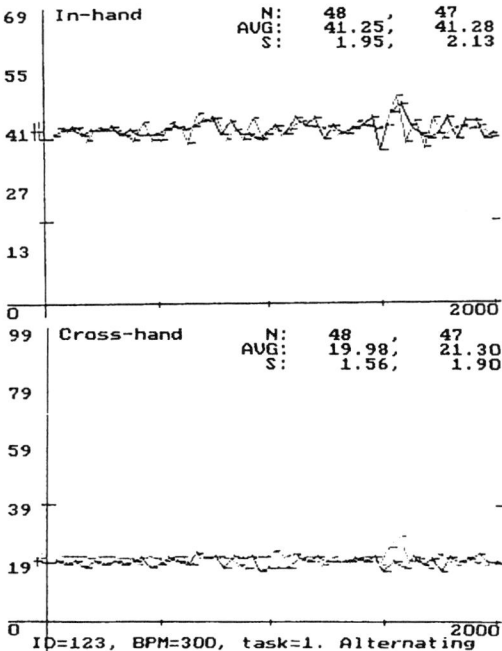

FIGURE 5. Graphic display of IRI on a bimanual alternation task. Normal adult. Response frequency 5 Hz (2.5 Hz for each finger). **Top panel:** IRI within finger. **Bottom panel:** IRI between fingers.

prescribed rate of 4 Hz for the leading finger. FIGURE 8 indicates that the dyslexic subject, by contrast (1) tapped with a substantially greater variability of IRI with each finger; (2) could not maintain the prescribed 2:1 pattern even at the slow rate of 3 Hz; (3) the two fingers intermittently tapped at the same frequency instead of in the prescribed 2:1 ratio; (4) the response frequency of the nonleading (slower) finger was intermittently pulled into the frequency range of the leading finger; and (5) the tapping ratio (leading/nonleading finger) shifted from the expected value of 2.00 to 1.70. A graphic display of IRI *between* the fingers on this trial (not reproduced here) indicated that the dyslexic subject intermittently switched back and forth between the prescribed asymmetric and an *alternation* pattern. There were, however, considerable individual differences in the novel pattern to which a subject shifted after exceeding the critical frequency threshold on this task. Other dyslexic individuals, for example, could not maintain the 2:1 pattern at all, and instead switched back and forth between the *alternation* and *synchronous* patterns. Still others produced more complex patterns that could not be reduced to simple harmonics.

Kelso *et al.*[25] and Yamanishi *et al.*[32] have demonstrated similar phase transitions on the bimanual alternation task as the response frequency was systematically scaled up in steps throughout one trial. Their subjects, in contrast to ours, generally maintained the new relative phase once they had switched to a new pattern, whereas our subjects made repeated efforts at self-correction. However, their subjects had been

98   ANNALS NEW YORK ACADEMY OF SCIENCES

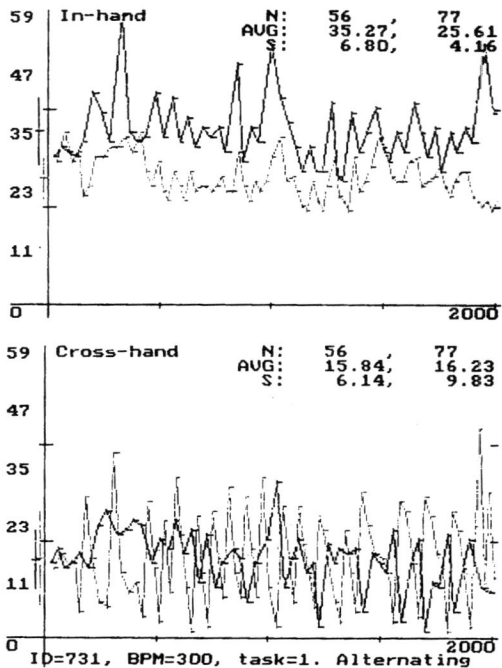

FIGURE 6. Graphic display of IRI on a bimanual alternation task. Severely dyslexic adult. Response frequency 5 Hz (2.5 Hz for each finger). **Top panel:** IRI within finger. **Bottom panel:** IRI between fingers.

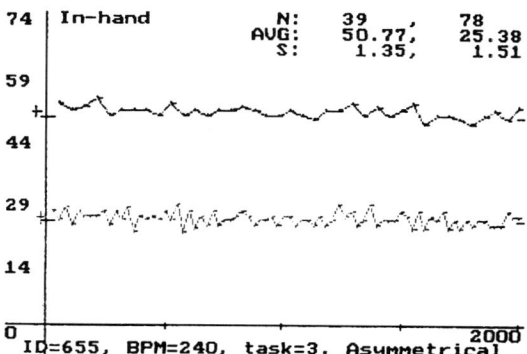

FIGURE 7. Graphic display of IRI on an asymmetric 2:1 tapping task. Normal adult. Response frequency 4 Hz for leading finger, 2 Hz for nonleading finger. IRI within finger.

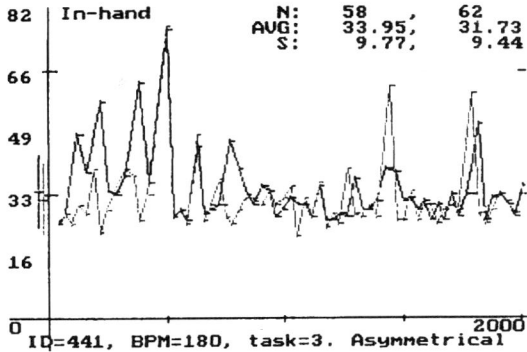

FIGURE 8. Graphic display of IRI on an asymmetric 2:1 tapping task. Severely dyslexic adult. Response frequency 3 Hz for leading finger, 1.5 Hz for nonleading finger. IRI within finger.

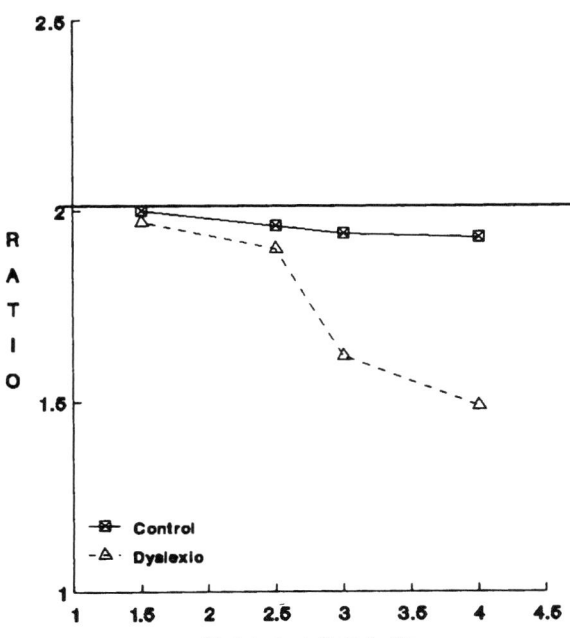

FIGURE 9. Changes in tapping on an asymmetric 2:1 tapping task, as a function of response frequency. Ratio computed as number of responses, leading finger/number of responses, nonleading finger.

trained in preliminary trials and were specifically instructed not to self-correct. Moreover, the response frequency in those studies was increased in graded steps during the course of a single trial, while we examined the effects of response frequency on bimanual coordination in separate trials.

The fact that both dyslexic subjects and controls made repeated efforts at self-correction despite instructions to the contrary, made it difficult to analyze phase transitions and "relaxation times" by formal methods. As a compromise, we first compared the response ratios between the left and right fingers across asymmetric tapping trials. In each case, the expected ratio of leading/nonleading fingers was 2.00. We predicted that whenever subjects switched from the prescribed pattern, they would shift to either the alternation or synchronous tapping pattern, whose theoretical tapping ratio in both cases was 1.00. A failure to maintain the prescribed 2:1 pattern should therefore result in lower ratios that approached 1.00 as a limit. Consistent with the prediction, the tapping ratios of dyslexic individuals decreased progressively as the response frequency was scaled up (see FIG. 9).

Despite the fact that the subjects attempted to self-correct throughout a trial, we were able to apply more detailed quantitative measures in small samples of dyslexic individuals and controls. These pilot studies indicated that the variability in relative phasing between the fingers increased as subjects approached their critical frequency threshold, and before they actually switched to a novel pattern.[33] However, contrary to predictions,[25,32] the variability of relative phase did not decrease after the transition to a new (and presumably more stable) phase pattern, probably because subjects made constant efforts at self-correction and therefore switched back and forth between different patterns of bimanual coordination throughout the trial.

TEMPORAL RESOLUTION AND DEVELOPMENT DYSLEXIA

A comparison of motor performance by dyslexic individuals and controls on various bimanual coordination tasks at different response frequencies has identified a developmentally invariant deficit of temporal resolution that is consistently greater at high than low frequencies. There was, however, no discrete frequency threshold that discriminated the timing precision or temporal resolution of dyslexic subjects and controls categorically. For one thing, the frequency for making such discriminations varied as a function of age, dyslexic children showing the effect of response rate on timing precision at lower response frequencies than adolescents or adults. For another thing, the effects of response frequency on timing precision varied with the nature of the bimanual task. Thus, the frequency threshold was lower on "complex" bimanual tasks that required the subject to maintain a relatively unstable relative phase between the fingers, whereas dynamically stable bimanual tasks that did not require an initial uncoupling of intrinsic synergies or a suppression of mirror movements (e.g., tapping in synchrony) were nondiscriminating except in very young dyslexic children. Finally, all dyslexic individuals, including young children, performed the analogous unimanual tapping tasks with the same timing precision as controls. In short the temporal resolution deficits in DD could not be reduced to deficiencies in any single or "basic" timing mechanisms dedicated to the processing of temporal information in the high-frequency range,[11] or a single behavioral score or discrete physiological parameter.

Reading groups differed most consistently on bimanual tasks that required the integration of asynchronously timed responses of the left and right index fingers, and that presumably depended on the coordination of movements between the right and left sides of the body. The essential differences between reading groups on tasks of bimanual coordination may therefore best be described in terms of (1) variations in the ability to uncouple intrinsic behavioral synergies (unintended bilateral coactivation of homotopic muscles on the two sides of the body; mirror movements), and (2) difficulties in reassembling the dissociated behavioral units into various flexible coalitions that were required for the various asynchronous bimanual tasks.

The findings reported here are largely limited to a single paradigm of bimanual coordination. Nevertheless, they raise the more general theoretical question whether the temporal resolution deficits of dyslexic individuals in clinically more relevant patterns of behavioral coordination such as reading and language processing are at all definable in terms of isolated behavioral variables, or whether instead the core difficulties of dyslexic individuals may reside in their difficulties with assembling component units of behavior into temporally ordered larger ensembles, not only in motor action but also in language performance and reading. During the early stages of learning to read, the components that contribute to fluent reading are themselves often impaired in dyslexic children. However, clinical work with such children suggests that the basic components of skilled reading are relatively susceptible to improvement with appropriate remedial instructions. Yet, even after the deficiencies at a basic level have been corrected, severely impaired dyslexic students typically continue to show an impaired capacity to organize these elements into coordinated ensembles.

The outcome variable of primary interest in our studies was timing precision in motor action, and response frequency turned out to be an important control parameter. The asymmetric, asynchronous 2:1 tasks of bimanual coordination could, however, be construed as depending both on serial order control and timing precision, and our findings indicated that in the analyses of the more complex motor patterns, timing precision, serial ordering, and response frequency were consistently interactive in the apparent coordination failures of dyslexic students. While it is both possible and necessary to decompose temporal resolution in motor action into component variables of timing precision, serial ordering, and frequency for purposes of experimental investigation, it may be theoretically meaningless to reduce the temporal resolution "deficit" of dyslexic individuals to a single temporal variable, or to localize this deficit in any specific and neuroanatomically defined region of the central nervous system.

Neuroscientists are expressing similar concerns at a more fundamental level, by calling attention to the fact that the enormous advances in our knowledge about cellular, subcellular, and synaptic phenomena have shed little, if any, light on the operating principles by which large collections of cells cooperate to induce behavior patterns whose properties cannot be reduced to, or deduced from the properties of the cooperating units.[29,30] They have proposed a number of qualitatively different perspectives for rationalizing human brain behavior relations as an alternative to traditional solutions in terms of hard-programmed or hard-wired central executive agencies. Their long-range goal is to provide a coherent and plausible account for the enduring issues of emergent properties and self-organization in terms of abstract formal operating principles,[24,34,35] and to resolve the otherwise intractable "degrees of freedom problem"[36] that inevitably surface when one attempts to relate brain functions at a microscopic level to behavioral coordination at a macroscopic level.

Some of these models have been translated into hypotheses from which follow concrete predictions that can and have been tested experimentally on behavioral coordination in humans. For the most part, however, the experiments motivated by these perspectives have been limited to narrowly defined motor skills examined in carefully trained normal adults,[25] or to species-typical patterns of locomotion in developing infants.[37] Whether the same formal models can be fruitfully applied to the study of complex behavioral variations in DD remains an empirical question that can only be answered by research. Our descriptive studies suggest that the perspectives may eventually provide a theoretically coherent framework for experimental investigation on many of the unresolved and basic issues concerning the etiology and natural history of DD. Even if the new models can, at this time, only be applied as a metaphor, they will nevertheless serve as an important heuristic for reexamining the phenomenology of DD from a point of view that differs radically from traditional hierarchic models that have long dominated neuropsychological research on the many puzzles of DD, but that have not led to theoretically coherent or clinically useful answers.

REFERENCES

1. Ellis, A. W. 1985. The cognitive neuropsychology of developmental (and acquired) dyslexia: A critical survey. Cogn. Neuropsych. **26:** 169–205.
2. Jorm, A. F. 1979. The cognitive and neurological basis of developmental dyslexia. A theoretical framework and review. Cognition **7:** 19–33.
3. Denckla, M. B. D. 1979. Childhood learning disabilities. *In* Clinical Neuropsychology, K. M. Heilman and E. Valenstein, Eds. Oxford Univ. Press. New York.
4. Geschwind, N. & A. M. Galaburda. 1985. Cerebral lateralization: Biological mechanisms, associations and pathology. Arch. Neurol. **42:** 428–459.
5. Kinsbourne, M., *et al.* 1991. Neuropsychological deficits in adults with dyslexia. Develop. Med. Child Neurol. **33:** 763–775.
6. Shaywitz, S. E., *et al.* 1992. Evidence that dyslexia may represent the lower tail of a normal distribution of reading ability. New Eng. J. Med. **326:** 145–150.
7. Hulme, C. 1988. The implausibility of low-level visual deficits as a cause of children's reading difficulties. Cogn. Neuropsychol. **5:** 369–374.
8. Mann, V. A. 1986. Why some children encounter reading problems: The contribution of difficulties with language processing and phonological sophistication to early reading disability. *In* Psychological and Educational Perspectives on Learning Disabilities, J. K. Torgesen and B. Y. L. Wong, Eds.: 133–149. Academic Press. New York.
9. Coltheart, M., *et al.* 1983. Surface dyslexia. Q. J. Exp. Psychol. **35A:** 469–495.
10. Tallal, P., R. Stark & D. Mellits. 1985. The relationship between auditory temporal analysis and receptive language development. Neuropsychologia **23:** 527–534.
11. Livingston, M. S., G. D. Rosen, F. W. Drislane & A. M. Galaburda. 1991. Physiological and anatomical evidence for a magnocellular defect in developmental dyslexia. Proc. Natl. Acad. Sci. **88:** 7943–7947.
12. Lovegrove, W. J., R. P. Garzia & S. B. Nicholson. 1990. Experimental evidence for a transient system deficit in specific reading disability. J. Am. Optomet. Assoc. **61:** 137–146.
13. Hanes, M. L. 1986. Rhythm as a factor of mediated and nonmediated processing reading. *In* Rhythm in Psychological, Linguistic and Musical Processes, J. R. Evans and M. Clynes, Eds. Thomas. Springfield, Ill.
14. Hammond, G. R. 1982. Hemispheric differences in temporal resolution. Brain Cogn. **1:** 95–118.
15. Tzeng, O. J. L. & W. S.-Y. Wang. 1984. Search for a neurocognitive mechanism for language and movements. Am. J. Physiol. **246:** R904–R911.
16. Wolff, P. H., C. Cohen & C. Drake. 1984. Impaired motor timing control in specific reading retardation. Neuropsychologia **22:** 587–600.
17. Wolff, P. H., G. F. Michel, M. Ovrut & C. Drake. 1990. Rate and timing precision of motor coordination in developmental dyslexia. Dev. Psychol. **26:** 349–359.

18. WOLFF, P. H., G. F. MICHEL & M. OVRUT. 1990. The timing of syllable repetitions in developmental dyslexia. J. Speech Hear. Res. **33:** 281–289.
19. OJEMANN, G. 1984. Common control and thalamic mechanisms for language and motor function. Am. J. Physiol. **246:** R901–R903.
20. KELSO, J. A. S. & B. TULLER. 1987. Intrinsic time in speech production: Theory, methodology and preliminary observations. *In* Motor and Sensory Processes of Language, E. Keller and M. Gopnik, Eds.: 203–221. Lawrence Erlbaum. Hillsdale, N.J.
21. BAKKER, D. J. 1972. Temporal Order in Disturbed Reading: Developmental and Neuropsychological Aspects in Normal and Reading Retarded Children. Rotterdam Univ. Press. Rotterdam, the Netherlands.
22. KEELE, S. W. & R. IVRY. 1990. Does the cerebellum provide a common computation for diverse tasks? Ann. N.Y. Acad. Sci. **608:** 179–211.
23. HOPF, H. C., H. J. SCHLEGEL & K. LOWITZSCH. 1974. Irradiation of voluntary activity to the contralateral side in movements of normal subjects and patients with central motor disturbances. Eur. Neurol. **12:** 142–147.
24. FENTRESS, J. C. 1991. The role of timing in motor development. *In* The Development of Timing Control and Temporal Organization in Coordinated Action, J. Fagard and P. H. Wolff, Eds.: 341–366. North-Holland. Amsterdam, the Netherlands.
25. KELSO, J. A. S., K. G. HOLT, P. RUBIN & P. N. KUGLER. 1981. Patterns of interlimb coordination emerge from properties of non-linear, limit cycle oscillatory processes: Theory and data. J. Mot. Behav. **13:** 226–261.
26. PREILOWSKI, B. F. B. 1972. Possible contributions of the anterior forebrain commissures to bilateral motor coordination. Neuropsychologia. **10:** 267–277.
27. GLADSTONE, M., C. T. BEST & R. J. DAVIDSON. 1989. Anomalous bimanual coordination among dyslexic boys. Dev. Psychol. **25:** 236–246.
28. SCHOENER, G. & J. A. S. KELSO. 1988. Dynamic pattern generation in behavioral and neural systems. Science **239:** 1513–1520.
29. DAVIES, P. 1988. The Cosmic Blueprint. Simon & Schuster. New York.
30. TINBERGEN, N. 1950. The hierarchical organization of nervous mechanisms underlying instructive behavior. Symp. Soc. Exp. Biol. **14:** 305–312.
31. KELSO, J. A. S. & B. TULLER. 1981. Toward a theory of apractic syndromes. Brain Lang. **13:** 224–245.
32. YAMANISHI, J., M. KAWATO & R. SUZUKI. 1980. Two coupled oscillators as a model for the coordinated finger tapping by both hands. Biol. Cybern. **37:** 219–225.
33. ROUSSELLE, C. & P. H. WOLFF. 1991. The dynamics of bimanual coordination in developmental dyslexia. Neuropsychologia **29:** 907–924.
34. LLINAS, R. R. 1988. The intrinsic electrophysiological properties of mammalian neurons: Insights into central nervous system function. Science **242:** 1654–1664.
35. JORDAN, M. I. 1990. Motor learning and the degrees of freedom problem. *In* Attention and Performance XIII, M. Jeannerod, Ed.: 796–836. Lawrence Erlbaum. Hillsdale, N.J.
36. BERNSTEIN, N. 1967. The Co-ordination and Regulation of Movements. Pergamon. New York.
37. THELEN, E., K. D. SKALA & J. A. S. KELSO. 1987. The dynamic nature of early coordination: Evidence from bilateral leg movements in young infants. Dev. Psychol. **23:** 179–186.

Neural Representation of Stimulus Times in the Primary Auditory Cortex[a]

DENNIS P. PHILLIPS

Departments of Psychology[b] and Otolaryngology
Dalhousie University
Halifax, Nova Scotia, Canada, B3H 4J1

INTRODUCTION

By definition, sounds are physical events that are distributed in time. It follows from this that the faithful neural encoding of a sound requires that the nervous system in some way preserve or "represent" the relevant time structure of the signal in the cadence of spike discharges evoked by the sound. By the same line of argument, it may come as no surprise that demonstrable[1-3] or presumed[4] pathologies of the central auditory nervous system commonly give rise to impoverished perceptual performance on tasks based on temporal auditory processing. It is becoming increasingly clear, however, that "temporal auditory processing" may be an umbrella term for what are in fact quite heterogeneous time-dependent auditory analyses.[2,5,6] In particular, the fashion in which acoustic events are distributed in time may have important consequences both for the identity of the neural mechanisms that encode them, and for the nature of the percepts they generate.

The purpose of the present paper is to examine the fashion and fidelity with which the time structure of sounds is represented in the activity of neurons of the primary auditory cortex. It is likely that of all the cortical auditory fields, the primary one has the most precise neural representation of sound time structure. This is an important point, because higher level, cortically based perceptual or language processors probably derive their acoustic input directly or indirectly from the primary field;[7] the temporal grain of the primary field's output is thus a limiting factor on the temporal grain of the information available to higher level processors. Accordingly, knowledge of the temporal grain of sound representation in the primary auditory cortex may provide us with insights into the kinds of auditory perceptual deficits to be expected in listeners with pathologies of forebrain auditory processing mechanisms.

We begin by sketching two kinds of sound time structure, the percepts they generate, and the neural mechanisms thought to encode them. We then examine the expression of these codes in the activity of primary auditory cortex neurons, and briefly compare the representation of sounds at that locus with that which exists in the auditory brainstem. Finally, we shall examine evidence on the consequences of cortical lesions on percepts based on these two kinds of sound time structure.

---

[a]Some of the research described here was supported by grants from the Natural Sciences and Engineering Research Council of Canada.
[b]Where correspondence should be addressed.

KINDS OF SOUND TIME STRUCTURE

In what follows, we focus on two forms of sound time structure, loosely labeled *periodic* and *transient* (FIG. 1). Both of these features of a sound serve to identify what the signal is (as opposed to where it is relative to the listener). At the outset, it should be emphasized that these are by no means exhaustive of the temporal processes in hearing. The *binaural* processing of stimulus event times used in sound localization[8] is mentioned only in passing: it can be thought of as a running temporal cross-correlation of the signals at the two ears, of which the perceptual consequence is a spatial locus for the perceptually identified sound. Additionally, the concept of the ear's "temporal window,"[5,9,10] that is, a narrow time window through which auditory perceptual mechanisms sample the incoming stream of sound, is simply taken for granted.

Strictly periodic (i.e., repetitive) acoustic events, even broad-band ones, are quite capable of generating a pitch percept. For example, broad-band noise that is periodically interrupted with a 50 percent duty cycle may evoke a percept whose pitch can be matched to that of a tone, and for interruption rates up to at least 250 Hz.[11] The tonal quality of the percept cannot be related to the spectral content of the sound, because the signal is inherently broad-band. Rather, the apparent pitch of the signal is related to the sound's temporal properties, such that the pitch is dependent on the period of the modulation. Now, if the repetitive signal giving rise to the pitch percept is intrinsically broad-band in spectral content, then it follows that the neural mechanisms generating the percept must be based on neuronal timing. In some fashion, the brain must have neuronal responses entrained to the periodicities in the signal, such that the intervals between neuronal responses accurately indicate the signal's periodicity [FIG. 1(a)]. This issue has been explored in physiological studies of the auditory brainstem[12,13] where it is apparent that individual neurons can entrain spike action potential responses to periodicities well in excess of 2000 Hz. In practice, such responses are steady state, and while neurons may not discharge a spike in response to every stimulus period, the intervals between the spikes that are discharged are typically integral multiples of the stimulus period. Failure to entrain to the stimulus periodicity is revealed either in the inter-spike interval distribution becoming continuous and random with respect to the stimulus periodicity, or in response failure (i.e., no spikes).

There are a number of cases of pitch percepts arising from a stimulus periodicity for which the neural code might be either spectral or temporal: one is the pitch of the human voice. This pitch is determined in large part by the rate of glottal pulses. Each glottal pulse is a relatively noisy signal, but the voice pitch is shaped as much by their repetition rate (*temporal* frequency) as by the spectral content of any one of them. In adult males, the rate of glottal pulses in near 128 Hz, while in adult females, the rate is closer to 220 Hz.[14] These are the fundamental frequencies: the laryngeal tone consists in the fundamental and the higher harmonics, with the final amplitude spectrum being shaped by the filter function of the upper vocal tract. The rate of glottal pulsing is under voluntary control, and it is largely by voluntary modulation of the pulsing rate that a speaker sings or produces intonation contours (inflexions) in speech.

A second, and perhaps related, case is that of the missing fundamental percept evoked by tone complexes.[15,16] Briefly, if a listener is presented with a complex of tonal signals in which the elements are equally spaced in the frequency domain (e.g., 400, 600, 800 Hz), then she or he typically perceives the stimulus as a complex with a pitch equal to the fundamental (200 Hz), whether or not the signal contains spectral

A. Periodic, steady-state case

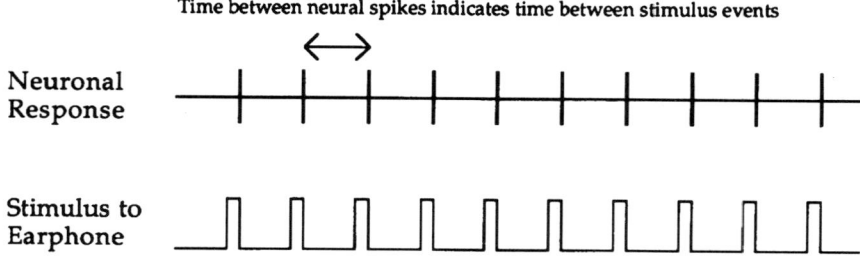

B. Transient case

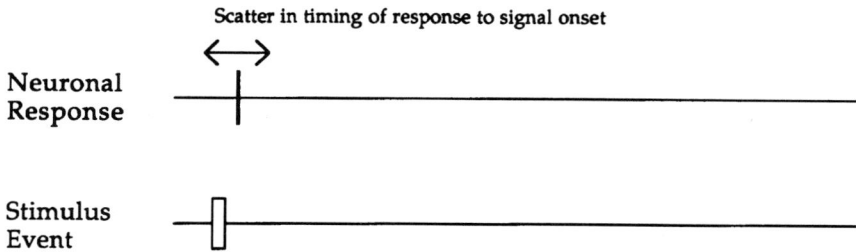

FIGURE 1. Schematic diagram depicting two types of sound time structure, and the principles of the neural codes thought to encode them. In the periodic, steady-state case (**A**), repetitive, discontinuous brief sounds evoke periodic neuronal responses, in which the timing of the neuronal discharges reflects the timing of the events in the stimulus. Such sounds often give rise to a pitch percept, with the perceived pitch being determined by the periodicity of the signal. In the transient case (**B**), which underlies the perceptual skill of temporal resolution, the limitation on the brain's ability to exhibit temporally separated responses to successive stimulus events resides in the precision with which the responses to the onsets of the stimulus events are timed.

energy at the fundamental frequency. Although such signals may contain no energy at the fundamental, the time waveform of the sound has a periodicity at the fundamental frequency, so there is the possibility of a temporal neural code underlying the percept. On the other hand, a case can be made for a spectral code based on the *pattern* of neural elements excited by the elements of the tone complex, since the harmonic relations of the elements precisely specify the fundamental. In most naturally occurring harmonic complexes, the fundamental is actually present, and so it is also possible that the pitch of the harmonic complex lacking the fundamental is in some sense based on familiarity, that is, a learned response.[17] Indeed, most recent accounts of pitch perception, especially in the cases of complex sounds, are expressed in purely psychological terms and assume a central pattern recognition process that operates on both spectral pitch (i.e., percepts driven directly by the tonal content of the sound) and virtual pitch (i.e., percepts driven by recognition of a familiar pattern of spectral content).[17] The perceived pitch of human voices might be recognized in part on these principles. Thus, voices heard over the telephone often appear to have characteristic pitches, even though the telephone transmits little or no energy at the pitch frequency.

A quite different set of temporal processes pertains in the case of the perceptual task of temporal resolution. Consider the task of being presented with two brief sounds and being required to make a judgment about them; for example, which one came first? The ability to perform this task requires the listener to perceptually segregate the two sounds (or, minimally, their onsets) in time, which in turn requires that the brain have temporally segregated responses to the two events (or their onsets). There is no burden on neurons to respond in a steady fashion, or even for individual neurons to respond to both events, since the two sounds may be so different (in spectral content or spatial location) that they activate nonoverlapping populations of neurons. One limiting factor on the brain's ability to support temporally segregated responses to successive sounds is obviously the temporal precision with which *transient* responses indicate the timing of the sounds [FIG. 1(b)]. This jitter in transient response timing is typically measured using the standard deviation of the first-spike latency.[14,18]

At a strictly introspective level, it may be noteworthy that the periodic/transient distinction being made here has another corollary. In the case of repetition pitch, one typically has little conscious perceptual access to the individual acoustic events generating the pitch percept. Thus, in the case of a train of transients presented at, say, 200 Hz, what one experiences is a single perceptual event (a buzz), which happens to have a pitch (near 200 Hz). Likewise, in sound localization, there is no sense in which we perceive the signal arriving at one ear and then at the other, and deduce from that interaural time difference the spatial location of the source: rather, we perceive a single stimulus event that happens to have a spatial location. These instances are quite in contrast to the temporal resolution case, which is virtually defined by conscious access to temporally segregated percepts driven by the individual acoustic events.

CORTICAL CODING OF STIMULUS PERIODICITIES

The primary auditory cortex is one of a number of adjacent cerebral territories in direct receipt of afferents from the auditory thalamus. Most of its neurons are narrowly tuned to tone frequency, and these tuned elements are spatially arrayed in striplike assemblies ("isofrequency lines"[19]). The isofrequency lines are themselves typically arrayed according to the tone frequencies (cochlear places) they represent, which likely span the audible range. Overlaying this "tonotopic" map are patchily distributed territories specialized for the representation of spatial or bandwidth parameters of sounds.[5] These territories do not respect each other's boundaries, with the result that different neurons within isofrequency lines may be variously sensitive to the center frequency, bandwidth, and/or spatial location of a stimulus.

The ability of primary auditory cortical neurons to encode stimulus periodicities on a temporal basis, that is, by time-locking spike action potentials to the stimulus cycles, has been studied for over a decade, and using a variety of stimulus configurations. Steinschneider *et al.*[20] recorded both multiple-unit and intracortical evoked potential responses to low-frequency tones in the auditory cortex of the alert monkey. They found that both kinds of neuronal responses showed observable time locking to the stimulus periodicities only for signal frequencies less than about 200 Hz. Other authors[21–23] have studied individual cortical cells ("single units") with amplitude-modulated tones or noise. In such studies, the animal is typically presented with long-duration stimuli that contain many cycles of the modulation; the response train is then "folded" on the period of the modulation cycle, and the extent to which the distribution of action potentials is restricted within the cycle is measured using circular statistics. These studies have been in agreement that cortical neurons are very poor at entraining spikes to the modulating waveform when its frequency exceeds about 50 Hz.

Two groups have studied cat cortical neurons with repetitive click stimuli.[24,25] These experiments differ from the foregoing in that the physical stimulus is, in principle, discontinuous, because the clicks are separated by periods of silence. The more quantitative study is perhaps that of Eggermont[24] in the lightly (ketamine-) anesthetized adult animal. He showed that irrespective of how neuronal responses were measured, limiting click rates were usually less than 32/s. He argued that the failure of cortical neurons to entrain spikes to clicks at higher rates likely reflected the development of a short-duration inhibitory feedback response immediately following the spike discharge. This line of argument is compatible with the independent observation that the temporal precision with which transient responses are locked to the onset of a brief tone pulse is typically sufficient to support spike entrainment to stimulus rates far in excess of those to which the neuron actually does entrain.[26] An earlier study[25] in the awake cat's cortex reported that a small proportion of neurons discharged time-locked spikes to click stimuli presented at up to 250 Hz, although the criteria for "time-locking" used in that study were perhaps less stringent than the response measures used by others.[24,27]

Two other recent studies merit attention. Schwarz and Tomlinson[15] studied neurons in the primary auditory cortex of awake monkeys with harmonic tone complexes that lacked fundamental frequencies. The monkeys used in the study had previously been trained in a psychophysical pitch matching task, and two of the three animals had presented evidence that they perceived missing fundamentals. (The monkeys were not, however, performing any psychophysical task at the time of the physiological recordings.) Schwarz and Tomlinson found no evidence for cortical cells selective for combinations of harmonic components, nor for cortical cells whose spike behavior might reflect the output of a periodicity pitch detector. Thus, cortical cells tuned to low (spectral) frequencies did not respond to the low-frequency missing fundamentals generated by higher frequency harmonic complexes.

Reale and Brugge[28] studied cat cortical neurons with binaural beat stimuli. These are long-duration (usually 3–5 s), low-frequency, binaural tones in which the signal frequencies at the two ears differ by a small amount, for example, 5 Hz. This frequency disparity creates a continuously changing interaural phase difference, and the perceptual consequence of the auditory nervous system's tracking of that change is a spatial image that moves around the head toward one ear (that receiving the higher frequency signal), and then jumps back to repeat the cycle. The rate of this "beating" equals the frequency difference between the tones at the ears. Reale and Brugge[28] presented evidence that some cortical neurons could synchronize their spike discharges to the binaural beat, but only for beat frequencies less than about 40 Hz.

Most of the stimuli used in the foregoing studies have previously been applied in the study of auditory brainstem neurons. This is an important point because a direct comparison of the fidelity of the temporal representations of signal periodicities at the two levels provides us with information about whether the afferent pathways to the cortex have preserved those temporal codes. If the input to the cortex has *not* preserved a code developed in the brainstem, or some transformation of it, then the cortex likely contains little or no information about the relevant stimulus property, and it would therefore follow that we have little reason to believe that the cortex is implicated in the neural processes that underlie perception of that property. On the other hand, if the cortex *does* contain information about a stimulus property, then we do have reason to believe that the cortex is involved with behavioral responses to that stimulus dimension.

The studies of stimulus periodicity coding in cortical auditory neurons revealed that spike entrainment to the stimulus cycles was generally very poor for temporal frequencies in excess of about 30 to 50 Hz, and was only rarely observed above 100 Hz. This is more than an order of magnitude poorer than the time locking to periodicities seen in the cochlear nerve and cochlear nucleus of the caudal auditory brainstem.[12,13] Likewise, whereas Reale and Brugge[28] found only the occasional cortical neuron that phase-locked spike discharges to binaural beat frequencies in excess of 30 Hz, an earlier study[29] of the auditory midbrain found the upper limit of such responses to be closer to 80 Hz. In the repetition pitch domain, the performance of cortical neurons does not even match behavioral performance, since the pitch percept extends at least to 250 Hz.[11] The fact that the cortex's steady-state temporal coding is, by comparison with that seen in the auditory brainstem, also impoverished for binaural beat stimuli, suggests that it is the coding of periodicities *per se,* and not just those related to pitch percepts that is not faithfully preserved at the level of cortical output.

TRANSIENT RESPONSES OF AUDITORY CORTICAL NEURONS

Neurons of the primary auditory cortex respond briskly and transiently to the onset of a steady tonal or other stimulus, largely irrespective of the duration of the signal.[30] The neurons are sensitive to both the carrier frequency of a tone pulse and its rise ("attack") time, which contributes significantly to the short-term spectrum at signal onset.[31] The brevity of the response is thought to be shaped by the development of a postonset inhibitory response and by neural adaptation.[24,30] Sensitivity to the carrier frequency is simply the expression of the neurons' excitatory frequency tuning. Sensitivity to the bandwidth and the gross shape of the signal's onset spectrum reflect the presence, disposition, and strength of inhibitory inputs in frequency-intensity domains that flank the excitatory one ("lateral" inhibition). Taken together, these observations suggest that primary auditory cortex neurons are specialized to respond to brief stimulus events, and to be sensitive to the spectral content of those events.[31]

FIGURE 2 illustrates some of the general properties of these transient responses. The upper panel is a conventional peristimulus time histogram that depicts the summed responses of neuron RR408 to 100 repetitions of a preferred-frequency, 25-ms-duration tone pulse presented at 40-dB sound pressure level (SPL). The repetition rate of the pulses was 1/s, which means that the stimulus off-time was so much longer than the stimulus on-time that the responses to the separate presentations of the tone pulse can be treated as independent. Even a casual inspection of this histogram reveals that the response was quite time locked to the stimulus onset (which occurred at time zero on the abscissa), and that, on average, it consisted of about 3 to 4 spikes per stimulus trial.

The lower panels of FIGURE 2 show the same response, but plotted in two different ways to illustrate the fine time structure of the response. On the right, spike response times have been measured not from the time of stimulus onset, but from the time of the first spike of the response to the stimulus. What is apparent from such plots is that the timing of the later spikes in the response is highly nonrandom. In many neurons, these "normalized response histograms" show deep periodicities, indicating that when a neuron discharges a burst of spikes in response to tone onset, there are preferred interspike intervals in the response.[32] Two things make this

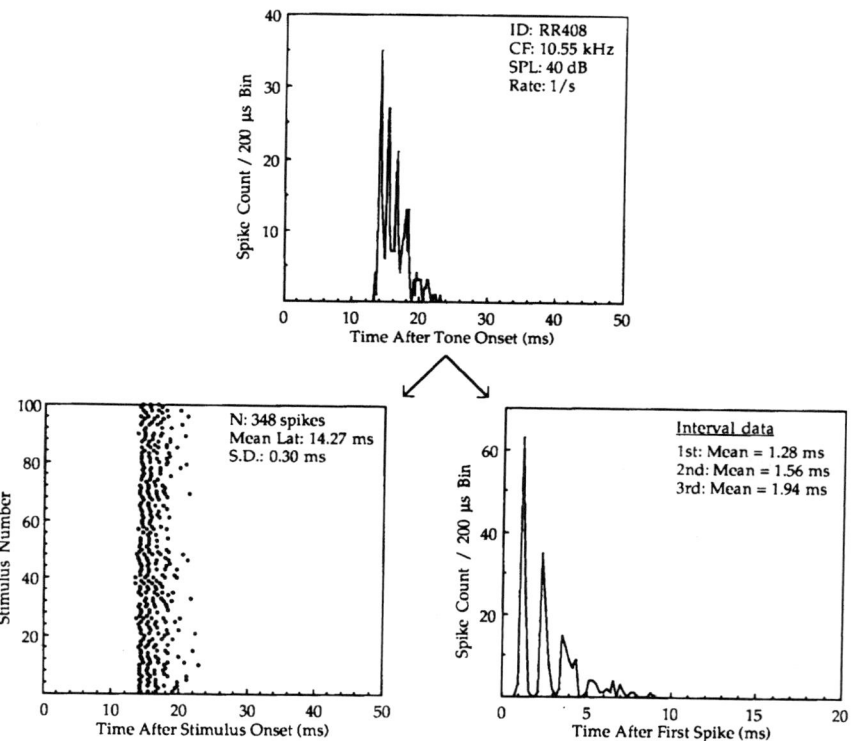

FIGURE 2. Properties of the transient responses of cat primary auditory cortex neurons. **Upper panel** shows a conventional peristimulus time histogram, which depicts the time at which the indicated neuron discharged spike action potentials, measured from the time of stimulus onset, are summed across 100 presentations. **Right panel** shows the same responses, but in this case with the time of the second, third (and later) spikes measured from the time of the first spike in the response. Note that the resulting histogram is deeply periodic, and that the time between successive peaks is very short. **Left panel** again is based on the same responses, but this time shows them as a raster, where *each row of dots* indicates the response to a single stimulus trial. Note that the timing of response initiation is extremely regular, that is, the response indicates the timing of the stimulus event with great precision.

periodic spike timing behavior particularly interesting. One is that the lengths of the intervals between the spikes are largely independent of the stimulus condition, that is, they contain little information about the stimulus. The second is that the mean interspike intervals are typically very short, generally less than 2 ms, and often as short as 1 ms.[32] This is about as short as neuronal biophysics will permit. It has the consequence that the neuronal response to the onset transient is very salient, that is, because the interspike intervals are so short, these responses have a high signal-to-noise ratio against the background of spontaneous spike discharges in which the interspike intervals are typically very much longer.

The left panel of FIGURE 2 shows the response of the same neuron presented as a dot raster. In this plot, the time of occurrence of each spike, measured from the start of the stimulus (abscissa), is shown separately for each of the 100 stimulus trials (ordinate). Again, the burst nature of the response is evident as a train of spikes on each stimulus trial, and the regularity of the interspike intervals is revealed by the orderliness with which the second (and sometimes third) spike of the response tracks the timing of the first spike. The further point that this depiction of the response illustrates, however, is the temporal precision with which the response is initiated. The jitter in the timing of the first spike is usually measured in the form of the standard deviation of the first-spike latent period.[13,18] As indicated in the raster, for this stimulus condition in this neuron, the jitter was around a third of a millisecond.

Unlike the interspike intervals of the transient response of cortical cells, the jitter in the timing of the first spike (i.e., the temporal precision with which a stimulus event is timed), does vary with the stimulating condition. In general, the standard deviation (s.d.) of the first-spike latency varies linearly with the mean latent period, which itself is a sensitive function of the spectral content and amplitude of a brief sound.[18,27,31,33] FIGURE 3 shows the effect of tone pulse amplitude on the spike timing of one neuron. Each panel shows the peristimulus time histogram representing the responses of neuron RR412 to 100 repetitions of a preferred frequency tone pulse of the amplitude specified for each panel. Note that as the signal amplitude is increased, that is, as one scans from the lower to the upper panels of FIGURE 3, there are two consequences for the timing of the discharges in the neuron's response. One is that the histogram shifts leftward along the abscissa, reflecting a shortening of the mean latent period (specified in the legend of each panel). The second is that the histograms, which on average are based on only about one spike per stimulus trial, become more peaked, indicating an increase in the temporal precision with which the response is initiated. The s.d.'s for the responses depicted in FIGURE 3 are indicated in the legends. Note that with increasing stimulus level, these decline toward an asymptote, which for this neuron, was near 0.5 ms.

Using stimulus paradigms of this kind, Phillips and Hall[18] tracked the minimal s.d.'s of cat primary auditory cortical neurons, and presented population data on them. The histogram presented in FIGURE 4 shows the distribution of minimal s.d.'s found in that study. It is apparent that in most neurons, minimal s.d.'s were less than 1.0 ms, and for about a third of the sample, minimal s.d.'s were less than 0.5 ms. What makes this distribution of special interest is the extent to which it matches with the same measurements made on neurons of the cochlea and auditory brainstem. Rhode and Smith[13] have presented data on the cochlear nerve and cochlear nucleus, and the curve in FIGURE 4 is derived from their report. It represents the s.d.'s measured from cochlear nerve fibers studied with tone bursts. It is clear that the distributions for the cochlear nerve and the auditory cortex are very similar, indicating that the afferent pathways onto cortical neurons have preserved this aspect of stimulus timing. This finding thus stands in marked contrast to the observations on

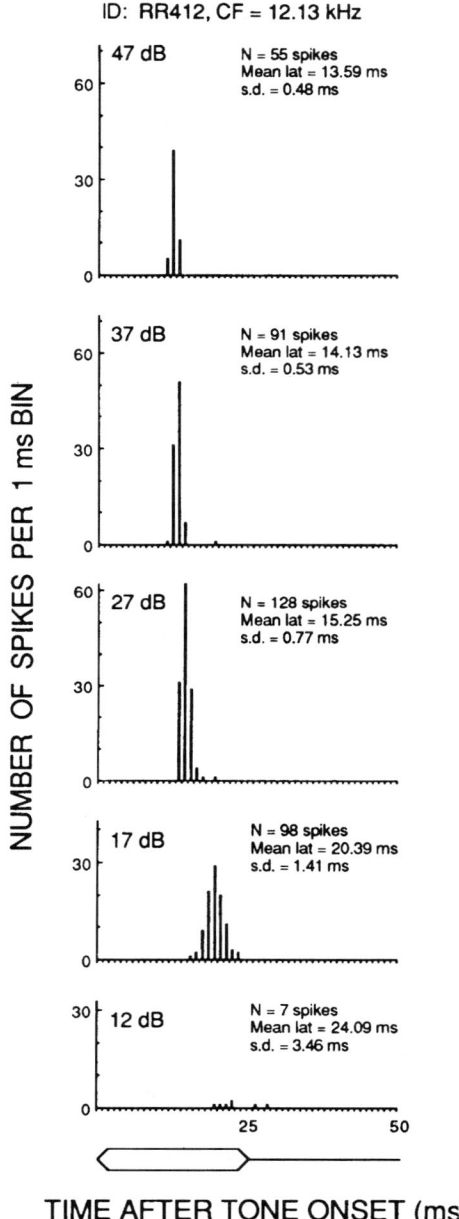

FIGURE 3. Variation of transient response timing with stimulus amplitude. Each panel shows the peristimulus time histogram of the summed responses of the neuron to 100 presentations of a preferred frequency tone pulse of the amplitude specified for each panel. Note that as the stimulus amplitude is increased, the mean response latency shortens, and the histogram becomes more peaked.

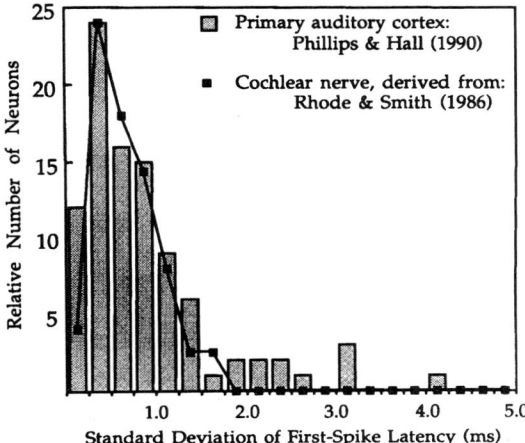

FIGURE 4. Histogram shows the distribution of minimal standard deviations of mean first-spike latencies obtained from cat primary auditory cortex neurons. (Redrawn from Phillips and Hall.[18]) *Solid line* shows comparable data obtained from cochlear nerve fibers. (Derived from Rhode and Smith.[13]) Note that the two distributions are very similar.

the cortical coding of stimulus periodicities, where the fidelity of the cortex's temporal code is grossly impoverished by comparison with that of the cochlear nerve.

The sensitivity of cortical neurons to the transient content of sounds is also expressed in the temporal patterning of spikes evoked by much more complex signals, viz., vocalizations.[34-36] Wollberg and Newman[36] were early to report experiments on the auditory cortex of alert monkeys studied with conspecific vocalizations. They showed that the timing of the spike discharges evoked by these sounds was highly nonrandom, and presumably tied to the transient content of the vocalizations. In this regard, reversing the vocalization (i.e., playing it backward) often had little effect on whether the stimulus was effective in evoking spike discharges *per se*, but it not uncommonly had the effect of reversing the cadence of spike discharges evoked by the sound.[37] Note that this observation has the further implication that what drives the responses of primary auditory cortical neurons is the acoustic content of the sound, and not its behavioral significance (although the latter may modify the strength and/or lability of responses).[38]

The fact that cortical auditory neurons can time stimulus event times with better than millisecond accuracy likely means that the timing mechanisms of the cortex could support temporal resolution at the limits of behavioral performance,[18] which is probably close to 2-3 ms.[39,40] This being the case, we have reason to suspect that the primary auditory cortex might be involved at some level in the perceptual elaboration of sounds with durations or spacings with this temporal grain. The most obvious such perceptual task is, of course, speech recognition, since the acoustic signal contains elements as brief as a few milliseconds (e.g., consonantal burst). In this regard, the temporal precision of transient responses in the primary field is demonstrably capable of indicating the timing of the phonetically important elements of speech signals, for example, voice onset times.[41] The spectral identity of the elements will likely be represented in which neurons of the tonotopic array are activated.[5,42] These observations, and the position of the auditory sensory cortex in the chain of processors required for speech recognition,[5,7] are quite compatible with the activation of the human primary field seen in positron emission tomography during speech processing.[43] The further conceptual point is that, insofar as stimulus representation in the primary auditory cortex is concerned, speech may be "special"[5,6,44,45] only in the sense that spoken language is the most obvious stimulus in which the identification of the elements is so heavily dependent on temporal resolution.

Data on the cortical auditory fields surrounding the primary one are much less complete than those reviewed earlier for the core field. Some of the fields are tonotopically organized, while others contain neurons that are broadly tuned to frequency.[46] Onset latencies to brief sounds are typically longer than those for neurons in the primary field,[46–48] and to the extent that the precision of transient response timing is related to mean latency (both within and across neurons[18]), this suggests that the behavioral temporal resolution that the "secondary" fields are capable of supporting is likely poorer than that supported by the primary field. One study[23] has provided a preliminary survey of several fields for their ability to encode periodic amplitude modulations of preferred-frequency carrier tones, and found the temporal response of that coding to be, in most cases, even poorer than that seen in the primary field.

EFFECTS OF PRIMARY AUDITORY CORTEX LESIONS

The foregoing paragraphs have sketched an overview of two kinds of temporal coding in auditory cortical neurons, and found that the temporal coding of periodicities is grossly impoverished in the primary field, both by comparison with the coding seen in the auditory brainstem, and by comparison with normal behavioral performance. In contrast, the precision of transient response timing appears to be at least as good as that seen in the cochlea, and apparently maps well onto normal behavioral performance. This differential preservation of transient response timing has relatively direct implications for the effects of primary auditory cortex lesions on auditory behavior, viz., that one would anticipate more profound deficits in auditory discriminations based on temporal resolution than in those based on periodicity coding.

Most of the evidence on these issues has come from studies of patients with a syndrome termed *pure word deafness* (acquired auditory verbal agnosia).[5–7,49,50] Briefly, these patients have relatively intact reading, writing, and speech production, but they are unable to comprehend spoken language; any audiological deficit is insufficient to account for the speech comprehension problem, and the recognition of nonverbal sounds is typically thought to be preserved. These patients usually have either a unilateral left-sided lesion, or bilateral lesions that involve Heschl's gyri (or adjacent white matter) on the superior temporal plane within the Sylvian fissure. In man, the primary auditory cortex is located on the transverse gyri of Heschl,[51,52] and so the diagnosis of pure word deafness has become a neurological marker for those patients whose auditory perceptual skills (or deficits in them) are likely to provide insight into the role of the primary field in man. In the broader context, lesions of Heschl's gyri deprive the cerebral language processor of acoustic input, and since the agnosia for sounds in these patients often appears superficially to be restricted to spoken language, pure word deafness has for some time been thought of as a disconnection syndrome.[7] As in the case of the visual agnosias,[53] however, there is increasing evidence that the speech recognition deficit is simply the most obvious expression of a more general perceptual processing disorder.[1,5,6,54] It is the nature of any such disorder that is of interest here.

Although the available data on the psychoacoustic skills of these patients might properly be regarded as preliminary, two lines of this evidence suggest that at a strictly phenomenological level, the kinds of auditory processing deficits (in the time domain) shown by patients with word deafness might map quite well onto those functions in which the primary field has been implicated by the neurophysiological studies. The first line of evidence comes from studies of speech recognition. Studied for their ability to identify phonemes (usually by sound-print matching), these patients typically are more impaired for the stop consonants than for steady-state vowels[54–57] (and more often than not, this extends to patients with more generalized auditory agnosias[58,59]). What makes the differential loss of stop consonant discrimination of special interest is that the acoustic signals for the stops are quite temporally differentiated and aperiodic (e.g., burst, aspiration, voicing onset) and the timing of the components is important for phoneme identification (e.g., voice onset times). In contrast, steady vowels have no phonetically important acoustic time structure (unless one were to argue that the neural code for vowel identity was a periodic, temporal one based on phase locking to the individual formant frequencies[60,61] rather than a spectral one residing in tonotopy). Moreover, the temporal grain of the acoustic events in stop consonants, that is, element durations or spacings in the milliseconds to tens-of-milliseconds range, is "within range" of the transient timing mechanisms of the primary field, but quite possibly not within range of those in the cerebral territories further removed from the thalamic input.

The consonant *identification* errors made by word-deaf patients can be for voicing and/or place (of articulation).[54–57,59,62] Errors in voicing are perhaps unsurprising, since this is a temporal distinction: viz., between short and long voice onset times. Identification errors in place of articulation are, however, also to be expected.[5] In the absence of a fully functioning primary auditory field, the cerebral cortex is deprived of an acoustic representation of signals with the required temporal grain for normal speech recognition: rather than neuronal responses being locked in time to the successive events in the signal, neuronal responses may well be more temporally "smeared," that is, less temporally differentiated. We might speculate that such an impoverished sensory representation could support only a temporally "blurred" speech percept, and perhaps one unusually dominated by the representation of the vowels, since these speech elements have the greater acoustic energy. Interestingly, when these patients have been studied with synthetic speech sound continua for the integrity of their *discrimination* functions for voicing or place, either or both may be unusually flattened.[54,55,59] This suggests that the percepts evoked by speech sounds, and presumably by other sounds of comparable temporal grain, might indeed be less temporally differentiated in these listeners.

A second line of evidence on this issue comes from studies attempting to measure temporal resolution directly in these patients using nonverbal sounds. Three studies[1,54,57] have measured click fusion thresholds (i.e., the minimum time between two transients required for them to be perceptually separated in time) in patients with pure word deafness. In contrast to normal listeners in the same laboratories, who had fusion thresholds between 1 and 3 ms, word-deaf patients had fusion thresholds between 15 and 30 ms. Patients with larger lesions appear to have still poorer temporal resolution.[62,63] Again, while these data must be regarded as preliminary, they point to a temporal resolution defect whose grain matches that with which an intact primary auditory field may be uniquely capable of representing the timing of aperiodic, transient acoustic events in the timing of neuronal discharges.

In the present context, the apparent preservation of nonverbal sound recognition in word deafness[1,50,54,55,57] might now be viewed in a new light. The acoustic discriminations required to perform these tasks (often sound-picture matching) simply do not challenge temporal auditory processes in the same way that speech recognition does. As a task, distinguishing a telephone ringing from a hand clap or an animal vocalization might succeed in eliminating the contribution of strictly verbal processes, but in doing so, it may also have succeeded in providing the listener with a perceptual task that does not tax the auditory sensory–perceptual mechanisms to the degree that speech discrimination does.

Interestingly, the discrimination of voice gender often survives in patients who have even severe impairment in the recognition of the phonetically important components of the speech signal.[56,57,59,62,64,65] Some authors further report that their patients retain the ability to discriminate intonation contours, that is, slow variations in voice pitch.[50,57] Recall that the principal acoustic cue to voice gender is the rate of (periodic) glottal pulsing, since this is higher in females than males, and that the perceptual distinction between the two lies in the pitch domain. As mentioned in the Introduction, there are at least two different ways of thinking about how the perceptual system might represent this pitch difference. One is in a strictly periodic, temporal code, in which the timing of the laryngeal pulses is preserved in the timing of spike discharges in steady-state responses, as must presumably be the case in repetition pitch. If we take that view, then the survival of voice gender discriminations in patients lacking the primary auditory cortex suggests that this cerebral region is not critically involved in the processes mediating that discrimination. Such a conclusion is compatible with the neurophysiological evidence (given earlier) since those studies revealed that neurons of the primary field did not have a steady-state temporal response capable of encoding periodicities of the rates occurring in human speech. A second account of voice pitch (and therefore voice gender) discrimination is couched in purely psychological terms, that is, based on the operation of some form of central pattern recognizer.[17] To the extent that voice gender discrimination may indeed be a higher level pattern-recognition process, it is perhaps unsurprising that the patients in whom the discrimination appears not to survive have bilateral lesions that are often larger in the right hemisphere than in the left.[62,66,67] This finding may map quite well onto independent evidence on the role of a number of right hemisphere mechanisms in the discrimination of the pitch of complex sounds.[16,43]

CONCLUSIONS

The purpose of this paper has been to draw a distinction between two forms of temporal auditory processing. The two types of processing are involved in the perceptual events driven by different types of acoustic signals, and are likely mediated by different neuronal mechanisms. In one of them (the "transient" case), what emerges from the temporal analysis is a perceptual resolution or segregation in the time domain, while in the other (the "periodic, steady-state" case), what emerges is a pitch (or other) percept, but not an obvious segregation in the time domain. The afferent pathways to the primary auditory cortex have preserved the neural timing of transient stimulus events; in contrast, the fidelity of the periodic temporal response is grossly impoverished by comparison with that seen in the auditory periphery. Cortical lesions that involve the primary field appear to have a profound effect on perceptual performance in tasks requiring temporal resolution, and in particular, of the grain in which the neurophysiological studies have directly implicated the primary field. In contrast, there is some evidence that percepts based on steady-state periodicities survive in listeners with lesions of the primary auditory cortex.

The evidence reviewed here has told us about the temporal grain with which acoustic events are represented in the spike activity of neurons of the primary auditory cortex. That is, it has told us about the temporal grain of information available to cortically based perceptual or cognitive processors operating on the output of the primary auditory field. What we should recall, however, is that the operation of those higher level processors itself takes time.[68] The perceptual processes of detecting, discriminating or recognizing an auditory event are not instantaneous. One of the principal challenges confronting research into developmental or acquired disorders of "rapid auditory temporal processing" is that of teasing out where in the chain of time-dependent auditory processes the deficit lies. The present paper has simply identified one possibility: the representation of the stimulus time structure in the sensory cortex.

ACKNOWLEDGMENTS

Special thanks are due to Drs. P. A. McMullen and R. Parncutt for helpful discussions of some of the issues covered in this paper.

REFERENCES

1. ALBERT, M. L. & D. BEAR. 1974. Brain **97**: 373–384.
2. HENDLER, T., N. K. SQUIRES & D. S. EMMERICH. 1990. Ear Hear. **11**: 403–416.
3. SWISHER, L. & I. J. HIRSH. 1972. Neuropsychologia **10**: 137–152.
4. TALLAL, P. & R. E. STARK. 1981. J. Acoust. Soc. Am. **69**: 568–574.
5. PHILLIPS, D. P. 1993. J. Exp. Psychol. Hum. Percept. Perform. In press.
6. PHILLIPS, D. P. & M. E. FARMER. 1990. Behav. Brain Res. **40**: 85–94.
7. GESCHWIND, N. 1965. Brain **88**: 237–294.
8. PHILLIPS, D. P. & J. F. BRUGGE. 1985. Annu. Rev. Psychol. **36**: 245–274.
9. MOORE, B. C. J., B. R. GLASBERG, C. J. PLACK & A. K. BISWAS. 1988. J. Acoust. Soc. Am. **83**: 1102–1116.
10. VIEMEISTER, N. F. & G. H. WAKEFIELD. 1991. J. Acoust. Soc. Am. **90**: 858–865.
11. MILLER, G. A. & W. G. TAYLOR. 1948. J. Acoust. Soc. Am. **20**: 171–182.
12. MØLLER, A. R. 1969. Acta Physiol. Scand. **75**: 542–551.
13. RHODE, W. S. & P. H. SMITH. 1986. J. Neurophysiol. **56**: 261–286.
14. DANILOFF, R., G. SCHUCKERS & L. FETH. 1980. The Physiology of Speech and Hearing. Prentice-Hall. Englewood Cliffs, N.J.
15. SCHWARZ, D. W. F. & R. W. W. TOMLINSON. 1990. J. Neurophysiol. **64**: 282–298.
16. ZATORRE, R. J. 1988. J. Acoust. Soc. Am. **84**: 566–572.
17. PARNCUTT, R. 1989. Harmony: A Psychoacoustical Approach. Springer-Verlag. Berlin/New York.
18. PHILLIPS, D. P. & S. E. HALL. 1990. J. Acoust. Soc. Am. **88**: 1403–1411.
19. MERZENICH, M. M., P. L. KNIGHT & G. L. ROTH. 1975. J. Neurophysiol. **38**: 231–249.
20. STEINSCHNEIDER, M., J. AREZZO & H. G. VAUGHAN. 1980. Brain Res. **198**: 75–84.
21. CREUTZFELDT, O., F.-C. HELLWEG & C. E. SCHREINER. 1980. Exp. Brain Res. **39**: 87–104.
22. MÜLLER-PREUSS, P. 1986. Eur. Arch. Psychiat. Neurol. Sci. **236**: 50–55.
23. SCHREINER, C. E. & J. V. URBAS. 1988. Hear. Res. **32**: 49–64.
24. EGGERMONT, J. J. 1991. Hear. Res. **56**: 153–167.

25. RIBAUPIERRE, F. DE, M. H. GOLDSTEIN & G. YENI-KOMSHIAN. 1972. Brain Res. **48:** 205–225.
26. PHILLIPS, D. P. 1989. Hear. Res. **40:** 137–146.
27. PHILLIPS, D. P., S. E. HALL & J. L. HOLLETT. 1989. J. Acoust. Soc. Am. **85:** 2537–2549.
28. REALE, R. A. & J. F. BRUGGE. 1990. J. Neurophysiol. **64:** 1247–1260.
29. YIN, T. C. T. & S. KUWADA. 1983. J. Neurophysiol. **50:** 1000–1019.
30. PHILLIPS, D. P. 1985. Hear. Res. **19:** 253–268.
31. ———. 1988. J. Neurophysiol. **59:** 1524–1639.
32. PHILLIPS, D. P. & S. A. SARK. 1991. Hear. Res. **53:** 17–27.
33. BRUGGE, J. F., N. A. DUBROVSKY, L. M. AITKIN & D. J. ANDERSON. 1969. J. Neurophysiol. **32:** 1005–1024.
34. NEWMAN, J. D. & Z. WOLLBERG. 1973. Brain Res. **54:** 287–304.
35. SOVIJARVI, A. R. A. 1975. Acta Physiol. Scand. **93:** 318–335.
36. WOLLBERG, Z. & J. D. NEWMAN. 1972. Science **175:** 212–214.
37. GLASS, I. & Z. WOLLBERG. 1983. Hear. Res. **9:** 27–33.
38. PHILLIPS, D. P. 1988. *In* Sensory Processing in the Mammalian Brain. Neural Substrates and Experimental Strategies, J. S. Lund, Ed.: 172–203. Oxford Univ. Press. New York.
39. HIRSH, I. J. 1959. J. Acoust. Soc. Am. **31:** 759–767.
40. PATTERSON, G. E. & D. M. GREEN. 1970. J. Acoust. Soc. Am. **48:** 894–905.
41. STEINSCHNEIDER, M., J. AREZZO & H. G. VAUGHAN. 1982. Brain Res. **252:** 353–365.
42. ———. 1990. Brain Res. **519:** 158–168.
43. ZATORRE, R. J., A. C. EVANS, E. MEYER & A. GJEDDE. 1992. Science **256:** 846–849.
44. LIBERMAN, A. M., F. S. COOPER, D. P. SHANKWEILER & M. STUDDERT-KENNEDY. 1967. Psych. Rev. **74:** 431–461.
45. SCHOUTEN, M. E. H. 1980. Acta Psychologica **44:** 71–98.
46. REALE, R. A. & T. J. IMIG. 1980. J. Comp. Neurol. **192:** 265–291.
47. PHILLIPS, D. P. & S. S. ORMAN. 1984. J. Neurophysiol. **51:** 147–163.
48. SCHREINER, C. E. & M. S. CYNADER. 1984. J. Neurophysiol. **51:** 1284–1305.
49. ELLIS, A. W. & A. W. YOUNG. 1988. Human Cognitive Neuropsychology. Erlbaum. Hove, England.
50. COSLETT, H. B., H. R. BRASHEAR & K. M. HEILMAN. 1984. Neurology **34:** 347–352.
51. GALABURDA, A. & F. SANIDES. 1980. J. Comp. Neurol. **190:** 597–610.
52. MUSIEK, F. M. & A. G. REEVES. 1990. J. Am. Acad. Audiol. **1:** 240–245.
53. FARAH, M. J. 1990. Visual Agnosia. Disorders of Object Recognition and What They Tell Us About Normal Vision. MIT Press. Cambridge, Mass.
54. AUERBACH, S. H., T. ALLARD, M. NAESER, M. P. ALEXANDER & M. L. ALBERT. 1982. Brain **105:** 271–300.
55. PRAAMSTRA, P., P. HAGOORT, B. MAASSEN & T. CRUL. 1991. Brain **114:** 1197–1225.
56. SAFFRAN, E. M., S. M. MARIN & G. YENI-KOMSHIAN. 1976. Brain Lang. **3:** 209–228.
57. YAQUB, B. A., G. G. GASCON, M. AL-NOSHA & H. WHITAKER. 1988. Brain **111:** 457–466.
58. KAZUI, S., H. NARITOMI, T. SAWADA & N. INOUE. 1990. Brain Lang. **38:** 476–487.
59. MICELI, G. 1982. Neuropsychologia **20:** 5–20.
60. YOUNG, E. D. & M. B. SACHS. 1979. J. Acoust. Soc. Am. **66:** 1381–1403.
61. CARNEY, L. H. & C. D. GEISLER. 1986. J. Acoust. Soc. Am. **79:** 1896–1914.
62. TANAKA, Y., A. YAMADORI & E. MORI. 1987. Brain **110:** 381–403.
63. BUCHTEL, H. A. & J. D. STEWART. 1989. Brain Lang. **37:** 12–25.
64. ADAMS, A. E., K. ROSENBERGER, H. WINTER & C. ZÖLLNER. 1977. Arch. Psychiatr. Neurol. Sci. **224:** 213–220.
65. HORENSTEIN, S. & K. BEALMEAR. 1973. Trans. Am. Neurol. Assoc. **98:** 264–267.
66. SHOUMAKER, R. D., E. T. AJAX & T. SCHENKENBERG. 1977. Dis. Nerv. Syst. **38:** 293–299.
67. VON STOCKERT, T. R. 1982. Brain Lang. **16:** 133–146.
68. MASSARO, D. W. 1972. Psych. Rev. **79:** 124–145.

Temporal Analysis in Normal and Impaired Hearing

BRIAN C. J. MOORE

Department of Experimental Psychology
University of Cambridge
Downing Street
Cambridge CB2 3EB, England

INTRODUCTION

In characterizing temporal analysis in the auditory system, it is essential to take account of processes that take place in the peripheral part of the auditory system. The cochlea contains an array of filters (called the "auditory filters") that separate the components in a complex signal into "channels" tuned to different center frequencies.[1,2] The resulting tonotopic organization is preserved throughout the auditory system. Temporal analysis can be considered as resulting from two main processes: analysis of the time pattern occurring within each frequency channel, and comparison of the time patterns across channels. This paper considers each of these processes in turn.

A major difficulty in measuring the temporal resolution of the auditory system is that changes in the time pattern of a sound are generally associated with changes in its magnitude spectrum—the distribution of energy over frequency. Thus, the detection of a change in time pattern can sometimes depend not on temporal resolution *per se*, but on the detection of the spectral change. Sometimes, the detection of spectral changes can lead to what appears to be extraordinarily fine temporal resolution. For example, a single click can be distinguished from a pair of clicks when the gap between the two clicks in a pair is only a few tens of microseconds.[3] Although spectrally based detection of temporal changes is interesting, and does occur in everyday life, this paper concentrates on experimental situations that avoid the confounding effects of spectral cues.

WITHIN-CHANNEL TEMPORAL ANALYSIS USING BROAD-BAND SOUNDS

The experiments described next all use broad-band sounds whose long-term magnitude spectrum is unaltered by the temporal manipulation being performed. For example, interruption or amplitude modulation of a white noise does not change its long-term magnitude spectrum.

The Detection of Gaps in Broad-Band Noise

The threshold for detecting a gap in a broad-band noise provides a simple and convenient measure of temporal resolution. Although white noise excites many different frequency channels in the auditory system, it is generally assumed that this task depends primarily on within-channel processes, rather than on comparisons across channels (although the fact that the gap occurs synchronously in all channels may well be important, and information may be combined across channels at some level higher than the cochlea). The gap threshold is typically 2–3 ms.[4,5] The threshold increases at very low sound levels when the level of the noise approaches the absolute threshold, but is relatively invariant with level for moderate to high levels.

The Discrimination of Time-Reversed Signals

The long-term magnitude spectrum of a sound is not changed when that sound is time reversed (played backward in time). Thus, if a time-reversed sound can be discriminated from the original, this must reflect a sensitivity to the difference in time pattern of the two sounds. This was exploited by Ronken,[6] who used as stimuli pairs of clicks differing in amplitude. One click, labeled A, had an amplitude greater than that of the other click, labeled B. Typically the amplitude of A was twice that of B. Subjects were required to distinguish click pairs differing in the order of A and B: either AB or BA. The ability to do this was measured as a function of the gap between A and B. Ronken found that subjects could distinguish the click pairs for gaps down to 2–3 ms. Thus the limit to temporal resolution found in this task is similar to that found for the detection of a gap in broad-band noise. It should be noted that, in this task, subjects do not hear the individual clicks within a click pair. Rather, each click pair is heard as a single sound with its own characteristic quality. For example, the two click pairs AB and BA might sound like "tick" and "tock."

Temporal Modulation Transfer Functions

The experiments described previously each give a single value to describe temporal resolution. A more general approach is to measure the threshold for detecting changes in the amplitude of a sound as a function of the rapidity of the changes. In the simplest case, white noise is sinusoidally amplitude modulated, and the threshold for detecting the modulation is determined as a function of modulation rate. The function relating threshold to modulation rate is known as a temporal modulation transfer function (TMTF).[7] An example of the results is shown in FIGURE 1.[8] The thresholds are expressed as $20 \log m$, where m is the modulation index ($m = 0$ corresponds to no modulation and $m = 1$ corresponds to 100 percent modulation). For low modulation rates, performance is limited by the amplitude resolution of the ear, rather than by temporal resolution. Thus, the threshold is independent of modulation rate for rates up to about 16 Hz. As the rate increases beyond 16 Hz, temporal resolution starts to have an effect; performance worsens, and for rates above about 1000 Hz the modulation cannot be detected at all. Thus, sensitivity to modulation becomes progressively less as the rate of modulation increases. The modulation frequency at which sensitivity has fallen by 3 dB (in units of $20 \log m$) gives a measure of temporal resolution known as the "cutoff frequency." The shapes of TMTFs do not vary much with overall sound level, but the ability to detect the modulation does worsen at low sound levels. Although it is generally assumed that this task depends primarily on within-channel processes, it is possible that across-channel processes play a role at high modulation rates.[9]

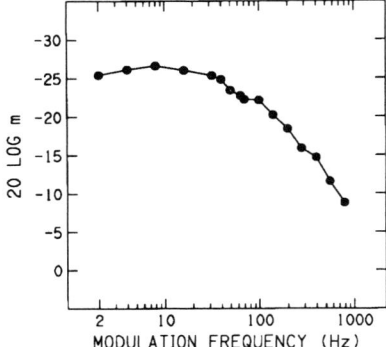

FIGURE 1. A TMTF, showing the threshold for detecting sinusoidal amplitude modulation of white noise as a function of modulation rate. Thresholds are expressed as 20 log m, where m is the modulation index. The higher the sensitivity to modulation, the more negative is this quantity. (Adapted from Bacon and Viemeister[8] by permission.)

WITHIN-CHANNEL TEMPORAL ANALYSIS USING NARROW-BAND SOUNDS

The experiments described previously all used broad-band stimuli. It has often been assumed that the results depend primarily on within-channel processes, but there is no guarantee that this is the case. In addition, these experiments provide no information regarding the question of whether the temporal resolution of the ear varies with center frequency. This issue can be examined by using narrow-band stimuli that excite only one, or a small number, of auditory channels.

It has often been suggested that temporal resolution might be limited by the response time of the auditory filters. For example, if a stimulus is turned off and on again to form a temporal gap, ringing in the auditory filters might partially fill in the gap, so that the output of the auditory filters would show only a small dip. This is illustrated in FIGURE 2. The narrower the bandwidth of a filter, the longer is its response time. The auditory filters have narrower bandwidths at low center frequencies than at high.[1] Thus, if the responses of the auditory filters limit temporal resolution, resolution should be worse at low frequencies than at high. The experiments described next provide an initial test of this idea.

Discrimination of Time-Reversed Sinusoids

Green[10] used time-reversed stimuli where each stimulus consisted of a brief pulse of a sinusoid in which the level of the first half of the pulse was 10 dB different from that of the second half. Subjects were required to distinguish two signals, differing in whether the half with the high level was first or second. Green measured performance as a function of the total duration of the stimuli. The threshold was similar for center frequencies of 2 and 4 kHz, and was between 1 and 2 ms. However, the

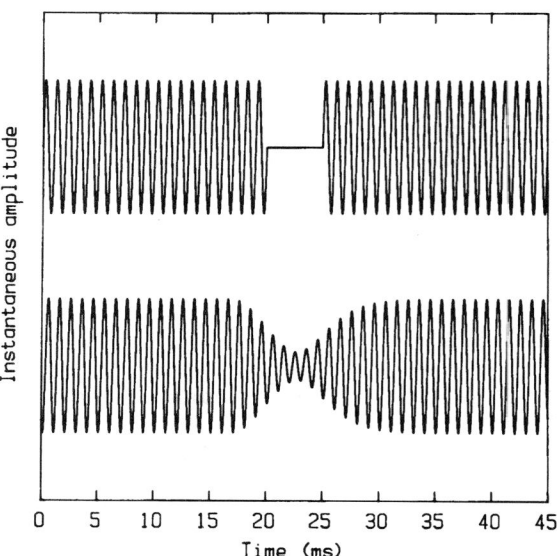

FIGURE 2. The response of a simulated auditory filter to a 1-kHz sinusoid containing a 5-ms gap. The *upper trace* shows the input to the filter, and the *lower trace* shows the output. The filter was centered at 1 kHz and its characteristics were chosen to simulate those of a human auditory filter with the same center frequency. Only the portions of the waveforms immediately before and after the gap are shown. Note that the gap is partially filled in by the ringing in the filter.

threshold was slightly higher for a center frequency of 1 kHz, being between 2 and 4 ms. Thus, these data suggest that the response time of the auditory filters was not important above 2 kHz, but may have played a role below that.

It is interesting that performance in this task was actually a nonmonotonic function of duration. Performance was good for durations in the range 2–6 ms, worsened for durations around 16 ms, and then improved again as the duration was increased beyond 16 ms. For the very short durations, subjects listened for a difference in quality between the two sounds—rather like the "tick" and "tock" described earlier for Ronken's stimuli. At durations around 16 ms, the tonal quality of the bursts became more prominent, and the quality differences were harder to hear. At much longer durations the soft and loud segments could be separately heard, in a distinct order. It appears, therefore, that performance in this task was determined by two separate mechanisms, one based on timbre differences associated with the difference in time pattern, and the other based on the perception of a distinct succession of auditory events.

Detection of Temporal Gaps in Narrow-Band Noise

When a temporal gap is introduced into a narrow-band sound, the spectrum of the sound is altered. Energy "splatter" occurs outside the nominal frequency range of the sound. To prevent the splatter being detected, the sounds are presented in a background sound, usually a noise, designed to mask the splatter.

Several researchers have measured thresholds for detecting gaps in narrow-band noises.[11-13] An example of the results[12] is shown in FIGURE 3. The stimulus containing the gap was a noise with bandwidth one-half of the center frequency, and a continuous background noise with a notch of the same width was used to mask splatter. The gap thresholds are large (about 22 ms) at the lowest center frequency used (200 Hz) and decrease monotonically with increasing center frequency. The gap thresholds for the highest center frequency (8 Hz) are similar to those found with broad-band noise (about 3 ms). This suggests that the results obtained with broad-band noise reflect the use of information from the higher frequency regions of the spectrum.

One problem in interpreting this experiment is that the bandwidth of the stimuli used increased with increasing center frequency; the bandwidth was always one half of the center frequency. Noise bands have inherent fluctuations in amplitude, and the rapidity of these fluctuations increases with increasing bandwidth. Gap thresholds for noise bands may be partly limited by the inherent fluctuations in the noise.[12,14,15] Randomly occurring dips in the noise may be "confused" with the gap to be detected. The confusion would be maximal for dips comparable in duration to the gap. In practice, this means that noise with a narrow bandwidth, and hence slow fluctuations, would create the greatest confusion and give the largest gap thresholds. The data are consistent with this view: gap thresholds for narrow-band noises increase with decreasing noise bandwidth.[12,14] Furthermore, gap thresholds measured with very narrow noise bands show little effect of center frequency.[14,16,17]

Gap thresholds for narrow-band noises tend to decrease with increasing sound level for levels up to about 30 dB above absolute threshold, but remain roughly constant after that.

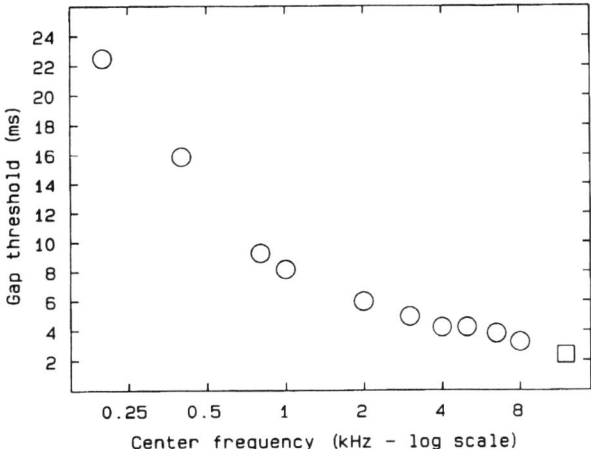

FIGURE 3. Gap thresholds for noise bands plotted as a function of center frequency. The bandwidth of the noise was 0.5 times the center frequency. The *square* at the right-hand side shows the gap threshold for wideband noise. (Adapted from Shailer and Moore[12] by permission.)

Detection of Temporal Gaps in Sinusoids

Shailer and Moore[18] studied the ability of subjects to detect a temporal gap in a sinusoid. To mask "splatter" associated with the introduction of the gap, the sinusoid was presented in a continuous noise with a spectral notch at the frequency of the sinusoid. The results were strongly affected by the phase at which the sinusoid was turned off and on to produce the gap. Only the simplest case will be considered here, called "preserved phase" by Shailer and Moore. In this case, the sinusoid was turned off at a positive-going zero crossing (i.e., as the waveform was about to change from negative to positive value), and it started (at the end of the gap) at the phase it would have had if it had continued without interruption. Thus, for the preserved-phase condition it was as if the gap had been "cut out" from a continuous sinusoid. For this condition, the detectability of the gap increased monotonically with increasing gap duration.

Shailer and Moore[18] found that the gap threshold was roughly constant at about 5 ms for center frequencies of 400, 1000, and 2000 Hz. Recently, gap thresholds for sinusoids have been measured for center frequencies of 100, 200, 400, 800, 1000, and 2000 Hz using a condition similar to the preserved-phase condition of Shailer and Moore.[19] The gap thresholds were almost constant over the frequency range 400–2000 Hz, but increased somewhat at 200 Hz, and increased markedly, to about 18 ms, at 100 Hz. Individual variability also increased markedly at 100 Hz.

Overall, the results of experiments using narrow-band stimuli indicate that the auditory filter does not play a major role in limiting temporal resolution, except perhaps at very low frequencies (200 Hz and below).

MODELING TEMPORAL RESOLUTION BASED ON WITHIN-CHANNEL PROCESSES

As described earlier, the response of the auditory filter does not seem to be a limiting factor in most tasks involving temporal resolution. This has led to the idea that there is a process at a level of the auditory system higher than the auditory nerve that is "sluggish" in some way, thereby limiting temporal resolution. Models of temporal resolution are especially concerned with this process. The models assume that the internal representation of stimuli is "smoothed" over time, so that rapid temporal changes are lost but slower ones are preserved. Although this smoothing process almost certainly operates on neural activity, the most widely used models are based on smoothing a simple transformation of the stimulus, rather than its neural representation. This is done for simplicity and mathematical convenience, even though it is not very realistic.

Models Based on a Lowpass Filter

A popular model of temporal resolution[7,20,21] is illustrated in FIGURE 4. There is an initial stage of bandpass filtering, reflecting the action of the auditory filters. For simplicity, only one filter is shown; in reality there would be an array of parallel channels, each like that shown in the figure. The filter is followed by a nonlinear device; the figure shows a half-wave rectifier. This rectifier passes portions of the waveform of one polarity (say, the positive parts), but does not pass portions of the

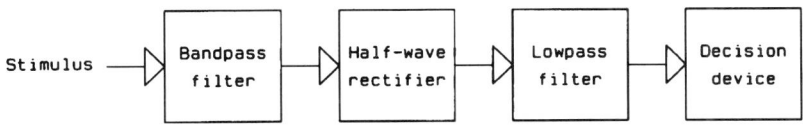

FIGURE 4. A block diagram of a model of temporal resolution. See text for details.

opposite polarity. This resembles the way that neural spikes tend to occur for a particular polarity of the stimulating waveform. The output of the rectifier is fed through a lowpass filter, which has the effect of smoothing the output of the rectifier. In effect, the output of the lowpass filter resembles the amplitude envelope of the output of the bandpass filter. However, rapid envelope fluctuations are reduced in magnitude, while slower ones are preserved. The output of the lowpass filter is fed to the final stage of the model, a decision device.

Models Based on a Sliding Temporal Integrator

A variation of this type of model is illustrated in FIGURE 5. As before, the initial stages are a bandpass filter and a nonlinear device. However, the nonlinear device in this case has a square-law characteristic. This device gives a quantity that is related to the instantaneous power at the output of the bandpass filter. The next stage is a temporal integrator that sums the energy occurring within a certain time interval or "window." The window is assumed to slide in time, so that the output of the temporal integrator is like a running average of the input. This has the effect of smoothing rapid fluctuations while preserving slower ones. The temporal integrator is equivalent to the lowpass filter in FIGURE 4, except that the smoothing is applied to a powerlike quantity rather than an amplitudelike quantity. Finally, as before, the output of the temporal integrator is fed to a decision device.

In the simplest form of this model, all the power within the window is weighted equally to determine the output. The window in this case is described as "rectangular," and the window is completely defined by its duration. However, it is more realistic to consider the window as a weighting function, having a particular mathematical form.[22,23] The form of this weighting function is called the "shape" of the temporal window. FIGURE 6 shows estimates of this shape obtained by measuring the combined effects of forward and backward masking.[24,25] The shape of the temporal window is almost invariant with center frequency, except for a slight broadening (associated with poorer temporal resolution) at low center frequencies. The temporal window broadens somewhat as the sound level decreases.

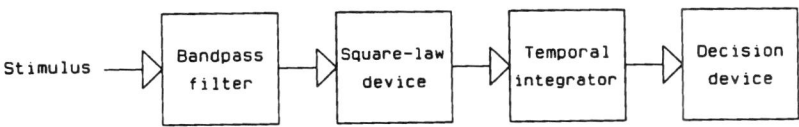

FIGURE 5. A variation of the type of model shown in FIGURE 4.

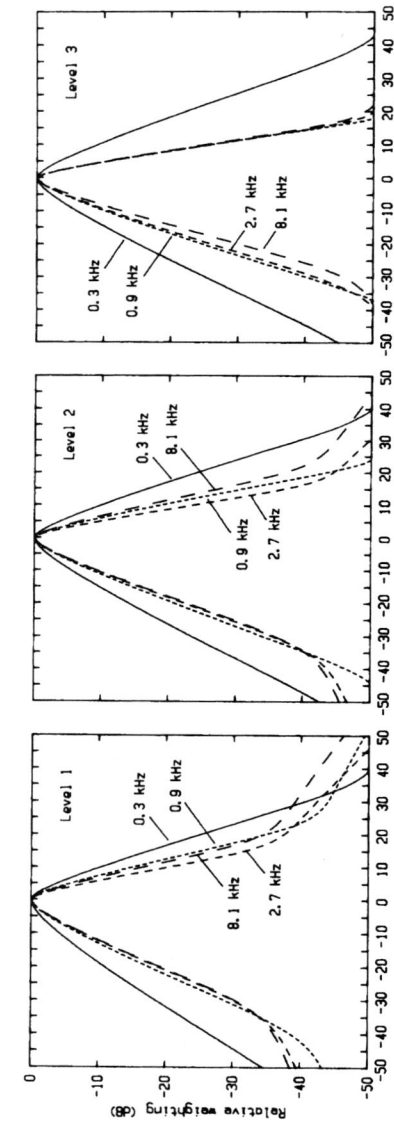

FIGURE 6. Some examples of temporal window shapes at different center frequencies and levels. The three levels used were each separated by 10 dB, with level 3 being the highest.

Models Incorporating Compressive Nonlinearities

The models described earlier assume that a simple transformation of the stimulus magnitude is integrated over time. However, it seems more realistic to assume that neural activity is integrated.[26,27] Unfortunately, it is much more difficult to construct a model based on this assumption, since we do not know the level in the auditory system at which the integration takes place, and since it would be necessary to include a variety of complex phenomena such as neural saturation and adaptation. An intermediate step is to model one or more of the basic properties of the transformation from stimulus magnitude to neural activity. One such property is the fact that the number of neural spikes evoked by a stimulus is not directly proportional to the stimulus intensity. Rather it is a nonlinear, compressive function of stimulus intensity; the number of spikes grows more slowly than the stimulus intensity.

Several workers have suggested models of temporal resolution in which there is a compressive nonlinearity prior to the temporal integrator.[27-29] In these models, temporal resolution is determined by the type of nonlinearity assumed, as well as by the temporal integrator and the sensitivity to changes in the output of the integrator.

WITHIN-CHANNEL TEMPORAL ANALYSIS IN HEARING-IMPAIRED SUBJECTS

Temporal Analysis in Subjects with Cochlear Hearing Loss

A common type of hearing loss results from impaired functioning of the cochlea. There is some controversy as to whether temporal resolution is affected by cochlear hearing loss; some measures appear to show reduced temporal resolution, while others do not.

One important factor influencing the results is the degree to which the stimuli contain random fluctuations in amplitude. For stimuli that have marked slow fluctuations, such as narrow bands of noise, subjects with cochlear impairment often have larger than normal gap-detection thresholds.[13,30-32] Gap detection, however, is not usually worse than normal when the stimuli are sinusoids.[33,34] Glasberg et al.[32] and Moore and Glasberg[33] suggested that the poor gap detection for narrow-band noise stimuli might be a consequence of abnormal loudness perception. For most people with cochlear hearing loss, the loudness of sounds grows more rapidly than normal with increasing sound level, once the sounds are above threshold. This is called *loudness recruitment*.[35] The effects of loudness recruitment can be incorporated in models of temporal resolution by assuming a less compressive nonlinearity prior to the temporal integration mechanism. For a person with recruitment, the inherent fluctuations in a narrow-band noise would result in larger-than-normal loudness fluctuations from moment to moment, so that inherent dips in the noise might be more confusable with the gap to be detected. To assess this idea, Glasberg and Moore[36] simulated the effects of loudness recruitment by processing the envelopes of narrow bands of noise so as to magnify the envelope fluctuations. As predicted, the ability of normally hearing subjects to detect gaps in the bands of noise was adversely affected by the magnified envelope fluctuations.

A second important factor influencing measures of temporal resolution is the sound level used. Many measures of temporal resolution show that performance in normally hearing subjects worsens at low sensation levels (SLs).[4,7,8,11,12,37] It is not generally possible to test hearing-impaired subjects at high SLs, because of their loudness recruitment. Thus, hearing-impaired subjects sometimes appear to have worse temporal resolution than normal subjects when tested at the same SPLs, but at equal SLs they perform as well as or better than normal.[30,32-34,38]

A final important consideration is the bandwidth available to the listeners. For example, several studies measuring TMTFs for broad-band noise showed that impaired listeners were generally less sensitive to high rates of modulation than normal listeners.[8,39,40] However, this may have been largely a consequence of the fact that high frequencies were inaudible to the impaired listeners;[8] most of the subjects used had greater hearing losses at high frequencies than at low.

Bacon and Gleitman[37] measured TMTFs for broad-band noise using subjects with relatively flat hearing losses. They found that at equal (high) sound pressure levels (SPLs) performance was similar for hearing-impaired and normally hearing subjects. At equal (low) SLs, the hearing-impaired subjects tended to perform better than the normally hearing subjects. Moore et al.[9] controlled for the effects of listening bandwidth by measuring TMTFs for an octave-wide noise band centered at 2 kHz, using subjects with unilateral and bilateral cochlear hearing loss. Over the frequency range covered by the noise, the subjects had reasonably constant thresholds as a function of frequency, both in their normal and their impaired ears. They found that performance was similar for the normal and impaired ears, both at equal SPL and equal SL, although there was a slight trend for the impaired ears to perform better at equal SL.

The overall pattern of results from subjects with cochlear hearing loss can be interpreted in the following way. The central temporal integration mechanism (low-pass filter or sliding temporal window) is probably normal. However, the nonlinearity preceding the integrator is less compressive in ears with a cochlear impairment than in normal ears (reflecting the loudness recruitment in the impaired ears). For stimuli with inherent slow amplitude fluctuations (such as narrow bands of noise) this can lead to poorer gap detection in impaired ears, since the inherent fluctuations become more confusable with the gap to be detected. For deterministic stimuli (such as sinusoids), however, or for broad-band noise stimuli, it can actually lead to better performance in impaired than in normal ears, when the comparison is made at equal SLs. In practice, hearing-impaired subjects often show poor performance on measures of temporal resolution because the stimuli are at low SLs and/or because the audible bandwidth of the stimuli is restricted.

Temporal Resolution in Subjects with Retrocochlear Hearing Loss

There have been relatively few studies of temporal resolution in subjects with retrocochlear hearing loss. Formby[41] measured TMTFs using a broad-band noise carrier for six subjects with eighth-nerve tumors. All of the subjects showed poorer sensitivity to modulation and lower cutoff frequencies for the TMTFs than normal listeners. In four of the subjects, the poor temporal resolution might have been caused by their markedly elevated absolute thresholds at high frequencies. However, two subjects had relatively small elevations in absolute threshold, and their absolute thresholds did not vary markedly with frequency. One of these subjects showed normal modulation thresholds at low modulation rates but higher-than-normal modulation thresholds at high modulation rates. The other subject showed poor modulation thresholds at all rates, but with especially poor performance at high rates; that subject could not detect modulation in his impaired ear for rates above 100 Hz. Thus, it appears that eighth-nerve tumors can lead to marked impairment of temporal resolution. The mechanisms underlying this impairment are not, at present, understood.

TEMPORAL ANALYSIS BASED ON ACROSS-CHANNEL PROCESSES

The Discrimination of Huffman Sequences

Patterson and Green[42] and Green[10] have studied the discrimination of a class of signals that have the same long-term magnitude spectrum, but that differ in their short-term spectra. These sounds are called *Huffman sequences*. They are brief broad-band sounds, like clicks, except that the energy in a certain frequency region is delayed relative to that in other regions. The amount of the delay, the center frequency of the delayed frequency region, and the width of the delayed frequency region can all be varied. If subjects can distinguish a pair of Huffman sequences differing, for example, in the amount of delay in a given frequency region, this implies that they are sensitive to the difference in time pattern. Green[10] measured the ability of subjects to detect differences in the amount of delay in three frequency regions: 650 Hz, 1900 Hz, and 4200 Hz. He found similar results for all three center frequencies: subjects could detect differences in delay time of about 2 ms regardless of the center frequency of the delayed region.

It should be noted that subjects did not report hearing one part of the sound after the rest of the sound. Rather, the differences in time pattern were perceived as subtle changes in sound quality. Further, some subjects required extensive training to achieve the fine acuity of 2 ms, and even after this training the task required considerable concentration.

Detection of Onset and Offset Asynchrony in Multicomponent Complexes

Zera and Green[43] measured thresholds for detecting asynchrony in the onset or offset of complex signals composed of many sinusoidal components. The components were either uniformly spaced on a logarithmic frequency scale, or formed a harmonic series. In one stimulus, the standard, all components started and stopped synchronously. In the "signal" stimulus, one component was presented with an onset or offset asynchrony. The task of the subjects was to discriminate the standard stimulus from the signal stimulus. They found that onset asynchrony was easier to detect than offset asynchrony. For harmonic signals, onset asynchronies of less than 1 ms could generally be detected, whether the asynchronous component was leading or lagging the other components (although in the latter case, thresholds increased markedly for delays in the higher harmonics, presumably because for the higher harmonics several harmonics fall within the passband of a single auditory filter and produce a masking effect on the asynchronous component). Thresholds for detecting offset asynchronies were larger, being about 3–10 ms when the asynchronous component ended after the other components, and 10–30 ms when the asynchronous component ended before the other components. Thresholds for detecting asynchronies in logarithmically spaced complexes were generally two to fifty times larger than for harmonic complexes.

The difference between harmonically and logarithmically spaced complexes may be explicable in terms of perceptual grouping. The harmonic signal was perceived as a single sound source. The logarithmically spaced complex was perceived as a series of separate tones, like many notes being played at once on an organ. It seems that it is difficult to compare the timing of sound elements that are perceived as coming from different sources, a point that will be expanded later. The high sensitivity to onset asynchronies for harmonic complexes is consistent with the finding that the perceived timbres of musical instruments are partly dependent on the exact onset times and rates of rise of individual harmonics within each musical note.[44]

Judgment of Temporal Order

The ability to judge the temporal order of a sequence of sounds depends strongly on whether the task requires actual *identification* of the order of individual elements or whether it can be performed by *discrimination* of different orders or by attaching well-learned labels to different orders. In the latter case, resolution can be rather fine. With extended training and feedback subjects can learn to distinguish between and identify orders within sequences of nonrelated sounds lasting only 10 ms or less.[45] For sequences of tones, the component durations necessary for labeling different orders may be as low as 2–7 ms.[46] This is the type of acuity that would be expected for speech sounds, since these consist of well-learned sequences to which consistent labels have been attached.

When the task is to identify the order of sounds in a sequence, performance is generally markedly worse. For example, Hirsh[47] found that, for pairs of unrelated items, trained subjects required durations of about 20 ms per item for correct order identification.

THE ROLE OF PERCEPTUAL GROUPING IN TEMPORAL ANALYSIS

The Formation of Perceptual Streams

A fast sequence of sounds (say 10 sounds per second) may not be perceived as a coherent whole. Rather, the sounds may be "grouped" according to their attributes, for example, their pitches, timbres, loudnesses, or subjective locations. Van Noorden[48] investigated this grouping using a tone sequence where every second B was omitted from the regular sequence ABABAB..., producing a sequence ABA ABA.... He found that this sequence could be perceived in two ways, depending on the frequency separation of A and B. For small separations, a single rhythm, resembling a gallop, was heard. For larger separations, two separate tone sequences could be heard, one of which (A A A) was running twice as fast as the other (B B B). This latter effect has been referred to as "stream segregation." Thus, the perceived rhythm was completely altered by the different perceptual groupings.

The Role of Perceptual Grouping in Judgments of Temporal Order

Sometimes, judgments of temporal order can be markedly poorer than described earlier. Poor performance seems to occur especially when the individual items in the sequence are not heard as coming from a single source, but instead form several perceptual streams. For example, Bregman and Campbell[49] investigated temporal order judgment for rapid tone sequences. They used untrained subjects, so that performance presumably depended on the subjects actually perceiving the sounds as a sequence, rather than on their learning the overall sound pattern. In a repeating cycle of mixed high and low tones their subjects could discriminate the order of the high tones relative to one another, or of the low tones among themselves, but they could not order the high tones relative to the low ones. Bregman and Campbell suggested that this was because the high and low tones split into separate perceptual streams, with judgments across streams being difficult.

Ladefoged and Broadbent[50] reported that extraneous sounds in sentences were grossly mislocated, so that a click might be reported as occurring a word or two away from its actual position. Also, untrained subjects are remarkably poor at judging the temporal order of three or four unrelated items, such as a hiss, a tone, and a buzz.[51,52] Most subjects cannot identify the order when each successive item lasts 150–200 ms. Overall, it seems that we are rather good at judging the temporal order of sounds that form a single perceptual stream, but poor at judging the order of items that are assigned to different perceptual streams.

Sometimes, perceptual grouping processes can improve temporal order judgments by "stripping away" irrelevant stimulus elements. Bregman and Rudnicky[53] presented subjects with a sequence of four brief tones in rapid succession. Two of the tones, labeled X, had the same frequency, but the middle two, A and B, were different. The four-tone sequence was either XABX or XBAX. The subjects had to judge the order of A and B. This was harder than when the tones AB occurred in isolation [FIG. 7(a)] because A and B were perceived as part of a longer four-tone pattern, including the two "distractor" tones, labeled X (FIG. 7(b)]. They then embedded the four-tone sequence into a longer sequence of tones, called *captor* tones [FIG. 7(c)]. When the captor tones had frequencies close to those of the distractor tones, they "captured" the distractors into a separate perceptual stream, leaving the tones AB in a stream of their own. This made the order of A and B easy to judge.

Bregman and Dannenbring[54] investigated the perception of tone sequences containing high- and low-frequency tones in which successive tones were connected by frequency glides. They found that these glides reduced the tendency for the sequences to split into high and low streams, while at the same time order perception was easier.

The effects of frequency glides and other types of transitions in preventing stream segregation are probably of considerable importance in the perception of speech. Speech sounds may follow one another in very rapid sequences, and the glides and partial glides observed in the acoustic components of speech may be a strong factor in maintaining the speech as a unified perceptual stream.

Change Detection and Contrast Effects

The auditory system seems particularly well suited to the analysis of changes in the sensory input. When part of a complex stimulus is changed, the changed aspect stands out perceptually from the rest. For example, a white noise heard in isolation may be described as "colorless"; it has no pitch and has a neutral sort of timbre. However, when a white noise follows soon after a stimulus with spectral structure, the noise sounds "colored." The coloration corresponds to the inverse of the spectrum of the preceding sound. If the preceding sound is a noise with a spectral notch [FIG. 8(a)], the white noise [FIG. 8(b)] has a pitchlike quality, with a pitch value corresponding to the center frequency of the notch.[55] It sounds like a noise with a

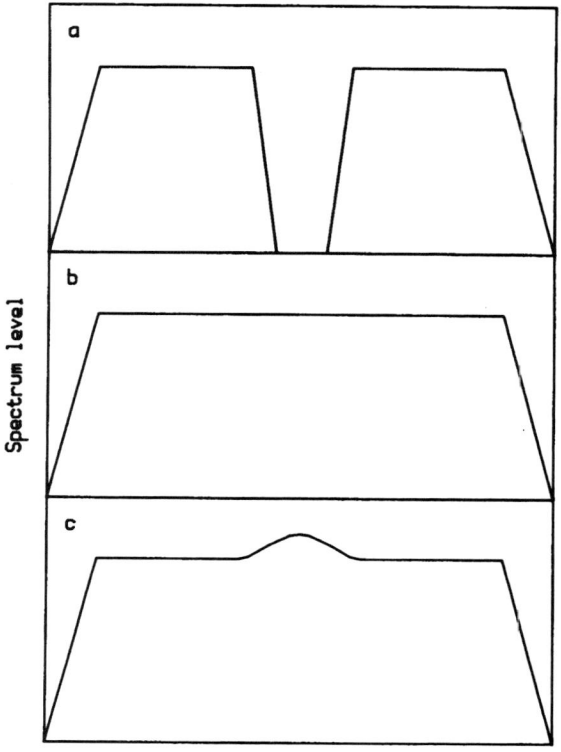

FIGURE 7. Schematic illustration of the spectra of stimuli used to demonstrate the effect of contrast with previous sounds. **(a)** A noise with a spectral notch is presented first. **(b)** The stimulus is then changed to a noise with a flat spectrum. Normally this noise is perceived as "colorless." **(c)** Following the noise with the spectral notch, however, it sounds like a noise with a spectral peak, such as that shown here.

small spectral peak [FIG. 8(c)]. A harmonic complex tone with a flat spectrum may be given a speechlike quality if it is preceded by a harmonic complex having a spectrum that is the inverse of that of a speech sound, such as a vowel.[56]

The Role of Coherent Changes in Perceptual Grouping

The different frequency components arising from a single sound source usually vary in a highly coherent way. They tend to start and finish together, to change in intensity together, and to change in frequency together. This fact is exploited by the auditory system: if two or more components in a complex sound undergo the same kinds of changes at the same time, then they tend to be grouped and perceived as part

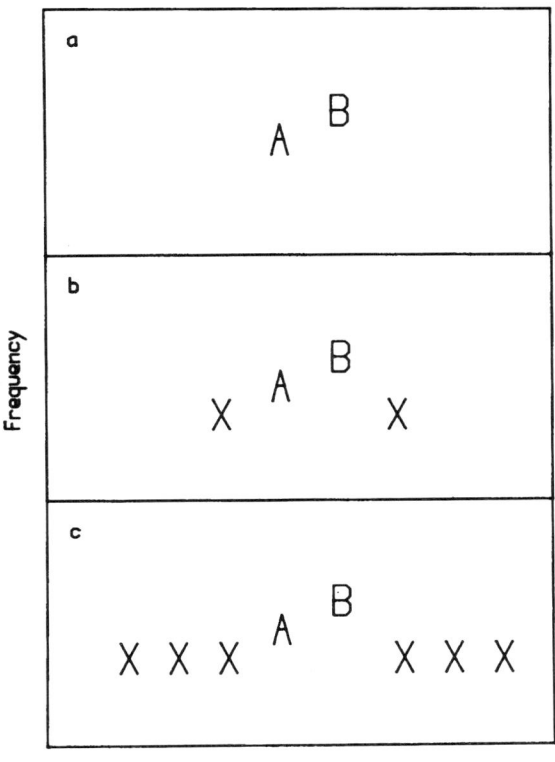

FIGURE 8. Schematic illustration of the stimuli used by Bregman and Rudnicky.[53] (a) When the tones A and B are presented alone, it is easy to tell their order. (b) When the tones A and B are presented as part of a four-tone sequence XABX, it is more difficult to tell their order. (c) If the four-tone sequence is embedded in a longer sequence of X tones, the Xs form a separate perceptual stream, and it is easy to tell the order of A and B.

of the same source. Asynchronies in the onsets of sounds provide a powerful example of this. The components in a complex sound tend to be grouped together if they start synchronously; otherwise they form separate streams. The onset asynchronies necessary to allow the separation of two complex tones are not large, about 30 ms being sufficient,[57] although such a small asynchrony will not usually give the impression that the sounds started at different times.

SUMMARY

The ear contains an array of filters that separate the components of a complex signal into "channels" tuned to different center frequencies. Temporal analysis can be considered as two processes: analysis of the time pattern occurring within each channel, and comparison of the time patterns across channels. Within-channel acuity can be characterized by tasks such as gap detection, or by the ability to detect amplitude modulation as a function of modulation rate. The smallest detectable gap duration for a white noise stimulus is 2–3 ms. The results can be modeled by an array of filters, with each filter followed by a nonlinearity and a (central) sliding temporal integrator.

Hearing impairment of cochlear origin can have adverse effects on temporal resolution because it often reduces the audible bandwidth of the stimuli, and because it results in a reduced sensation level of the stimuli. The sliding temporal integrator appears to be unaffected by hearing loss, although the nonlinearity preceding the integrator may be abnormal, and this can lead to reduced temporal resolution for sounds with slowly fluctuating envelopes. Hearing impairment of more central origin may also adversely affect temporal resolution, but the mechanisms responsible for this are not known.

The acuity of across-channel temporal analysis depends on whether the task is one of discrimination or of identification of temporal order. The finest acuity (1–2 ms) occurs for discrimination tasks. Identification of temporal order is an order of magnitude worse. When the elements of a sequence of sounds are perceived as more than one source (more than one perceptual stream), the ability to judge the order of the elements can be very poor. Perceptual grouping processes can also have dramatic effects on the perceived temporal structure of sound. Conversely, temporal structure can have a powerful influence on perceptual grouping.

ACKNOWLEDGMENTS

I thank Sid Bacon, Michael Shailer, and Michael Stone for helpful comments on an earlier version of this paper.

REFERENCES

1. MOORE, B. C. J., Ed. 1986. Frequency Selectivity in Hearing. Academic Press. London.
2. MOORE, B. C. J. 1989. An Introduction to the Psychology of Hearing, 3rd ed. Academic Press. London.
3. LESHOWITZ, B. 1971. Measurement of the two-click threshold. J. Acoust. Soc. Am. **49:** 426–466.
4. PLOMP, R. 1964. The rate of decay of auditory sensation. J. Acoust. Soc. Am. **36:** 277–282.
5. PENNER, M. J. 1977. Detection of temporal gaps in noise as a measure of the decay of auditory sensation. J. Acoust. Soc. Am. **61:** 552–557.
6. RONKEN, D. 1970. Monaural detection of a phase difference between clicks. J. Acoust. Soc. Am. **47:** 1091–1099.
7. VIEMEISTER, N. F. 1979. Temporal modulation transfer functions based on modulation thresholds. J. Acoust. Soc. Am. **66:** 1364–1380.
8. BACON, S. P. & N. F. VIEMEISTER. 1985. Temporal modulation transfer functions in normal-hearing and hearing-impaired subjects. Audiology **24:** 117–134.
9. MOORE, B. C. J., M. J. SHAILER & G. P. SCHOONEVELDT. 1992. Temporal modulation transfer functions for band-limited noise in subjects with cochlear hearing loss. Br. J. Audiol. **26:** 229–237.
10. GREEN, D. M. 1973. Temporal acuity as a function of frequency. J. Acoust. Soc. Am. **54:** 373–379.

11. FITZGIBBONS, P. J. 1983. Temporal gap detection in noise as a function of frequency, bandwidth and level. J. Acoust. Soc. Am. **74**: 67–72.
12. SHAILER, M. J. & B. C. J. MOORE. 1983. Gap detection as a function of frequency, bandwidth and level. J. Acoust. Soc. Am. **74**: 467–473.
13. BUUS, S. & M. FLORENTINE. 1985. Gap detection in normal and impaired listeners: The effect of level and frequency. *In* Time Resolution in Auditory Systems, A. Michelsen, Ed.: 159–179. Springer-Verlag. New York/Berlin.
14. SHAILER, M. J. & B. C. J. MOORE. 1985. Detection of temporal gaps in band-limited noise: Effects of variations in bandwidth and signal-to-masker ratio. J. Acoust. Soc. Am. **77**: 635–639.
15. GREEN, D. M. 1985. Temporal factors in psychoacoustics. *In* Time Resolution in Auditory Systems, A. Michelsen, Ed.: 122–140. Springer-Verlag. New York/Berlin.
16. DE FILIPPO, C. L. & K. B. SNELL. 1986. Detection of a temporal gap in low-frequency narrow-band signals by normal hearing and hearing-impaired listeners. J. Acoust. Soc. Am. **80**: 1354–1358.
17. EDDINS, D. A., J. W. HALL & J. H. GROSE. 1992. Detection of temporal gaps as a function of frequency region and absolute noise bandwidth. J. Acoust. Soc. Am. **91**: 1069–1077.
18. SHAILER, M. J. & B. C. J. MOORE. 1987. Gap detection and the auditory filter: Phase effects using sinusoidal stimuli. J. Acoust. Soc. Am. **81**: 1110–1117.
19. MOORE, B. C. J., R. W. PETERS & B. R. GLASBERG. 1993. Detection of temporal gaps in sinusoids: Effects of frequency and level. J. Acoust. Soc. Am. In press.
20. RODENBURG, M. 1977. Investigation of temporal effects with amplitude modulated signals. *In* Psychophysics and Physiology of Hearing, E. F. Evans and J. P. Wilson, Eds.: Academic Press. London.
21. GREEN, D. M. & T. G. FORREST. 1988. Detection of amplitude modulation and gaps in noise. *In* Basic Issues in Hearing, H. Duifhuis, H. P. Wit, and J. P. Horst, Eds.: Academic Press. New York.
22. MUNSON, W. A. 1947. The growth of auditory sensation. J. Acoust. Soc. Am. **19**: 584–591.
23. ZWISLOCKI, J. J. 1969. Temporal summation of loudness: An analysis. J. Acoust. Soc. Am. **46**: 431–441.
24. MOORE, B. C. J., B. R. GLASBERG, C. J. PLACK & A. K. BISWAS. 1988. The shape of the ear's temporal window. J. Acoust. Soc. Am. **83**: 1102–1116.
25. PLACK, C. J. & B. C. J. MOORE. 1990. Temporal window shape as a function of frequency and level. J. Acoust. Soc. Am. **87**: 2178–2187.
26. DIVENYI, P. & R. V. SHANNON. 1983. Auditory time consonants unified. J. Acoust. Soc. Am. **Suppl 174**: S10.
27. SHANNON, R. V. 1986. Temporal processing in cochlear implants. *In* The Scott Reger Memorial Conference. Iowa Univ. Press. Iowa City.
28. PENNER, M. J. 1980. The coding of intensity and the interaction of forward and backward masking. J. Acoust. Soc. Am. **67**: 608–616.
29. PENNER, M. J. & R. M. SHIFFRIN. 1980. Nonlinearities in the coding of intensity within the context of a temporal summation model. J. Acoust. Soc. Am. **67**: 617–627.
30. FITZGIBBONS, P. J. & F. L. WIGHTMAN. 1982. Gap detection in normal and hearing-impaired listeners. J. Acoust. Soc. Am. **72**: 761–765.
31. FLORENTINE, M. & S. BUUS. 1984. Temporal gap detection in sensorineural and simulated hearing impairment. J. Speech Hear. Res. **27**: 449–455.
32. GLASBERG, B. R., B. C. J. MOORE & S. P. BACON. 1987. Gap detection and masking in hearing-impaired and normal-hearing subjects. J. Acoust. Soc. Am. **81**: 1546–1556.
33. MOORE, B. C. J. & B. R. GLASBERG. 1988. Gap detection with sinusoids and noise in normal, impaired and electrically stimulated ears. J. Acoust. Soc. Am. **83**: 1093–1101.
34. MOORE, B. C. J., B. R. GLASBERG, E. DONALDSON, T. MCPHERSON & C. J. PLACK. 1989. Detection of temporal gaps in sinusoids by normally hearing and hearing-impaired subjects. J. Acoust. Soc. Am. **85**: 1266–1275.
35. FOWLER, E. P. 1936. A method for the early detection of otosclerosis. Arch. Otolaryngol. **24**: 731–741.

36. GLASBERG, B. R. & B. C. J. MOORE. 1992. Effects of envelope fluctuations on gap detection. Hear. Res. **64:** 81–92.
37. BACON, S. P. & R. M. GLEITMAN. 1992. Modulation detection in subjects with relatively flat hearing losses. J. Speech Hear. Res. **35:** 642–653.
38. TYLER, R. S., A. Q. SUMMERFIELD, E. J. WOOD & M. A. FERNANDES. 1982. Psychoacoustic and phonetic temporal processing in normal and hearing-impaired listeners. J. Acoust. Soc. Am. **72:** 740–752.
39. FORMBY, C. 1982. Differential sensitivity to tonal frequency and to the rate of amplitude modulation of broad-band noise by hearing-impaired listeners. Ph.D. Thesis, Washington University, St. Louis, Mo.
40. LAMORE, P. J. J., C. VERWEIJ & M. P. BROCAAR. 1984. Reliability of auditory function tests in severely hearing-impaired and deaf subjects. Audiology **23:** 453–466.
41. FORMBY, C. 1986. Modulation detection by patients with eighth-nerve tumors. J. Speech Hear. Res. **29:** 413–419.
42. PATTERSON, J. H. & D. M. GREEN. 1970. Discrimination of transient signals having identical energy spectra. J. Acoust. Soc. Am. **48:** 894–905.
43. ZERA, J. & D. M. GREEN. 1993. Detecting temporal onset and offset asynchrony in multitonal complexes. J. Acoust. Soc. Am. In press.
44. RISSET, J. C. & D. L. WESSEL. 1982. Exploration of timbre by analysis and synthesis. *In* The Psychology of Music, D. Deutsch, Ed.: 25–58. Academic Press. New York.
45. WARREN, R. M. 1974. Auditory temporal discrimination by trained listeners. Cognitive Psychol. **6:** 237–256.
46. DIVENYI, P. L. & I. J. HIRSH. 1974. Identification of temporal order in three-tone sequences. J. Acoust. Soc. Am. **56:** 144–151.
47. HIRSH, I. J. 1959. Auditory perception of temporal order. J. Acoust. Soc. Am. **31:** 759–767.
48. VAN NOORDEN, L. P. A. S. 1975. Temporal coherence in the perception of tone sequences. Ph.D. Thesis, Eindhoven Univ. of Technology, Eindhoven, the Netherlands.
49. BREGMAN, A. S. & J. CAMPBELL. 1971. Primary auditory stream segregation and perception of order in rapid sequences of tones. J. Exp. Psychol. **89:** 244–249.
50. LADEFOGED, P. & D. E. BROADBENT. 1960. Perception of sequence in auditory events. Q. J. Exp. Psychol. **12:** 162–170.
51. BROADBENT, D. E. & P. LADEFOGED. 1959. Auditory perception of temporal order. J. Acoust. Soc. Am. **31:** 151–159.
52. WARREN, R. M., C. J. OBUSEK, R. M. FARMER & R. P. WARREN. 1969. Auditory sequence: Confusion of patterns other than speech or music. Science **164:** 586–587.
53. BREGMAN, A. S. & A. RUDNICKY. 1975. Auditory segregation: Stream or streams? J. Exp. Psychol.: Hum. Percept. Perform. **1:** 263–267.
54. BREGMAN, A. S. & G. DANNENBRING. 1973. The effect of continuity on auditory stream segregation. Percept. Psychophys. **13:** 308–312.
55. ZWICKER, E. 1964. 'Negative afterimage' in hearing. J. Acoust. Soc. Am. **36:** 2413–2415.
56. SUMMERFIELD, A. Q., A. S. SIDWELL & T. NELSON. 1987. Auditory enhancement of changes in spectral amplitude. J. Acoust. Soc. Am. **81:** 700–708.
57. RASCH, R. A. 1978. The perception of simultaneous notes such as in polyphonic music. Acustica **40:** 21–33.

Temporal Auditory Processing in Infancy

SANDRA E. TREHUB

Centre for Research in Human Development
University of Toronto
Erindale Campus
Mississauga, Ontario, Canada L5L 1C6

INTRODUCTION

One of the most intriguing aspects of our perceptual system is its ability to derive relatively accurate and useful percepts of the world from sensory information, particularly when such information underspecifies the distal stimulus.[1] In such situations, organizing processes necessarily play a prominent role. Perceptual organization in the temporal domain is particularly critical because most, if not all, meaningful auditory signals undergo change over time. Nevertheless, research on auditory development in general and on temporal auditory processing in particular tends to focus on the perception of relatively simple stimuli, mostly single, unchanging sounds.

TEMPORAL RESOLUTION

The pulselike nature of natural sounds in the environment has drawn attention to the need to distinguish continuous signals from interrupted signals, or those with gaps. In the typical study of gap detection, the experimenter attempts to determine the minimum silent interval necessary for an adult or child to report hearing two sounds rather than one.[2,3] In the only investigation of this phenomenon with infants, Lynne Werner and her associates[4] had 3-month-olds, 6-month-olds, and 12-month-olds discriminate interrupted from uninterrupted broad-band noise. The minimum detectable gap, or gap-detection threshold, was considerably larger for infants than for adults. Although there were suggestions of minor improvement in temporal resolution for 12-month-olds, such improvement likely continues until at least 6 years of age.[3,5]

A related ability is auditory fusion, or the perception of two successive repetitions of the same waveform as a single sound. If such fusion did not regularly occur, we would hear many more separate echoes in enclosed spaces than we actually do. It is only when the repetition follows the original sound by 30 ms or more that we hear such echoes.[6] As is the case with gap detection, auditory fusion has a prolonged developmental course, with improvement still evident at 9 years of age.[7]

Another echo-suppression phenomenon that has been investigated developmentally is the precedence effect.[8] When two identical sounds are presented from different locations, with one sound delayed relative to the other, listeners hear a single sound emanating from the leading loudspeaker. Perception of the lagging sound is suppressed until the delay between sounds is somewhere between 4 and 40 ms, depending on the nature of stimulation, beyond which sounds are localized at their true locations.[8,9] To place this finding in context, one must understand that adults detect much shorter onset-time differences when the sounds originate from the same location. Newborn infants, in contrast to adults, respond to precedence-effect stimuli as if the sounds from both sources were audible.[10,11] By 6 months of age, and perhaps before, infants experience the precedence effect, but they continue to hear only the leading sound at onset-time differences well beyond those perceived as two successive sounds by children and adults.[12] Consistent with these reports of temporal processing delays in early life is evidence of relatively poor discrimination of signal and silence durations by infants and 5-year-old children.[13]

The factors presumed responsible for infants' poor resolution of such signals include immature temporal coding in the primary auditory pathways,[4] elevated thresholds for the detection of auditory stimuli,[14,15] and difficulties with selective attention.[16] Does this mean that the auditory temporal world of infants is unlike that of adults? If auditory temporal organization depends on reasonably adequate resolution of component sounds, then the infant's temporal world would differ considerably. If, however, *patterns* of sounds can be recognized and distinguished from other patterns, even with limited resolution, then infants would have the potential to engage in adultlike temporal processing.

GLOBAL PROCESSING

Warren[17] claims that adults perceive many auditory sequences, including speech and music, as temporal compounds or wholes, without resolving these patterns into ordered sequences of sounds. He argues, further, that our ability to identify the components of speech, for example, does not provide the basis for speech perception but rather is a consequence of such perception. In other words, auditory patterns are more than the sum of their parts, exhibiting unique emergent properties.

A number of recent studies indicate that infants also engage in global or relational processing of auditory patterns. For the most part, these studies have used a conditioned head turn procedure originally developed for evaluating infants' discrimination of single sounds.[18,19] Briefly, infants listen to repetitions of a tone sequence presented from a loudspeaker to one side. On half of the test trials, the repeating pattern is replaced with another pattern that is altered in some respect. On the remaining trials, the repetitions continue without change, the change and no-change trials being presented in random order. When the pattern repetitions are identical, listeners can use absolute cues to guide performance. When the patterns repeat with variations, however, listeners must use relational cues to solve the task.[20] The experimenter, who is unaware of the identity of the trials (change or no-change), records any head turns to the loudspeaker. Whenever a turn occurs within 4 seconds of a sound change, the attending computer automatically delivers reinforcement, illuminating and activating an animated toy near the loudspeaker. A significantly greater incidence of responding on change than on no-change trials indicates that infants can detect the change in question.

The term "temporal" is used here in a broad as well as a narrow sense. In the narrow sense, temporal patterning refers to arrays of relative sound and silence durations, or timing. In another sense, however, all auditory events or sequences are necessarily temporal because they unfold over time. In this latter sense, manipulations of the relative pitch or loudness of pattern elements would alter the temporal structure of those patterns.

Classification of Auditory Sequences by Rhythmic Structure

The pattern of relative onset times in a sequence of sounds confers a distinct temporal or rhythmic identity,[21] just as the pattern of relative pitches in a sequence of notes confers a distinct melodic identity.[22] In neither case are the absolute values critical. Leigh Thorpe and I evaluated infants' ability to extract the temporal organization of a tone sequence and to generalize this organization across variations in tempo.[23] Specifically, we trained infants to discriminate between three- or four-tone sequences with contrasting rhythmic structure, for example, a 1,2 (X XX) versus 2,1 (XX X) pattern or a 2,2 (XX XX) versus 3,1 (XXX X) pattern. Subsequently, we evaluated their ability to perform the same rhythm discrimination when the tempo, or rate of presentation, varied across repetitions. Infants succeeded in this task (see FIG. 1), indicating that they could categorize auditory sequences on the basis of their temporal structure or rhythm. Presumably, this skill should enable infants to make perceptual compensations for differences in speaking rate,[24] to selectively direct their attention to running speech on the basis of temporal marking,[25,26] and to perceive the invariance of songs like "Twinkle, Twinkle Little Star," whether the tempo is fast or slow.

Temporal Grouping

When we listen to auditory sequences, we tend to group subsets of elements within the overall stimulus, the resulting groups being influenced by the relative duration of elements and by other parameters such as the frequency, intensity, and timbre of elements. Our disposition to group stimuli is so compelling that we even group successive tones or clicks that are identical in all respects.[27,28] Some of these grouping processes may be primitive in the sense that they are relatively impervious to experience.[29] In such cases, our knowledge of the world or of the actual stimulus situation does not stop us from perceiving certain auditory events in a nonveridical manner.

Leigh Thorpe and I examined infants' propensity to impose temporal organization on isochronous tone sequences.[30,31] We generated six-tone patterns in which the first three tones differed from the last three in fundamental frequency, spectral structure

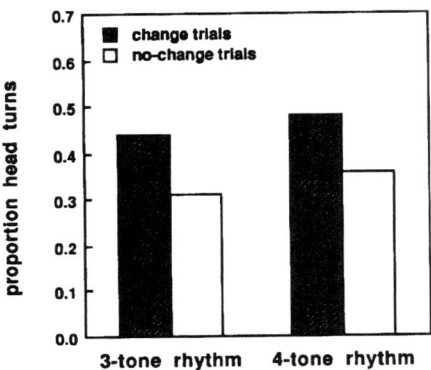

FIGURE 1. Mean proportion of head turns on change and no-change trials for the 3-tone and 4-tone rhythms. (Data from Trehub & Thorpe, 1989.[23])

(sawtooth versus sine waves), or intensity (schematic representation: XXXOOO). We reasoned that if infants organized such sequences into two groups of three tones, as we do, then they would have greater difficulty detecting temporal perturbations *between* groups of tones compared with identical perturbations *within* a tone group. The standard patterns consisted of isochronous sequences and the comparison patterns had one intertone interval extended by 75 ms or more. An extended intertone interval or pause between groups (XXX OOO) would preserve the presumed structure of the original pattern, making such a change less noticeable. By contrast, a pause at another location (XXXO OO) would generate a new temporal structure, which would enhance the salience of this otherwise equivalent durational cue. In fact, infants more readily detected the temporal alterations when they occurred within a tone group, implying that they had grouped the original patterns of isochronous tones on the basis of similar pitch, loudness, or timbre. Moreover, greater disparities in the grouping parameter (e.g., fundamental frequency) promoted stronger grouping effects.

We have labeled this phenomenon the *duration illusion,* referring to the misperception of silent intervals at critical locations in a stimulus sequence. Perceptual "errors" or distortions such as these are clear manifestations of perceptual organization, guiding the listener's parsing of auditory stimuli into manageable chunks, highlighting key structural aspects of stimulation, and promoting useful interpretations of stimulus input. Similar temporal organizational processes may be schema based or dependent on experience. One such example is the perception of pauses between words,[32] an illusion that operates only for familiar languages.

Other research on infants' perception of extended passages of speech and music indicates comparable sensitivity to the temporal organization of such sequences. In one study,[33] the investigators altered samples of maternal speech by inserting pauses (silent intervals) either between clausal units or within such clauses. The versions with intact clauses and those with temporally altered clauses were made available at different loudspeakers. After a period of familiarization, infants could activate one or the other version by looking at the appropriate spatial location, and could keep listening to such speech by remaining oriented to that location. Infants as young as 6 months of age looked longer at the loudspeaker delivering intact clauses, which presumably reflected their sensitivity to the temporal organization of clauses. More recently, 9-month-old infants have exhibited similar listening preferences for intact phrases.[34]

Phrase boundaries in music are marked by some of the same features that mark clause boundaries in speech, for example, drops in pitch and increased duration of the last word or note.[35] It would not be surprising, then, if infants showed comparable sensitivity to the temporal integrity of musical phrases. To evaluate this possibility, Krumhansl and Jusczyk[35] altered Mozart minuets by adding one-second pauses either at the end of each musical phrase or within the phrases. As was the case for speech, infants looked significantly longer at the loudspeaker emitting intact phrases than at the one with temporally distorted phrases. Collectively, these studies indicate that infants segment complex auditory stimuli in structurally significant ways. In fact, they exhibit parsing strategies that resemble those used in mature speech comprehension and reading.

Classification of Auditory Sequences by Pitch Contour

The contour of a melody refers to its pitch configuration, or the manner in which the component pitches change or do not change over time (i.e., whether they rise, fall, or stay the same). Such configural information plays a prominent role in the perception and retention of unfamiliar melodies, with adults remembering little about the actual pitch distance (i.e., number of semitones) between adjacent notes.[36] Even with familiar melodies, adults remember detailed information about the relations between notes (i.e., intervals), but little about the absolute pitch level of any notes.[37] On the whole, then, our representation of melodies is abstract and relational, much like that of speech.

In recent years, it has become apparent that infants readily discriminate between melodies with contrasting contour, whether the contour change was accomplished by simply reordering the component notes[38] or by the addition of a single new note.[39] Moreover, infants can be trained to classify melodies on the basis of contour alone, ignoring discriminable differences in absolute pitch and pitch distance.[20] Specifically, they learned not to respond to melodies with a simple up–down contour, responding only to melodies with a different contour configuration (see FIGS. 2 and 3). Infants accomplished this task in a context in which each melody was presented

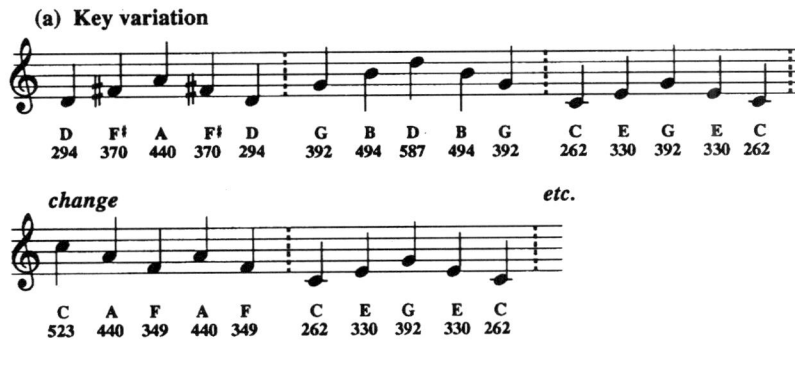

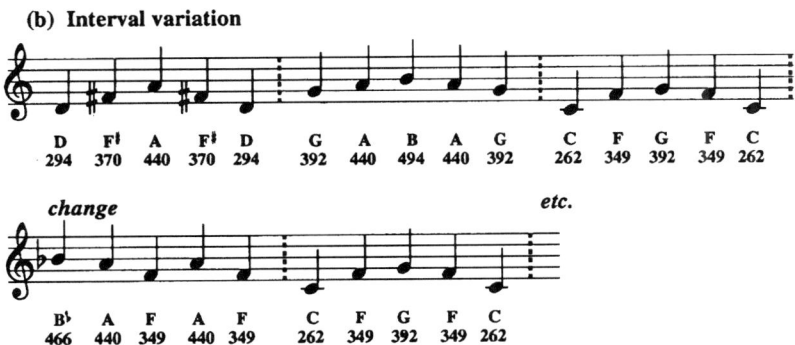

FIGURE 2. Examples of repeating stimuli for the key variation (**a**) and interval variation (**b**) conditions. Each example depicts three successive presentations of the standard melody followed by a change and subsequent return to the standard melody. (Stimuli from Trehub et al., 1987.[20])

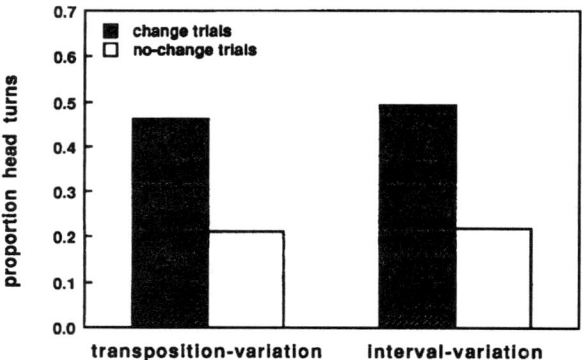

FIGURE 3. Mean proportion of head turns on change and no-change trials for the transposition-variation (i.e., key-variation) and interval-variation conditions. (Data from Trehub et al., 1987.[20])

at a different pitch level than the immediately preceding or following melody, precluding the use of absolute pitch cues. Infants' global or relational pitch processing strategy parallels that of adults, but is in marked contrast to the local pitch strategy typically used by nonhuman species.[40,41]

In short, when infants hear a melody that exceeds their immediate memory span, they encode and retain a summary description that enhances contour information at the expense of pitch and interval information. Their pitch-contour strategy can be viewed as yet another perceptual organizational device, one that provides an effective means of parsing complex auditory sequences. In all likelihood, infants use pitch-contour processing in conjunction with temporal grouping or rhythm processing to generate a powerful contour/rhythm parser.

Pitch and duration have correlated patterns of occurrence in speech[42] and music.[43] Indeed, Carlson and his associates[44] contend that speech and music performance have common codes for marking structural constituents. Moreover, they suggest that this situation arises from the importation of acquired speech decoding skills into the domain of music. The findings of research with infants favor an alternative scenario, which is that both speech and music capitalize on inherent or universal principles of auditory pattern processing. This is not to say that nothing needs to be learned, but rather that not everything does. It is likely that we begin with structured or organized percepts[45,46] that we later fine-tune to the requirements of our linguistic and musical culture.

Classification of Auditory Sequences by Interval Structure

In music, as in speech, adults' perception of important structures is thought to be based not only on fundamental grouping processes but also on the progressive internalization of observed regularities.[47,48] It is possible, however, that some regularities in our musical culture and in others might reflect relative ease of initial processing or relative ease of mastery. If this were the case, then infants should perform better on highly conventional or prototypical patterns than on atypical patterns.

In a series of studies,[49–51] my colleagues and I attempted to determine whether infants could detect very subtle changes to conventional and unconventional melodies. The conventional melodies were based on a frequently occurring pattern that is considered central to Western music, notably the major triad. The unconventional melodies were identical in contour (up–down) and temporal structure (isochronous), having one or more wrong notes in terms of conventional Western scales. The infant's task was to detect a semitone change in one position of each of the melodies. This would constitute an interval change or a change in pitch distance between adjacent notes. Because such a change would conserve the contour of the melody and because infants are primarily contour processors,[20] the task would be a particularly difficult one for them. As before, the repeating melodies were always transposed so that absolute pitch cues were unavailable. The outcome was that infants were generally able to detect the interval change in the context of the highly conventional melody, but were generally unable to do so in the context of the unconventional pitch patterning (see FIGS. 4 and 5).

Why might this be the case? Psychoacoustically, intervals that approximate simple frequency ratios are considered more consonant than those with complex frequency ratios.[52] The notes of the major triad (C E G in the key of C major) approximate very simple ratios (4:5:6), and the outer notes of the triad (C G), in particular, are related by a ratio approximating 2:3, which is prevalent in natural sounds, including the simultaneous components of vowels. Just as attractive faces (from an adult's perspective) are preferred by infants,[53] and, just as some vowels are especially good exemplars of a particular phonetic category for infants and adults,[54–56] so some patterns of intervals may be inherently easier to perceive or remember than others. Although early experience seems to play an important role in

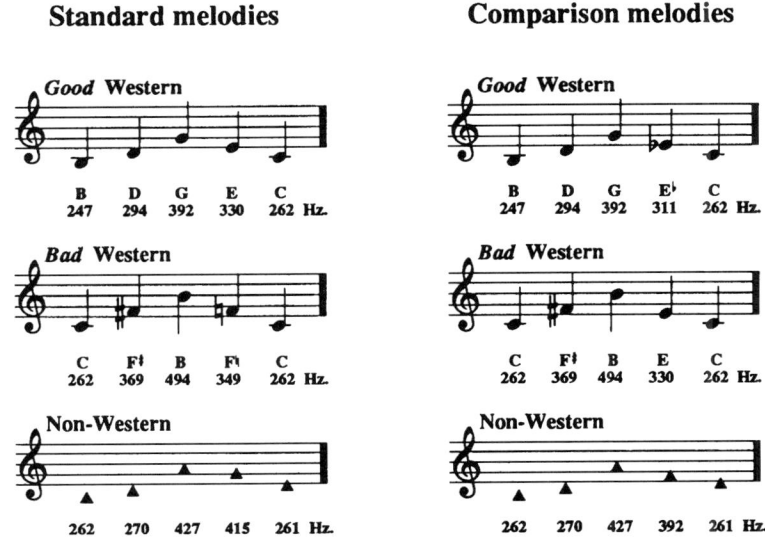

FIGURE 4. Standard and comparison melodies for three conditions, *good* Western, *bad* Western, and *non*-Western. (Non-Western melodies cannot be written in conventional music notation.) (Stimuli from Trehub *et al.*, 1990.[50])

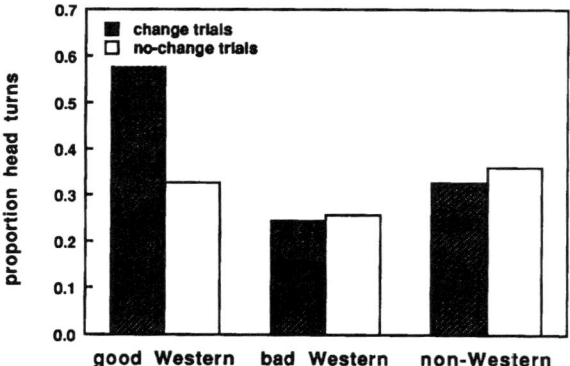

FIGURE 5. Mean proportion of head turns on change and no-change trials for the *good* Western, *bad* Western, and *non*-Western melodies. (Data from Trehub et al., 1990.[50])

the formation of vowel categories,[56] this does not rule out the possibility that prototypic vowels in foreign languages would be more learnable than nonprototypic vowels.

It is important to bear in mind that the infants in the foregoing melody-perception studies were 6 months of age or older, making it possible that previous exposure to music, however limited, had been responsible for the effects observed. Nevertheless, research on American infants' perception of foreign melodies is at odds with an experiential interpretation.[57] Although North American adults were able to detect more subtle differences to Western than to Javanese melodies, infants performed equivalently on both. This finding indicates that culture-specific exposure can narrow listeners' interval categories,[58] as is the case for their phonetic categories.[59]

Classification of Auditory Sequences by Number of Sounds

The foregoing research indicates that infants, despite the relative poverty of their temporal resolution, exhibit a variety of seemingly sophisticated skills for auditory pattern processing. These pattern processing skills are likely to be activated more or less automatically, whether or not learning is involved. Other pattern-processing skills may depend on focused attention, which may be absent in infants. However, it may be difficult to determine, on an *a priori* basis, which tasks require such focused attention and which do not.

We know that prelinguistic infants can extract information related to the number of elements in simple visual displays. For example, they can differentiate displays of two items from those with three,[60,61] and can also detect numerical correspondences across modalities, matching displays of two or three items to equivalent numbers of sounds.[62] This is not to suggest that infants can count, but rather that they apprehend some quality associated with two-ness or three-ness. Nevertheless, this ability seems to be limited to small number displays. On the basis of infants' precocity in auditory pattern processing, their apprehension of qualities associated with number might be superior in the auditory domain.

To explore this possibility, my colleagues and I evaluated the ability of 7- to 10-month-old infants to discriminate between sets of auditory sequences differing in number.[63] The sequences in each set were characterized by a common number of tones, but varied in tempo (rate), overall pattern duration, pattern density, and the frequency of tones. Tones within each sequence were identical in frequency, but tonal frequency varied randomly across patterns (12 possible frequencies). Infants listened to a series of variable exemplars from one set, which was defined by an invariant number of tones (three, four, or five), and were rewarded for responding (i.e., turning) to exemplars from a different set (i.e., different number of elements). Infants discriminated four-tone comparison patterns from a three-tone standard set, three-tone comparisons from a four-tone standard, and five-tone comparisons from a four-tone standard. In short, numerical information processing in infancy does not seem to be restricted to very small number sets, as has been suggested previously. Nevertheless, the limits of this ability may be reached with sequences of five or more elements.

The sequential processing that characterizes audition may highlight or enhance numerical information, in contrast to visual perception where simultaneity may pose special difficulties. For example, the first or last element of a pattern is considerably more ambiguous for visual than for auditory patterns, creating a need for strategic enumeration processes in the latter. In any case, these findings indicate that infants have some prerequisite skills for concepts as abstract as number.

Infant Movement Responses to Complex Sound Sequences

It is clear that infants perceive important aspects of temporal patterning in complex auditory sequences such as music and speech. In laboratory settings, moreover, they exhibit distinctive patterns of responding such as turning to one type of pattern but not another, or looking longer in the direction of a preferred type of pattern. Such differential responding is usually preceded by highly structured and artificial training regimens. In some research contexts, however, the simple presentation of auditory stimulation has resulted in differential affective responses to contrasting speech samples such as infant-directed versus adult-directed speech[64] or maternal-approving versus -disapproving speech.[65] It is worth noting that the speech samples in these situations were highly contrastive in pitch and temporal patterning. In fact, the speech that induced positive affect was characterized by smooth, simple pitch contours and slow tempo in contrast to the less preferred speech, which had many more abrupt changes.

Gabrielsson[66] has drawn attention to some of the perceptual consequences of timing in music performance such as the listener's experience of motion, whether or not this "motional" experience results in overt movements like tapping or dancing. For example, when performed appropriately, a march has a motion character distinct from that of a Viennese waltz. Also of interest is the fact that some cultures do not have verbal distinctions between movement and music, movement being considered intrinsic to musical performance and to listening. It is possible, then, that natural movement patterns to music would be more readily observable in listeners with imperfect knowledge of our social conventions.

To gain insight into this issue, my colleagues and I videotaped infants 9–13 months of age as they listened to different musical materials. The infants sat in a chair (walker with wheels removed) and listened to a series of excerpts from commercial recordings of "McNamara's Band" (band and chorus), which was lively and rhythmic, and "Traumeri" (pan flute and orchestra), which was slow and melodic. Each infant heard five 45-s excerpts from each recording in random order. Adults subsequently watched the videotapes without sound and attempted to guess which music had been presented on each trial, receiving immediate feedback after each guess. Adults performed significantly above chance levels, but they were unable to specify the features that guided their judgments. To isolate a possible basis for adults' success, we had independent observers code the videotapes for the duration of bouncing, defined as vertical motion of the head or torso. Presumably, bouncing would be an appropriate and interpretable response to lively, rhythmic music. Indeed, the mean duration of bouncing to "McNamara's Band" (29.3 s) significantly exceeded the duration of bouncing to "Traumeri" (7.7 s). This differential pattern of movement responses provides evidence that the temporal patterning of complex auditory sequences is not only noticed by infants but has demonstrable effects on their behavior.

GLOBAL PROCESSING AND ATTENDING

Warren[17] has identified two fundamentally different means by which we recognize auditory sequences and distinguish different arrangements of their components. He contends that one of these means, the recognition of unresolved patterns or temporal compounds, is much more important in daily life than is the other, the analysis of component sounds. Auditory analysis not only involves the resolution of individual components but also their identification and appropriate sequencing. The terms "higher level" and "lower level" seem to be less appropriate designations for these auditory processes than the alternative terms "global" and "local." In any case, infants are remarkably adultlike in global processing at the same time as they are notably deficient in local processing. What are the likely consequences of infants' global mode of processing?

According to Jones and Boltz,[43] the temporal patterning of words, pitches, and other information affects our attention to such information. Highly coherent events, such as speech or musical patterns, are structurally predictable, at least in part, exhibiting distinct rhythmic patterns. Events with low coherence, such as word lists or traffic noise, have little structural predictability. When listeners are exposed to highly coherent or rhythmically patterned sounds, they can track information efficiently, without the requirement of continuous monitoring,[26] and can engage in future-oriented attending.[43] The result of such future-oriented or dynamic attending is the generation of expectancies about what is likely to happen and when. From this perspective, listening to rhythmically patterned sounds is a rhythmic activity itself, with listeners sharing and becoming attuned to the rhythmic pattern of stimulation.[43] On the basis of the research presented here, infants seem to inhabit an auditory temporal world that is similar, in many respects, to that of adults. Thus, they may well engage in dynamic listening, effectively deploying their limited attentional resources well before they acquire linguistic knowledge. Indeed, such listening strategies may facilitate the acquisition of language.

Some individuals, even after joining the linguistic world, may have difficulty engaging in and capitalizing on this dynamic mode of attending. Potential consequences of such difficulty include deficits in the processing of speech presented at rapid rates or deficient application of speech processing strategies to secondary language tasks like reading and writing. Exploring individual differences in the temporal organization of auditory patterns and the short- and long-term correlates of such differences represent important challenges for future research.

REFERENCES

1. POMERANTZ, J. R. & M. KUBOVY. 1986. Theoretical approaches to perceptual organization: Simplicity and liklihood principles. *In* Handbook of Perception and Human Performance, Vol. II, Cognitive Processes and Performance, K. R. Boff, L. Kaufman, and J. P. Thomas, Eds. Wiley-Interscience. New York.
2. FITZGIBBONS, P. J. 1983. Temporal gap detection in noise as a function of frequency, bandwidth, and level. J. Acoust. Soc. Am. **70:** 955–965.
3. IRWIN, R. J., A. K. R. BALL, N. KAY, J. A. STILLMAN & J. ROSSER. 1985. The development of auditory temporal acuity in children. Child Dev. **56:** 614–620.
4. WERNER, L. A., G. C. MAREAN, C. F. HALPIN, N. B. SPETNER & J. M. GILLENWATER. 1992. Infant auditory temporal acuity: Gap detection. Child Dev. **63:** 260–272.
5. WIGHTMAN, F., P. ALLEN, T. DOLAN, T. KISTLER & D. JAMIESON. 1989. Temporal resolution in preschool children. Child Dev. **60:** 611–624.
6. SCHUBERT, E. D. 1980. Hearing: Its Function and Dysfunction. Springer-Verlag. Wien, Austria.
7. DAVIS, S. M. & R. L. MCCROSKEY. 1980. Auditory fusion in children. Child Dev. **51:** 75–80.
8. CLIFTON, R. K. 1985. The precedence effect: Its implications for developmental questions. *In* Auditory Development in Infancy, S. E. Trehub and B. A. Schneider, Eds. Plenum. New York.
9. GREEN, D. M. 1976. An Introduction to Hearing. Erlbaum. Hillsdale, N.J.
10. CLIFTON, R. K., B. A. MORRONGIELLO, J. W. KULIG & J. W. DOWD. 1981. Newborns' orientation toward sound: Possible implications for cortical development. Child Dev. **52:** 833–838.
11. MORRONGIELLO, B. A., R. K. CLIFTON & J. W. KULIG. 1982. Newborn cardiac and behavioral orienting responses to sound under varying precedence effect conditions. Infant Behav. Dev. **5:** 249–259.
12. MORRONGIELLO, B. A., J. W. KULIG & R. K. CLIFTON. 1984. Developmental changes in auditory temporal perception. Child Dev. **55:** 461–471.
13. MORRONGIELLO, B. A. & S. E. TREHUB. 1987. Age-related changes in auditory temporal perception. J. Exp. Child Psychol. **44:** 413–426.
14. SCHNEIDER, B. A. & S. E. TREHUB. 1992. Sources of developmental change in auditory sensitivity. *In* Developmental Psychoacoustics, L. A. Werner and E. W. Rubel, Eds. American Psychological Association. Washington, D.C.
15. TREHUB, S. E., B. A. SCHNEIDER & M. ENDMAN. 1980. Developmental changes in infants' sensitivity to octave-band noises. J. Exp. Child Psychol. **29:** 282–293.
16. WERNER, L. A. & J. Y. BARGONES. 1991. Sources of auditory masking in infants: Distraction effects. Percept. Psychophys. **50:** 405–412.
17. WARREN, R. M. 1993. Perception of global properties of sound sequences. *In* Thinking in Sound: Cognitive Aspects of Human Audition, S. McAdams and E. Bigand, Eds. Oxford Univ. Press. Oxford, England.
18. EILERS, R. E., W. R. WILSON & J. M. MOORE. 1977. Developmental changes in speech discrimination in infants. J. Speech Hear Res. **20:** 766–780.
19. KUHL, P. K. 1985. Methods in the study of infant speech perception. *In* Measurement of Audition and Vision in the First Year of Postnatal Life: A Methodological Overview, G. Gottlieb and N. A. Krasnegor, Eds. Ablex. Norwood, N.J.
20. TREHUB, S. E., L. A. THORPE & B. A. MORRONGIELLO. 1987. Organizational processes in infants' perception of auditory patterns. Child Dev. **58:** 741–749.
21. WHITE, B. W. 1960. Recognition of distorted melodies. Am. J. Psychol. **73:** 100–107.

22. DOWLING, W. J. 1978. Scale and contour. Two components of a theory of memory for melodies. Psychol. Rev. **85:** 341–354.
23. TREHUB, S. E. & L. A. THORPE. 1989. Infants' perception of rhythm. Categorization of auditory sequences by temporal structure. Can. J. Psychol. **43:** 217–229.
24. EIMAS, P. D. & J. L. MILLER. 1980. Contextual effects in infant speech perception. Science **209:** 1140–1141.
25. BAILEY, P. J. 1983. Hearing for speech: The information transmitted in normal and impaired speech. *In* Hearing Science and Hearing Disorders, M. E. Lutman and M. P. Haggard, Eds. Academic Press. London.
26. MARTIN, J. G. 1972. Rhythmic (hierarchical) versus serial structure in speech and other behavior. Psychol. Rev. **79:** 487–509.
27. FRAISSE, P. 1982. Rhythm and tempo. *In* The Psychology of Music, D. Deutsch, Ed. Academic Press, New York.
28. WOODROW, H. 1909. A quantitative study of rhythm. Arch. Psychol. **18:**(1).
29. BREGMAN, A. S. 1990. Auditory Scene Analysis. MIT Press. Cambridge, Mass.
30. THORPE, L. A. & S. E. TREHUB. 1989. Duration illusion and auditory grouping in infancy. Dev. Psychol. **25:** 122–127.
31. THORPE, L. A., S. E. TREHUB, B. A. MORRONGIELLO & D. BULL. 1988. Perceptual grouping by infants and preschool children. Dev. Psychol. **24:** 484–491.
32. STUDDERT-KENNEDY, M. 1975. From continuous signal to discrete message: Syllable to phoneme. *In* The Role of Speech in Language, J. F. Kavanaugh and J. E. Cutting, Eds. MIT Press. Cambridge, Mass.
33. HIRSH-PASEK, K., D. G. KEMLER NELSON, P. W. JUSCZYK, K. WRIGHT CASSIDY, B. DRUSS & L. KENNEDY. 1987. Clauses are perceptual units for young infants. Cognition **26:** 269–286.
34. JUSCZYK, P. W., K. HIRSH-PASEK, D. G. KEMLER NELSON, L. KENNEDY, A. WOODWARD & J. PIWOZ. 1992. Perception of acoustic correlates of major phrasal units by young infants. Cog. Psychol. **24:** 252–293.
35. KRUMHANSL, C. L. & P. W. JUSCZYK. 1990. Infants' perception of phrase structure in music. Psychol. Sci. **1:** 70–73.
36. BARTLETT, J. C. & W. J. DOWLING. 1980. Recognition of transposed melodies: A key-distance effect in developmental perspective. J. Exp. Psychol.: Hum. Percept. **6:** 501–515.
37. ATTNEAVE, F. & R. K. OLSON. 1971. Pitch as a medium: A new approach to psychophysical scaling. Am. J. Psychol. **84:** 147–166.
38. TREHUB, S. E., D. BULL & L. A. THORPE. 1984. Infants' perception of melodies: The role of melodic contour. Child Dev. **55:** 821–830.
39. TREHUB, S. E., L. A. THORPE & B. A. MORRONGIELLO. 1985. Infants' perception of melodies: Changes in a single tone. Infant Behav. Dev. **8:** 213–223.
40. D'AMATO, M. R. 1988. A search for tonal pattern perception in cebus monkeys: Why monkeys can't hum a tune. Music Percept. **5:** 453–480.
41. HULSE, S. H., S. C. PAGE & R. F. BRAATEN. 1990. An integrative approach to serial pattern learning: Music perception and comparative acoustic perception. *In* Comparative Perception, Vol. II, Communication, W. C. Stebbins and M. Berkley, Eds. Wiley. New York.
42. ALLEN, G. D. 1975. Speech rhythm: Its relation to performance universals and articulatory timing. J. Phon. **3:** 75–86.
43. JONES, M. R. & M. BOLTZ. 1989. Dynamic attending and responses to time. Psychol. Rev. **96:** 459–491.
44. CARLSON, R., A. FRIBERG, L. FRYDÉN, B. GRANSTRÖM & J. SUNDBERG. 1989. Speech and music performance: Parallels of contrasts. Contemp. Music Rev. **4:** 391–404.
45. TREHUB, S. E. 1985. Auditory pattern perception in infancy. *In* Auditory Development in Infancy, S. E. Trehub and B. A. Schneider, Eds. Plenum. New York.
46. TREHUB, S. E. & L. J. TRAINOR. 1993. Listening strategies in infancy: The roots of language and musical development. *In* Thinking in Sound: Cognitive Perspectives on Human Audition, S. McAdams and E. Bigand, Eds. Oxford Univ. Press. London.

47. JONES, M. R. 1982. Music as a stimulus for psychological motion, Part II, An expectancy model. Psychomusicology **2:** 1–13.
48. KRUMHANSL, C. L. 1990. Cognitive Foundations of Musical Pitch. Oxford Univ. Press. New York.
49. COHEN, A. J., L. A. THORPE & S. E. TREHUB. 1987. Infants' perception of musical relations in short transposed tone sequences. Can. J. Psychol. **41:** 33–47.
50. TREHUB, S. E., L. A. THORPE & L. J. TRAINOR. 1990. Infants' perception of *good* and *bad* melodies. Psychomusicology **9:** 5–15.
51. TRAINOR, L. J. & S. E. TREHUB. Musical context effects in infants and adults: Key distance. J. Exp. Psychol.: Hum. Percept. In press.
52. RAKOWSKI, A. 1990. Intonation variants of musical intervals in isolation and in musical contexts. Psychol. Music **18:** 60–72.
53. LANGLOIS, J. H. & L. A. ROGGMAN. 1990. Attractive faces are only average. Psychol. Sci. **1:** 115–121.
54. GRIESER, D. L. & P. K. KUHL. 1989. Categorization of speech by infants: Support for speech-sound prototypes. Dev. Psychol. **25:** 577–588.
55. KUHL, P. K. 1991. Human adults and human infants show a "perceptual magnet effect" for the prototypes of speech categories, monkeys do not. Percept. Psychophys. **50:** 93–107.
56. KUHL, P. K., K. A. WILLIAMS, F. LACERDA, K. N. STEVENS & B. LINDBLOM. 1992. Linguistic experience alters phonetic perception in infants by 6 months of age. Science **255:** 606–608.
57. LYNCH, M. P., R. E. EILERS, D. K. OLLER & R. C. URBANO. 1990. Innateness, experience, and music perception. Psychol. Sci. **1:** 272–276.
58. TRAINOR, L. J. & S. E. TREHUB. 1992. A comparison of infants' and adults' sensitivity to western musical structure. J. Exp. Psychol.: Hum. Percept. **18:** 394–402.
59. WERKER, J. F. & C. E. LALONDE. 1988. Cross-language speech perception: Initial capabilities and developmental change. Dev. Psychol. **24:** 672–683.
60. STARKEY, P. & R. G. COOPER. 1980. Perception of numbers by human infants. Science **210:** 1033–1035.
61. STRAUSS, M. S. & L. E. CURTIS. 1981. Infant perception of numerosity. Child Dev. **52:** 1146–1152.
62. STARKEY, P., E. S. SPELKE & R. GELMAN. 1983. Detection of 1-1 correspondences by human infants. Science **222:** 79–81.
63. TREHUB, S. E., L. A. THORPE & A. J. COHEN. 1991. Infants' auditory processing of numerical information. Paper presented at the Society for Research in Human Development, Seattle, Wash.
64. WERKER, J. F. & P. J. MCLEOD. 1989. Infant preference for both male and female infant-directed talk: A developmental study of attentional and affective responsiveness. Can. J. Psychol. **43:** 230–246.
65. FERNALD, A. Approval and disapproval: Infant responsiveness to vocal affect in familiar and unfamiliar languages. Child Dev. In press.
66. GABRIELSSON, A. 1988. Timing in music performance and its relations to music experience. *In* Generative Processes in Music: The Psychology of Performance, Improvisation, and Composition, J. A. Sloboda, Ed. Clarendon Press. Oxford.

Temporal Order Determinants in a Somesthetic Frequency Discrimination: Sequential Order Coding

VERNON B. MOUNTCASTLE

Philip Bard Laboratories of Neurophysiology
Department of Neuroscience
The Johns Hopkins University School of Medicine
Baltimore, Maryland 21215

INTRODUCTION

We address in this symposium the questions of temporal information processing in the nervous system, and temporal dynamics in behavior and in brain activity. One can suppose that the organizers of our meeting intended these questions to be discussed from different points of view, as witness the diversity of our individual scientific cultures. We consider the problem along time scales that differ by two orders of magnitude, from serial order in behavior to serial order in neural activity. The problem of the former has long been of major interest in psychology. It was treated by Karl Lashley in a famous address at the Hixon symposium in 1948.[1] Many of you are concerned, as was Lashley, with the problem of serial order in language and its disturbances. Of that I shall say nothing.

Instead, I present some experimental evidence concerning the question of serial order in neuronal activity in the brain, the time series composed by the sequential order in which central neurons discharge impulses. This is an old, persistent, and still vexed question in central nervous system (CNS) physiology.[2-5] I indicate briefly some aspects of the problem by the following questions: (1) Is information carried uniquely by the sequential order of impulse discharge in neurons? (2) If so, how is that temporal order "processed" in the nervous system, particularly when it is clear that complex operations are carried out on short samples?[6] (3) Can streams of impulses carry discriminably different sets of information embedded in different sequential orders, even when overall frequencies are the same? (4) Do populations of active neurons transmit information embedded uniquely in the relations between their independent sequential orders?[7] (5) Is there a special significance when the parallel streams of action potentials in adjacent elements are "coherent" versus when they are not?[8-10] (6) Can spatially distributed stimuli be signaled by the serial order of impulse discharges, instead of or in addition to the spatially distributed patterns of activity in the population of peripheral and central neurons driven by the stimuli?[11] (7) And, what sort of neural apparatus/mechanism could measure and hold in working memory the sequence of time intervals between incoming nerve impulses, compare that sequence with a slightly different one arriving later over the same input channels at the same overall frequency, and generate an output signal of discrimination between the two? This last question is at the center of what I have to say. I present evidence in that which follows that the answer is yes to the first and to the third questions; answers to the remainder are uncertain.

I chose for this study frequency discrimination in the somesthetic sense of flutter, for which stimuli are sinusoidal and thus perfectly periodic, leaving aside for the present the more general case of temporal order referred to before. I provide evidence that the sequential orders of nerve impulses in first-order afferents of the somatic afferent system innervating the hand, under drive by mechanical sinusoids, and the postcentral cortical neurons upon which they project, do transmit discriminable signals based upon the serial orders of impulse discharges, when the overall frequencies of neural activity are not discriminable.[12] I then illustrate how code changes in the populations of neuronal activity occur in the multinoded, multiply interconnected, distributed system that links the afferent input level, the sensory area of the hemisphere receiving the input signals, to the motor cortex of the opposite hemisphere, which controls the differential motor response.[13]

The Sense of Flutter Vibration

The low-frequency component of the compound somesthetic sense of flutter vibration is that faint, quivering sensation evoked when low-frequency mechanical sinusoids are delivered to the skin; for example, to the glabrous skin of the hand. This subjective quality of flutter is determined uniquely by the periodic nature of the adequate proximal stimuli, and the perfectly periodic trains of impulses evoked at stimulus frequencies in one particular set of primary afferent fibers, the quickly adapting Meissner afferents.[14] The quality of the sensation depends upon the temporal order in the relevant streams of neural impulses. The deep, penetrating hum of vibration evoked by higher stimulus frequencies, 50–400 Hz, depends uniquely upon similarly entrained activity set in motion in a different set of fibers, the Pacinian afferents.

The Nature of the Tasks

The tasks for our human and monkey subjects are outlined in FIGURE 1, and a drawing of a working monkey is shown in FIGURE 2. The detection task is simple, but that of frequency discrimination is not, as witness the experience of our human subjects and the 100+ days of training required for monkeys to learn the task and reach asymptotic limens. The subject in this latter task must do the following: (1) detect probe indentation of the skin of one hand and in response close a signal gate with the other hand; (2) identify the frequency of the base stimulus and store that information in some form of short-term memory; (3) identify the frequency of the comparison stimulus, compare it with the stored frequency of the first stimulus, and make a discrimination whether the two differ, and whether the second is higher or lower in frequency than the first; (4) hold that decision in memory for the full second of the comparison stimulus; absent that requirement for delay correct responses are made with reaction times of 400–450 ms after onset of the comparison stimulus; this hold requirement is a difficult part of the task for both humans and monkeys; (5) detect withdrawal of the probe from the skin at the end of the comparison stimulus; and (6) generate the arm trajectory to the correct target.

Primate Capacities for Detection and Discrimination in the Sense of Flutter Vibration

Monkeys and humans detect mechanical stimuli delivered to the glabrous skin of palm or fingers over a frequency range from 5 Hz to about 400 Hz. Thresholds are

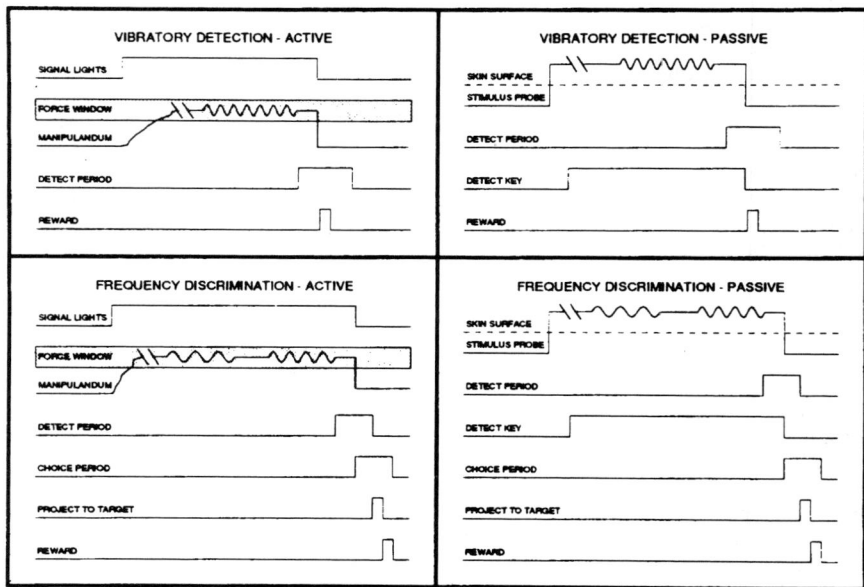

FIGURE 1. Schematic outline of the active and passive forms of the frequency discrimination tasks for monkeys and for humans. The force window and force cursor in the active task were indicated by visual signals, not shown. The sinusoidal signals shown are for illustrative purposes, and are not frequencies used. (From Mountcastle et al.[12] Reproduced by permission.)

nearly identical for the two primates; they are minimal at about 250 Hz [FIG. 3(a)]. Moreover, thresholds are similar whether stimuli are acquired by active manipulation of a vibrating object, or received passively in the manner of FIGURE 2, as shown in FIGURE 3(b). The two primates possess virtually identical capacities to discriminate between mechanical sinusoids of the same frequency but different amplitudes,[15] and between sinusoids of equal subjective magnitude but different frequencies.[12,15] Psychometric functions for humans working in the frequency discrimination task over the range from 20 Hz to 200 Hz are shown in FIGURE 4, and functions for monkeys and humans working in the range of flutter are shown for comparison in FIGURE 5. The Weber fractions for both intensity and frequency are about 10 percent.

Neural Signals in the Somatic Afferent Pathway Evoked by Flutter Stimuli[12,14–16]

The First-Order Input

Stimuli at the detection thresholds for monkeys (FIG. 3) evoke minimal but untuned activity in small sets of quickly adapting (Meissner) afferents innervating the glabrous skin of the hand. Monkeys and humans can detect sinusoidal stimuli at

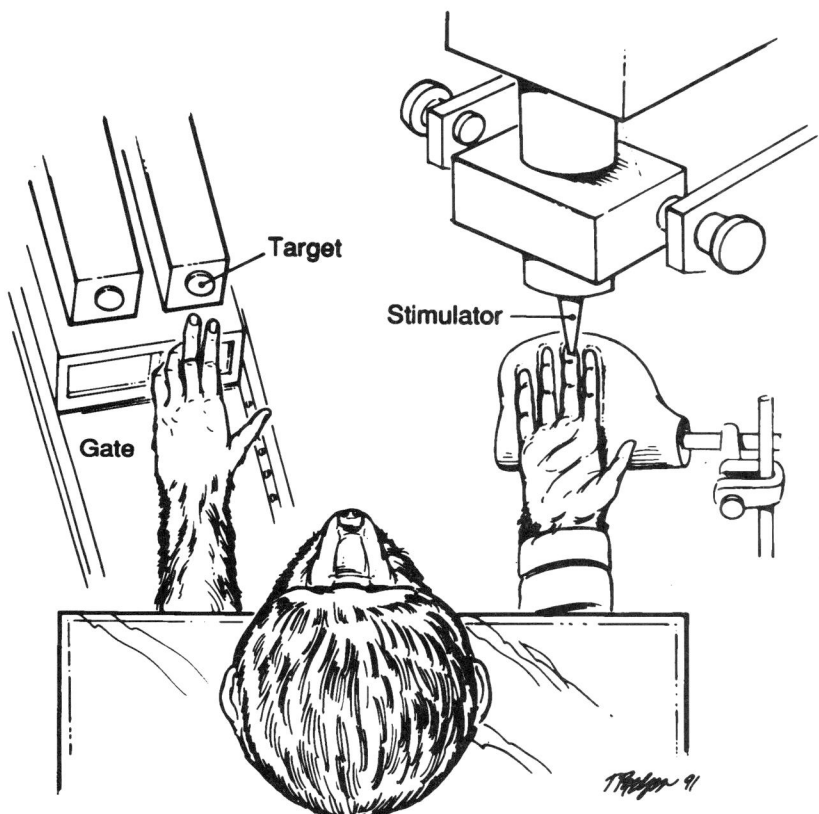

FIGURE 2. Drawing of a monkey working in the discrimination task. The right hand is fitted to a custom mold, and taped or glued in place. Stimuli are delivered via a probe with rounded, 2-mm-diameter tip. The two target switches are placed at comfortable arm's length for arm trajectories that differ by 20–30° in the horizontal dimension. (From Mountcastle et al.[13] Reproduced by permission.)

these magnitude levels, but cannot identify or discriminate between their frequencies. Increases in stimulus magnitudes by 6–8 dB reach the tuning thresholds, at which frequency discriminations can be made, and at which the Meissner afferents are entrained to discharge one impulse per cycle of sinusoidal stimuli, in the frequency range of flutter (5–50 Hz). The magnitude interval between absolute and tuning thresholds, in which frequency discriminations cannot be made, is called the *atonal interval*. A similar magnitude interval in which tones can be detected but frequencies not discriminated characterize the human performance in audition. Analyses of responses of a single QA fiber innervating the glabrous skin of the monkey hand are shown in FIGURE 6(a). The results of studies of this sort over a wide range of frequencies are shown for populations of both the Meissner and the Pacinian

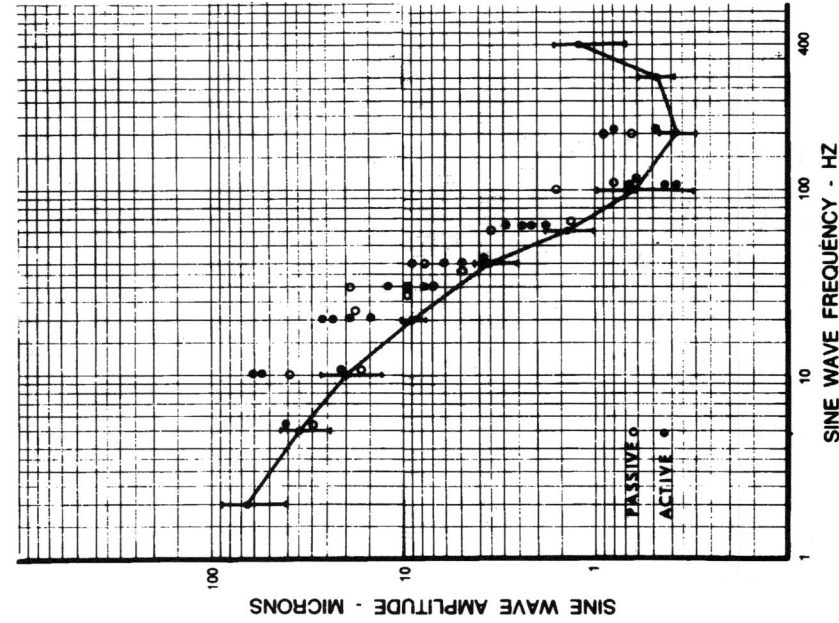
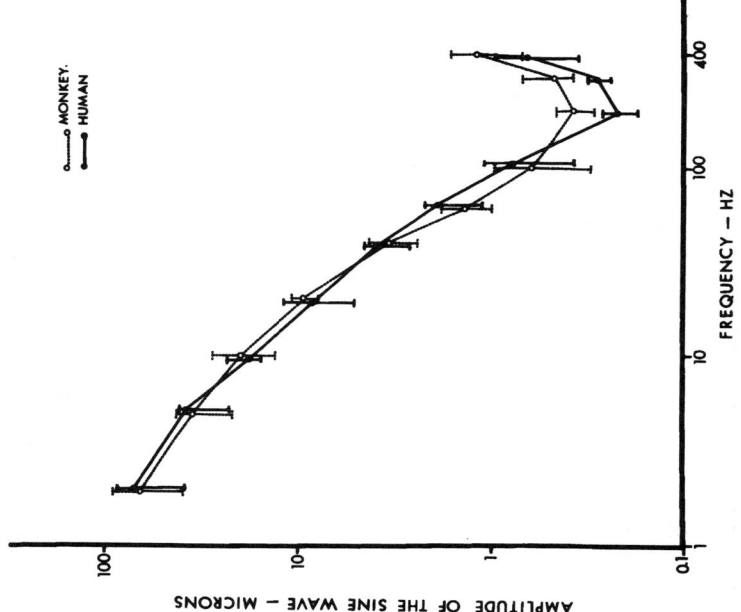

FIGURE 3. (a) Averaged frequency threshold functions for five human and six monkey subjects; values for each frequency obtained in the passive detection function outlined in FIGURE 1. Each point is the average 50 percent detection made at the indicated frequency; *vertical lines* are ±1 SE of means. (From Mountcastle et al.[14] Reproduced by permission.) (b) The standard monkey function repeated from (a). *Dots* are results of a later study comparing monkey detection capacity in the active (*filled*) and passive (*empty*) modes of the detection task of FIGURE 1. The task in the later study differs from the earlier in that subjects were required to withhold response for the full 1 s of the comparison stimulus, thus accounting for the slightly higher thresholds.

afferents in FIGURE 6(b). The most sensitive elements of the two sets of fibers outline the monkey detection function. The dual nature of the subjective sense of flutter vibration is matched by the two sets of peripheral afferent fibers relevant for it.

Further increases in stimulus magnitude recruit additional Meissner afferents to the active population engaged by the stimuli, and this spatial recruitment is linear in nature,[17] as is the subjective magnitude estimation in humans. However, over a wide range of increasing stimulus magnitudes there is no change in the periodic discharge in individual fibers, until stimuli at many times tuning thresholds evoke two or more impulses per stimulus cycle [see FIG. 6(a)]. This characteristic makes the somesthetic mode of flutter ideal for study of central neural discriminations based upon the temporal order in neural activity. This is so because when stimulus amplitudes are adjusted to equal subjective magnitudes, along the curves of FIGURE 3, one can be

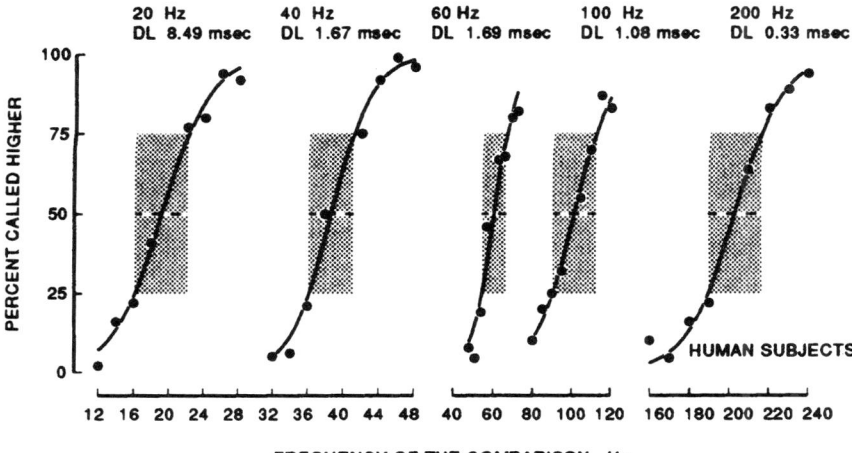

FIGURE 4. Psychometric functions for humans working in the passive frequency discrimination task of FIGURE 1. Averaged results are shown for three experienced male subjects, aged 25, 34, and 71 years, with base frequencies as shown. *Data points* are means of 60–70 trials each, and indicate percent of trials on which the comparison stimulus was identified as higher in frequency than the base. *Curves* are logistic functions fitted to those points. DLs calculated as one-half the interquartile ranges. Weber fractions in cycle lengths are 18, 7.5, 6.7, 10.2, 10.1, and 6.6 percent for base frequencies shown from 20 to 200 Hz, respectively. (From Mountcastle et al.[12] Reproduced by permission.)

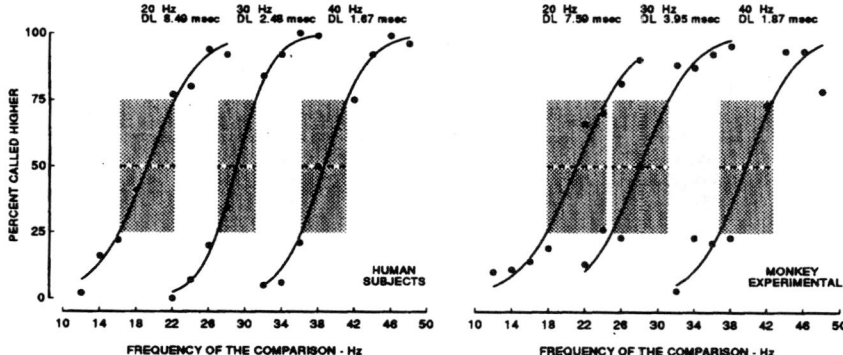

FIGURE 5. Comparison of capacities of human and monkey for frequency discriminations in the sense of flutter; passive test of FIGURE 1. (**a**) data for human subjects from FIGURE 4; (**b**) performance of a well-trained monkey in recording sessions. He performed slightly better in final pre-experimental sessions. (From Mountcastle et al.[12] Reproduced by permission.)

reasonably certain that two mechanical sinusoids between which discrimination is sought (e.g., 30 vs. 32 Hz), delivered sequentially in the pattern of FIGURE 1, evoke successively two tuned trains of impulses in the same single set of first-order fibers, and two successive periods of activity in the same set of postcentral neurons upon which those afferents project. Thus central discrimination must be based upon the serial order in which impulses are discharged and not upon a spatial shift in the cortical neural field.

Postcentral Cortical Signals

The Meissner afferents project over the lemniscal component of the somatic afferent system upon sets of neurons in areas 3b, 1, and 2 (somatic area I, SI) of the contralateral postcentral gyrus, neurons that possess functional properties similar to those of the Meissner afferents: they are cortical quickly adapting (QA) neurons. The convergence common in sensory systems occurs predominantly between neural elements serving one somesthetic mode, rather than between modes (e.g., not between QA and Pacinian elements for flutter and vibration, respectively). This iso-

---

FIGURE 6. (**a**) Interval and cycle histograms for responses of a Meissner quickly adapting afferent innervating the glabrous skin of a monkey's hand. Fiber isolated by microdissection of the median nerve in the forearm, in anesthetized monkey. Mechanical sinusoids of 1-s duration and 40 Hz superimposed upon 500-μm step indentation of the skin. Peak-to-peak amplitudes of the sine wave stimuli indicated on each histogram; 0.5-ms bins for the interval histograms, 0.25-ms bins for the cycle histograms. Stimuli weaker than those producing perfect tuning evoked impulses phase locked to the stimulus at nearly equal integral multiples of the stimulus period. This is the atonal interval.[21] (From Talbot et al.[21] Reproduced by permission). (**b**) Correlation between the monkey detection function and tuning thresholds for quickly adapting and pacinian afferents innervating the glabrous skin of the monkey hand. (From Mountcastle et al.[14] Reproduced by permission.)

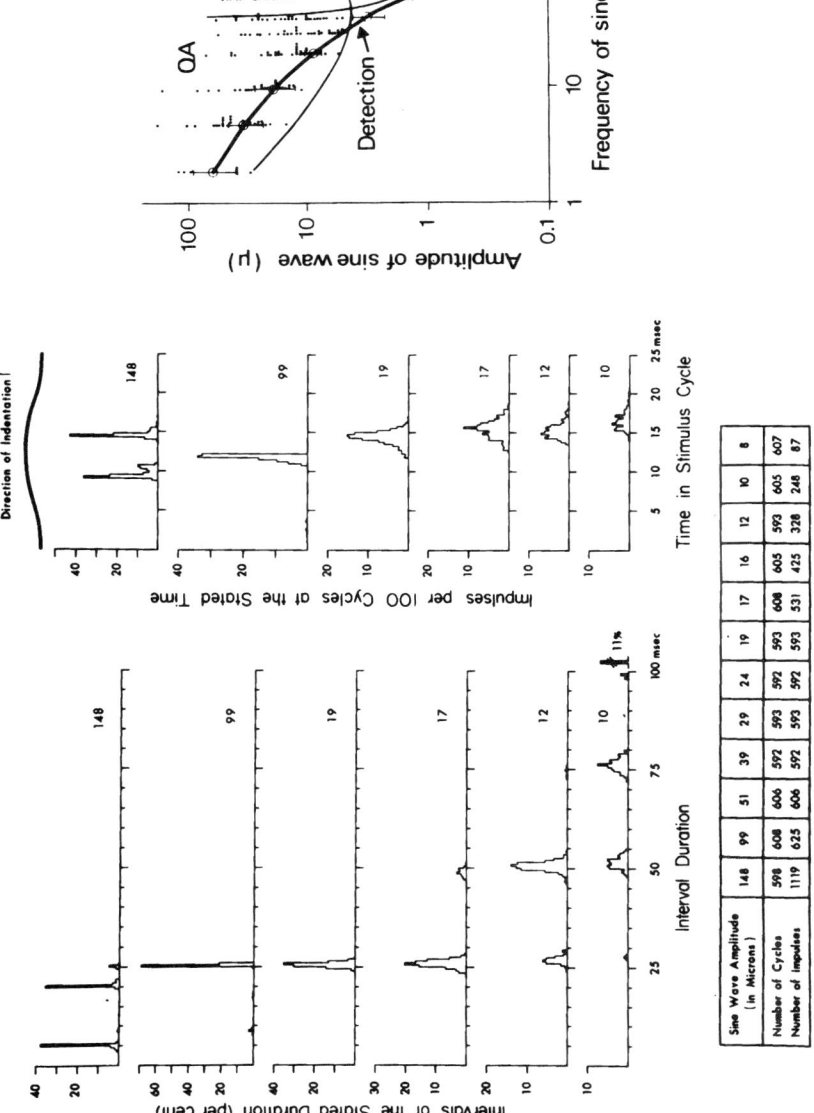

lation depends upon both a strict anatomical segregation and the powerful afferent or collateral inhibition operating at each synaptic level of the system. Indeed this isolation has been proved in a remarkable series of experiments carried out in Sweden, in which it was shown that isolated electrical stimulation of single identified Meissner afferent fibers in human peripheral nerves evoked a pure sense of flutter.[18–20] Moreover, changes in stimulus frequency elicited changes in the subjective sense of frequency. It seems certain that under these circumstances the several mechanoreceptive afferent channels innervating the glabrous skin of the hand secure isolated channels to the central perceptual mechanisms, through and beyond the primary sensory area in the postcentral gyrus.

The responses of a cortical quickly adapting neuron (a QA neuron) of a waking monkey driven by 20-Hz mechanical sinusoids at different magnitudes, delivered to the glabrous skin of his contralateral hand, are analyzed in FIGURE 7.[21] Several features are notable: (1) The cortical response at detection threshold (about 5 µ) is not periodically ordered, and in this range of stimulus magnitudes monkeys and humans can detect but not discriminate between the frequencies of mechanical sinusoids; (2) with increasing stimulus magnitudes there is an increasingly strong cyclic entrainment of the QA neuronal discharge, at stimulus frequency; (3) there is

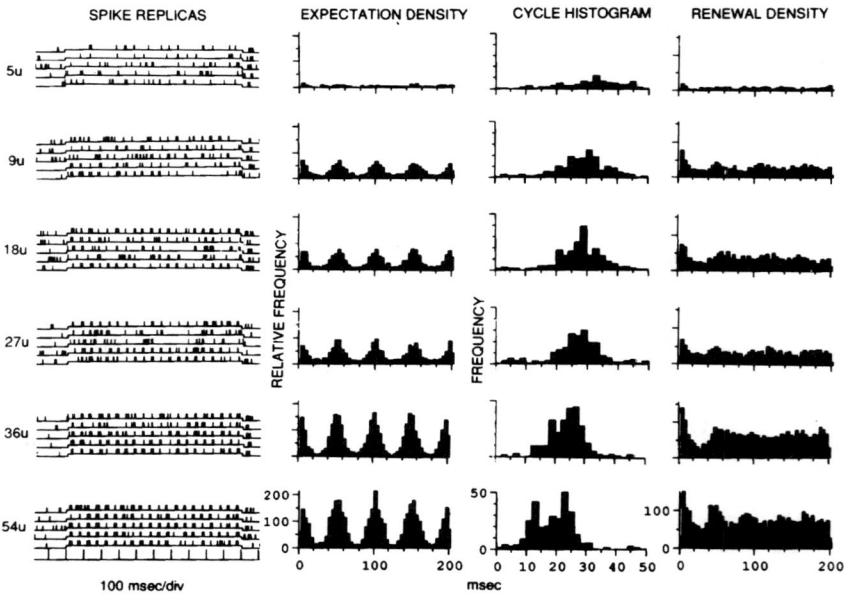

FIGURE 7. Results of a stimulus magnitude study of a QA neuron of the somesthetic cortex of a waking monkey working in the passive detection task of FIGURE 1. *Spike replicas* of responses evoked by stimuli of increasing sine wave peak-to-peak amplitude shown to the left. Each *line* represents a single trial, each *short upstroke* the instant of neuronal discharge. Behavioral detection threshold at 4–5-µ stimulus amplitude. The cycle histograms and the expectation density (autocorrelation) analyses show the strong periodic entrainment evoked by stimuli above threshold. The periodicity depends upon the sequential order in which the neuron discharged impulses, for it is destroyed after a random shuffle of impulse interval sequences, as shown the renewal density histograms, far right.

no sign of the perfect periodicity characteristic of first-order QA fibers activated by these stimuli; (4) the periodic signal is produced by a serial order code, the sequential order in which impulses occur (see expectation density analysis, column 2 of FIG. 7); and (5) this periodicity is destroyed by a random shuffle of that sequential order (see renewal density, column 4 of FIG. 7). Thus a change in the code for frequency has occurred between periphery and cortex, from the perfect periodicity at the first-order level in which each impulse interval signals stimulus cycle length, to a serial order code in which no impulse interval signals cycle length, which is embedded in the serial order. Such a change is predictable from the convergence at the intervening synaptic levels, between first-order fibers all periodically entrained, but with some phase shifts and interfiber jitter.

Postcentral Cortical Mechanisms in Frequency Discrimination

This knowledge of the primate capacity for frequency discrimination and of the relevant peripheral and cortical neural events evoked by flutter stimuli allowed us to plan and execute experiments in which discriminative behavior and the brain events evoked by the stimuli discriminated could be observed simultaneously (for technical details, see reference 12). Typical results obtained in such an experiment are given in FIGURE 8, for a neuron of area 3B of the postcentral gyrus of a monkey working in the "passive" task of FIGURE 1. Replicates of the neural impulses evoked by the pairs of flutter stimuli between which the animal discriminated are shown in columns 1 and 2; the psychometric function for his discrimination in this run is shown to the right. It is not possible, at least for me, to discriminate by visual inspection between sets of neural impulses evoked by stimuli between which the animal readily discriminated; for example, 20 versus 22 Hz, or 20 versus 18 Hz. Analyses for another neuron responding to similar sets of stimuli are shown in columns 1 and 2 of FIGURE 9. The expectation density analyses (the autocorrelation functions) shown in columns 3 and 4 reveal what can be discriminated, that is, the strong periodic entrainment with perfect matches between periods in the neuronal discharge and the cycle lengths of the stimuli evoking them. It is my proposition that it is these differences in period lengths that are the essential neural discriminanda for frequency discrimination in the sense of flutter. This periodicity depends upon the serial order in which impulses are discharged, for it is destroyed by a random shuffle of impulse intervals, as shown by the results of the renewal density analyses of column 5, FIGURE 9. Moreover, periodicity is due to the sequential order of predominantly short intervals, and not by a predominance of impulse intervals equal to or close to stimulus cycle lengths, as shown by the inset interval histograms of column 5, FIGURE 9. Other candidate discriminanda can be eliminated: (1) the pairs of discriminable stimuli evoke overall frequencies of discharge that cannot themselves be discriminated (FIG. 10); a simple "frequency code" will not suffice; (2) a spatial shift in the neural populations activated by the two stimuli cannot provide a discriminandum, for the two stimuli activate the same single population, as discussed earlier. How strong the power of these periodic neuronal signals is in the population of QA postcentral neurons is shown by the Fourier analyses of FIGURE 11.

LaMotte and I observed some years ago[22] that monkeys could no longer make frequency discriminations like those of FIGURE 5, after removal of the postcentral gyrus contralateral to the stimulated hand. I have recently confirmed that finding in a monkey with a much smaller lesion, one confined to the representation of the glabrous skin of the hand in areas 3b an 1 of the contralateral postcentral gyrus. It

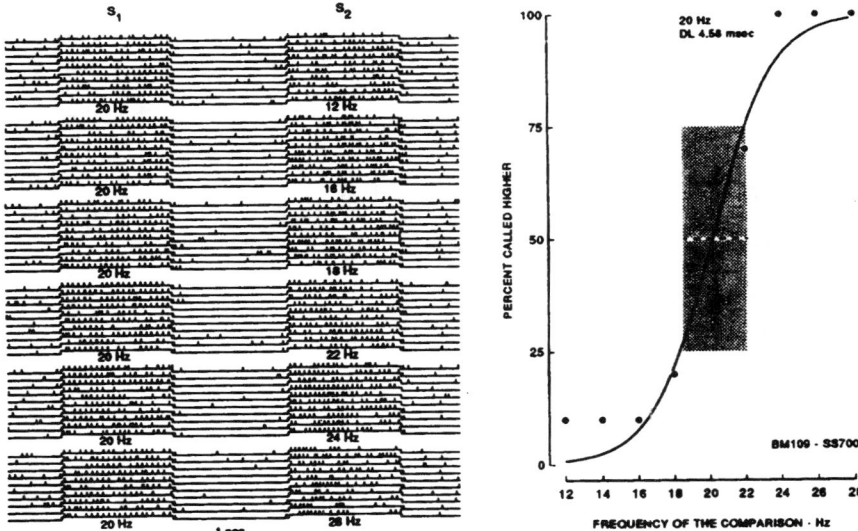

FIGURE 8. Data obtained as a monkey worked in the passive frequency discrimination task of FIGURE 1. The psychometric function to the **right** shows the behavioral performance: *data points* indicate percent of trials in which the comparison stimulus was identified as higher in frequency than that of the base stimuli, here 20 Hz; the *curve* is a logistic function fitted to those points. Weber fraction, 9 percent. The *spike replicas* to the **left** are those for a postcentral neuron observed simultaneously, and driven by the stimuli (delivered to the glabrous skin of the contralateral third finger) between which the animal discriminated. Each *line* represents a single trial, each *short upstroke* the instant of neuronal discharge. Steps indicate stimulus times. Expectation density analyses like that of FIGURE 9 and harmonic analyses showed periodic entrainment by both the base and the comparison stimuli. (From Mountcastle et al.[12] Reproduced by permission.)

was therefore surprising to observe for many hundreds of postcentral QA neurons, *no sign whatsoever of the discrimination operation itself.*[12] Indeed, we observed in many control experiments that postcentral QA neurons responded with exactly the same patterns to stimulus sequences as those of FIGURE 1, whether monkeys used those stimuli to make frequency discriminations, or whether the stimuli were delivered to monkeys in the alert but idling state, and thus were irrelevant for behavior. This was the case for the neuron of FIGURE 9.

We concluded from these observations that SI of the postcentral gyrus is the essential input funnel through which afferent signals initiate the chain of neural events leading to sensory discrimination and to generation of a differential output signal from the brain. However, our observations suggested that the discrimination operation is not local to that sensory cortex. This led to the general proposition I now wish to pursue, that *the discrimination operation is not localized in the usual sense, but is embedded in the dynamic operations in the multiply noded and multiply interconnected distributed system linking the postcentral somesthetic area of the sensory hemisphere with the precentral motor cortex of the opposite hemisphere.* It is in that motor cortex that population signals are generated that drive the arm in a

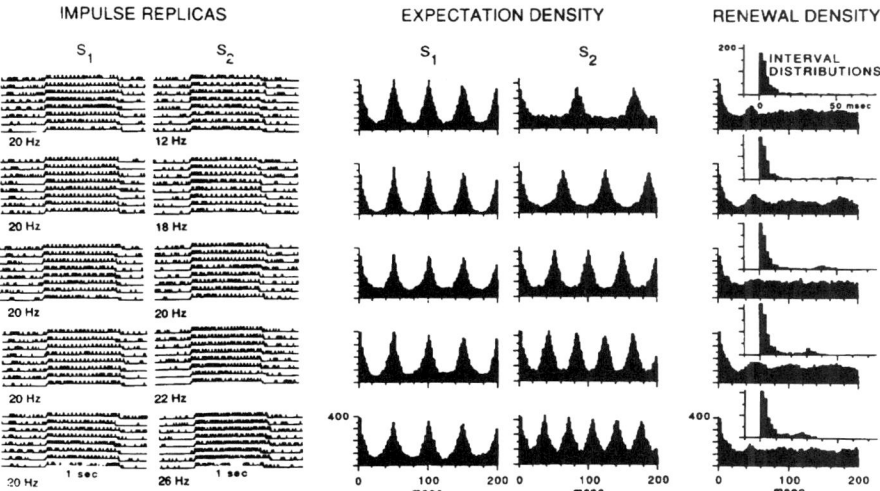

FIGURE 9. Results obtained in study of a neuron of area 1 of the postcentral gyrus of an alert monkey, not working in any task. Stimulus sequences as for the passive task of FIGURE 1, delivered to distal pad of contralateral second finger. **Columns 1 and 2,** *spike replicas* of responses evoked by the base (S1) and comparison (S2) stimuli; only 5 of the 8 classes presented are shown. Each *line* is record for a single trial, each *short upstroke* the instant of neuronal discharge. Expectation density histograms show the strong periodic entrainment of neural activity, with periods that match exactly the cycle lengths of the stimuli that evoked them, as shown by harmonic analyses, not illustrated. The renewal density histograms of **column 5** for the neural responses of **column 2** show that the periodic nature of the discharge depends upon the serial order in which impulses are discharged, for the periodicity is eliminated by a random shuffle of impulse interval sequences. The *inset histograms* of impulse interval distributions in **column 5** show that the periodicity is not due to the presence of large numbers of intervals at or near stimulus cycle lengths. (From Mountcastle et al.[12] Reproduced by permission.)

differential projection to one of two targets (FIG. 2). We then turned directly to a study of the precentral cortex of the motor hemisphere, that ipsilateral to the stimulated hand and contralateral to the projecting arm.

Selective Output Signals in the Motor Cortex Opposite the Responding Arm

We have recently completed a study of area 4 of the precentral motor cortex opposite the projecting arm, in monkeys as they worked in the "passive" task of FIGURE 1.[13] Eight hundred nineteen of the 1137 neurons studied were active in the task, 635 of them selectively so for one of the two arm projections. The majority of these (436/635 = 69 percent) discharged during the reaction and/or the movement times, in patterns well known from many earlier studies of the motor cortex in waking monkeys. The remaining 199 neurons displayed unusual properties. They began to discharge 200 to 300 ms after onset of the 1-s-duration comparison stimuli, and commonly reached peak rates of discharge before movement began. They were

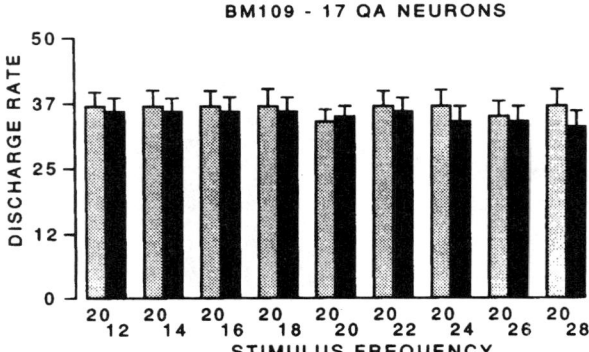

FIGURE 10. Results of rate analysis for 17 QA neurons of postcentral areas 3b/1 of a monkey as he worked in the passive frequency discrimination task of FIGURE 1. Discharge rates are expressed as impulses per second and are the averages of the mean discharge rates for each neuron, themselves the averages of 5–10 trials per class. *Shaded columns* plot discharge rates in responses evoked by the base stimuli (20 Hz for all classes); *solid columns* plot discharge rates of the responses to comparison stimuli. The evidence suggests that the capacity of monkeys to make frequency discriminations in the sense of flutter cannot be made on the basis of a neural rate code. (From Mountcastle et al.[12] Reproduced by permission.)

highly discriminative as regards the correct outcome of the discrimination operation. An example is given in FIGURE 12, for a neuron with an absolutely discriminative signal for stimuli lower in frequency than that of the base stimuli. The analysis to the right of FIGURE 12 shows what was true for all discriminative motor cortical neurons; that is, they are not periodically entrained by the sinusoidal stimuli. This contrasts with the strongly periodic entrainment of neurons of SI of the sensory hemisphere by these same stimuli.

Control experiments showed that area 4 neurons of the motor hemisphere were active only when stimuli were delivered to animals in the working state. Otherwise, these neurons were inactive, as shown by the histograms of FIGURE 13. The timing of the onset and peak rates of discharge for all the discriminative neurons studied in the motor cortex of a single hemisphere are shown in FIGURE 14. This illustrates the rising crescendo of discriminative activity in the motor cortex that signals the upcoming correct movement. A histogram of the onset times for all selective neurons studied in the motor cortex is given in FIGURE 15. The dual distribution is obvious. The mean lead time for the discriminative component of the population is 691 ± 18.4 ms (SEM) before the end of the 1-s comparison stimulus. That is, the afferent, sensory processing, discriminative operations, and interhemispheric transfer produce within 200 to 300 ms a surging discriminative signal in the motor cortex.

Discriminative neurons of the sort described were observed in all cellular layers throughout the broad expanse of the exposed portion of area 4; we did not explore the anterior bank of the central sulcus. Electromyogram (EMG) recordings showed that the muscles of the contralateral projecting arm were silent during the period of the comparison stimuli. Almost equal numbers of neurons discriminative for high- and low-frequency comparison stimuli were encountered.

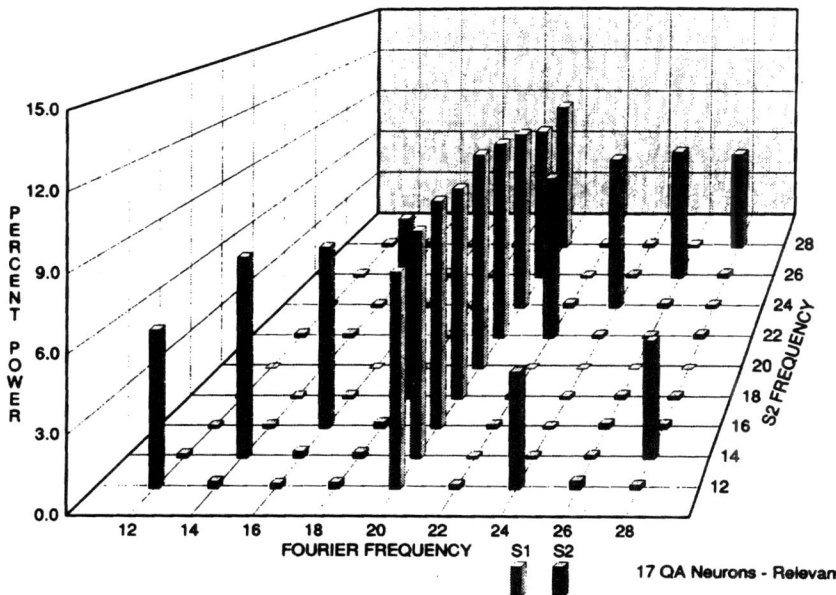

FIGURE 11. Results of spectral analysis of the responses of the 17 postcentral QA neurons of FIGURE 10. *Light columns* indicate the percent of total spectral power (range 1–500 Hz) evoked at the frequency of the base stimuli. *Dark columns* show percent total spectral power evoked at the frequencies of the comparison stimuli, from 12 to 28 Hz, in different rows. Power at second harmonics significant at comparison frequencies of 12 and 14 Hz, but not at others, did not interfere with frequency discrimination. The differences in the power spectra for the responses to base and comparison stimuli is regarded as the neural discriminandum at the level of the postcentral somesthetic cortex. (From Mountcastle et al.[12] Reproduced by permission.)

Studies of the Intervening Nodes of the System

I give here the results of some preliminary studies of intervening nodes in the sensory–motor distributed system, as follows.

1. Many QA neurons of area 2 of the somesthetic sensory cortex, which subtend multifingered receptive fields on the contralateral hand, are readily driven by the stimuli of the discrimination task. They are not activated in a selective manner, and rarely are periodically entrained by mechanical stimuli delivered to their receptive fields (only 11/89 neurons). Almost all area 2 QA neurons are selectively sensitive to the direction of stimulus motion across the skin.

2. Thirty of 129 neurons of area 2/5 of the postcentral gyrus of the motor hemisphere were active in the task. On these, 11 discharged in a discriminative way during the periods of the comparison stimuli without periodic entrainment, like many neurons of the motor cortex of the same hemisphere.

These neurons of area 2/5 do not respond to cutaneous stimuli directly, and of course have no receptive fields on the ipsilateral hand, even when active in the task.

3. Twenty-one of 35 neurons studied in area 6 of the motor hemisphere were active in task, and 12 of the 21 showed strongly discriminative discharges during comparison stimuli either higher or lower in frequency than that of the base stimuli.

Taken together, all our results lead to the hypothesis given earlier. Namely, that the discriminative operation is not local to any cortical area, but is embedded in the dynamic activity of the distributed system linking the sensory cortex of one hemisphere and the motor cortex of the other.

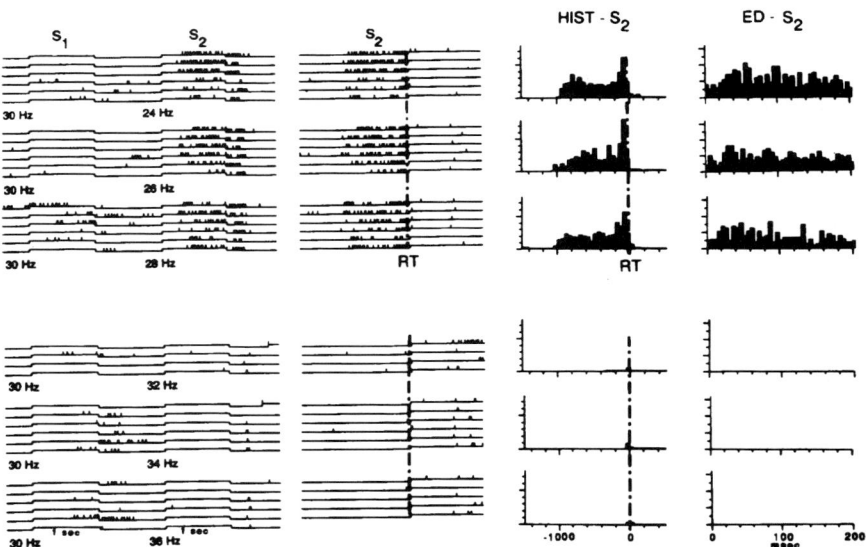

FIGURE 12. Results of study of a neuron of area 4 of the motor cortex ipsilateral to the stimulated hand and contralateral to the projecting arm, as a monkey worked in the passive discrimination task of FIGURE 1. Each *line* is a replica of a single trial, each *short upstroke* the instant of cell discharge. Trials with comparison stimuli of different frequencies were sequenced randomly. The *replicas* are oriented in time to the end of the comparison stimuli in the first columns to the left, and to the end of the reaction times (RT) in columns next right. Peristimulus time histograms for the latter are shown in the column next right (Histogram S2), and the same data are shown after the expectation density analysis in the column far right (ED S2). This neuron discharged selectively in an absolutely discriminative pattern for comparison stimuli lower in frequency than the base stimulus, ceased to discharge abruptly at the end of the RT, and was not periodically entrained by the stimuli. Ordinate scales: for frequency histograms, 50 impulses/s/large-scale division; for ED, 10 impulses/s/large-scale division. (From Mountcastle et al.[13] Reproduced by permission.)

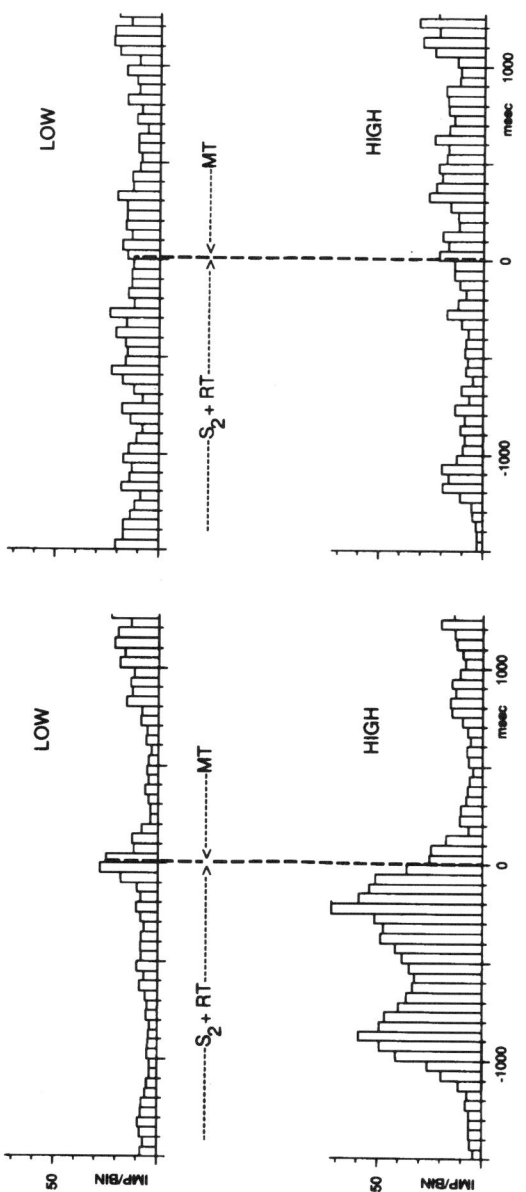

FIGURE 13. Results of study of a neuron of area 4 of the precentral gyrus of the motor hemisphere in a monkey working in the passive discrimination task of FIGURE 1, shown in (**a**) and (**b**) when the same patterns of stimuli were delivered to the alert but idling monkey. Peristimulus time histograms of the neuronal activity before, during, and after delivery of the comparison stimuli (S2), oriented to the end of the reaction time (RT), the start of the movement time (MT). The neuron was highly discriminative for comparison stimuli higher in frequency than the 20 Hz of the base stimulus, but did not discharge at a level significantly above background rates when stimuli were delivered in the nonworking state.

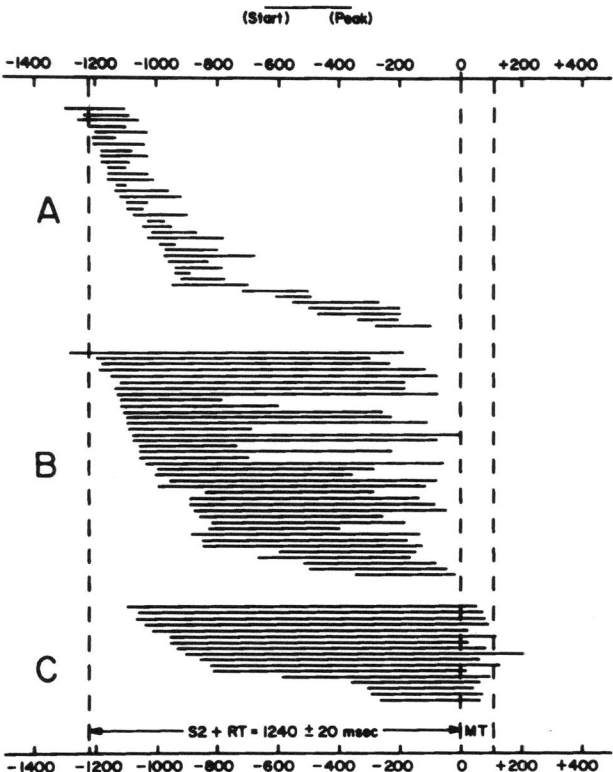

FIGURE 14. Time courses of the discharges of all discriminative neurons studied in area 4 of the precentral motor cortex of a single monkey, as he worked in the passive task of FIGURE 1. The *left end* of each line indicates onset of significant discharge, the *right end* the instant of peak frequency of discharge. Group A neurons discharged briefly, but different cells discharge at different delays after onset of the comparison stimuli. Neurons of groups B and C discharged continuously; C differed from B by reaching peak discharge during the movement time. The illustration shows the surging crescendo of discriminative neuronal population activity in the motor cortex ipsilateral to the stimulated hand during the discrimination task. That activity is regarded as the output to the motor cortex of the discrimination operations in the distributed system linking the sensory cortex of one hemisphere with the motor cortex of the other. (From Mountcastle et al.[12] Reproduced by permission.)

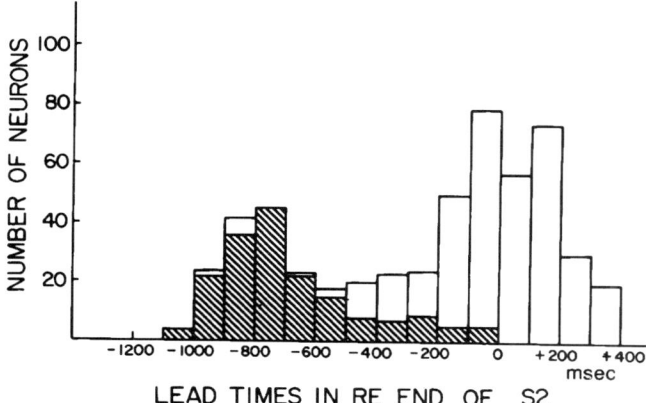

LEAD TIMES IN RE END OF S2

FIGURE 15. Histogram of the lead times for all selective neurons of the motor cortex studied in monkeys as they worked in the passive frequency discrimination task of FIGURE 1, plotted as times from significant onsets of discharge to the end of the comparison stimuli, S2. *Cross-hatching* indicates lead times for neurons discharging in a discriminative manner during the S2 period: mean lead times 691 ±18 ms (SEM); $ne = 180$. *Empty cells* indicate lead times for standard motor cortical neurons discharging selectively during the RT and/or the MT periods: mean lead times = 19 ±13 ms (SEM; $n = 356$. The latter group displayed the well-known behavior of motor cortical neurons during reaching of the contralateral hand to target. (From Mountcastle et al.[13] Reproduced by permission.)

DISCUSSION

Temporal Order Coding and Code Changes in the Distributed Sensory–Motor System

I define a neural code for a sensory system in a colloquial sense as a set of neural signals reflecting the physical characteristics of proximal peripheral stimuli, *and* that can be shown on other grounds to be used in perception and/or behavioral response. Such signals link the physical order of the world to the neural order of the brain.

For the sense of flutter, the mechanical sinusoids of the physical order are transformed and signaled to the brain by the perfectly periodic discharge in one particular set of peripheral fibers, the Meissner or quickly adapting afferents (QA), in a code in which inter-impulse intervals equal more or less exactly the cycle lengths of the sinusoidal peripheral stimuli. The code is more than that, however, for it is combined with the code of the labeled line, for periodic activity in the QA afferents evokes the sense of flutter whether driven by the natural physical stimuli or by direct electrical stimulation of single fibers in humans.[18–20] This last fact emphasizes that such labeled lines in the somesthetic afferent system can have, under some circumstances, isolated and private lines for the perceptual operation.

The nearly perfect periodic code in the QA afferent fibers is projected centrally over this private labeled line through the lemniscal component of the somatic afferent system to the QA neurons of the somesthetic cortex of the postcentral gyrus. There is a code change in that passage, however, for at the cortical level periodicity depends upon a serial order code, in which no individual intervals match the cycle lengths of the physical stimulus. This is easily predicted from the convergence between adjacent elements of the QA system, and some phase jitter between adjacent neural elements in the initial entrainment.

The evidence I presented previously makes a strong case for the conclusion that the neural discriminandum between physical stimuli of different frequencies is the difference in the period lengths of the powerfully entrained cortical QA activity. However, we have learned nothing of how a discrimination "apparatus," itself composed of neurons, could: (1) recognize and hold in a short-term memory the period lengths in the activity evoked by the base stimulus; (2) compare that length with the slightly different period lengths in the activity evoked in the same set of neural elements one second later by the comparison stimulus; and, (3) generate an output signal that discriminates between physical stimuli higher or lower in frequency than the base stimuli.

That discriminative signal is exactly what we have seen at the output level of the system in the precentral motor cortex of the contralateral—the motor—hemisphere. Here 30 percent of the cortical neurons differentially active during projected arm movements begin to discharge during one or the other of the set of comparison stimuli, either higher or lower in frequency than the base stimuli. This discriminative discharge begins within 200 ms after onset of the comparison stimuli and 800–1000 ms before movement begins. The signals are selective for that set of motor cortical neurons driving the contralateral area to the correct target. No periodicity has ever been observed in that discriminative signal. The seminal work of Georgopoulos and his colleagues[23,24] suggests that what is selected is that set of motor cortical neurons whose directional vectors sum to a population vector pointing in the direction of the correct projection movement.

The Distributed Processing System and Interhemispheric Transfer

The corpus callosum is necessary for the transfer of learned, complex tasks from one hemisphere to the other, both in monkeys[25–28] and in humans.[29] What is required for the task of FIGURE 1 is not transfer of the learned discrimination itself, but of an output signal from the discrimination operation adequate to bring to action a set of motor cortical neurons that will drive the arm to the correct target. The hand and finger representation zones of areas 3b, 1, and 2 of the somesthetic cortex are virtually free of connections to the other hemisphere.[30–32] Several pathways lead from the hand/finger area of SI to areas in both the parietal and frontal lobes of the brain, all of which are reciprocally connected with homologous areas of the opposite hemisphere (for review, see reference 33): (1) from SI posteriorly to area 5, and from 5 to 7b; (2) from areas 2, 5, and 7b forward to areas in the premotor cortex of the frontal lobe; (3) from SI to SII of the parietal lobe, both contra- and ipsilaterally.[24] The output from SI in the discriminative task is likely to activate all of these pathways, which suggests that more than one pathway may be open to the opposite hemisphere.

Studies of the remaining capacities for frequency discrimination in monkeys in the sense of flutter after cortical lesions are currently incomplete; the evidence available lends some support to the system concept.[22]

1. Lesions restricted to the input funnel for the task, SI of the sensory hemisphere, eliminate frequency discrimination. The remaining somesthetic areas

of the parietal lobe cannot sustain such a discrimination, even after extensive attempts at retraining.
2. Removal of the output funnel for the task, area 4 of the motor hemisphere, eliminates frequency discrimination: the animal cannot then generate accurate arm trajectories to correct targets.
3. Removal of all parietal areas behind the central sulcus in the motor hemisphere does not impair performance in the discrimination task. Thus the interhemispheric pathways between the two parietal lobes are not essential for success in the task. The inference is that after such a lesion transfer to the motor hemisphere occurs between areas of the premotor cortex, but this has not yet been tested in monkeys with lesions of the premotor cortex.

The tentative conclusion is that either the posterior or the premotor routes between hemispheres will suffice for transfer in the task. This idea fits with our preliminary observations that discriminative signals occur in the posterior parietal and premotor areas of the motor hemisphere, during execution of the task. Indeed, one characteristic of a distributed processing system is that information can flow through the system over more than one pathway.

REFERENCES

1. LASHLEY, K. S. 1951. The problem of serial order in behavior. *In* Cerebral Mechanisms in Behavior, L. A. Jeffress, Ed.: 112–136. Wiley. New York.
2. MOORE, G. P., D. H. PERKEL & J. P. SEGUNDO. 1966. Statistical analysis and functional interpretation of neuronal spike trains. Annu. Rev. Physiol. **28**: 493–522.
3. PERKEL, D. H. & T. H. BULLOCK. 1969. Neural coding. *In* Neurosciences Research Symposium Summaries, Vol. 3, F. O. Schmitt, T. Melnechuk, G. C. Quarton, and G. Adelman, Eds.: 405–528. MIT Press. Cambridge, Mass.
4. KLEMM, W. R. & C. J. SHERRY. 1981. Serial order in spike trains: What's it "trying to tell us"? Intern. J. Neuroscience **14**: 15–33.
5. ———. 1982. Do neurons process information by relative intervals in spike trains? Neurosci. Biobehav. Rev. **6**: 429–437.
6. BIALEK, W., F. RIEKE, R. R. DE RUYTER VAN STEVENICK & D. WARLAND. 1991. Reading a neural code. Science **252**: 1824–1827.
7. GERSTEIN, G. L. 1987. Information flow and state in cortical neural networks: Interpreting multi-neuron experiments. *In* Organization of Structure and Function in the Brain, W. Seelen, X. X. Leinhos, and G. Shaw, Eds. VCH Verlagsgesellshaft. Weinheim, Germany.
8. GERSTEIN, G. L., P. BEDENBAUGH & M. H. AERSTEN. 1989. Neuronal assemblies. IEEE Trans. Biomed. Eng. **BME-36**: 4–14.
9. GRAY, C. M., A. K. ENGEL, P. KONIG & W. SINGER. 1992. Mechanisms underlying the generation of neuronal oscillations in cat visual cortex. *In* Induced Rhythms in the Brain, E. Kosar and T. H. Bullock, Eds.: 29–46. Birkhauser. Boston.
10. ECKHORN, R., T. SCHANZE, M. BROSCH, W. SALEM & R. BAUER. 1992. Stimulus-specific synchronizations in cat visual cortex: Multiple microelectrode and correlation studies from several cortical areas. *In* Induced Rhythms in the Brain, E. Basar and T. H. Bullock, Eds.: 47–82. Birkhauser. Boston.
11. RICHMOND, B. J., L. M. OPTICAN, M. PODELL & H. SPITZER. 1987. Temporal encoding of two-dimensional patterns by single units in primate inferior temporal cortex. I. Response characteristics. J. Neurophysiol. **57**: 132–146.
12. MOUNTCASTLE, V. B., M. A. STEINMETZ & R. ROMO. 1990. Frequency discrimination in the sense of flutter: Psychophysical measurements correlated with postcentral events in behaving monkeys. J. Neurosci. **10**: 3031–3044.

13. MOUNTCASTLE, V. B., P. P. ATLURI & R. ROMO. 1992. Selective output discriminative signals in the motor cortex of waking monkeys. Cereb. Cortex **2:** 277–294.
14. MOUNTCASTLE, V. B., R. H. LAMOTTE & G. CARLI. 1972. Detection thresholds for stimuli in humans and monkeys: Comparison with threshold events in mechanoreceptive afferent nerve fibers. J. Neurophysiol. **35:** 122–136.
15. LAMOTTE, R. H. & V. B. MOUNTCASTLE. 1975. Capacities of humans and monkeys to discriminate between vibratory stimuli of different frequency and amplitude: A correlation between neural events and psychophysical measurements. J. Neurophysiol. **38:** 539–559.
16. MOUNTCASTLE, V. B., W. H. TALBOT, H. SAKATA & H. HYVARINEN. 1969. Cortical neuronal mechanisms studied in unanesthetized monkeys. Neuronal periodicity and frequency discrimination. J. Neurophysiol. **32:** 452–484.
17. JOHNSON, K. O. 1974. Reconstruction of population response to a vibratory stimulus in quickly adapting mechanoreceptive afferent fiber population innervating the glabrous skin of the monkey. J. Neurophysiol. **37:** 48–72.
18. TOREBJORK, H. E., W. SHADY & J. OCHOA. 1984. Sensory correlates of somatic afferent fibre activation. Hum. Neurobiol. **3:** 15–20.
19. TOREBJORK, H. E., A. B. VALLBO & J. L. OCHOA. 1987. Intraneural microstimulation in man. Its relation to specificity of tactile sensations. Brain **110:** 1509–1529.
20. VALLBO, A. B., K. A. OLSSON, K. G. WESTBERG & F. J. CLARK. 1984. Microstimulation of single tactile afferents from the human hand. Sensory attributes related to unit type and properties of receptive fields. Brain **107:** 727–749.
21. TALBOT, W. H., I. DARIAN-SMITH, H. H. KORNHUBER & V. B. MOUNTCASTLE. 1969. The sense of flutter-vibration: Comparison of the human capacity with response patterns of mechanoreceptive afferents from the monkey hand. J. Neurophysiol. **31:** 301–334.
22. LAMOTTE, R. H. & V. B. MOUNTCASTLE. 1979. Disorders of somesthesis following lesions of parietal lobe. J. Neurophysiol. **42:** 400–419.
23. GEORGOPOULOS, A. P. 1986. On reaching. Ann. Rev. Neurosci. **9:** 147–170.
24. GEORGOPOULOS, A. P., M. D. CRUTCHER & A. B. SCHWARTZ. 1989. Cognitive spatial-motor processes. 3. Motor cortical prediction of movement directions during an instructed delay period. Exp. Brain Res. **75:** 183–194.
25. EBNER, F. F. & R. E. MYERS. 1962. Corpus callosum and the interhemispheric transmission of tactual learning. J. Neurophysiol. **25:** 380–391.
26. HUNTER, M., G. ETTLINGER & J. J. MCCABE. 1975. Intermanual transfer in the monkey as a function of amount of callosal sparing. Brain Res. **93:** 223–240.
27. MANZONI, T., P. BARBARESI & F. CONTI. 1984. Callosal mechanism for the interhemispheric transfer of hand somatosensory information in the monkey. Behav. Brain Res. **11:** 155–170.
28. MANZONI, T., F. CONTI & M. FABRI. 1986. Callosal projections from area SII to SI in monkeys: Anatomical organization and comparison with association projections. J. Comp. Neurol. **252:** 245–263.
29. GAZZANIGA, M. S., J. E. BOGEN & R. W. SPERRY. 1963. Laterality effects in somesthesis following cerebral commissurotomy in man. Neuropsychologia **1:** 209–215.
30. JONES, E. G. & S. H. HENDRY. 1980. Distribution of callosal fibers around the hand representation in monkey somatic sensory cortex. Neurosci. Lett. **19:** 167–182.
31. KILLACKY, H. P., H. J. GOULD III, C. G. CUSICK, T. P. PONS & J. H. KAAS. 1983. The relation of corpus callosum connections to architectonic fields and body surface maps in sensorimotor cortex of new and old world monkeys. J. Comp. Neurol. **218:** 384–419.
32. SHANKS, M. F., R. C. PEARSON & T. P. S. POWELL. 1985. The callosal connexions of the primary sensory cortex in the monkey. Brain Res. **356:** 43–65.
33. JONES, E. G. 1984. Connectivity of the primate sensory-motor cortex. *In* Cerebral Cortex, Vol. 5, Sensory-Motor Areas and Aspects of Cortical Connectivity, E. G. Jones and A. Peters, Eds.: 113–175. Plenum. New York.

Temporal Processing in the Visual Brain

RALPH M. SIEGEL[a] AND HEATHER L. READ

Center for Molecular and Behavioral Neuroscience
Rutgers University
Newark, New Jersey 07102

INTRODUCTION

The dynamical aspects of brain function have once again become a focus of attention in the neuroscience community. Oscillations of many different frequencies in electrical or magnetic measurements from the brain have been proposed to be involved in a myriad of cortical and subcortical functions. However, this is not a novel concept. In the 1940s, and 1950s, researchers primarily utilizing the electroencephalogram had already spoken of the role of oscillation and temporal dynamics in various brain states.[1,2] These early brain scientists were stymied in their attempts to develop these ideas because both the technical and theoretical substrates for an attack on these issues were lacking.

In the 1980s and 1990s, the technical expertise has evolved through the methods of single-unit, local-field-potential, and multiple-site recording methods. The new techniques allow us to measure the activity of single neurons and small groups of neurons with fine temporal and spatial resolution. However, the theoretical approaches, with some notable exceptions,[3-6] are still mired in the 1950s. But now, an entire field of mathematics and physics has been developed that bears directly on how large numbers of neurons can interact both spatially and temporally. This field is called nonlinear dynamical theory—popularly known to the laity as chaos theory.[7] This theory explores the range of interactions and dynamics that may occur in systems composed of nonlinear elements. These interactions can range from a nothing (i.e., a system at rest) to oscillations to chaotic activity (i.e., activity that is irregular and apparently noisy in space and time, but actually is predictable). In this review, we present some examples of experimental and theoretical studies to demonstrate the possible application of nonlinear dynamical theory to neurons in the visual system.

EXPERIMENTAL SINGLE-UNIT RECORDING IN CAT VISUAL CORTEX

Typically, when a neuron in the primary visual cortex is studied, its response is averaged over multiple presentations of a visual stimulus. However, this practice

---

[a]To whom correspondence should be addressed.

ignores the fact that the projective neuron (i.e., the cell that receives input from active cells) can only process the input from a cell once. It is *not* able to repetitively sample the interspike intervals[b] from its neighbors. This objection is normally addressed by considering that the projective neuron receives input from a gaggle of neurons and that some simple averaging of the spatially disparate inputs occurs. Here we will take a different point of view. We will consider what can be gleaned from the individual interspike intervals. Then in the theoretical portion, we will ask what dynamical process or set of processes might give rise to these temporal patterns.

Nonlinear dynamical theory utilizes a graphical representation of time sequences of data called the phase plot. In this representation of the data, the activity of the system at some time is plotted as a function of the activity of the system some time later. Certain theorems[8] state that this plot actually allows a reconstruction of the entire dynamics of the system. This permits the construction of a mathematical entity called the Poincaré section of the data, which when "read" appropriately, specify the underlying dynamics. Unfortunately the interspike intervals are not continuous in time and some modification of this method is needed. Accordingly, we will construct an *interspike interval return map,* which is similar in concept to the phase plot, by plotting each interspike interval against the next one.

Single-unit recordings were made in the primary visual cortex of anesthetized, paralyzed cats[9] using standard methodology. The interspike intervals were collected with a temporal precision of 0.1 ms. The optimal orientation of a bar for each cell was determined, and then a rectangular bar was flashed on and off with the stimulus on for one-half the time at a fixed stimulus rate. Typically, when recording from the brain in this way, an audible monitor is used to "listen" to the occurrence of neural activity. Under these experimental conditions, one can hear patterns in the interspike intervals that sound like a cantering or galloping horse, suggesting the presence of a complex temporal dynamic.

We can use the interspike interval return map previously discussed to graphically display these patterns. FIGURE 1 demonstrates such a plot for a cat primary visual cortex neuron. The temporal patterns are revealed in this plot as clusters of dots; repetitive visual stimulation often results in such clusters in the return maps. In the absence of visual stimulation, spontaneous activity has no clusters in the interspike interval return map. Those clusters arising from stimulation have specific relationships with each other. One can discern particular orders and shapes in the interspike interval return map. The variation in the densities of the clusters by themselves may give us new information about how the temporal patterns arise.[10] In particular, there are some clusters that have unique asymmetric shapes. These asymmetries suggest that the neuronal output and intervening interspike intervals are not all phase locked to the sensory stimulus in a simple and linear fashion. This is an interesting phenomenon, as it reflects complex interactions between either (1) the sensory stimulus rhythm and the single neuron's output cycle, or (2) the sensory stimulus rhythm and the chain of events preceding the neuron's output.

What is the source of these complex interactions? Presumably the interspike interval, and their temporal pattern, arise from the summed synaptic input to the cell and represent some order in this input. This assumption can be explicitly tested by modeling the single neuron and examining the effect of different inputs.

---

[b]An interspike interval is the time between temporally successive spikes (or action potentials) recorded from a neuron.

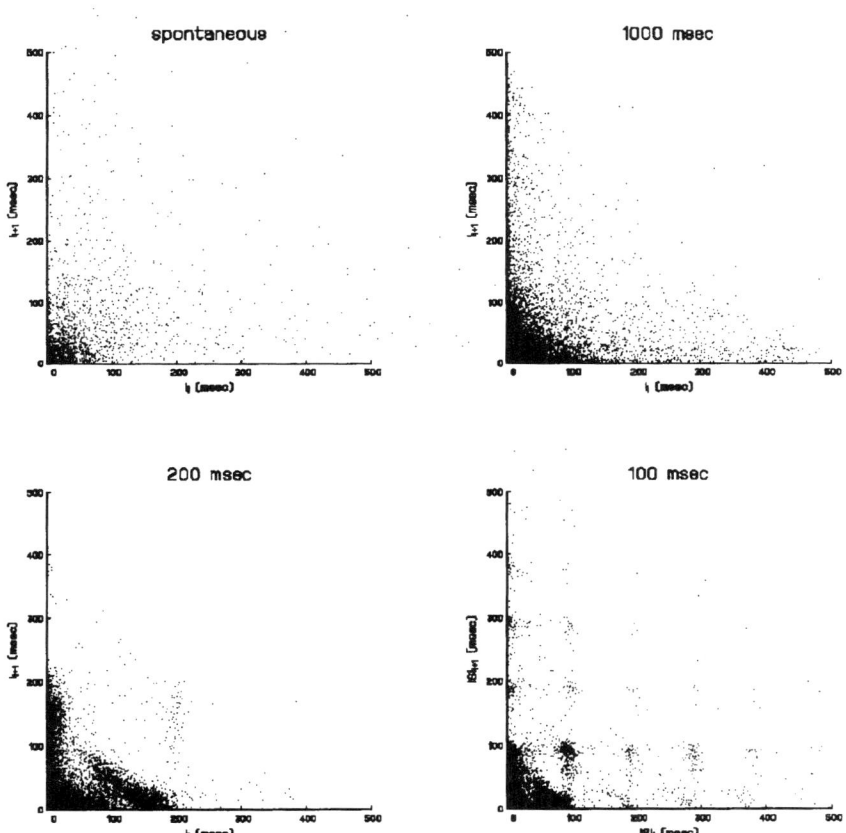

FIGURE 1. Interspike interval return maps for spontaneous and three different stimulus periods of a cat visual neuron. (**A**) Spontaneous activity. The spikes occur in bursts, but there is no pattern to the sequence of bursts that occur. (**B**) The 1000-ms stimulus period. At this stimulus period, there begins to be some structure in the return map. Most of the points fall below the line $I_{i+1} - I_i = T_s/2$, where T_s is the stimulus period. (**C**) The 200-ms stimulus period. The temporal pattern has become more complex; an attracting cluster at around (175, 25 ms) emerges. As well the cell begins to have longer interspike intervals at multiples of the stimulus period. (**D**) The 100-ms stimulus period. More complex patterns are seen. The attracting cluster stays at the same position in the graph relative to the driving period. Longer multiples of the driving period are seen. (From Siegel.[9] Reproduced by permission.)

A SIMPLE MODEL OF THE DYNAMICS OF A SINGLE NEURON

In 1965, Gerstein and Mandelbrot[3] proposed a simple model for the single neuron in which the membrane potential was subjected to a fluctuating input as a result of synaptic input. When the membrane potential reached threshold, a spike was deemed to occur and the membrane potential was reset back to its resting value. This model was quite good at replicating the interspike intervals of the spontaneously active neuron recorded *in vivo* (FIG. 2A). When subject to periodic input, the model responded with a somewhat periodic, yet irregular sequence of interspike intervals.[10] We examined the output of this model using the interspike interval return map and found that a simple periodic input was not sufficient to explain all the features in the interspike interval return map recorded *in vivo* in cat. Some of the clusters of dots in the data could be explained by a periodic input (FIG. 2B), but the more complex clusters were not.

We then tried using more complex input to the modeled neuron. We chose an input, not from a simple oscillator, but from a chaotic temporal sequence derived from the Duffing equation for a nonlinear pendulum. We found that under these conditions that a reasonable approximation to the *in vivo* data could be achieved (FIG. 2C). Since the chaotic input to the model represented the sum synaptic input to the actual neuron, these results raise the possibility that the summed synaptic input to the neuron *in vivo* is complex but ordered, and possibly chaotic. Thus by considering the fine temporal details in the recording study, we see evidence for the most complex type of activity described by nonlinear dynamical theory. The simpler dynamical behavior of an oscillation has been reported as strongly periodic local field potentials at 40 Hz by other groups in the visual cortex.[11] This finding provides us with evidence that the range of dynamics typically found in nonlinear dynamical systems are found in neural systems. But this leaves us no closer to the origins of these signals *in situ*. Therefore we have simply presented a phenomenon without presenting an explanation or cause. One possibility is that complex dynamics do not arise from extrinsic inputs, but arise from interaction between the neural elements.

SELF-ORGANIZING DYNAMICS IN A MODEL OF CORTEX

What process can give rise to these two types of dynamics (oscillation and putative chaos) reported in the primary visual cortex of the cat? The theoretical results summarized below suggest that these dynamics arise as a result of the neurons in the primary visual cortex interacting with each other and self-organizing into these temporal patterns.

In order to develop this idea further, we must present a model for collections of neurons—one that *could* in principle embody or evolve into some self-organized behavior. We will model a layer of neurons in the primary visual cortex of the cat. The neurons in layer II have a simple functional architecture which has been studied in detail by Gilbert and his colleagues.[12-14] These cells project laterally to neurons in two or three adjacent orientation columns that have matched orientation. The connections are excitatory. To simplify the model further, we will make all the synaptic connections equal in strength. Lastly, we will add a propagation delay between neurons that arises from the time needed for the action potential from one neuron to travel down the axon and cross the synaptic cleft. One thus has an array of these neurons in a line or on a surface. Each neuron was modeled by the

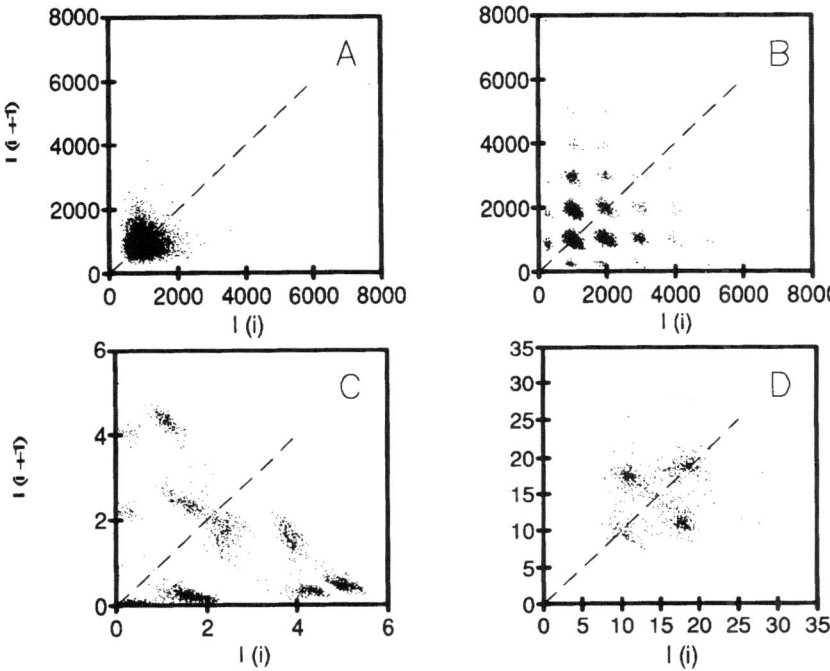

FIGURE 2. Interspike interval return maps for two different models of neural activity. Panels A–C are computed using the Gerstein–Mandelbrot integrate-and-fire model with a random walk to threshold. Panel **D** is derived from a collection of interconnected Hodgkin–Huxley neurons. (**A**) Interspike interval return map with spontaneous activity. Under these conditions there is no input to the model. (**B**) Periodic sinusoidal input to the model. Note the clusters of points similar to those seen in FIGURE 1D indicating a periodic component to the evoked activity. (**C**) Duffing oscillator input to the model. Note the asymmetry about $I_{i+1} = I_i$ in the interspike interval return map that is similar to that seen in the *in situ* neural data (FIG. 1C and 1D). These asymmetries were not found when a simple periodic input was presented to the model. This model suggests that the neuron in visual cortex is subject to a synaptic barrage that has both orderly and disorderly components (i.e., a putative chaotic input). The Duffing equation $\ddot{y}+a\dot{y}+y^3=c\sin(2\pi t)$ was integrated with fourth-order Runga-Kutta. (**D**) Interspike interval return map from a single neuron within a modeled collection of neurons. This map has similar asymmetries to those found *in situ*. This temporal sequence was taken from a set of twenty-five Hodgkin–Huxley neurons in a row. The pattern is nonrepeating. Each neuron was connected to five neighbors on each side. All synapses had the same value (0.140 mS/cm^2) and the time delay per neuron was 4.35 ms. (Panels A–C after Figure 3 of Siegel and Read.[10] Reproduced by permission.)

Hodgkin–Huxely equations to explicitly and realistically simulate the properties of neurons *in situ*.

Will this collection of neurons self-organize to generate some spatial–temporal patterns after being stimulated? Simulation of this collection of neurons with different settings of the two free parameters (synaptic strength and propagation delay) indicates that the answer to this question is emphatically "Yes!" Depending on these two parameters the network can either rapidly cease activity, oscillate, or behave in a seemingly random manner in space and time. This suggests that the population is self-organizing into the types of dynamics predicted by nonlinear dynamical theory (FIG. 3). The oscillatory behavior resembles standing waves in water. The more complex behaviors appear like patterns of spirals, rolls, or grids. They resemble those seen in other spatially distributed nonlinear systems. For example, the Belousov–Zhabotinsky reaction is a well-known dynamical system in which there is a spatial self-organization of the reaction product bromide into spirals and repeating grids on a surface.[15] The underlying mechanisms of the Belousov–Zhabotinsky reaction are well understood[16] and can be explained in terms of Universal mathematical laws of nonlinear dynamical theory. There are other such systems that have these behaviors, such as the slime mold and heat convection in a volume. The similarity in behavior between these other natural systems and the neural model is quite amazing when one considers that they are all *not* built of similar materials, nor do they have similar underlying chemical or physical substrates. This similarity in behavior result leads us to propose as a working hypothesis that the neural population is subject to the same mathematical constraints as are these other natural systems. These mathematical constraints are Universal in nature and serve to delimit the behavior of the neural system.[17]

But what of the firing pattern of the single cell embedded in the modeled neural population? FIGURE 2D shows the interspike interval from a single neuron of this

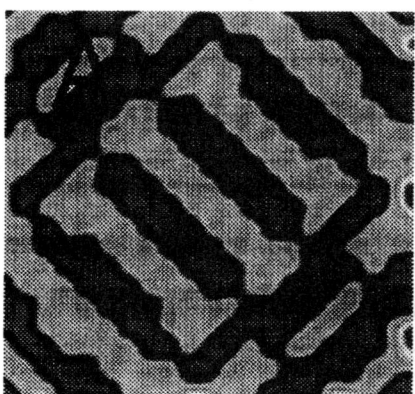 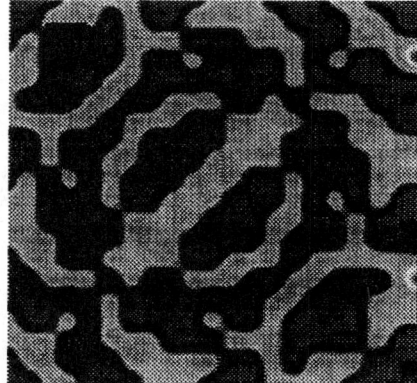

FIGURE 3. Spatial pattern of activity seen in a collection of neurons. (**A**) Rolls of activity, like waves in the ocean are seen. (**B**) More complex spatial patterns with geometric symmetry. These two simulations were run with different parameters. The view is looking down on a grid of four hundred neurons in a twenty-by-twenty grid. The darkness at each point in the image indicates the firing rate at each location. A clear geometrical pattern is seen that propagates in time and space. The implications of these patterns for visual hallucinations are discussed elsewhere.[18]

collection of neurons with parameter settings that lead to putatively chaotic activity. Note that we have replaced the terms "seemingly random" with "putatively chaotic." This is because we can now see clear order in the interspike intervals.

Let us now recall that the simple Gerstein and Mandelbrot model, taken in conjunction with the *in vivo* data, suggests that the input was chaotic in time. It is well nigh impossible to collect intracellular membrane potentials *in vivo* to test this theoretical prediction. But *in mechano* it is quite easy to compute the synaptic input to any cell. A return map of the modeled synaptic input shows clear order in terms of the looping structure (not illustrated). Such structures are also seen in known chaotic systems. This provides additional evidence that nonlinear dynamical behaviors are emerging in the population of neurons. The similarities are striking, more so because they emerged through a self-organizing process within the collection of neurons. There was nothing preprogrammed into this model that "forced" the system to behave in this way.

SUMMARY

In conclusion these three results taken together—the single-unit data, the Gerstein and Mandelbrot model, and the modeled collection of neurons—suggest that the analysis of the temporal dynamics of neural systems can be furthered by the application of nonlinear dynamical theory. Furthermore, it appears that the range of temporal dynamics possible in visual cortex is quite broad, encompassing simple oscillations and more complex, perhaps chaotic, dynamics. Lastly, it appears that there are powerful principles at work that are leading to the organized behavior of a population of neurons. We suggest that these principles are constrained not only by the biological properties of the nervous system, but by profound mathematical principles that have already been described in many physical nonlinear systems under the aegis of chaos theory. If such constraints exist, we may have available to us mathematical and physical constructs that will allow us to study, model, and predict the behaviors of large collections of neurons that ultimately underlie the neural functioning of the brain.

ACKNOWLEDGMENTS

We are grateful to Oliver Sacks and Charles Tresser for fruitful discussion of this work. We also thank Kathy Anderson for a critical reading of the manuscript.

REFERENCES

1. BEURLE, R. L. 1956. Properties of a mass of cells capable of regenerating pulses. Philos. Trans. R. Soc. London, Ser. B **240**: 55–94.
2. GASTAUT, H. 1954. Brain Mechanisms and Consciousness, H. H. Jasper, Ed.: 247–279. Blackwell. Oxford.
3. GERSTEIN, G. L. & M. MANDELBROT. 1964. Random walk models for the spike activity of a single neuron. Biophys. J. **4**: 41–68.
4. OPTICAN, L. M. & B. J. RICHMOND. 1987. Temporal encoding of two dimensional patterns by single units in primate inferior temporal cortex. III. Information theoretic analysis. J. Neurophysiol. **57**: 162–178.

5. RICHMOND, B. J. & L. M. OPTICAN. 1987. Temporal encoding of two dimensional patterns by single units in primate inferior temporal cortex. I. Response characteristics. J. Neurophysiol. **57:** 132–146.
6. SKARDA, C. A. & W. J. FREEMAN. 1987. How brains make chaos to make sense of the world. Behav. Brain Sci. **10:** 161–173.
7. CVITANOVIĆ, P. 1986. Universality in Chaos. Adam Hilgar. Bristol, England.
8. TAKENS, F. 1981. Geometry Symposium: Utrecht 1980, L. S. Young, Ed. Springer-Verlag. Berlin/New York.
9. SIEGEL, R. M. 1990. Non-linear dynamical system theory and primary visual cortical processing. Physica D **42:** 385–395.
10. SIEGEL, R. M. & H. L. READ. 1993. Models of temporal dynamics of visual processing. J. Stat. Phys. **70:** 297–308.
11. GRAY, C. M., A. K. ENGEL, P. KNIG & W. SINGER. 1990. Stimulus-dependent neuronal oscillations in cat visual cortex. I. Receptive field properties and feature dependence. Eur. J. Neurosci.
12. GILBERT, C. D. & T. N. WIESEL. 1985. Intrinsic connectivity and receptive field properties. Vis. Res. **25:** 365–374.
13. TS'O, D. Y., C. D. GILBERT & T. N. WIESEL. 1986. Relationships between horizontal interactions and functional architecture in cat striate cortex. J. Neurosci. **6:**1160–1170.
14. MCGUIRE, B. A., C. D. GILBERT & T. N. WIESEL. 1985. Ultrastructural characterization of long-range clustered horizontal connections in monkey striate cortex. Soc. Neurosci. Abstr. **11:** 17.
15. HUDSON, J. L. & J. C. MANKIN. 1981. Chaos in the Belousov-Zhabotinski reaction. J. Chem. Phys. **74:** 6171–6177.
16. PRIGOGINE, I. 1984. Order Out of Chaos. Bantam. New York.
17. FEIGENBAUM, M. J. 1980. Universal behavior in non-linear systems. Los Alamos Sci. **1:** 4–27.
18. SACKS, O. W. & R. M. SIEGEL. 1992. Migraine. O. W. Sacks, Ed. Univ. of California Press. Berkeley.

Spatiotemporal Motor Processing[a]

JAMES ASHE AND APOSTOLOS P. GEORGOPOULOS[b]

Brain Sciences Center
Veterans Affairs Medical Center
One Veterans Drive
Minneapolis, Minnesota 55417
and
Departments of Physiology and Neurology
University of Minnesota Medical School
Minneapolis, Minnesota 55455

INTRODUCTION

Many studies of motor function deal with essentially static aspects of motor control; for example, the representation of motor output in maps,[1] the encoding of motor parameters in the discharge of single cells,[2,3] and the effect of behavioral context on neuronal activity.[4] These questions do not encompass time as a crucial variable. However, actual motor performance always evolves in time. Moreover, daily activities, from eating to playing, depend critically on efficient processing of sensorimotor information. The devastating effect of a general slowness of this processing can be seen in patients with Parkinson's disease who, without medication, are quite incapacitated in practically all everyday activities. In this paper we focus on the spatiotemporal processing of sensory–motor information in the motor cortex and the basal ganglia within the context of simple motor acts, such as movements to a target, as well as in more complicated tasks, such as mental rotation. Moreover, we treat the temporal processing of movements more formally within the context of information theory.

BASAL GANGLIA

Perhaps the most striking example of abnormality in temporal sensory motor processing is seen in the clinical syndrome exhibited by patients with Parkinson's disease. Simple movements of the limb take much longer than normal, while simultaneous or sequential movements are particularly impaired.

Simple Limb Movements

A reduction in speed, of even the most simple movements, is one of the most consistent findings in Parkinson's disease.[5–8] Although movements of small amplitude are often completed within a time comparable to normal subjects, those of larger amplitude take significantly longer. Normal subjects tend to take the same amount of time to perform small- and large-amplitude movements, and achieve this by

---

[a]This research was supported by the U.S. Public Health Service under Grants NS17413 and PSMH48185.
[b]To whom correspondence should be addressed.

increasing the speed proportionately to the amplitude of the movement.[9] There are a number of possible explanations why this strategy is not used in Parkinson's disease.

(1) Patients with Parkinson's disease rely substantially on visual information, and when making movements to a visual target they perform "closed-loop," continually comparing the progress of the movement to the position of the target, thus reducing the speed.[7] In tasks where the movements are to be performed as quickly as possible, thus not allowing time for modification of motor output based on sensory feedback, Parkinson's disease patients are very inaccurate, particularly in larger movements. When there are no temporal restrictions, the large movements are performed as accurately as those of controls. In Parkinson's disease the speed–accuracy tradeoff is exaggerated, with the result that movements of a given accuracy take a longer time, and, conversely, attempted fast movements are very inaccurate.[7,10] In terms of the formulation of this question by Fitts,[11] Parkinson's disease patients show very low rates of information transmitted by their movements (see below).

(2) The initial burst of electromyographic (EMG) activity in agonist muscles is reduced, thus requiring a number of additional bursts of activity in order to reach the target.[9] Some scaling of initial agonist EMG activity does occur for movements of increasing amplitude, but the overall amount consistently falls short of that required to execute the movement at normal speed.[12] The temporal sequence and the duration of activation of agonist and antagonist muscles is normal.

(3) There is perhaps an impairment in planning or predicting upcoming motor behavior in Parkinson's disease. When given a set of visual and other sensory cues, normal subjects are able to predict or plan a movement in advance, so that it can then be generated quickly and accurately. Is it perhaps the inability to predict in this fashion in Parkinson's disease that leads to continuous monitoring of movement during its execution, with the inevitable slow or inaccurate result? This possibility has been tested in Parkinson's disease by assessing the ability to predict movement or motion in the external world. Patients were asked to follow a target that moved across a screen at a constant speed and changed directions in a predictable fashion. The target disappeared from the screen at certain points and the subjects had to move the cursor as if the target were still visible. Patients with Parkinson's disease had difficulty in accurately predicting the rate of target movement and the changes in direction.[13] However, it was found in other studies that Parkinson's disease patients were similar to controls in the continuous tracking of predictable or unpredictable target movement.[14,15]

The studies just reviewed have examined simple movements, usually across a single joint, and that they do not accurately reflect the disability experienced by patients is perhaps no surprise. We normally perform unconstrained movements using multiple joints in three-dimensional space. Abnormalities in the performance of simultaneous and sequential movements more closely reflect the degree of disability experienced by patients with Parkinson's disease, and underline the fact that deficits in the temporal processing of motor output is a major feature of the disease.

Simultaneous Movements

We normally perform simultaneous movements effectively and efficiently: indeed this is a normal part of our everyday motor repertoire. When driving a car, for example, it is vital to be able to engage the clutch with the left leg while moving the gear stick with the right hand. This ability to perform simultaneous movements is impaired in Parkinson's disease, and can lead to interference between two simultaneous tasks, so that the time taken to perform each task increases compared to the time for each task performed separately. In some cases the interference is such that one task stops completely. Schwab et al.[16] had patients draw with the nondominant hand while squeezing a bulb with the other hand, and found that the patients resisted doing the tasks simultaneously. In another study[17] patients were asked to press a counter with one hand while using a tweezers to pick up beads with the other; in this case, the patients avoided the counter press and concentrated on the beads. More recently Benecke et al.[18] have studied patients with Parkinson's disease, using tasks of equal complexity (elbow flexion, squeezing of an isometric force transducer, and finger flexion) executed by the same or different arms. There was an increase in movement time during the simultaneous performance of any two tasks, and this was most marked when the two tasks were combined in the same arm.

Sequential Movements

Many of our movements are part of a movement sequence, such as the sequential movements required to rise from a sitting position. In fact very few of our movements occur in isolation. These movement sequences, which are performed "automatically" by most people, cause great difficulty for patients with Parkinson's disease. The possible reasons for this were examined by Benecke et al.[19] in an experiment where patients with Parkinson's disease were required to perform three simple movements sequentially in various combinations. The interval between movements in the sequence was twice that seen in controls. The separate movements within a sequence were executed more slowly than when performed in isolation. The problem with sequential movements in Parkinson's disease is threefold: (1) the component movements are slower than normal when performed in isolation, (2) within a movement sequence the time taken to perform each component is increased, and (3) the time interval between each component in the sequence is also increased.

Neural Studies

Most neurons in the basal ganglia neurons change activity after the onset of EMG activity,[3,20–22] and have probably little to do with the initiation of movement in reaction-time (RT) tasks. Georgopoulos et al.[3] studied the relations between neural activity in the globus pallidus and the subthalamic nucleus, and parameters of movement in a task constrained to one dimension but allowing movements of different amplitudes in two directions. Significant relations were found for the direction, amplitude, and peak velocity of the movement. For movements in a particular direction, the discharge of many cells was related in a linear fashion to the amplitude of the movement. In these cases, given the rate of cell discharge, it would be possible to predict the amplitude of the movement. This relation was most significant during the movement, but was also evident in the discharge rate of the cells during 100 ms immediately prior to the movement. It appears that there was a gain in information after the beginning of the movement, resulting in a greater number of cells having a relation to movement amplitude. This relation of neuronal activity in the basal ganglia to the amplitude of movement is somehow the positive image of the negative condition in Parkinson's disease, namely the inability to produce large movements in a single step.

MOTOR CORTEX

Cells in the motor cortex typically change activity well before the beginning of the movement. Therefore, this structure, together with the cerebellum,[23] is involved in the initiation of movement in RT tasks. Studies of motor cortical cell activity during two- or three-dimensional reaching movements have shown a clear relation to the direction of movement in space,[2,24] and less so to its amplitude.[25-29]

Coding of Directional Information

The investigation of the relations of neural activity to direction is complicated by the fact that direction is not a linear variable but a closed circular (or spherical) variable. There are basically two ways to represent direction: one is to allocate specific cells to represent specific directions, and the other is to represent direction in an ensemble of cells. In the first case, reaching in the intended direction would be initiated by recruiting cells possessing the appropriate directionality, whereas in the second case the whole ensemble would be engaged in such a way that direction would be represented unambiguously in the ensemble. The results of experimental studies[2,24] proved the second idea to be correct. Indeed, most cells are active with movements in different directions, which means that for a movement in a particular direction a whole neuronal population is engaged; therefore, the direction of an intended movement is represented in the population. The question then is what is the nature of this representation and whether it is unambiguous and operationally useful.

A clue for the solution of this problem came from the directional tuning function of single-cell activity. This function has three basic characteristics: (a) it is broad, which means that cell activity varies throughout the range of directions, in both two-dimensional and three-dimensional space; (b) it is orderly and can be described well by a cosine function,[2,24] and (c) it is symmetric and unimodal, which means that there is a direction for which cell activity will be highest (the cell's "preferred direction"); the preferred directions differ for different cells and range throughout the whole directional continuum.[24] It follows from these characteristics of the directional tuning curve that, except at the peak, the directional information provided by cell activity is ambiguous, for the same discharge rate can correspond to two different directions.

The broad directional tuning of single-cell activity indicates that a given cell participates in movements of various directions and that, conversely, a movement in a particular direction will involve the activation of a whole population of cells: how, then, is the direction of reaching represented in a unique fashion in a population of neurons each of which is directionally broadly tuned? An unambiguous population code was proposed[30-32] that regarded the motor cortical command for the direction of reaching as an ensemble of vectors. Each vector represents the contribution of a directionally tuned cell. A particular vector points in the cell's preferred direction and has length proportional to the change in cell activity associated with a particular movement direction: then the vector sum of these weighted cell vectors (the "neuronal population vector") points at or near the direction of the movement.[30-32] Therefore, information concerning the direction of movement can be unambiguously obtained from the neuronal ensemble. This provides a tool with which to monitor the processing of directional information in time, that is, while the movement is intended.

Temporal Processing of Directional Information

There are several aspects of intending a movement: (a) The commonest case is when a movement is produced as soon as a stimulus appears. Under these circumstances there is a time interval between the occurrence of the stimulus and the beginning of the movement that is the traditional RT. The RT then can be regarded as a time during which the movement is *intended*. (b) In other cases a delay can be imposed so that the movement will be initiated after a period of waiting, while the stimulus is still present. These *instructed delay paradigms* probe further the representation of intended movements, in the sense that there is not an immediate motor output while the representation is being kept active. (c) In some cases of delayed movement tasks, the movements are produced on the basis of information kept in *memory*. The difference between these and the instructed delay task is that now the stimulus defining the direction of the movement is turned off after a short period of presentation and the movement is triggered after a delay by a separate "go" signal. Thus information concerning the intended movement has to be retained during the memorized delay.

In all three cases the representation of information about the intended movement can be studied under different conditions that impose different constraints on the system. It would be interesting to know whether this representation could be identified and visualized during the RT, the instructed delay, and the memorized delay periods. Since the information assumed to be represented is about direction, the neuronal population vector could be a useful tool by which to identify this representation. For that purpose we computed the population vector every 20 ms (a) during the RT,[32,33] (b) during an instructed delay period,[34] and (c) during a memorized delay period.[35] The results were clear: in all these cases the population vector pointed in the direction of the intended movement during the cited time periods. These findings (a) underscore the usefulness of the population vector analysis as a tool for visualizing representations of the intended movement, and (b) show that in the presence or absence of an immediate motor output, as well as when the directional information has to be kept in memory, the direction of the intended movement is represented in a dynamic form at the ensemble level. These results also document the involvement of the motor cortex in the representation of intended movements under various behavioral conditions.

Spatiotemporal Processing in a Directional Transformation

In the delayed-movement tasks previously described, the movement to be made is unequivocally defined in the sense that its direction is determined by the location of a stimulus relative to the starting point. In that situation the visual information concerning direction is used to generate the appropriate motor command to implement a movement in that direction; truly, this movement direction has to be generated and kept available during the delay period, but it is defined from the beginning; therefore, the direction of the intended movement is the same throughout the various times previously considered. A very different situation was created in an experiment[36] in which the direction of the movement to be made had to be determined freshly at every trial according to a certain rule, namely that the movement direction be at a clockwise (CW) angle from the stimulus direction. This experiment takes us away from the idea of a *fixed* motor intention: instead, this intention has now to be derived as the solution to the problem. Subjects performed eight sets of twenty consecutive trials each; one set for moving in the stimulus direction and seven for moving in directions at an angle from it. The angles were 5°, 10°, 15°, 35°, 70°, 105°, and 140°. The direction of the movement in two-dimensional space and the RT were measured. The major finding was that the RT increased as a linear function of the amplitude of the angle; the slope of the line was (2.37 ms/degree). This finding suggested that performance in the task may involve a mental rotation of the imagined movement vector about its origin. The rotation would begin from the stimulus direction and end when the required angle was judged to have been reached; in addition, corrections of this angle at the end of the rotation could be made; the slope of 2.37 ms/degree observed then would correspond to a rotation rate of 422 degrees/s.

The neural mechanisms underlying the process of mental rotation in the movement domain were investigated by training monkeys to perform a task in which they made a movement in a direction 90° counterclockwise (CCW) from a stimulus direction. We supposed that if a mental rotation of an imagined vector was taking place, the neuronal population vector could reveal it. Indeed, the population vector rotated during the RT from the stimulus to the movement direction through the 90° CCW angle.[37,38] Interestingly, the rotation rates (direction of population vector versus time) observed[38] were very similar to the rates (increase in RT versus angle) observed in the human studies.[36] Thus, the dynamic processing of a directional transformation was successfully visualized using the neuronal population vector analysis. The crucial aspect of this analysis is the consideration of neuronal populations as the meaningful level of synthesis of motor cortical events.

INFORMATION THEORETICAL ANALYSIS OF TEMPORAL MOTOR PROCESSING

When a pointing movement to a target has to be made, there usually intervenes a RT of approximately one-third of a second during which the movement is planned and its initiation implemented. The time from the onset until the end of the movement is the movement time that varies with the amplitude of the movement and the accuracy of the target.[11] Both of these times, then, reflect processing loads and can be used to derive rates of processing, given that these loads can be quantified. An accurate and convenient way is to quantify processing loads within the context of information theory. For targeted movements, Fitts[11] defined the processing load (I_d, index of difficulty) in bits, as

$$I_d = \log_2 \frac{2A}{W}, \qquad (1)$$

where W is the diameter of the target window (target accuracy) and A is the amplitude of the movement. The *rate* of information processing (I_p, index of performance) is in bits/second:

$$I_p = \frac{1}{T} \log_2 \frac{2A}{W}, \qquad (2)$$

where T is the movement time.

Rate of Information Processing in Reaching Tasks

Reaching movements have been studied in various tasks. With respect to the movement itself, these tasks can be distinguished between those that allowed unconstrained, free reaching in three dimensions, and those in which the reaching movement was constrained in one or two dimensions. Since constraining the movement is likely to have an effect on information processing, we discuss these tasks separately below.

Unconstrained Three-dimensional Reaching Movements

In a three-dimensional free-reaching task[24] monkeys made movements of amplitude $A = 12.5$ cm to visual targets of width $W = 1.6$ cm. Under these conditions the I_d was 3.97 bits, obtained by substitution of the preceding values in (**1**). The average movement time was 431 ms, which yields an I_p of 9.2 bits/s [from (**2**)]. It is noteworthy that this value is the same as that obtained in a previous three-dimensional reaching experiment (unpublished observations from Mountcastle et al.[39]). In that experiment monkeys had to reach to a target in front of them; first they depressed a key and when the target dimmed, they released the key and hit the target. The target was stationary or was moving at 12 or 21°/s when it dimmed. The I_p calculated from that experiment was 9.2 bits/s for the stationary target, and 8.3 and 8.4 bits/s for the 12 and 21°/s target motion, respectively. Thus these values of 8–9 bits/s are well established for three-dimensional reaching tasks.

In a different experiment, Sanes[10] studied normal human subjects and subjects with Parkinson's disease during repetitive movements between two targets. There was a consistent reduction in the rate of information processing in the parkinsonian group. In the case with the most pronounced difference in which movements of 32 cm were made between targets of 0.5 cm width, the I_d was 7 bits. The average movement time for this condition was 764 and 1118 ms, for the normal and parkinsonian subjects, respectively (estimated from data in [10, fig. 3]). This yields an I_p of 9.2 bits/s in the normal group and 6.3 bits/s in the parkinsonian group. The normal I_p is again the same as that obtained from monkeys in three-dimensional reaching tasks, but the parkinsonian I_p is much lower, by almost 3 bits. This attests in a formal way to the major defect in Parkinson's disease, namely the reduction in the rate of spatiotemporal motor processing.

Constrained Reaching Movements

Two-dimensional Movements: In a two-dimensional reaching task[40] monkeys and normal human subjects moved an articulated manipulandum in various directions to visual targets on a planar working surface. They first held the manipulandum in the center of the plane and then moved to radially arranged targets in a reaction-time task. The average I_p was 7.25 bits/s and was very similar in monkeys and human subjects.[40] This value is lower than that of 9.2 bits/s obtained for unconstrained movements (see earlier). This reduction probably reflects the constraint imposed on the two-dimensional movements.

One-dimensional Movements: Monkeys were trained to move a very low friction manipulandum along one dimension in response to a visual target.[3] The display consisted of two rows of 128 light-emitting diodes (LEDs). The two rows were placed one below the other, and the distance between adjacent LEDs in a row was 2.54 mm. The upper row indicated the target of the movement, whereas the lower indicated the current position of the manipulandum. The monkey had to move the manipulandum so that the lower (feedback) LED would be aligned to the upper (target) LED in a reaction-time task. Movements of three amplitudes (2.5, 6.25, and 10 cm) were performed. We calculated the I_p for the largest movements that were also the fastest. For these data (unpublished observations from Georgopoulos *et al.*[3]), A and W were 10 cm and 0.676 cm, respectively, and the average movement time was 770 ms; therefore, $I_d = 4.89$ bits and $I_p = 6.99$ bits/s.

This task was performed during recordings of single-cell activity in the basal ganglia of behaving monkeys.[3] The neural rate of movement information processing was estimated as follows: (a) For a given cell, the mean and standard deviation (SD) of the discharge rate during the movement time was calculated from 15 trials of movements made for each of the three amplitudes, as mentioned earlier. (b) A linear regression analysis was performed to determine the relations between the discharge rate and the amplitude of movement. It was found that for a number of cells a statistically significant relation existed of the following form:

$$D = K + Ba, \tag{3}$$

from which

$$A = \frac{D - K}{b}, \tag{4}$$

where D is the frequency of discharge, K is a constant, b is a regression coefficient, and A is the movement amplitude. (c) The W' predicted by a single cell's discharge was estimated for the 10-cm movement from the difference

$$W' = A_{high} - A_{low}, \tag{5}$$

where A_{high} and A_{low} are the predicted movement amplitudes obtained from (4) when D is substituted by the corresponding mean ±SD; that is, by a high and low discharge rate. Then, the I_d and I_p were calculated from those values; the average movement time was also available. Ten cases of cells recorded in the internal segment of the globus pallidus were analyzed; these cells had statistically significant relations to movement amplitude [(3)]. The mean (±SD) I_p was 1.57±0.83 bits/s. This value is appreciably lower than the I_p of 6.99 bits/s transmitted behaviorally by the movement (see earlier). Similarly low values were obtained for cells recorded in the external segment of the globus pallidus and the subthalamic nucleus. These results indicate that single cells do not carry enough information to fully account for the behavioral performance. This is not surprising, for the motor performance is the result of processing by the whole neuronal ensemble that should carry, as an ensemble, the requisite information. Indeed, this has been shown to be the case for the ensemble coding of the direction of movement (see below).

Rate of Information Processing in a Movement Sequence

In this task two-dimensional reaching movements were made in quick succession in response to a target shift.[40] Subjects were instructed to point with their hand to a visual target as soon and as quickly as possible. During various times following the appearance of the first target (50–400 ms) the target shifted, and the subject had to move to the new target. It was found that the rate of information processing increased substantially (by as much as twofold) during the second movement. The highest rate (14.4 bits/s) was attained when the target shifted 150 ms after its first appearance. These results show that it is possible to increase the rate of information processing of the motor system, that is, to increase the speed of the movement without degrading its accuracy. In a way, of course, this characterizes skilled motor performance. For example, a good tennis player is frequently both fast and accurate, especially so if one considers that the accuracy required under these circumstances extends to several aspects of movement, that is, orientation of the hand, force of hitting the ball, precise timing, and so forth. How is that increase in information processing being accomplished? We suggest that a key factor responsible for the improved performance in motor skills that involve a sequence of movements may be a parallel motor processing. It seems that, under certain conditions, generating a movement while another one is evolving or being generated "primes" the perceptual–motor system so that, instead of being constrained, it actually processes information more efficiently and emits movements that are faster than, and as accurate as, movements produced in isolation. A correlate of this increased efficiency in information processing was described by Soechting and Lacquaniti,[41] namely that when responding to a target change there is a reduction in the degrees of freedom of the movement; this is achieved by imposing constraints on the kinematic variables (angular deceleration at the shoulder and elbow joints), and by generating more stereotyped patterns of activity in the muscles acting on these two joints.

Rate of Motor Information Processing in Mental Rotation

The studies discussed previously concerned information processing during actual movements. We wish now to consider this question for a case that seemed to involve a mental movement, namely a mental rotation of movement direction. Some of the results of these studies were summarized earlier; we provide below the results of an information–theoretical analysis. In these experiments[36] human subjects were asked to make movements in directions at various angles from a stimulus direction that varied in two-dimensional space from trial to trial in a pseudorandom fashion. Under these conditions, the RT increased as a linear function of the angle; this suggested that subjects rotated mentally an imagined movement direction. Assuming this model of internal motion, we analyzed the amplitude-accuracy relations using Fitts's[11] approach described previously: for this case, we considered the RT as a mental movement time during which the imagined movement vector rotated. Indeed, we found that the increase in RT was a linear function of task difficulty that was calculated from the angle achieved and its variability. This indicates that Fitts's law holds for the hypothesized rotary motion of the imagined movement vector, and suggests that both real and imagined movements might be governed by similar amplitude–accuracy relations. The average I_p in this task was 4.21 bits/s, which is almost one-half the information processing rate for straight movements (I_p = 7.25 bits/s). This is probably due to the cognitive load in this task and also to the fact that rotation involves operating on direction, which is known to be a time-consuming process.[42]

The neural mechanisms underlying this mental rotation were studied by recording single-cell activity in the motor cortex of two monkeys who made movements at an angle 90° CCW from a stimulus direction.[37,38] The neuronal population vector (see earlier) was calculated as a measure of the directional tendency of the neuronal ensemble. It was found that during the RT it rotated CCW from the direction of the stimulus to the direction of the movement. These results provided a direct visualization of the mental rotation hypothesized previously in this task on the basis of the results obtained from human subjects, summarized in the preceding section. There were eight stimulus directions available, and therefore eight time-series of population vectors rotating during the RT; summary data are shown in [38, tables 4 and 5]. From these data, the estimated I_p was 4.785 bits/s. This is the estimate of the rate of processing of directional information by the neuronal ensemble during the mental rotation. The I_p of the behavioral performance in the same monkeys was also calculated as follows. The rotation angle required was 90°, with an allowance of ±30°, and therefore the angular "target" width was 60°; the average RT was 413.7 ms. From these data, I_p = 3.832 bits/s. There are two noteworthy points here. First, this last behavioral I_p by the monkeys is close to the value of 4.21 bits/s calculated from the human data given earlier. And second, the neural I_p of 4.785 bits/s was approximately 1 bit higher than the behavioral one of 3.832 bits/s calculated for the same conditions in the same animals. This validates further this analysis and suggests, as probably was expected, that there is some loss of information from motor cortical processing to behavior, as suggested previously.[43]

CONCLUSIONS

We have reviewed the general features of temporal sensory–motor processing in the basal ganglia and motor cortex. We have further quantified this processing within the context of formal information theory and evaluated the rate of information processing in various types of reaching movements. An important result of this analysis is that the highest processing rate (9.2 bits/s) is observed in unconstrained three-dimensional movements, and that this rate is appreciably reduced to about 7 bits/s in movements constrained to one or two dimensions. This shows that higher degrees of freedom in movement are processed more efficiently, and that the processing of "simpler," that is, constrained, movements is more difficult. One explanation for this could be the fact that three-dimensional movements are very practiced, which could result in more efficient information processing. This efficient processing of complex, multidimensional movements is reflected in their control by the central nervous system, as evidenced by the orderly variation of cell activity with movement parameters and the preferential disruption of multi- but not single-joint movements by reversible inactivation of central motor structures.[44]

Finally, the importance of considering neural information processing at the neuronal population level was discussed within the context of temporal processing of directional information and its transformation in a mental rotation task.

REFERENCES

1. WATERS, R. S., D. D. SAMULAK, R. W. DYKES & P. A. MCKINLEY. 1990. Topographic organization of baboon primary motor cortex: Face, hand, forelimb, and shoulder representation. Somatosens. Motor Res. **7**: 485–514.
2. GEORGOPOULOS, A. P., J. F. KALASKA, R. CAMINITI & J. T. MASSEY. 1982. On the relations between the direction of two-dimensional arm movements and cell discharge in primate motor cortex. J. Neurosci. **2**: 1527–1537.
3. GEORGOPOULOS, A. P., M. R. DELONG & M. D. CRUTCHER. 1983. Relations between parameters of step-tracking movements and single cell discharge in the globus pallidus and the subthalamic nucleus of the behaving monkey. J. Neurosci. **3**: 1586–1598.
4. MUIR, R. B. & R. N. LEMON. 1983. Corticospinal neurons with a special role in precision grip. Brain Res. **261**: 312–316.
5. WILSON, S. A. K. 1925. Disorders of motility and muscle tone, with special reference to the corpus striatum. Lancet **2**: 1–10.
6. DRAPER, I. T. & R. J. JOHNS. 1964. The disordered movement in Parkinsonism and the effect of drug treatment. Bull. Hopkins Hosp. **115**: 465–480.
7. FLOWERS, K. A. 1976. Visual 'closed-loop' and 'open-loop' characteristics of voluntary movement in patients with Parkinsonian and intention tremor. Brain **99**: 269–310.
8. EVARTS, E. V., H. TERAVAINEN & D. B. CALNE. 1981. Reaction time in Parkinson's disease. Brain **104**: 167–186.
9. HALLETT, M. & S. KHOSHBIN. 1980. A physiological mechanism of bradykinesia. Brain **103**: 301–314.
10. SANES, J. N. 1985. Information processing deficits in Parkinson's disease during movement. Neuropsychologia **23**: 381–392.
11. FITTS, P. M. 1954. The information capacity of the human motor system in controlling the amplitude of movement. J. Exp. Psychol. **47**: 381–391.
12. BERARDELLI, A., J. P. R. DICK, J. C. ROTHWELL, B. L. DAY & C. D. MARSDEN. 1986. Scaling of the size of the first agonist burst during rapid wrist movements in patients with Parkinson's disease. J. Neurol. Neurosurg. Psychiatry. **49**: 1273–1279.
13. FLOWERS, K. A. 1978. Lack of prediction in the motor behavior of Parkinsonism. Brain **101**: 35–52.
14. DAY, B. L., J. P. R. DICK & C. D. MARSDEN. 1984. Patients with Parkinson's disease can employ a predictive motor strategy. J. Neurol. Neurosurg. Psychiat. **47**: 1299–1306.
15. BLOXHAM, C. A., T. A. MINDEL & C. D. FRITH. 1984. Initiation and execution of predictable and unpredictable movements in Parkinson's disease. Brain **107**: 371–384.
16. SCHWAB, R. S., M. E. CHAFETZ & S. WALKER. 1954. Control of two simultaneous voluntary motor acts in normals and in parkinsonism. Arch. Neurol. Psychiatry **72**: 591–598.
17. TALLAND, G. A. & R. S. SCHWAB. 1964. Performance with multiple sets in Parkinson's disease. Neurology **9**: 65–72.
18. BENECKE, R., J. C. ROTHWELL, J. P. R. DICK, B. L. DAY & C. D. MARSDEN. 1986. Performance of simultaneous movements in patients with Parkinson's disease. Brain **109**: 739–757.
19. ———. 1987. Disturbance of sequential movements in patients with Parkinson's disease. Brain **110**: 361–379.
20. CRUTCHER, M. D. & M. R. DELONG. 1984. Single cell studies of the primate putamen. II. Relations to direction of movements and pattern of muscular activity. Exp. Brain Res. **53**: 244–258.

21. ANDERSON, M. E. & F. B. HORAK. 1985. Influence of the globus pallidus on arm movements in monkeys. III. Timing of movement related activity. J. Neurophysiol. **54:** 433–448.
22. MINK, J. W. & W. T. THACH. 1991. Basal ganglia control. II. Late pallidal timing relative to movement onset and inconsistent pallidal coding of movement parameters. J. Neurophysiol. **65:** 301–329.
23. THACH, W. T. 1978. Correlation of neural discharge with pattern and force of muscular activity, joint position, and direction of intended next movement in motor cortex and cerebellum. J. Neurophysiol. **41:** 654–676.
24. SCHWARTZ, A. B., R. E. KETTNER & A. P. GEORGOPOULOS. 1988. Primate motor cortex and free arm movements to visual targets in three-dimensional space. 1. Relations between single cell discharge and direction of movement. J. Neurosci. **8:** 2913–2927.
25. SCHWARTZ, A. B. & A. P. GEORGOPOULOS. 1987. Relations between the amplitude of 2-dimensional arm movements and single cell discharge in primate motor cortex. Soc. Neurosci. Abstr. **13:** 244.
26. GEORGOPOULOS, A. P. 1990. Neurophysiology and reaching. *In* Attention and Performance XIII, M. Jeannerod, Ed.: 227–263. Erlbaum. Hillsdale, N.J.
27. PARK, S.-K., J.-J. WANG, J. H. KIM & T. J. EBNER. 1987. Movement fields of neurons in the premotor cortex of the primate. Soc. Neurosci. Abstr. **13:** 1095.
28. PARK, S.-K., J. H. KIM & T. J. EBNER. 1988. Evaluation of motor parameters in the premovement discharge of premotor cortical neurons during two-dimensional movements. Soc. Neurosci. Abstr. **14:** 343.
29. KARLUK, D. & T. J. EBNER. 1989. Spatial representation of movement distance and direction in the premotor cortex. Soc. Neurosci. Abstr. **15:** 787.
30. GEORGOPOULOS, A. P., R. CAMINITI, J. F. KALASKA & J. T. MASSEY. 1983. Spatial coding of movement: A hypothesis concerning the coding of movement direction by motor cortical populations. Exp. Brain Res., Suppl. **7:** 327–336.
31. GEORGOPOULOS, A. P., A. B. SCHWARTZ & R. E. KETTNER. 1986. Neuronal population coding of movement direction. Science **233:** 1416–1419.
32. GEORGOPOULOS, A. P., R. E. KETTNER & A. B. SCHWARTZ. 1988. Primate motor cortex and free arm movements to visual targets in three-dimensional space. II. Coding of the direction of movement by a neuronal population. J. Neurosci. **8:** 2928–2937.
33. GEORGOPOULOS, A. P., J. F. KALASKA, M. D. CRUTCHER, R. CAMINITI & J. T. MASSEY. 1984. The representation of movement direction in the motor cortex: Single cell and population studies. *In* Dynamic aspects of neocortical function, G. M. Edelman, W. M. Cowan, and W. E. Gall, Eds.: 501–524. Wiley. New York.
34. GEORGOPOULOS, A. P., M. D. CRUTCHER & A. B. SCHWARTZ. 1989. Cognitive spatial motor processes. 3. Motor cortical prediction of movement direction during an instructed delay period. Exp. Brain Res. **75:** 183–194.
35. SMYRNIS, N., M. TAIRA, J. ASHE & A. P. GEORGOPOULOS. 1992. Motor cortical activity in a memorized delay task. Exp. Brain Res. **92:** 139–151.
36. GEORGOPOULOS, A. P. & J. T. MASSEY. 1987. Cognitive spatial-motor processes. 1. The making of movements at various angles from a stimulus direction. Exp. Brain Res. **65:** 361–370.
37. GEORGOPOULOS, A. P., J. T. LURITO, M. PETRIDES, A. B. SCHWARTZ & J. T. MASSEY. 1989. Mental rotation of the neuronal population vector. Science **243:** 234–236.
38. LURITO, J. L., T. GEORGAKOPOULOS & A. P. GEORGOPOULOS. 1991. Cognitive spatial-motor processes. 7. The making of movements at an angle from a stimulus direction: Studies of motor cortical activity at the single cell and population levels. Exp. Brain Res. **87:** 562–580.
39. MOUNTCASTLE, V. B., J. C. LYNCH, A. GEORGOPOULOS, H. SAKATA & C. ACUNA. 1975. Posterior parietal association cortex of the monkey: Command functions for operations within extrapersonal space. J. Neurophysiol. **38:** 871–908.
40. MASSEY, J. T., A. B. SCHWARTZ & A. P. GEORGOPOULOS. 1986. On information processing and performing a movement sequence. Exp. Brain Res. Suppl. **15:** 242–251.
41. SOECHTING, J. F. & F. LACQUANITI. 1983. Modification of a pointing movement in response to a change in target location. J. Neurophysiol. **49:** 548–564.

42. ROSENBAUM, D. A. 1980. Human movement initiation: Specification of arm, direction, and extent. J. Exp. Psychol.: General **109:** 444–474.
43. GEORGOPOULOS, A. P. & J. T. MASSEY. 1988. Cognitive spatial motor processes. 2. Information transmitted by the direction of two-dimensional arm movements and by neuronal populations in primate motor cortex and area 5. Exp. Brain Res. **69:** 315–326.
44. COOPER, S. E., H. J. MARTIN, E. SYBIRSKA, J. BRENNAN & C. GHEZ. 1989. Effects of motor cortex inactivation on forelimb motor control in the cat. Soc. Neurosci. Abstr. **15:** 789.

Neural Disorders of the Linguistic Use of Space and Movement[a]

HOWARD POIZNER[b] AND JUDY KEGL

Center for Molecular and Behavioral Neuroscience
Rutgers, The State University of New Jersey
197 University Avenue
Newark, New Jersey 07102

INTRODUCTION

Since sign languages utilize a transmission modality different from that of spoken languages, their study offers a unique opportunity for insight into the nature of neural mechanisms for language. We have been combining new techniques of three-dimensional computergraphic analysis of movement with linguistic analysis to illuminate neural mechanisms underlying signing from a striking new perspective: that of contrasting the processing deficits of signers with distinct language and movement disorders. Unilateral lesions in the left but not in the right cerebral hemisphere in Deaf signers produce sign language aphasias. These aphasias affect core grammatical components within a visual–gestural language despite the reliance of such components on the utilization of space. Thus, it would appear that the left cerebral hemisphere in man has an innate predisposition for language, independent of language modality. Our ability to create digital records of the spatiotemporal patterns of signing allows us to investigate signing not only as linguistic behavior, but also as motor behavior. In contrast to the representational–linguistic deficits of signers with aphasia, signers with Parkinson's disease show a unique set of signing alterations involving disturbed joint use, flattening of phonological distinctions, and timing disruptions. Analysis of patterns of breakdown of linguistic structure and motor control for sign language following brain damage in Deaf signers is allowing us to begin to map the neural substrate underlying the linguistic use of limb movement.

Understanding Brain Function for Language

Human language is a particularly important and promising vehicle for investigating brain and behavior relationships, since language is one of the highest of man's cognitive abilities and forms a major readout system of the brain. Our studies of language take a unique point of departure in that they explore brain organization for sign languages used by Deaf individuals. We are naturally led to the study of sign languages, since through their study we can begin to solve the problem of brain organization for language in general.

---

[a]This work was supported in part by National Institutes of Health Grant DC01664, and in part by National Science Foundation Grants DBS 92-13110 and BNS-9000407 to Rutgers, The State University of New Jersey.
[b]To whom correspondence should be addressed.

The left cerebral hemisphere provides the neural substrate for language in hearing–speaking individuals. Ninety-nine percent of right-handed, hearing subjects with aphasia have lesions in the left hemisphere.[1] Dichotic listening and tachistoscopic half-field studies confirm left-hemisphere specialization for spoken language in brain-intact hearing subjects.[2] Furthermore, the planum temporale, a portion of auditory association cortex thought to mediate language, is larger in the left hemisphere than in the right.[3] In addition, prelingual hearing infants show left-hemisphere specialization for the perception of speech sounds.[4,5] The underlying basis of the specialization of the left hemisphere for language, however, has not been clearly understood. How dependent is this left-hemisphere specialization for language on hearing, speech, and on the signal properties of speech sounds?

The study of sign languages of Deaf individuals provides a special opportunity for investigating brain function for language, since sign language displays complex *linguistic* structure, but, unlike spoken languages, conveys much of its structure by manipulating *spatial* relations. Since the left hemisphere has been considered specialized for language and the right hemisphere specialized for processing spatial relations, sign language exhibits properties for which each of the hemispheres of hearing individuals shows an opposing specialization. Because of the dual attributes, the study of sign language offers a valuable opportunity for refining our concept of brain function for language.

The study of visual–gestural languages can not only inform us about brain function for language, but can also serve as a new vehicle for probing the intersection of the brain's control of language and of movement. Our ability to create digital records of the spatiotemporal patterns of signing allows us to investigate signing not only as linguistic behavior, but also as motor behavior. In order to understand the operation of the coalitions of brain structures that make sign language processing possible, it becomes critical to investigate disorders in the specific channels of language expression and reception, as well as in processing the central, abstract attributes of language. An important contrast to signers with aphasia comes from the study of signers with disorders in channels of expression, such as disorders in the programming of movement occurring in Parkinson's disease. Because spoken language articulators are not directly visible in most cases, it is often difficult to determine the nature of their disturbance strictly from the secondary effects that their movements have on the sound stream. Such inferences are not necessary with signing, however, since in sign language we can directly observe and measure disruptions in visible articulators that consist of rigid, jointed links, namely the limbs. We have been contrasting signers with distinct language and motor disorders in order to investigate disturbances at different levels of linguistic representation, spatial cognition, and motor control. Before presenting these data on disturbances in sign language following brain damage, we briefly describe aspects of the linguistic structure of American Sign Language (ASL).

THE NATURE OF LANGUAGE IN THE VISUAL–GESTURAL MODALITY

American Sign Language is the visual–gestural language that has arisen in Deaf communities in the United States. Although ASL utilizes manual–visual channels for expression and reception, it displays all the complex organizational properties found in spoken languages, as well as all of their expressive power.[6-9] ASL has a gestural phonology, complex morphology, and recursive syntactic processes. As is the case for all natural human languages, the analytic manipulation of abstract formational units characterizes ASL at each of these levels of linguistic organization.

Phonology and Phonetics in a Visual–Gestural Language

Signs are comprised of nonmeaningful, sublexical components that can be characterized in terms of four major parameters: handshape, movement, place of articulation, and palm orientation. Representatives from these parameters minimally contrast pairs of signs. Moreover, sign languages, like spoken languages, involve the complex coordination and sequencing of motor gestures. Signs in sequence are also subject to language-specific phonological rules that apply to natural classes of segments when they occur in particular environments (e.g., at word or phrase boundaries, before or after other natural classes of segments, in closed versus open syllables, or within particular stress domains). There are also modality-specific phonetic processes at work that serve to facilitate ease of articulation. Such processes include smoothing the transition from one segment to the next, maintaining center of gravity, or regularizing periodicity in rhythmic sequences. The articulators affected by these phonetic adjustments differ from those involved in speech production. However, there are motoric processes at work and there are trading relations engaged that maximize ease of articulation while maintaining crucial linguistic distinctions that are parallel in languages in the two modalities.

Three-dimensional Morphology

ASL has a rich set of inflectional and derivational morphemes that are conveyed, not by changes in hand configuration, but by modulation of movement along specific planes in space.[6] For example, the form of one plural marker in ASL involves iterated movement of the hand and arm along an arc in a plane horizontal to the torso of the signer. The imposition of movement dynamics, reduplication, and/or spatial contouring onto an already motorically complex inventory of baseforms yields a semantically and morphologically rich series of inflectional and derivational paradigms. It also provides a unique opportunity to study, in a controlled, systematic, and completely natural way, the motor effects on joint and limb coordination that follow from nesting movements within other movements. The combinatorial properties of this system are clearly evidenced from the fact that a nearly exhaustive set of meaningful movement combinations can be generated by successively applying inflectional and derivational processes to sign baseforms.

In order to investigate the nature and breakdown of these grammatical processes in ASL, we have developed new techniques for three-dimensional movement tracking and computergraphic analysis.[10–12] FIGURE 1 presents a variety of morphological processes in ASL, conveyed through patterns of movement, that were digitized in three-dimensional space. The best-fitting plane of the hand motion was computed for each form and plotted in FIGURE 1. Several clusterings of forms emerge in FIGURE 1. Movements conveying temporal aspect distinctions (points H, J, and K) are grouped together in a sagittal plane, whereas those for number and distributional aspects (points A, B, C, D, E, and L) cluster in either the horizontal or vertical plane relative to the body. The correspondence between these clusterings, based purely on the spatial properties of the movements, and the independent linguistic classifications of

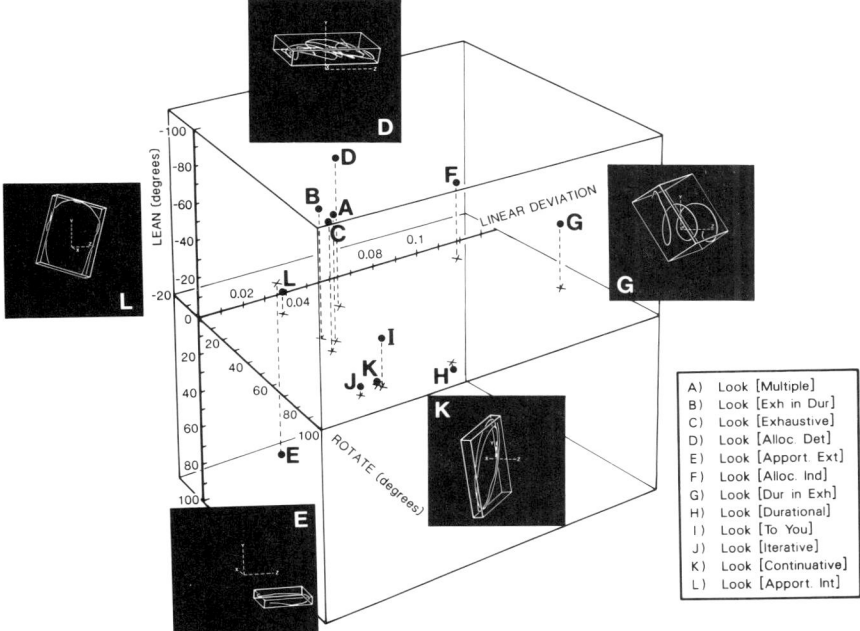

FIGURE 1. Three-dimensional visual-phonetics of the linguistic dimension *planar locus*. Best-fitting planes to hand motions were computed from digitized trajectories of a variety of morphological processes in ASL. The two axes *lean* and *rotate* provide two angles (elevation and azimuth) that specify the particular plane of motion. The third axis, *linear deviation*, specifies how planar a motion was. Clusters of morphological processes appear in the figure, based on this spatial property of plane of hand movement, that correspond to linguistic classifications of these forms. (Reprinted with permission from H. Poizner, U. Bellugi & E. S. Klima, 1991. Brain function for language: Perspectives from another modality. *In* Modularity and the Motor Theory of Speech Perception, I. Mattingly and M. Studdert-Kennedy, Eds.: 145–169. Erlbaum. Hillsdale, N.J.)

these same forms in ASL grammar is striking and attests to the spatial nature of ASL morphology.

Spatialized Syntax and Discourse

ASL syntax and discourse utilize a referential spatial network of points in space for purposes of verb agreement and pronominal reference both within sentences and across the sentences in a discourse.[13–17] Noun phrases introduced into ASL discourse are assigned to arbitrary loci in the horizontal plane of signing space that extends in an arc about a bent arm's length in front of the signer's torso. Pronoun signs directed to a specific locus (index point) on this plane clearly "refer back" to the previously mentioned noun. Verbs spatially agree with these preestablished reference points by moving from, by moving to, or being located at the same position in space. This spatial agreement not only signals within a sentence which roles or grammatical relations are borne by particular noun phrases, but also serves a discourse function. Because ASL is a language that freely omits independent noun phrases and pronouns once their reference has been established, it is the spatial agreement on verbs, sentence to sentence, that provides discourse cohesion. This spatial agreement allows a signer to track the relevant referent throughout a narrative.

FIGURE 2 presents a mininarrative illustrating aspects of ASL spatialized syntax and discourse processes. Two INDEX points, i, associated with the boy, and j, associated with his mother, are assigned distinct spatial loci. Once a position in space is linked to a noun phrase within a single sentence, that spatial locus is consistently used for reference to that same person throughout the discourse. Processing syntactic and discourse relations in ASL, thus also requires processing spatial relations among loci in particular planes in space. By investigating disturbances of signing under conditions of focal brain damage, we can analyze the extent to which the neural systems that underlie language are independent of modality, and the extent to which they are modality bound.

DIFFERENTIAL DISTURBANCES IN THE UTILIZATION OF SPACE IN BRAIN-LESIONED SIGNERS

We have been investigating the language, visual–spatial, and motor abilities of signers who have acquired lesions in either the left or the right cerebral hemisphere.[8,18–23] In addition, we have been contrasting the deficits of these signers with unilateral brain lesions with the deficits of signers with Parkinson's disease, a disorder that produces deficits in the control of movement.[24,25] We have been examining the effects of brain damage on the signing and nonlanguage spatial and motor capacities in Deaf signers from multiple perspectives. (1) Use of an adaptation for ASL of the Boston Diagnostic Aphasia Examination.[26] (2) Analysis of ASL production using three-dimensional computergraphic analyses. Our computergraphic techniques for motion analysis allow the visualization, manipulation, and graphic editing of digitized movement trajectories. The trajectory paths of each limb segment can be displayed simultaneously, and dynamically, with numeric and graphic displays of a variety of trajectory components. The simultaneous graphic and numeric display of data allow us to synchronize data around specific events. Numeric algorithms allow quantification of specific hand kinematic and joint kinematic features. (3) The linguistic analysis of free and elicited conversation and narratives. (4) Administration of the Supalla et al. ASL Test Battery,[27] which consists of an extensive series of tests of the production and comprehension of critical grammatical structures in ASL. (5) Tests of nonlanguage spatial processing and motor control.

To date, we have comprehensively analyzed six left-lesioned and four right-lesioned signers. Summary characteristics of these subjects appear in TABLE 1. Detailed case studies of left-lesioned GD, KL, and PD, and right-lesioned BI, SM, and GG may be found in Poizner et al.[18] and summarized in Bellugi et al.[19] A detailed case study of left-lesioned WL is reported in Corina et al.[20] Discussion of left-lesioned NS and right-lesioned AS may be found in Poizner and Kegl,[23] Kegl and Poizner,[21] and Kegl et al.[22]

TABLE 1 presents background information on the 10 signers with unilateral brain lesions. Nine of the 10 signers were Deaf; one was hearing. All the Deaf signers studied were right-handed, lifelong signers, who were members of the Deaf com-

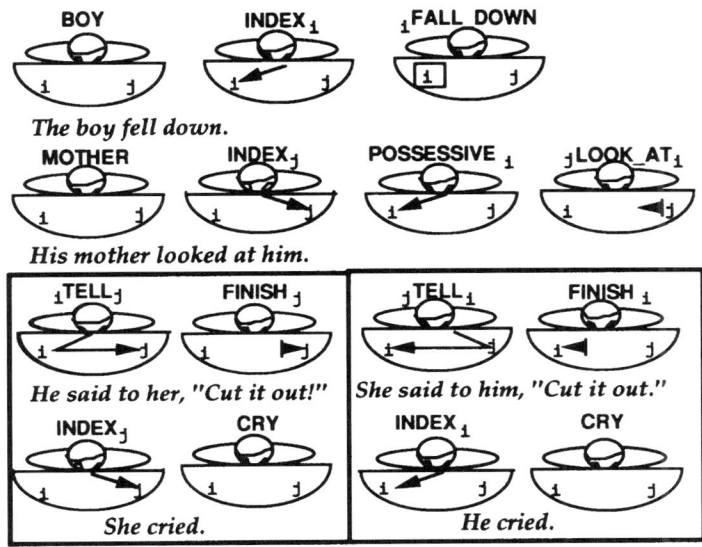
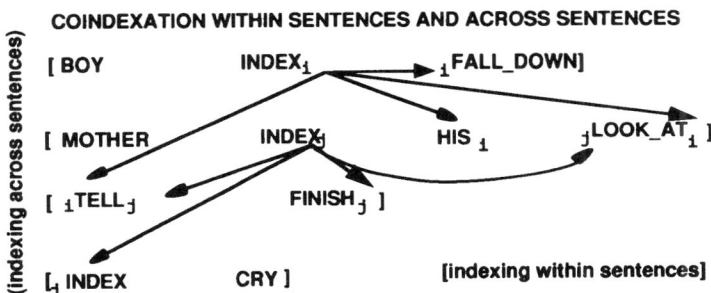

FIGURE 2. A mini ASL narrative illustrating the use of space in ASL for syntactic versus discourse processes. **Top Panel:** In the first sentence, the first two signs uniquely establish a relation between BOY and position i in the signing space. In the next sentence, a similar relation is established between MOTHER and position j. Signing FALL-DOWN at position i tells us who fell down, namely, the boy. Directing the possessive pronoun POSS(essive) toward position i while modifying the noun phrase MOTHER INDEXj, tells us that she is the boy's mother. The sign LOOK-AT, by means of its orientation toward position i indicates that the boy is the goal of the looking, while its positioning at point j tells us that it is the mother who does the looking. The two boxes indicate two alternate endings for the narrative. The signs for each are identical. They differ only in the INDEX points (i vs. j) with which they agree. **Bottom Panel:** *Arrows* indicate the original index associated with the noun phrases in the mininarrative and all subsequent references to those indices across the narrative. The individual sentences, bounded by *square brackets,* are arrayed vertically. (From H. Poizner and J. Kegl, Aphasiology, Vol. 6, 1992, pp. 219–256, Taylor and Francis, Inc., Washington, D.C. Reproduced with permission.)

TABLE 1. Summary Characteristics of the Brain-lesioned Signers

Patient	Age of Testing	Sex	Age Onset of Deafness	Handedness	Parents and Siblings	School	Spouse	Cultural Group	Hemiplegia	Lesion
Left-hemisphere Damaged Signers										
GD	38	F	Birth	Right	Older Deaf siblings	Residential Deaf school	Deaf	Deaf	Right hemiplegic	Most of convexity of left frontal lobe, including Broca's area
PD	81	M	5 yr.	Right	Hearing	Residential Deaf school	Deaf	Deaf	—	Left subcortical deep to Broca's area extending posteriorly beneath parietal lobe
KL	67	F	6 mo.	Right	Hearing	Residential Deaf school	Hard of hearing	Deaf	Right hemiplegic	Left parietal lobe in the region of the supramarginal and angular gyri, extending subcortically into middle frontal gyrus
WL	76	M	Birth	Right	Deaf siblings	Residential Deaf school	Deaf	Deaf	—	Left large frontotemporoparietal lesion; Broca's area and subsequent white matter, including arcuate fasciculus; considerable damage to white matter deep to left inferior parietal lobule
EN	81	F	5 yr.	Right	Deaf mother + 5 older Deaf siblings	Residential Deaf school	Deaf	Deaf	Right hemiplegic	Left posterior limb of the internal capsule, small portions of the posterior thalamus on the left and left mesial occipital cortex
NS	48	M	Birth	Right	Deaf sister + identical twin	Residential Deaf school	Deaf	Deaf	Right hemiplegic	Left posterior temporal lobe and large portions of the left supramarginal and angular gyri
Right-hemisphere Damaged Signers										
BI	75	F	Birth	Right	Hearing	Residential Deaf school	Deaf	Deaf	Left hemiplegic	Right hemisphere lesion (no scan)
SM	71	F	Birth	Right	Hearing	Residential Deaf school	Deaf	Deaf	Left hemiplegic	Right temporoparietal area; most of the territory of the right middle cerebral artery involved
GG	81	M	5 yr.	Right	Hearing	Residential Deaf school	Deaf	Deaf	—	Right superior temporal and middle temporal gyri extending into the angular gyrus
AS	38	F	Hearing	Right	Deaf grandparents	Public school; teaches in Deaf school	Hearing	Hearing	—	A wedge-shaped infarction extending from the right lateral ventricle to the cortex of the mesial portion of the right parietal lobe. The infarction involved substantial portions of Brodmann's areas 5, 7, 31, and 23 on the right, as well as the mesial portion of the right postcentral sulcus

munity. All were educated at residential schools for Deaf children and had used ASL as their primary form of communication throughout their lives. Three very recent cases that we are investigating add substantially to the small but accumulating set of signers with unilateral brain lesions. One right-lesioned signer, AS, was hearing, and thus was bilingual in ASL and English. She had Deaf grandparents, was a certified ASL interpreter, and continues to teach at a school for Deaf children. The other two very recent cases are left-lesioned, Deaf signers. Left-lesioned NS is a completely unique case, since he has an identical twin Deaf brother. The twin brother served as a virtually perfect control signer for this case. Left-lesioned EN comes from a large Deaf family. Her mother was Deaf, as were five of her siblings.

FIGURE 3 presents reconstructions of the brain lesions of the left-lesioned signers, and FIGURE 4 reconstructions of the lesions of the right-lesioned signers. The last column of TABLE 1 presents a brief description of each lesion.

Nonlanguage Spatial Cognition

We administered tests of nonlanguage spatial processing that maximally differentiate performance of left- as opposed to right-lesioned hearing subjects. These included tests of drawing, block design, visual neglect, perception of line orientation, and facial recognition. Across this range of tests, right-lesioned signers showed many of the classic visuospatial impairments seen in hearing patients with right-hemi-

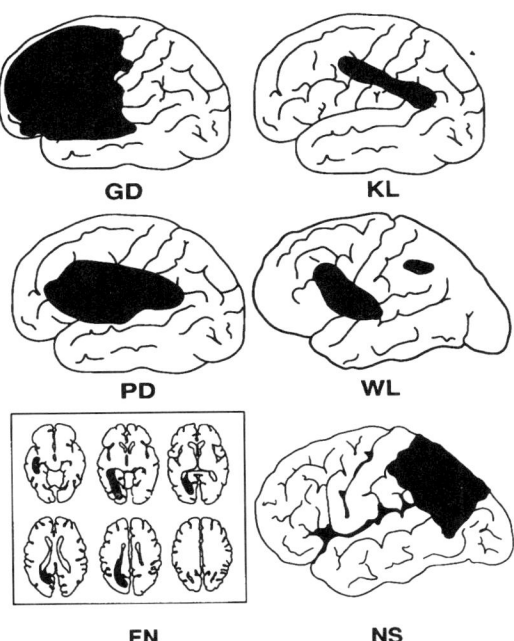

FIGURE 3. Reconstruction of brain lesions of the six left-lesioned signers. Lateral reconstructions of lesions are used except for the case of EN, where axial views are presented to best represent her subcortical lesion.

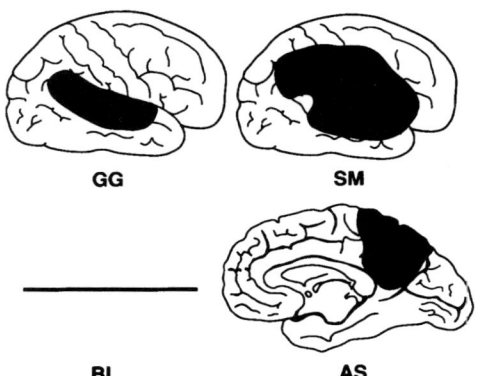

FIGURE 4. Reconstruction of brain lesions of the four right-lesioned signers. No CT scan was available for BI, so no reconstruction is presented. Lateral reconstructions are used for GG and SM, whereas a medial reconstruction of the lesion is used for AS.

sphere damage. In contrast, left-lesioned signers showed relatively preserved nonlanguage spatial functioning. The drawings of the right-lesioned signers, for example, showed severe spatial disorganization, including lack of perspective, neglect of the left side of space, and lack of preservation of the overall spatial configuration. The drawings of the left-hemisphere-damaged signers, although simplified, had coherent spatial organization, and did not exhibit the spatial distortions found in the drawings of the right-lesioned signers. These data on nonlanguage spatial processing indicate that the right hemisphere in Deaf signers can develop cerebral specialization for nonlanguage visuospatial functions.[18,28]

Linguistic Deficits in Brain-lesioned Signers

FIGURE 5 summarizes observed linguistic deficits across the left-lesioned and right-lesioned signers studied to date. A blackened box in FIGURE 5 indicates that a given subject showed some degree of deficit in the linguistic component indicated at the top of the column. FIGURE 5 makes no attempt to differentiate different degrees of deficits in each component, but rather indicates whether or not there was any disturbance in each of the specified language components.

The language components tabulated in FIGURE 5 reflect measures of the subjects' command of aspects of ASL phonetics, phonology, morphology, syntax, semantics, and discourse structure. Four of these components, phonology, morphology, syntax, and semantics,[c] are central levels of linguistic organization in ASL, since it is here

---

[c]The linguistic category labeled semantics straddles the line between core grammar and noncore. Logical form, or the level at which relations such as logical scope and coreference are interpreted, is part of core grammar. Word meaning, on the other hand, in the sense of lexical conceptual representations, constitutes a more noncore or more general cognitive knowledge about the world. Words (especially verbs) are core linguistic components that interface between core and noncore grammar by linking purely linguistic, hierarchical representations, such as the initial syntactic configuration of a verb and its required noun phrases, to a more generally cognitive conceptual representation of its meaning. A word's meaning can

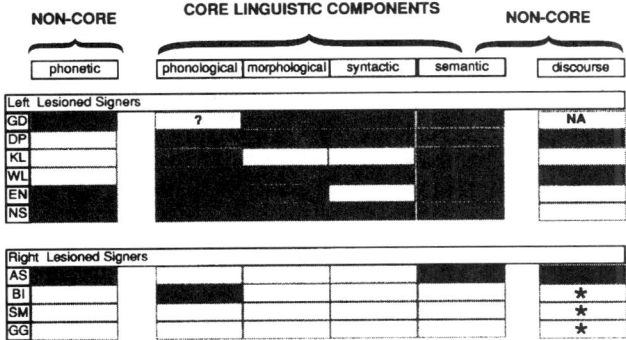

FIGURE 5. Linguistic deficits of the left-lesioned and right-lesioned signers. Deficits in core versus noncore components of ASL are presented. A *blackened box* indicates that a given subject showed some degree of deficit in the linguistic component indicated at the top of the column, but does not differentiate different degrees of deficits in each component. Note the differential involvement of core linguistic components in left as opposed to right-lesioned signers.

that the uniquely complex and highly constrained organizational properties of language are most clearly manifested. These organizational properties involve the recursive application of rules, hierarchical structure, and structure-dependent relationships. The other levels of language listed in FIGURE 5, phonetics and discourse, stand at the interface between strictly linguistic and extralinguistic aspects of human cognition. They are less constrained by universal principles that characterize core grammar, and are more influenced by nonlinguistic factors such as motor programming, physiological constraints on movement, memory factors, and general world knowledge or conceptual representations. However, they are still very much attributes of language.

By separately analyzing deficits at different levels of structure in ASL, we can analyze the representation of language in the brain not in terms of language as an undifferentiated entity, but rather in terms of subcomponents that have different formal properties and bear different functional loads.

FIGURE 5 reveals a number of important consequences of damage in anatomic structures in the left as opposed to structures in the right cerebral hemisphere on use of the components of ASL structure. First of all, FIGURE 5 clearly reveals that there is substantially greater disturbance in the components of language following lesions in the left as opposed in the right hemisphere in deaf signers. There are marked deficits in various linguistic categories for each of the left-lesioned signers, while right-lesioned signers exhibit relatively few deficits. Interestingly, the deficits that do

actually be considered its location within a highly complex semantic network—namely, a word's meaning is equivalent to the links or semantic relations that a given word holds to other words (meronymy (part/whole), synonymy, antonymy, ISA relations, etc.). Semantic field errors or anomia (word-finding difficulty) reflect noncore linguistic deficits that nonetheless can have massive repercussions for other aspects of language production or comprehension. The semantic deficits indicated in FIGURE 5 reflect primarily problems in noncore aspects of semantics, such as lexical access and word choice, as well as specific problems in the expression of real-world relationships via language.

occur in right-lesioned signers are virtually always in the noncore grammatical components of ASL, for example, in phonetics, lexical choice, and discourse. The one right-lesioned signer who had a deficit in one of the core grammatical components of ASL, right-lesioned BI, showed spatial irregularities in the formation of some signs. The few phonological errors she did make involved the way the hand was oriented in space, and not in such nonspatial parameters as the configuration of the hand itself. Thus, her occasional phonological errors were likely a result of a more basic visuospatial deficit. The semantic deficits manifested by AS fall into the noncore rather than core aspects of semantic ability.

In contrast, the deficits of the left-lesioned signers encompass core grammar components in each case. Moreover, certain left-lesioned signers showed differential deficits within the grammar of ASL. Left-lesioned KL effortlessly produced long strings of signs that showed a wide range of correct morphological and syntactic forms. However, she showed impairment at the phonological level, making frequent errors in the selection of the correct hand configurations, movements, and places of articulation from which signs are formed. Left-lesioned GD's signing was reduced to single sign utterances of largely referential signs, without any of the required syntactic and morphological markings of ASL. Her language profile was, in fact, much like that of hearing patients classified as having Broca's aphasia, and her lesion was typical of those that produce Broca's or agrammatic aphasia for spoken language. Left-lesioned PD, like KL, had a fluent sign aphasia, producing long strings of motorically facile signs. However, the nature of his sign language breakdown was quite different from that of KL's. Whereas KL showed preserved morphology and syntax, and impaired phonology, PD exhibited marked impairments in ASL morphology and syntax, but only mild impairments in ASL phonology. Left-lesioned PD made selection errors with ASL morphology and erred in the spatialized syntax of the language. Left-lesioned WL was markedly disturbed throughout the range of core grammatical components of ASL, making selection errors within the phonology, and showing impairments in ASL morphology and syntax. Left-lesioned EN showed phonological, morphological, and semantic errors. Finally, left-lesioned NS showed morphological and syntactic deficits with relatively preserved ASL phonology.

These accumulating cases of Deaf signers with unilateral brain lesions consistently demonstrate a left-hemisphere specialization for sign language, particularly with respect to core components of the grammar. FIGURE 5 reveals a striking contrast between the preponderance of core grammatical deficits exhibited by left-lesioned signers as compared to preserved grammar in right-lesioned signers. The grammatical deficits of the left-lesioned signers reflect frank sign language aphasias. The right-lesioned signers are relatively unimpaired linguistically. Moreover, the occurrences of deficits in noncore grammatical components in right-lesioned signers appear to be attributable to a nonlinguistic deficit (such as neglect of left hemispace, deficits in spatial memory, or spatial processing) that can significantly hinder linguistic output. Distinguishing between the linguistic deficits that characterize sign language aphasias, and the ways in which nonlinguistic deficits in channels of spatial analysis and movement control can impinge upon linguistic output is a topic to which we turn next.

Factors Hindering the Linguistic Use of Space and Movement

It is indisputable that nonlinguistic factors such as deficits in memory, attention, vision, or audition can hinder language comprehension, even in the absence of any deep language deficit, simply by interfering with the transmission of linguistic information to those areas of the brain dedicated to its processing. Similarly, nonlinguistic deficits can have repercussions that affect language production.

This section brings to bear results from our intensive studies of five Deaf signers with motor control deficits resulting from Parkinson's disease[24,25,29,30] on the comparison and contrast of the differential effects that unilateral lesions in one hemisphere produce on language and spatial cognition in Deaf signers. We are finding that these Parkinsonian signers show a unique set of signing alterations, involving disturbed joint use, flattening of phonological distinctions, and timing disruptions. The motor deficits associated with Parkinson's disease appear to have across the board effects on sign production and nonlinguistic motor abilities alike. Within the language domain, articulatory precision, and consequently ease of perception, is sacrificed in favor of greater ease of articulation. There is a greater reliance on unmarked handshapes, namely, those that are motorically simpler and require less fine motor control, a minimization of such quantal distinctions as maximally closed versus maximally open handshapes, or maximally spread versus unspread handshapes, in favor of more laxed hand configurations that minimally maintain such distinctions. The amplitude of movements, particularly the path movements in signs, is greatly reduced. Moreover, precise contact with specific locations on the body or on the nondominant hand are relinquished in favor of minimal hand orientation changes used to signal the trajectory that a fully realized path movement would normally take. Finally, precise palm orientation in signs is neutralized in favor of the most unmarked orientation of the hand. The Parkinsonian subjects we are studying range in impairment from mild to severe. Although they share to varying degrees the same set of signing alterations mentioned previously, our examples here will be drawn from a single signer, Parkinsonian JH, who can be characterized as moderate to severe in his symptoms.

Rather than a comprehensive three-way comparison of left-lesioned, right-lesioned, and Parkinsonian signers, we present just a few points of comparison that illustrate the differential effects on language production, across the different linguistic components indicated in FIGURE 5, that these different disorders affect. Our examples are chosen to aid in teasing apart purely linguistic deficits from nonlinguistic deficits that interfere superficially with language production.

Deficits at the Formational Level: Phonetics and Phonology

Because some brain damaged signers may also exhibit nonlinguistic motor deficits, it is crucial to clearly demarcate those errors that we classify as *phonological*, and to clearly distinguish them from nonlinguistically relevant sign disturbances that result from more general motor or attentional problems (e.g., microkinesia or hemispatial neglect) that may affect the fine-grained details of the articulation, that is, the low-level phonetics.

Phonological Deficits: Sublexical Paraphasias

A clear phonological error is a sublexical sign paraphasia that results in the substitution of one linguistically relevant parameter value for another, yielding either another possible sign or a well-formed nonsense sign. Most of the left-lesioned signers had at least mild deficits of this sort. Left-lesioned KL, for example, although fluent in her sign production, produced frequent sublexical paraphasias where she would substitute one handshape, movement, or place of articulation for another—substituting a W for a V-handshape in CAREFUL, an up-and-down rather than a circular movement in ENJOY, and a chin rather than cheek place of articulation for the sign SEE. All of these substitutions resulted in nonsense signs. Left-lesioned WL also made frequent phonological paraphasias, creating many nonsense signs. For example, in the sign for SISTER, left-lesioned WL substituted an F for an L handshape, two visually dissimilar, but articulatorily similar handshapes differing in only a single distinctive feature (whether the index finger does or does not contact the thumb). This selection error cannot be considered phonetic, but must be considered phonological, since distinctive rather than redundant features of the phonology were substituted. Right-lesioned and Parkinsonian signers, in contrast, did not show sublexical paraphasias, reflecting intact phonological capacities in these subjects.

Nonlinguistic deficits can also affect the output of the phonology, more precisely, phonetic aspects of articulation. Interestingly, we have observed such interferences with sign production both from disorders of motor control and of spatial cognition. However, the deficits that do occur differ markedly from the phonological deficits seen in left-lesioned signers where there is misselection of phonological elements in the context of motorically facile signing. Pure motor disturbances can condition changes in the application of phonological rules by either destroying the environments in which a given rule would have applied, or by creating new conditions under which a specific rule will apply. Consider data from two neurologically impaired signers, one (AS) with damage to the right hemisphere affecting spatial memory, perception, and attention, and the other (JH), a signer with Parkinson's disease affecting sign timing and rhythm, movement amplitude, and articulatory precision. Neither of these signers was impaired with respect to core linguistic functions, yet both show the effects of nonlinguistic impairments on their sign production.

Motor Neglect and Phonetic Disturbances in a Right-lesioned Signer

Right-lesioned AS exhibited higher order visuospatial deficits, including defective performance on judging the angular orientation of lines and neglect of left hemispace. In the first few days following her surgery, right-lesioned AS was unable to recognize the left side of her body, but at the time of testing only a mild visual and motor neglect remained. In free conversation and elicited narratives, right-lesioned AS used her right hand for single-handed signs, and she showed timing and coordination problems in some of her two-handed signs (ENJOY, RIGHT, HARD, REMEMBER). In these signs, her left hand seemed to lag behind the right, a two-handed coordination problem that appears to have resulted from her motor neglect. With symmetrical signs not involving sequencing between the two hands, the effects of the left-hand lag were negligible. In a two-handed symmetrical sign like ENJOY, her left-handed movement was just slightly out of synchrony with her right hand. However, delay in the initiation of left-hand movement in two-handed signs involving sequencing of the two hands sometimes triggered sign internal sequencing, orienting, and coordination errors. For example, the sign RIGHT, meaning, "correct," is typically articulated as follows:

(1) Left hand: A 1-handshape, palm oriented sideways, fingertip forward moves to the center of the signing space about waist height in front of the signer.

(2) Right hand: The hand in the same configuration moves to a position above the left hand and then downward to contact with it. (Optionally, there can be a slight upward bounce at the end of the sign.)

In right-lesioned AS's articulation of RIGHT, the left hand was delayed in initiating its movement such that it actually followed rather than preceded the articulation of the right hand. This delay triggered a chain of sequencing, movement, and orientation changes that, taken as a whole, significantly distorted the sign. Right-lesioned AS's articulation was as follows:

(1) Right hand: A 1-handshape, palm oriented sideways and fingertip forward, moves to the center of the signing space slightly above waist height in front of the signer.
(2) Left hand: The hand in the same configuration moves to a position below the right hand and then upward to contact it from below.
(3) Right hand: Having been contacted, the right hand moves upward in center space to approximately chin height.

As can be seen, the delayed articulation of the left hand led to a reorganization and resequencing of the sign, producing phonetic distortions in the two-handed signing of this right-lesioned signer. Some changes, such as the reorienting of the movement of the right hand, might be thought to be phonological in nature, but actually are triggered responses that occur because low-level phonetic sequencing errors modify the linguistic environment in which downward movement can occur.

Phonetic Disturbances in Parkinsonian Signing

A sign like NEW, is typically articulated with two flat B-handshapes, palms upward, with the back side of the moving hand making contact with a scooping-type motion against the palm of the stationary nondominant hand. The articulation of this sign is quite altered by Parkinsonian JH, who signs NEW using two B-handshapes, but with fingers slightly spread and slightly laxed, and with both palm orientations rotated toward the signer's chest. The dominant (right) hand does not contact the palm of the nondominant left hand, but rather just minimally realizes a scooping motion about an inch away from it. The hand, which is typically stationary, mirrors slightly the movement of the dominant hand, but in the opposite direction in Parkinsonian JH's production. The sign looks as though the two hands were pulled about one inch apart and rotated 90 degrees. The sign movement, rather than being abrupt, is uniformly slowed and smoothed, thereby obscuring the boundaries between transition into and out of the sign and the actual articulation of the sign itself. The sign is still recognizable, but laxed. This is the hallmark of Parkinsonian signing—the relaxation or "schwa-ing" of all features of articulation toward some central/unmarked articulation, but never to the point of actually fully obliterating a linguistically relevant distinction.

In contrast with left-lesioned aphasic signers, who make selective linguistic substitution errors (paraphasias) that obliterate linguistically essential aspects of a sign, JH and the other Parkinsonian signers that we have studied compromise maximal linguistic contrasts that normally serve to facilitate ease of perception in favor of ease of articulation. However, they faithfully maintain relevant linguistic distinctions. As a consequence of the across the board lowering and shrinking of

Parkinsonian JH's signing space, signs like THINK and REMEMBER, typically made at the forehead, are lowered to the cheek; signs like LOOK-AT and SEE, normally made at eye-level, are lowered to chin level; and signs like DRINK and GRANDMOTHER, normally articulated at the chin, are lowered to mid-chest level. Still, the displacement of the signs is regular and systematic, relative distinctions are preserved, and the intended place of articulation can be recovered. In fact, Parkinsonian signing shares much in common with whispering in sign—a form of signing that intentionally lowers and shrinks the size of signs to prevent ease of perception to all but the intended recipient who knows to shift gaze so that the displaced and reduced sign space of the whisperer is accessible to foveal rather than peripheral vision.[d] As with whispering, systematic and recoverable shrinking of signs and the signing space demonstrates maintained sensitivity to, rather than the loss of, linguistically relevant distinctions.

Deficits at the Morphological Level

Morphological deficits can range from the underuse to the overuse of units at the morphological level. We find both types of deficits in the left-lesioned signers. Left-lesioned PD has a tendency to misuse or overuse certain morphological forms, signing, for example, LOOK [Habitual], meaning, "look regularly," in the context where LOOK [Multiple], meaning, "look at them," is required, or signing CARELESS [Predispositional], meaning, "characteristically careless," in a context where only the uninflected form CARELESS would be appropriate. Left-lesioned NS, in contrast, shows a markedly reduced inventory, sampling only minimally from the range of aspect markers depicted in FIGURE 1. Left-lesioned NS's inventory of forms marking differences in aspectual verb morphology is limited to a single, undifferentiated form involving repetition of the verb's movement. Moreover, this form is used inconsistently. His identical twin, however, uses a much more comprehensive range of morphological forms.

Left-lesioned EN is somewhat atypical, both in the sense that her lesion is subcortical, and that she exhibits a shrinking and lowering of the signing space that resembles that of Parkinsonian signers. Her case thus provides an interesting point of contrast with disturbances associated with Parkinsonian signing. Consider a complex sign like GIVE [Durational in Exhaustive], meaning "give continuously over time to each of them" (see FIGURE 1, G, for an illustration of the hand movement). The base sign GIVE normally is signed with a repeated circular motion ([Durational]) while moving to distinct points arranged in a horizontal arc from left to right ([Exhaustive]). Left-lesioned EN, however, would repeat this complex form using only the repeated circular motion, deleting the right-to-left motion. In fact, in free conversation, she would frequently replace repeated movements to distinct points along a horizontal arc (plural inflection) with repeated movements to a single point (what looks like aspectual morphology). Both of these articulations sacrifice

---

[d]This is not to say that Parkinsonian signing is identical to whispering. On the contrary, whispering maintains sign prosody, which is characteristically flattened in Parkinsonian signing. With respect to eye gaze, the sign receiver normally looks at an area centered on the signer's chin. This eye-gaze pattern allows one to use foveal vision for the complex marked signs and facial expressions. It also relegates signs made below chest height, which happen to select from only the most unmarked handshapes and movements, to one's peripheral vision.[31]

crucial linguistic information, and contrast with the reductions seen in Parkinsonian signers.

Correct Morphology but Spatial Reduction in Parkinsonian Signers

Parkinsonian JH, despite a severe motor deficit, makes use of a wide range of morphological forms marking temporal aspect, number, and distribution. His morphologically complex signs include such forms as GO-OUT [Habitual], meaning, "go out regularly," LOOK-AT [Durational], meaning, "look at continuously," CHALLENGE [Exhaustive], meaning, "challenge each of them to a fight," and JOURNEY [Exhaustive], meaning, "go to visit many places." Although these forms are greatly reduced in amplitude, and are realized with more distal joints, they are used regularly and appropriately. Furthermore, morphological distinctions are not lost due to his reductions.

Preserved Morphology in Right-lesioned Signers

Right-lesioned AS not only produces the full range of morphological forms, but does so with an articulation that, even put to the scrutiny of three-dimensional computergraphic analysis, is indistinguishable from that of neurologically intact control signers.

Deficits at the Syntactic and Discourse Levels

Syntactic Deficits in a Left-lesioned Signer

ASL has three verb classes: (a) plain verbs [no overt agreement, require SVO (subject-verb-object) word order—e.g., CRY in FIG. 2]; (b) person-agreeing verbs [spatial agreement with object and/or subject; restricted to persons—e.g., LOOK-AT, TELL in FIG. 2]; and (c) motion/location verbs [spatial agreement with locations established in the signing space—e.g., FALL-DOWN in FIG. 2]. As mentioned earlier, person agreement in ASL makes use of previously established points in the signing space that have been uniquely associated with specific individuals in the sentence or discourse. These points are generally established in a semicircular plane radiating about a bent elbow's length out from the signer's torso. The initial association of a particular index point with a particular person is arbitrary. Verbs move between these index points to indicate the grammatical relations borne by the relevant noun phrases in the sentence. Verbs of motion and location "agree" not with person, but with locations and objects established in the signing space. Frequently, these locative agreement points have a nonarbitrary relation to one another that approximates the real-world spatial relations held between the nouns to which they refer.

Left-lesioned NS, who exhibits a mild syntactic deficit, underuses the inflectional spatial morphology marking subject and object person agreement in ASL, heavily favoring uninflected, plain verb forms. As a consequence of his syntactic deficit, left-lesioned NS's sign production and comprehension are heavily dependent upon the use of SVO word order. Moreover, left-lesioned NS's comprehension drops when his interlocutors stray from this canonical order. Neither of these deficits is seen in his identical twin brother. Since these deficits occur for both left-lesioned NS's comprehension and production, they indicate the central and deep nature of his syntactic loss.

Correct Syntax but Spatial Reductions in a Parkinsonian Signer

Parkinsonian JH, on the other hand, uses a full array of spatially realized verb agreement. Despite the fact that the amplitude of his signing space is significantly reduced, Parkinsonian JH still uses space to establish agreement of verbs with locations and with person referents. His space, although shrunken, is not flattened. FIGURE 6 compares the articulation of 1st-person-ASK-3rd-person, meaning, 'I ask him,' by Parkinsonian JH versus a control signer. FIGURE 6 shows that although Parkinsonian JH's movement is very small and executed with the wrist rather than with the entire arm, his movement trajectory still serves to correctly mark morphological agreement with subject and object.

Parkinsonian JH, in fact, even preserves verb agreement in motorically complex "reversible" verbs like 3rd-person-INVITE-1st-person ("s/he invited me") that require a movement from the signer (object) to 3rd person (subject), a reversal of the typical pattern for other verb classes.

Correct Syntax but Impaired Discourse in a Right-lesioned Signer

As noted earlier, right-lesioned AS correctly used spatial agreement on verbs to indicate the grammatical relations held by specific noun phrases within sentences. In right-lesioned AS's free conversation, there were no within sentence errors either in person or in locative agreement. Yet, analysis of referential agreement across sentences in a discourse (see FIG. 2, panel B) revealed that right-lesioned AS did not consistently associate the same spatial index to the same noun phrase referent from

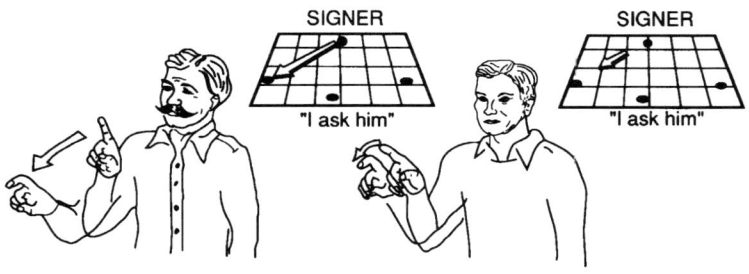

FIGURE 6. Correct syntax but spatial reductions in a Parkinsonian signer. The articulation of 1st-person-ASK-3rd-person, meaning, 'I ask him,' by Parkinsonian JH is compared to that of a control signer. Parkinsonian JH's movement correctly marks morphological agreement with subject and object, but is of very small amplitude and executed with the wrist as opposed to the shoulder and elbow.

sentence to sentence.[e] Instead, the locations of the referent points that she established in a discourse across sentences showed spatial drift and inconsistencies.[21] This was true for both the maintenance of person agreement and of the locative arrangement of entities established in the signing space. The fact that the mechanics and form of spatial indexing is so similar at both levels, makes this subject's differential maintenance of spatial agreement at the syntactic versus discourse levels all the more revealing. Since this signer had an intact left hemisphere, her case demonstrates the importance of left-hemisphere structures for mediating spatialized *syntax* (i.e., sentence level constraints on coreference) in ASL.

Deficits in Semantics

Most left-lesioned signers, including NS, exhibited semantic field errors, such as substituting FOX for WOLF (NS), or GRANDMOTHER for GRANDDAUGHTER (EN), but these errors are not spatial in nature and will not concern us here. Right-lesioned AS, on a portion of the Supalla *et al.* ASL Test Battery (in press) that elicited the production of motion and location verbs made numerous errors in orientation (like right-lesioned BI, mentioned earlier) and in classifier choice, particularly with respect to choosing the appropriate classifiers to reflect a given perspective (e.g., a close-up versus long shot). Her errors generally consisted of combining in one motion location verb, two classifiers that conflicted with respect to perspective—namely, using a classifier associated with a close-up view in conjunction with a classifier associated with a distant view. Parkinsonian JH, in contrast, did not show a semantic deficit.

DISTORTIONS OF THE SIGNING SPACE IN LEFT-LESIONED, RIGHT-LESIONED, AND PARKINSONIAN SIGNERS

We conclude our comparison of left-lesioned NS, right-lesioned AS, and Parkinsonian JH by considering the effect that their disorders had on the three-dimensional shape of their signing spaces. The signing space is the area that usually extends from the signer's forehead to about the waist extending outward in front of the signer about a bent arm's length in an arc. Each disorder manifested itself differently with respect to its effect on the topography of the signing space. FIGURE 7 illustrates the differential distortion in use of the signing space in these three brain-damaged signers. Left-lesioned NS shows a flattening, concurrent with a vertical and lateral enlargement of his signing space.[f] Right-lesioned AS shows an asymmetrical raising and favoring of the right side, primarily in situations where she is in too close proximity to her interlocutor. And, Parkinsonian JH shows a symmetrical shrinking and lowering of his signing space.

---

[e]AS compensates for inconsistent use of spatial indices across sentences in a discourse by reestablishing the indexing of noun phrases in practically every sentence, where the norm would be to establish a noun phrase once and thereafter refer back to it by pointing to its index point (pronoun reference) or allowing a verb to agree with its index point.

[f]The lack of enlargement on the right side of signing space is a consequence of NS's right hemiplegia.

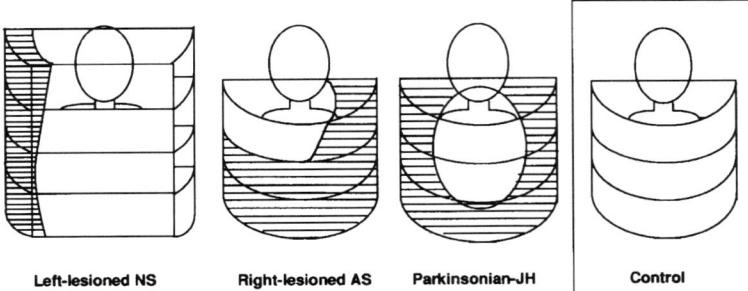

FIGURE 7. Differential distortions of signing space in a left-lesioned, a right-lesioned, and a Parkinsonian signer. The *whitened areas* of the figure indicate portions of the signing space used by each subject. Note that left-lesioned NS flattens and enlarges portions of his signing space, whereas right-lesioned AS uses only the upper right quadrant of her signing space. This distortion in right-lesioned AS's signing space occurs when she is signing a close distance away from her interlocutor. In contrast, Parkinsonian JH's sign space distortions involve a uniform shrinkage of the space utilized. All signers except Parkinsonian JH used the upper head area.

Reliance upon uninflected verb forms instead of spatial agreement to mark grammatical relations, and the absence of rich temporal aspect morphology in both the vertical and horizontal planes (see FIG. 1), results in an observable flattening of left-lesioned NS's signing space. This flattening is clearly evidenced when compared with the three-dimensional, sculpted signing space used by left-lesioned NS's identical twin brother. There is little variation in the orientation or movement path of NS's signs. In fact, one's first impression in looking from NS's signing to that of his twin brother approximates the effect of putting on special glasses and suddenly having a three-dimensional image pop out when looking at the signing of the twin brother. Left-lesioned NS's distorted signing space is the result of his linguistic deficits at the morphological and syntactic levels. The absence of syntactic agreement in left-lesioned NS's mildly agrammatic signing means that he does not set up noun phrases in space. Such spatial establishment allows pronominal references and verb agreement to link antecedent noun phrases with their anaphors (items that refer back to them) throughout the sentence and remaining discourse. The enlargement of left-lesioned NS's signing space vertically and horizontally appears to be the result of an increased use of nonlinguistic gestures (mime) to fill in where his syntax fails. These gestures are not constrained by the boundaries of the linguistic signing space.

Parkinsonian JH's signing space reflects the across the board effect of his motor deficit. His entire signing space is reduced in amplitude and lowered—systematically. If we were to plot classes of signs associated with specific places of articulations, we would see that, although the signs are displaced, they are still distinctly clustered, and are distinct in location from other signs differing in place features. If we were to look at this signing space from the side, we would see that unlike left-lesioned NS's space which favors body contact, Parkinsonian JH's space shrinks away from body contact. The distortions in Parkinsonian JH's signing space reflects his favoring ease of articulation over ease of perception. However, they nonetheless appear to be tempered by his linguistic sensitivity to crucial distinctive features and grammatical inflections.

Right-lesioned AS's signing space is normal in size but asymmetrical. Spatial agreement points are raised and favor the right side, a distortion that was likely related to his signer's left hemispatial neglect. Even within this distorted signing space, however, individual sentences are completely grammatical, having correct spatial agreement. The degree of distortion of AS's signing space varies as a factor of her proximity to her interlocutor. When an interlocutor is too close, AS has problems visually attending to signs made by her interlocutor that appear in the lower left quadrant of her (AS's) left hemispace. This is evidenced not only by AS's sign space distortion, but also by her unusual eye-gaze pattern. Rather than maintaining a characteristic gaze toward the area of the interlocutor's chin, while using peripheral vision to detect signs at the extremes of the signing space, right-lesioned AS tracks with her eye gaze any signs that move into her lower left quadrant. In the same way that the receiver of whispered signing shifts gaze to get the reduced and displaced signs into foveal vision, AS tracks signs moving to the lower left quadrant to keep them in view. However, this sporadic tracking of the hands as opposed to a single repositioning of gaze is a very unusual behavior that is quickly noted. The distortion of AS's signing space also appears to have nonlinguistic origins, reflecting her visuomotor neglect of left hemispace. Neglect of only the lower left hemispace is characteristic of patients with her medial and superior right parietal lesion. The particular ways in which right-lesioned AS's spatial deficits affected her signing space help illuminate the interplay that can occur between spatial and linguistic processing in sign language.

BRAIN, LANGUAGE, AND MODALITY

The nature of the signing deficits produced by different neural disorders of linguistic processing, spatial cognition, and motor control is providing new and unique information on the functional anatomy of language and its relation to modality. Patterns of language breakdown and preservation in left- as opposed to right-lesioned signers lead to the following conclusions. Because the left-lesioned signers show frank sign language aphasias and the right-lesioned signers show preserved core linguistic function, it appears that it is, indeed, the left cerebral hemisphere that is specialized for sign language. This provides support for the proposition that the left cerebral hemisphere in humans has an innate predisposition for language. Thus, there appear to be anatomical structures within the left hemisphere that emerge as special-purpose linguistic processors in persons who have profound and lifelong auditory deprivation and who communicate with a linguistic system that uses radically different channels of reception and transmission from that of speech. In this crucial respect, brain organization for language in Deaf signers parallels that in hearing, speaking individuals. Moreover, deficits in spatial cognition and in motor control are seen to disrupt the utilization of space in sign language, but at very different levels from the linguistic representational loss of signers with aphasia. Through the study of signers with differential disruption to the central processing/representation of language and in the channels of expression and reception, we are beginning to unravel the entwined strands of linguistic form and linguistic structure as determinants of brain organization for language.

ACKNOWLEDGMENTS

We thank the group at the Salk Institute in the Laboratory of Ursula Bellugi for their contributions to the initial groundbreaking work on sign aphasia upon which our current research program has built. We thank Hannah Damasio for reconstructing several of the brain lesions in FIGURE 3 and 4. Several individuals have been instrumental to our current projects, in particular Diane Brentari, Branch Coslett, Toni Fuller, Abhay Kothari, Joanne Lauser, Ruth Loew, and Vicki Joy Sullivan. We are also grateful to Ted Supalla and Elissa Newport, who made available a prepublication version of their ASL Sign Battery and scoring materials. Finally, of course, we are most grateful to the subjects who participated in all of these studies and to their families for their time, effort, and valuable insights.

REFERENCES

1. GESCHWIND, N. 1970. The organization of language in the brain. Science **170**: 940–944.
2. STUDDERT-KENNEDY, M. & D. SHANKWEILER. 1970. Hemispheric specialization for speech perception. J. Acoust. Soc. Am. **48**: 579–594.
3. GESCHWIND, N. & W. LEVITSKY. 1968. Human brain: Left-right asymmetries in temporal speech region. Science **161**: 186–187.
4. ENTUS, A. K. 1977. Hemispheric asymmetry in processing of dichotically presented speech and nonspeech stimuli by infants. *In* Language Development and Neurological Theory, S. J. Segalowitz and F. A. Gruber, Eds.: 63–73. Academic Press. New York.
5. MOLFESE, D. L., R. B. FREEMAN & D. S. PALERMO. 1975. The ontogeny of brain lateralization for speech and nonspeech stimuli. Brain Lang. **2**: 365–368.
6. KLIMA, E. & U. BELLUGI. 1979. The Signs of Language. Harvard Univ. Press. Cambridge, Mass.
7. LANE, H. & F. GROSJEAN. 1980. Recent Perspectives on American Sign Language. Erlbaum. Hillsdale, N.J.
8. POIZNER, H., U. BELLUGI & E. S. KLIMA. 1990. Biological foundations of language: Clues from sign language. *In* Annual Review of Neuroscience, Vol. 13, W. Maxwell Cowan, Ed.: 283–307. Annual Reviews. Palo Alto, Calif.
9. WILBUR, R. 1987. American Sign Language. Little, Brown. San Diego.
10. POIZNER, H., E. WOOTEN & D. SALOT. 1986. Computergraphic modeling and analysis: A portable system for tracking arm movements in three-dimensional space. Behav. Res. Methods, Instrum. Comput. **18**: 427–433.
11. JENNINGS, P. & H. POIZNER. 1988. Computergraphic modeling and analysis II: Three-dimensional reconstruction and interactive analysis. J. Neurosci. Methods **24**: 45–55.
12. KOTHARI, A., H. POIZNER & T. FIGEL. 1992. Interactive three-dimensional graphic analysis for studies of neural disorders of movement. SPIE Visual Data Interpretation **1668**: 83–92.
13. PADDEN, C. 1988. Interaction of morphology and syntax in American Sign Language. *In* Outstanding Dissertations in Linguistics, Series IV. Garland. New York.
14. LILLO-MARTIN, D. & E. S. KLIMA. 1990. Pointing out differences: American Sign Language pronouns in syntactic theory. *In* Theoretical Issues in Sign Language Research, P. Siple, Ed. Univ. of Chicago Press. Chicago.
15. KEGL, J. A. 1986. Clitics in American Sign Language. *In* The Syntax of Pronominal Clitics, H. Borer, Ed.: 285–309. Academic Press. New York.
16. ———. 1987. Coreference relations in American Sign Language. *In* Studies in the Acquisition of Anaphora: Applying the Constraints, Vol. 2, B. Lust, Ed.: 135–170. Reidel. Dordrecht, the Netherlands.
17. SHEPARD-KEGL, J. 1985. Locative relations in American Sign Language word formation, syntax, and discourse. MIT Working Papers in Linguistics, Cambridge, Mass.
18. POIZNER, H., E. S. KLIMA & U. BELLUGI. 1987. What the Hands Reveal about the Brain. Bradford Books/MIT Press. Cambridge, Mass.
19. BELLUGI, U., H. POIZNER & E. S. KLIMA. 1989. Language, modality and the brain. Trends Neurosci. **12**: 380–388.

20. CORINA, D., H. POIZNER, U. BELLUGI, L. BATCH, D. FEINBERG & D. DOWD. 1992. Dissociation between linguistic and non-linguistic gestural systems: A case for compositionality. Brain Lang. **43**: 414–447.
21. KEGL, J. & H. POIZNER. 1991. The interplay between linguistic and spatial processing in a right-lesioned signer. J. Clin. Exp. Neurophychol. **13**: 38–39.
22. KEGL, J., H. POIZNER & R. LOEW. 1992. Linguistic-specific processing deficits in a left-lesioned signer of ASL. Proceedings of the NIDCD Conference on Aging: The Quality of Life, Washington, D.C., Feb.
23. POIZNER, H. & J. KEGL. 1992. The Neural basis of language and motor behaviour: Evidence from American Sign Language. Aphasiology **6**: 219–256.
24. BRENTARI, D. & H. POIZNER. A phonological analysis of a deaf Parkinsonian signer. Lang. Cognitive Processes. In press.
25. LOEW, R., J. KEGL & H. POIZNER. 1992. Flattening of distinctions in a Parkinsonian signer. Proceedings of the Boston University Conference on Language Development, Boston, Oct.
26. GOODGLASS, H. & E. KAPLAN. 1983. The Assessment of Aphasia and Related Disorders, Lea and Febiger, Eds. Philadelphia.
27. SUPALLA, T., E. NEWPORT, J. SINGLETON, S. SUPALLA, G. COULTER & D. METLAY. American Sign Language Test Battery. Linstok Press. Silver Spring, Md. In press.
28. POIZNER, H., E. KAPLAN, U. BELLUGI & C. PADDEN. 1984. Visual-spatial processing in Deaf brain-damaged signers. Brain Cognition **3**: 281–306.
29. BRENTARI, D., H. POIZNER & J. KEGL. 1993. Differential depth of phonological disruption in aphasic and Parkinsonian signers. Unpublished manuscript.
30. KEGL, J. & H. POIZNER. The preservation of linguistic distinctions in a Parkinsonian signer. In preparation.
31. SIPLE, P. 1980. Visual constraints and the forms of signs. Sign Lang. Stud. **19**: 95–110.

Cerebellar Involvement in the Explicit Representation of Temporal Information[a]

RICHARD IVRY

Department of Psychology
University of California
Berkeley, California 94720

INTRODUCTION

In considering the neural bases of temporal information processing, two distinct questions should be kept in mind. First, it is important to distinguish between those tasks in which timing is explicitly represented and those tasks in which the temporal properties are an implicit, emergent property. For example, a baseball pitcher must rotate his shoulder forward before his hand releases the ball. While the time at which each of these events should occur may be explicitly represented, it is also possible that this temporal information is implicit: the actions needed to release the ball may be initiated once the forward action of the arm reaches a particular position or velocity. Even in repetitive movements, it may not be necessary to postulate an explicit timing mechanism. For example, when people repetitively swing their arm in a pendular motion, the preferred rate of oscillation can be predicted simply by consideration of biomechanical factors such as the length and mass of the arm.[1]

Nonetheless, it seems reasonable to assume that there are motor tasks in which timing is explicitly controlled. For example, while biomechanical analyses can predict the preferred rate of oscillation, people are capable of adjusting that rate. Indeed, an impressive feature of the literature on repetitive movements is that people are able to produce such movements over a wide range of frequencies.[2-4] Models of this phenomenon generally postulate an explicit timing mechanism with an adjustable rate parameter.[5] Explicit timing would also seem necessary for certain perceptual tasks, such as when people are asked to judge which of two tones is longer in duration. A variety of mechanisms have been proposed to account for performance on these tasks, all sharing the feature of an explicit timing device.[6]

Assuming that there are tasks in which timing is explicitly controlled, we can then turn to the second question. Specifically, does this set of tasks involve the operation of a common timing mechanism, or are there multiple timing mechanisms in the brain? Neuropsychological research has tended to favor the latter answer, with researchers pointing to the fact that damage to a wide range of neural systems can disrupt performance on tasks that involve temporal information processing.[7] These results have led Richelle *et al.*[8] to conclude that we should "admit that there are as many clocks as there are behaviors exhibiting timing properties" (p. 90). However, conclusions such as this may be ill-advised. As noted previously, behaviors that exhibit temporal regularities need not require the operation of an internal clock.

---

[a]The author was supported in part by National Institute of Neurological Disorders and Stroke Grant NS30256 and in part by a fellowship from the Sloan Foundation.

Moreover, the plethora of neural disabilities associated with impaired performance on timing tasks may simply reflect the fact that these tasks require the integration of a number of cognitive operations, only one of which may be devoted to the representation of temporal information.

These two questions have shaped the framework for our research strategy on timing. We have chosen tasks that not only appear to require explicit timing, but are also as simple as possible in order to reduce the importance of nontemporal processes. Our initial research with healthy young adults led to the hypothesis that these tasks involve the operation of a common internal clock, and our subsequent patient research indicated that the cerebellum is the critical neural structure associated with this timing mechanism. More recently, we have shifted our focus to investigate the generality of the cerebellar timing hypothesis. This issue can be approached on two fronts. First, we can use a new set of tasks to assess whether the integrity of the cerebellum is necessary for successful performance, thus indicating the role of timing in these tasks. Second, we can reexamine tasks that have been associated with the cerebellum to see whether the timing hypothesis provides a parsimonious interpretation of the data.

THE CEREBELLUM AS AN INTERNAL CLOCK

Two tasks have been central to our research. The first, a production of time task, is a repetitive finger-tapping task. Each trial begins with the presentation of a series of computer tones, separated by isochronous intervals. The intertone interval in our research has varied from 325 ms to 550 ms. By pressing a response key, the subject attempts to synchronize his or her responses with the tones. After a series of paced responses, the tones cease and the subjects' task is to continue tapping at the target rate until they have produced 30 unpaced intertap intervals (ITIs). Our primary measure is the variability of the standard deviation of the ITIs. Given that the target ITI is arbitrarily defined, we assume that this task requires explicit control of the timing of the response.

The second task is a perception of time task. On each trial two intervals are presented, a standard and a comparison interval. The intervals can be unfilled, marked at the beginning and end by either 50-ms tones or light flashes, or filled, in which case the interval is represented by the duration of a continuous tone or visual stimulus. The subjects' task is to indicate whether the comparison interval is shorter or longer than the standard interval. The duration of the comparison interval is varied, and responses to the different values are collected. From the obtained psychophysical function, a difference threshold can be estimated to provide a measure of temporal acuity on this task. For example, if the standard interval is 400 ms, a subject with good temporal acuity might have a difference threshold (1 standard deviation) of 25 ms, whereas a subject with poor acuity might have a difference threshold of 35 ms.

A significant correlation between performance on the motor and perception timing tasks is found in healthy young adults.[9] People who were consistent on the repetitive-tapping task also had lower difference thresholds on the time-perception task. Significant correlations were also obtained when subjects performed the repetitive-tapping task with different effectors (hand, foot, forearm), whereas little correlation was observed when comparing performance on this task with that measured on other motor tasks that did not require precise timing.[10] These results suggest that there is a common timing mechanism that is utilized in both perception and action, a result that meshes with our intuition. The lack of correlation between the repetitive-tapping and the nontiming motor tasks indicates that the correlations between the timing tasks cannot be attributed to general factors such as motivation.

Evidence of an internal clock that is shared by both motor and perceptual systems raises the possibility that this function might be dependent on a restricted set of neural structures. That is, if a common internal clock is associated with a certain neural structure, then lesions of this structure should disrupt performance on both motor and perceptual tasks that require precise timing. Positive results, of course, would not only provide converging evidence for a common timing mechanism, but would also be an important first step in identifying the neural bases of this form of timing.

To explore this issue, we tested three different patient groups on the repetitive-tapping and auditory time-perception tasks.[11] The three groups were (1) patients with lesions that included premotor cortical areas ($n = 8$), (2) patients with Parkinson's disease ($n = 30$), and (3) patients with cerebellar lesions ($n = 30$). While all of these patients had suffered a loss of coordination, the control of timing is presumably only one component of coordination. We were interested in whether the tapping task would yield any dissociations in performance. In particular, normal performance on the tapping task for one of these groups would suggest that the affected neural structures for that group are not part of an internal timing mechanism.

Two of the patient groups, the cortical patients and the cerebellar patients, were impaired on the tapping task in comparison to age-matched control subjects (FIG. 1). The mean standard deviation for these groups was approximately 50 percent higher than that obtained from the control subjects. In contrast, the Parkinson patients performed comparably to the control subjects. A subset of the Parkinson patients were tested in a second session after having skipped their L-DOPA medication for about 16 hours. While these patients showed a severe exacerbation of Parkinson symptoms in the *off* medication state, their performance on the tapping task was unchanged (but was significantly altered on a second motor task measuring their ability to produce isometric force pulses).

The finding that two patient groups were impaired on the tapping task is problematic. There are at least two interpretations of these results. One possibility is that timing may be a distributed process, dependent on the normal functioning of both cortical and cerebellar structures. Alternatively, since the tapping task may be disrupted by other functional deficits that do not involve timing, only one (or neither) of these structures may be involved in timing. For example, the patient may be able to time the movements, but may have difficulty in executing the movements. Thus, the perception task is critical in determining if the deficits on the tapping task truly reflected a deficit in timing, since there were no motor requirements in this task.

The results of the perception task supported the hypothesis that timing was not a distributed process. Only the patients with cerebellar lesions were impaired on this task (FIG. 2). Whereas the difference threshold for control, Parkinson, and cortical patients was about 30 ms, the value for the cerebellar group was 46 ms. An important control task emphasized that this deficit was specific to timing. When judging the loudness of a variable pair of tones in comparison to the loudness of a standard tone pair, the cerebellar patients performed as well as the control subjects. An unexpected, but important finding was that the cortical patients were impaired on this task (perhaps because some of the lesion extended into primary or secondary auditory areas). Thus, the two perception tasks yielded a double dissociation. The cerebellar patients were selectively impaired on the time-perception task, while the cortical patients were selectively impaired on the loudness-perception task. In neuropsycho-

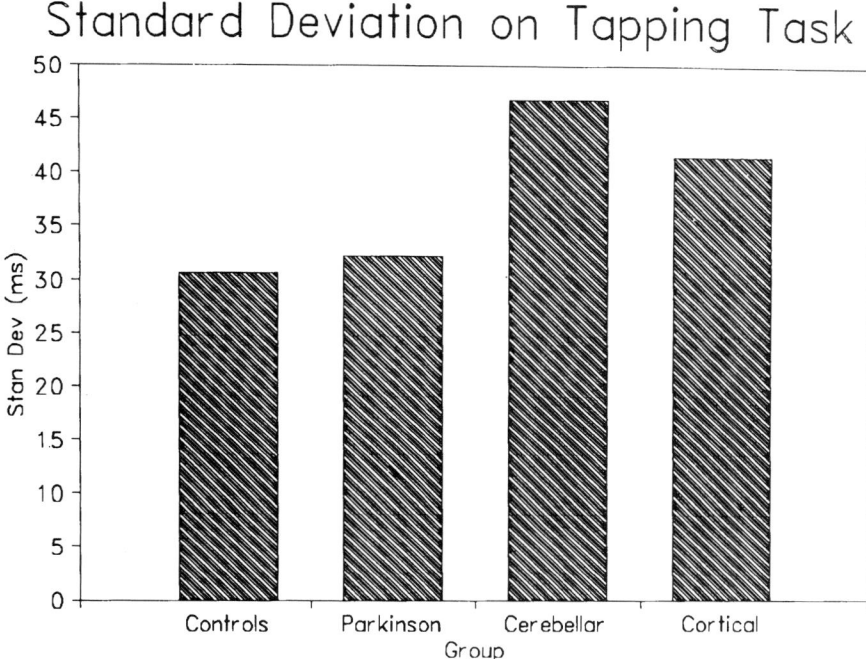

FIGURE 1. Mean standard deviation of intertap intervals on the repetitive tapping task for age-matched control subjects and three neurological groups with movement disorders. (From Ivry and Keele.[11] Reproduced by permission.)

logical research, double dissociations provide the strongest evidence that a particular mental operation (e.g., timing) is specifically associated with a neural system (e.g., the cerebellum).

Taken together, the impaired performance of the cerebellar patients on the repetitive-tapping and time-perception tasks provided evidence that the cerebellum could be characterized as an internal timing mechanism. A role for the cerebellum in temporally coordinating motoric events has been suggested by other researchers.[12,13] A timing hypothesis can also provide an account of many of the symptoms observed in cerebellar patients. For example, electromyography has indicated that intentional tremor and dysmetria result from abnormal timing of antagonist muscle activity to counteract the forces generated by agonist muscles.[14,15] The finding that cerebellar patients were impaired on a purely perceptual task was more surprising given the traditional association of this neural structure with motor control. Our hypothesis is that the prominent role of the cerebellum in motor control is because most coordinated actions require fine timing. More important, the computational capabilities of this structure are not restricted to the motor domain, but are also accessible to nonmotor tasks that are dependent on precise timing. In other words, the domain of cerebellar function is not defined in terms of tasks (e.g., motor control), but in terms of the computation performed by this structure (e.g., timing).

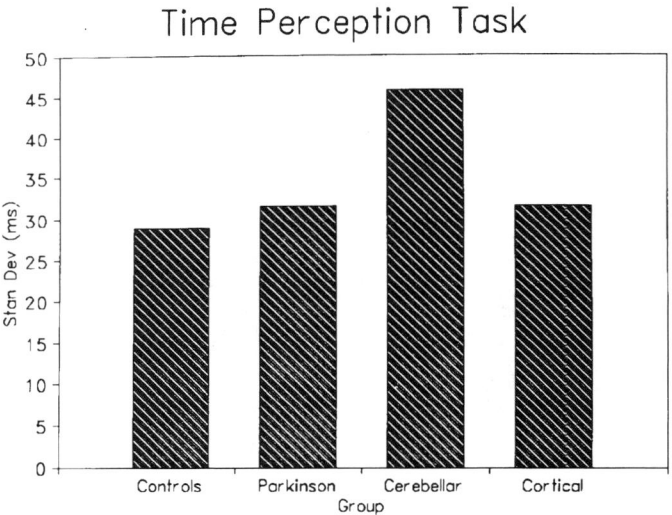
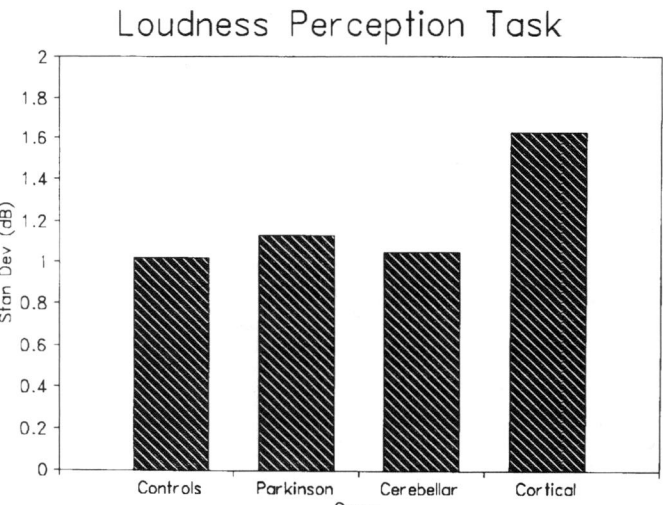

FIGURE 2. Mean standard deviation on a time perception (**top panel**) and a loudness perception (**bottom panel**) task. The scores were obtained using the parameter estimation by sequential testing procedure (PEST). (From Ivry and Keele.[11] Reproduced by permission.)

In subsequent research, we have sought to replicate these results, to identify those regions within the cerebellum that are most essential for timing, and to assess whether the cerebellum plays a role in other tasks that require timing. In one study, patients with focal cerebellar lesions, either in medial or lateral regions, were tested on the repetitive-tapping task.[16] Since the lesions were unilateral, each patient could serve as his or her own control by comparing performance when tapping with a finger on the impaired side with his or her performance when tapping with a finger on the unimpaired side. A mathematical model was used to determine whether the increased variability when tapping with the affected hand was due to a timing deficit or a problem in motor implementation.[4] A second double dissociation was found in this study. The model indicated that the source of the deficit for patients with medial lesions was due to problems in implementation, whereas the source of the deficit for patients with lateral lesions was due to a problem in timing. This result is consistent with the pattern of neural connectivity of the cerebellum.[17,18] Medial regions project primarily to spinal structures that are associated with motor execution. In contrast, lateral cerebellar regions project to regions of the cerebral cortex, including areas associated with motor planning.

In extensions of our perceptual results, patients with cerebellar lesions were tested on the time-perception task under various conditions (unpublished data). First, as in the original study, unfilled intervals were marked by 50-ms auditory clicks. In the second condition, the standard and comparison duration were continuous tones creating filled intervals. In the third condition, the temporal stimuli were signaled by the illumination of a light for a variable duration. The patients performed more poorly than control subjects in all three conditions. As before, no difference was found between the patients and control subjects on a nontemporal perception task, the loudness perception task.

A different population of subjects with coordination problems provided further evidence of the role of the cerebellum in timing. A significant proportion of children are diagnosed as developmentally clumsy. Clumsiness, however, can take many forms and there is some evidence that the symptoms may reflect subclinical neurological disorders. In our study, two groups of clumsy children were identified: those with soft neurological signs consistent with basal ganglia dysfunction and those with soft neurological signs of cerebellar dysfunction. Only the children with cerebellar symptoms were impaired on the repetitive-tapping and time-perception tasks.[19,20]

Given the inherent limitations in human neuropsychological research, we are currently developing an animal model to investigate the neural mechanisms of time perception. In our first experiment, twelve rats were trained on a time-discrimination task in which they were rewarded for pressing one lever following the presentation of a visual stimulus for 360 ms and a second lever following the presentation of a 670-ms visual stimulus. One of these two stimuli were presented on half of the trials. On the other trials, a range of probe durations were presented and responses to these stimuli were not rewarded. From the responses to the complete set of stimuli, a psychometric function can be plotted and used to estimate a point of subjective equality and a standard deviation for each rat. Following extensive training on this task, bilateral cerebellar lesions were made in eight of the animals. The lesions were targeted for the lateral cerebellar nuclei (dentate and interpositus) given that output from the neocerebellum must pass through these nuclei. Four other animals received sham lesions.

In this initial experiment, the lesioned animals were significantly impaired in comparison to either their presurgery performance or the postsurgery performance of the sham group (FIG. 3). As in our human studies, cerebellar lesions increased the variability of the rats' responses. In addition, the point of subjective equality, the 50 percent point in the psychometric functions, was shifted to an earlier point in time for seven of the eight rats with cerebellar lesions. For some of the animals, the deficits were relatively long lasting, extending throughout the two month postsurgery testing period. For others, recovery appeared to be complete by the end of the experiment.

In further studies, we plan to determine if the rate of recovery is correlated with the foci of the lesions. Furthermore, we also need to conduct some important control experiments, such as demonstrating that cerebellar lesions do not produce a general impairment in the rats' performance on psychometric testing. For example, if a stimulus parameter such as brightness was varied, we would not expect to observe any deficit following cerebellar lesions. Finally, we are attempting to identify the boundary conditions of the cerebellar timing system. Rats are being simultaneously trained on two duration discrimination tasks, a short-range timing task and a long-range timing task. In the short-range task, the durations are centered around 525 ms; for the long-range task, the durations are centered around 33 s. We predict that cerebellar lesions will selectively impair performance on the short-duration task and not the long-duration task. Such a result, coupled with previous findings implicating cholinergic systems in timing tasks on the order of 10–30 s[21,22] would begin to identify dissociable neural mechanisms of timing.

The tapping and time-perception results had led to the cerebellar timing hypothesis. Given this hypothesis, the role of the cerebellum in other tasks that require temporal information processing can be investigated. Ivry and Diener[23] found that patients with cerebellar lesions were impaired in judging the velocity of a moving

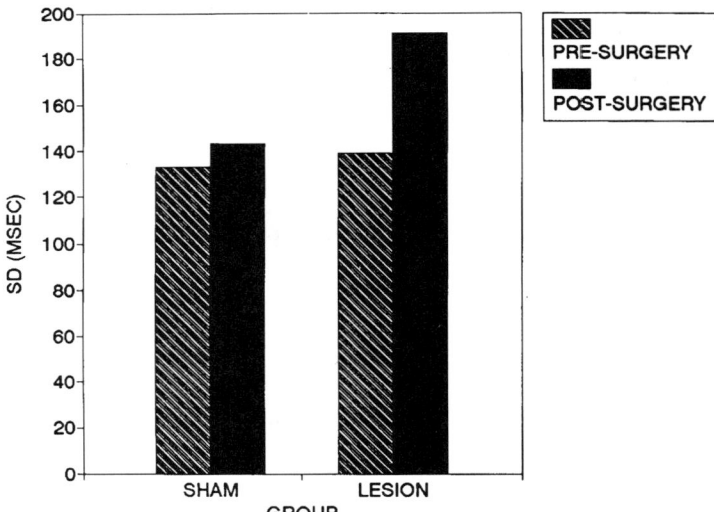

FIGURE 3. Mean standard deviation for experimental ($n=8$) and sham ($n=4$) rats on the time-perception task. The scores were obtained using the method of constant stimuli. (Unpublished data.)

visual stimulus (FIG. 4). In three experiments, subjects had to judge the relative speed of a display of moving dots. They were instructed to maintain fixation during the stimulus presentation to eliminate any effects that might be due to the aberrant eye movements observed in cerebellar patients. Performance on this task was similar for patients who were unable to maintain fixation. Moreover, errors on the perceptual task were not correlated with electroocular activity. These results suggest that the deficit in the velocity perception task are not the indirect consequence of a motor problem in controlling eye movements.

The velocity perception study provides an example of how the issue of implicit and explicit timing can be investigated. Velocity, by definition, requires an analysis of information over time. However, the temporal information need not be explicitly represented. Velocity detectors could be hardwired, with different activation thresholds being associated with inputs arising from neighboring spatial locations.

However, the timing capabilities of the cerebellum might be exploited for computing precise velocity information. The activity in some neocerebellar Purkinje cells is correlated with the speed of a moving visual stimulus, independent of the motion effects introduced by eye, head, and body motion.[24] These cells could thus be generating a viewer-independent representation of the stimulus motion that would be essential for generating predictive pursuit or saccadic eye movements, functions that are known to be impaired in cerebellar patients.[25-27] These findings suggest that problems in generating predictive eye movements following cerebellar lesions may arise from deficits in computing velocity information. If this hypothesis is correct, then on the basis of parsimony, we would infer that velocity perception requires the

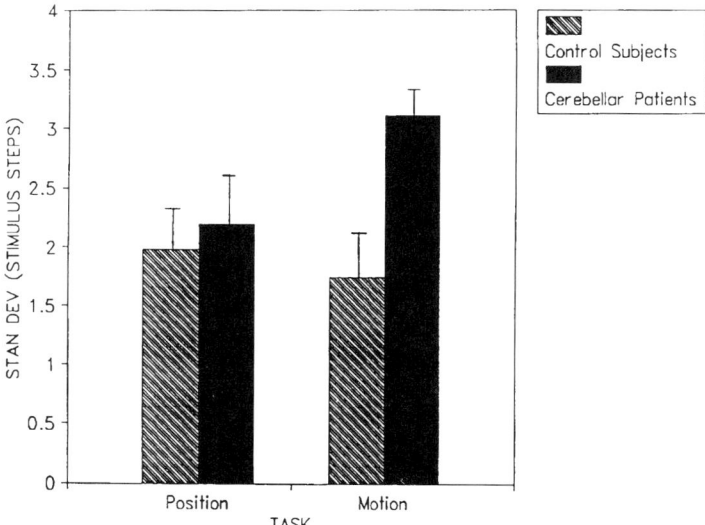

FIGURE 4. Mean standard deviation for age-matched control subjects and patients with cerebellar lesions on two visual-perception tasks. In the control task, the stimuli were similar to the motion task, but the position of the comparion stimulus was shifted relative to the position of the standard stimulus. Temporal information processing was assumed to only be required in the motion task. (From Ivry and Diener.[23] Reproduced by permission.)

explicit processing of temporal information and that because of this requirement, the cerebellum is an integral part of the process.

CEREBELLAR TIMING IN SPEECH PERCEPTION AND PRODUCTION

Speech perception and speech production are, of course, preeminent examples of tasks in which information must be processed over time. The logic that guided our research on velocity perception can also be applied to these task domains. We have investigated one speech phenomenon that might be expected to utilize an explicit timing mechanism: the perception and production of voicing in consonant–vowel syllables. In producing voiced phonemes such as /b/ and /d/, the vocal cords begin to vibrate at approximately the same time as the release of airflow. In contrast, the vocal-cord vibration is delayed in the production of unvoiced phonemes such as /p/ and /t/. The time between airflow release and vocal-cord vibration is referred to as *voice-onset time* (VOT). In English, the VOT for the syllable "ba" is approximately 0 ms, whereas the VOT for the syllable "pa" is about 40 ms.

Using a speech synthesizer to generate the formants associated with "ba" and "pa," a continuum of speech sounds can be created by varying VOT (done by deleting information in the vicinity of the fundamental and first formant). A seminal result in speech perception is that such continua are perceived categorically.[28] Below a critical VOT value, subjects consistently perceive "ba"; above that value, the percept is consistently "pa," and the boundary from one percept to the other is much steeper than that observed with nonspeech stimuli containing similar frequency information.

To determine if the cerebellar timing mechanism was involved in the perception of VOT, cerebellar patients were tested on a "ba-pa" continuum.[29] For control purposes, the patients were also tested on a "ba-da" continuum. For these stimuli, the synthetic manipulation is of the second and third formant transitions, with the temporal events being constant. On both continua, the performance of the cerebellar patients was similar to that of age-matched control subjects (FIG. 5). This null result was replicated in a second group of patients (unpublished data).

Different interpretations of these null results are raised when considering the issue of implicit versus explicit timing. On the one hand, VOTs may be explicitly computed. If so, the lack of a deficit would indicate that the requisite processing falls outside the domain of the cerebellar timing system. It has been argued that speech perception involves dedicated processors.[30] Perhaps one of these processors may be specialized for computing temporal information in the speech signal.

On the other hand, the timing differences between voiced and voiceless phonemes may only be represented implicitly. These differences may be correlated with a different acoustic cue, one that is exploited by psychological processors involved in speech perception. For example, there are marked spectral differences between voiced and voiceless phonemes, with the former having much greater power in the lower frequency region.[31,32] A psychological operation that analyzed the distribution of energy in the frequency spectrum at signal onset should be able to determine if a sound is voiced or voiceless without needing any explicit representation of temporal information (other than be able to note the onset of a signal). If this were the case, then the null results for the cerebellar patients could simply reflect the fact that precise timing is not needed for this speech-perception task.[33]

While we have not identified any speech-perception deficits in cerebellar patients, the timing hypothesis does offer a parsimonious account of certain aspects of the

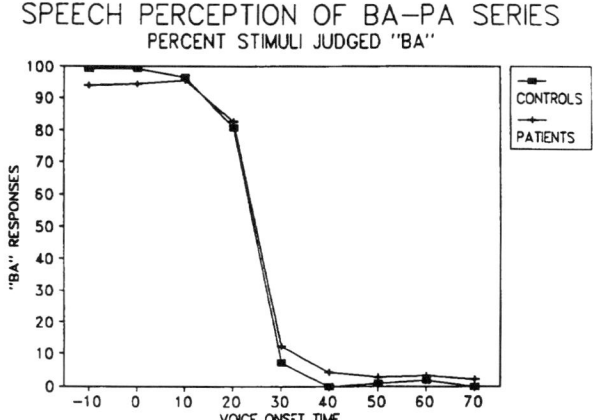

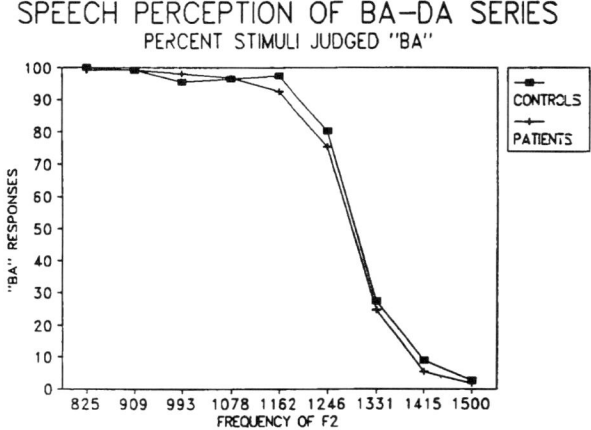

FIGURE 5. Identification functions for the speech-perception tasks for age-matched control subjects and patients with cerebellar lesions. **Top panel** is for the "ba-pa" continuum in which the stimuli vary in simulated VOT. **Bottom panel** is for the "ba-da" control continuum in which the stimuli vary in the trajectory of the simulated second and third formant transitons. (From Ivry and Gopal.[29] Reproduced by permission.)

speech disorders observed in these patients. Cerebellar dysarthria is characterized by inconsistency in the articulation of phonemes and heightened variability in the control of rate and stress.[34] We hypothesized that if cerebellar dysarthria were due to a selective deficit in temporally coordinating events across different articulators, then errors in articulation should conform to a predictable distribution. Specifically, errors should be distributed on the voicing dimension and not in terms of place of articulation ("ba" versus "da"). For example, if, due to poor temporal coupling, the initiation of vocal-cord vibration was delayed when attempting to say "ba," the percept might be "pa." A problem in temporally coordinating the actions underlying voicing and consonantal release would not lead a "ba" to be heard as a "da." The temporal structure of these two syllables is similar; they differ in terms of the configuration of the positioning of the lips and tongue.

These predictions were supported in two analyses.[29] When healthy subjects labeled the patients' productions, mispercepts were almost always along the VOT dimension and rarely along the control, spectral dimension (TABLE 1). For example, if the patient said "ba," the judge was much more likely to hear it as "pa" than "da." Of the 26 labeling errors in this task (13 percent of total productions), 88 percent were due to errors along the voicing dimension. Moreover, acoustic measurements of VOT in the productions of cerebellar patients were significantly more variable than those obtained from age-matched controls. Spectral events, measured during the steady-state vocalic portion of the syllables, revealed fewer differences between the patients and control subjects.

At first glance, the speech results might seem at odds with the claim that the cerebellum operates as an internal timing mechanism. The timing hypothesis was motivated by the finding that cerebellar patients show a dual deficit in both production and perception tasks that require precise timing. In the speech domain, the timing hypothesis can account for at least some aspects of the patients' production problems, but these same patients were unimpaired on the speech-perception task. While this discrepancy may indicate problems for the cerebellar timing hypothesis, it is also possible that the critical factor is that the cerebellum is only involved when the task re-

TABLE 1. Errors in Perceptual Classifications of Syllables Produced by Patients with Cerebellar Dysarthria

Stimulus	Response	Total
Controls		
Voiced	Voiceless	2
Voiceless	Voiced	0
Total Voicing Errors		2
Labial	Alveolar	3
Alveolar	Labial	1
Total Place Errors		4
Patients		
Voiced	Voiceless	12
Voiceless	Voiced	11
Total Voicing Errors		23
Labial	Alveolar	0
Alveolar	Labial	3
Total Place Errors		3

quires explicit timing. It seems reasonable to assume that this is the case in the repetitive-tapping task. As with other complex movements, the problems seen in the speech of cerebellar patients can be attributed to the need for precise temporal coordination between the activity of different muscle groups. However, even if timing is explicitly controlled in the production of actions such as speech, the perception of these actions need not involve the representation of temporal information.

CEREBELLAR TIMING AND SENSORIMOTOR LEARNING

The cerebellum has been assumed to play a major role in sensorimotor learning. While the first evidence came from studies examining adaptation of the vestibuloocular reflex,[35] recent work has involved a classical conditioning paradigm.[36,37] In this paradigm, a conditioned stimulus (CS), such as a tone, is repeatedly paired with an unconditioned stimulus (US), such as an airpuff, delivered to the cornea. The airpuff will trigger an unconditioned response (UR), the retraction of the nictitating membrane. Over trials, the tone will come to elicit a similar response (CR). Numerous studies have now demonstrated that acquisition and/or retention of the CR is severely disrupted or even abolished following cerebellar lesions. Since the UR remains intact, the effect is attributed to a learning deficit rather than a motor deficit. The learning hypothesis is further supported by studies indicating that the cerebellum is a plausible site for integrating information from pathways conveying signals associated with the US and CS.[38]

It is important to ask why the cerebellum is critical for the acquisition and retention of conditioned responses. A first proposal might be that the cerebellum is essential for learning the simple, reflexivelike responses elicited in conditioning paradigms. If this hypothesis were correct, then the cerebellum would be expected to play a role in all forms of classical conditioning. This hypothesis is refuted by the available evidence. In the eyeblink paradigm, the CS not only comes to elicit an eyeblink CR, but it also becomes associated with other fear-related CRs, such as a decrease in heart rate. Cerebellar lesions have no effect on the heart-rate response.[39]

The dissociation between the eyeblink and heart rate CRs indicate that only a subset of conditioned responses is dependent on the cerebellum. One hypothesis that would account for this dissociation would be that the cerebellar learning domain is restricted to responses dependent on the skeletal musculature. Autonomic responses (such as heart rate) are assumed to be mediated by other neural systems. An alternative hypothesis is that the cerebellum is essential when the task requires the animal to represent the temporal relations between different stimuli. That is, the cerebellum is critical for learning tasks that require explicit timing.

Consider the eyeblink paradigm. The conditioned eyeblink is only adaptive if it occurs prior to the airpuff, allowing the animal to reduce the negative effects of the aversive US. The animal must then learn the temporal relationship between the CS and US in order to be able to produce an anticipatory CR. That the animal is learning about the timing between the two stimuli rather than simply linking the CR to the first stimulus is shown by studies that manipulate the CS–US interval. Over a range of CS–US intervals, the peak amplitude of the CR occurs just prior to the onset of the US. Thus, the time at which the CR peaks is directly related to the CS–US interval.[40] In conditioning of autonomic responses, such as changes in heart rate, there is only a weak correlation between CR latency and the CS–US interval.

Thus, there are two different accounts of the cerebellar role in learning. One hypothesis focuses on the task domain, postulating that the cerebellum is essential for learning skeletal responses. The other hypothesis emphasizes a computational mechanism, postulating that the cerebellum will be required when the task requires the representation of precise temporal information. A recent unpublished study by Steinmetz provides an initial unconfounding of these two hypotheses.

Rats were trained on one of two operant conditioning tasks.[41] The stimulus and (overt) response was the same in both tasks. A 1-s tone was presented and the animal had to press a lever during that 1-s interval in order to receive a reinforcement. What differed between the two groups was the nature of the reinforcer. For the positive condition, rats received food if they responded prior to the termination of the tone. For the negative condition, rats were shocked if they failed to respond before the end of the tone.

Separate groups of rats were trained to comparable levels of performance on the positive and negative tasks. The animals in both groups were then given bilateral cerebellar lesions. A striking dissociation was evident during postsurgery testing. Whereas the lesions produced a marked impairment in performance on the negative task, performance on the positive task was unaffected. This result is at odds with predictions derived from a hypothesis emphasizing the importance of the cerebellum for learned skeletal responses. In both conditions, the response is a single lever press. The lesions, however, only disrupted learning in one condition.

Examination of the response topography suggests that the dissociation observed by Steinmetz may be accounted for by the timing hypothesis (FIG. 6). While the response is always a lever press, the time at which the response occurs is different for the two groups. Rats trained in the positive condition, appear to respond as quickly as possible: their response latencies are skewed toward the initial half of the 1-s tone interval and appear to form a simple reaction time distribution. In contrast, the distribution of response latencies in the negative condition are skewed toward the end of the 1-s tone interval. In this condition, the rats appear to be delaying their responses for as long as possible. It is unclear why there is this difference in the distribution of the response latencies. For whatever reason, in the positive condition, the rats obtain the reward as quickly as possible, and in the negative condition, they respond at the last possible moment. (Perhaps evolutionary pressures have acted to create this difference. If food is available, one must act fast to beat competitors. If punishment is imminent, delay taking avoidance action in the hope that an external agent will intervene.) These distributions suggest that the animal requires explicit timing in only the negative condition. Thus, the selective effects of cerebellar lesions may be the result of the timing demands in the negative condition. The null results for the positive condition would reflect the fact that the critical associative process for this group is not dependent on the explicit representation of temporal information.

Steinmetz's experiment may have inadvertently unconfounded the skeletal musculature and timing hypotheses. However, it is important to note that a second confound remains. All of the cases in which the cerebellum is associated with learning not only require precise timing, but also involve situations where the animal must learn an avoidance response. That is, in all of these conditions, the animal is able to use an external error signal (airpuff, retinal slip, or shock) to modify its behavior. Perhaps the cerebellum is essential for learning avoidance responses involving the skeletal musculature.[37] The cerebellum was not involved in the condition where the rat presses the lever in order to obtain a food reward, but here there is really no error signal (other than internal states associated with hunger or frustration).

What is needed are experiments that unconfound timing and error correction. Together with Steinmetz, we are currently conducting such an experiment. In the positive-timed condition, we are setting up a situation where the rat must time a

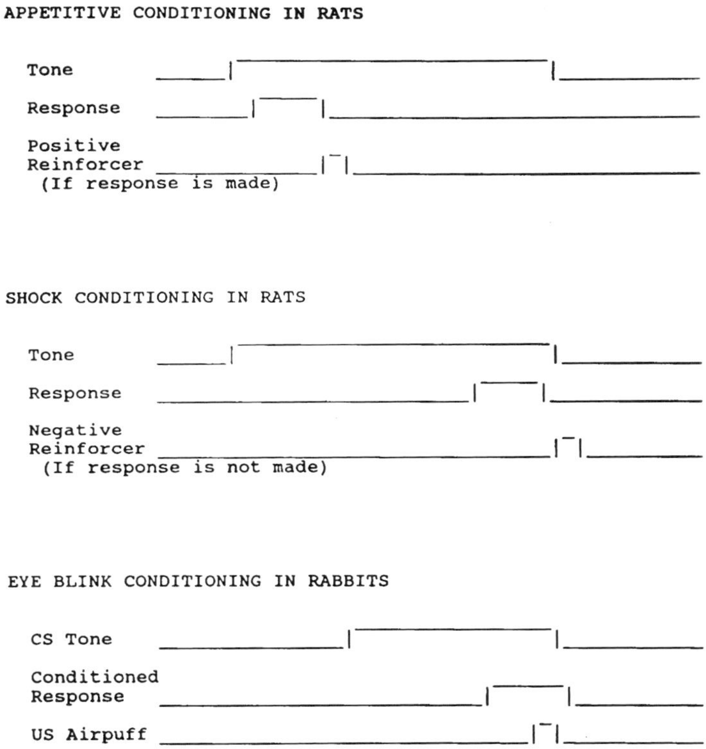

APPETITIVE CONDITIONING IN RATS

```
Tone                    ____|‾‾‾‾‾‾‾‾‾‾‾‾‾‾‾‾‾‾‾‾‾|____
Response                _____|‾‾‾|_____
Positive
Reinforcer              _____|⁻|_____
(If response is made)
```

SHOCK CONDITIONING IN RATS

```
Tone                    ____|‾‾‾‾‾‾‾‾‾‾‾‾‾‾‾‾‾‾‾‾‾|____
Response                _____|‾‾‾|____
Negative
Reinforcer              _____|⁻|____
(If response is not made)
```

EYE BLINK CONDITIONING IN RABBITS

```
CS Tone                 _____|‾‾‾‾‾‾‾‾‾‾‾‾|____
Conditioned
Response                _____|‾‾‾|____
US Airpuff              _____|⁻|____
```

FIGURE 6. Schematic diagram of the temporal relationship between the stimuli and response in three animal learning paradigms (see text). Note that the animals' responses are delayed until the end of the tone in the shock-conditioning and eye-blink-conditioning paradigms.

response in order to receive a food pellet. To do this, the stimulus is again a 1-s tone, but the rats are only reinforced when they respond during the last 300 ms of the stimulus. In a negative-untimed condition, the interval between the tone onset and shock is varied. We expect this variation will make the rats respond as quickly as possible, thus removing the need to do any timing. If timing is the critical factor, then lesioned animals should show a learning impairment in the positive-timed condition. If error correction is important, then the lesions should only disrupt performance in the negative-untimed condition.

CONCLUSIONS

The research reviewed in this chapter offers some resolutions to the two questions posed in the Introduction. Studies with healthy subjects indicated a correlation between performance on movement and perception tasks that required precise timing. This evidence bolstered our assumption that these tasks involve the explicit representation of temporal information. Neuropsychological studies indicated that the cerebellum was a critical neural structure for representing this information. Further patient and animal research has provided one means of assessing whether other tasks require the explicit representation of temporal information. These studies have demonstrated that the timing hypothesis can provide a parsimonious account of a number of seemingly disparate functions associated with the cerebellum.

Two points, however, should be kept in mind in considering the generality of the cerebellar timing hypothesis. First, it would be unreasonable to assume that the cerebellum is involved in all tasks that require the explicit representation of temporal information. This information occurs over a variety of scales, and the cerebellar timing system may be capable of representing this information over a limited temporal range. If the domain of the cerebellum was originally limited to the coordination of action, then its timing capabilities may have been constrained by evolutionary processes to a range relevant for motor control. Second, it cannot be inferred from the timing hypothesis that there is a single timing mechanism in the cerebellum. Rather, the hypothesis is offered as a general computational description of cerebellar function. It is reasonable to suppose that this computational capability is distributed throughout the cerebellum, with different regions representing the temporal information utilized in different tasks.

ACKNOWLEDGMENTS

Steven Keele, Eliot Hazeltine, and Art Shimamura provided useful comments in the preparation of this paper.

REFERENCES

1. TURVEY, M. T., L. D. ROSENBLUM, P. N. KUGLER & R C. SCHMIDT. 1986. Fluctuations and phase symmetry in coordinated rhythmic movements. J. Exp. Psychol.: Hum. Percept. Perform. **12:** 564–583.
2. IVRY, R. & D. CORCOS. Slicing the variability pie: Component analysis of coordination and motor dysfunction. *In* Variability and Motor Control, K. Newell and D. Corcos, Eds. In press.
3. KELSO, J. A. S. 1984. Phase transitions and critical behavior in human bimanual coordination. Am. J. Physiol. **15:** R1000–R1004.
4. WING, A. 1980. The long and short of timing in response sequences. *In* Tutorials in Motor Behavior, G. Stelmach and J. Requin, Eds. North-Holland. New York.
5. HAKEN, H., J. A. S. KELSO & H. BUNZ. 1985. A theoretical model of phase transitions in human hand movements. Biol. Cybern. **51:** 347–356.
6. IVRY, R. & R. HAZELTINE. 1992. Models of timing-with-a-timer. *In* Time, Action, and Cognition, F. Macar, V. Pouthas, and W. Freidman, Eds.: 183–189. Kluwer. Dordrecht, the Netherlands.
7. PASTOR, M. A., J. ARTIEDA, M. JAHANSHAHI & J. A. OBESO. 1992. Time estimation and reproduction is abnormal in Parkinson's disease. Brain **115:** 211–225.
8. RICHELLE, M., H. LEJEUNE, J. J. PERIKEL & P. FERY. 1985. From biotemporality to nontemporality: Toward an integrative and comparative view of time in behavior. *In* Time, Mind, and Behavior, J. A. Michon and J. L. Jackson, Eds.: 75–99. Springer-Verlag. Berlin/New York.

9. KEELE, S., R. POKORNY, D. CORCOS & R. IVRY. 1985. Do perception and motor production share common timing mechanisms? Acta Psychol. **60:** 173–193.
10. KEELE, S., R. IVRY & R. POKORNY. 1987. Force control and its relation to timing. J. Motor Behav. **19:** 96–114.
11. IVRY, R. B. & S. W. KEELE. 1989. Timing functions of the cerebellum. J. Cogn. Neurosci. **1:** 134–150.
12. HOUK, J. C., S. P. SINGH, C. FISHER & A. G. BARTO. 1990. An adaptive sensorimotor network inspired by the anatomy and physiology of the cerebellum. *In* Neural Networks for Control, W. T. Miller, R. S. Sutton, and P. J. Werbos, Eds.: 301–348. MIT Press. Cambridge, Mass.
13. PELLIONISZ, A. & R. LLINAS. 1982. Space-time representation in the brain: The cerebellum as a predictive space-time metric tensor. Neuroscience **7:** 2949–2970.
14. HORE, J., B. WILD & H. C. DIENER. 1991. Cerebellar dysmetria at the elbow, wrist, and fingers. J. Neurophysiol. **65:** 563–571.
15. VILIS, T. & J. HORE. 1980. Central neural mechanisms contributing to cerebellar tremor produced by limb perturbations. J. Neurophysiol. **43:** 279–291.
16. IVRY, R., S. KEELE & H. DIENER. 1988. Dissociation of the lateral and medial cerebellum in movement timing and movement execution. Exp. Brain Res. **73:** 167–180.
17. ASANUMA, C., W. THACH & E. JONES. 1983. Anatomical evidence for segregated focal groupings of efferent cells and their ramifications in the cerebellothalamic pathway of the monkey. Brain Res. Rev. **5:** 267–298.
18. ———. 1983. Brainstem and spinal projections of the deep cerebellar nuclei in the monkey with observations on the brainstem projections of the dorsal column nuclei. Brain Res. Rev. **5:** 299–322.
19. LUNDY-EKMAN, L., R. IVRY, S. W. KEELE & M. WOOLLACOTT. 1991. Timing and force control deficits in clumsy children. J. Cogn. Neurosci. **3:** 370–377.
20. WILLIAMS, H. G., M. H. WOOLLACOTT & R. IVRY. 1992. Timing and motor control in clumsy children. J. Motor Behav. **24:** 165–172.
21. MECK, W. H. 1983. Selective adjustment of the speed of internal clock and memory processes. J. Exp. Psychol.: Anim. Behav. Processes **9:** 171–201.
22. MECK, W. H. & R. M. CHURCH. 1987. Cholinergic modulation of the content of temporal memory. Behav. Neurosci. **101:** 457–464.
23. IVRY, R. B. & H. C. DIENER. 1991. Impaired velocity perception in patients with lesions of the cerebellum. J. Cogn. Neurosci. **3:** 355–366.
24. SUZUKI, D. & E. KELLER. 1988. The role of the posterior vermis of monkey cerebellum in smooth-pursuit eye movement control. II. Target velocity-related Purkinje cell activity. J. Neurophysiol. **59:** 19–40.
25. ASCHOFF, J. & B. COHEN. 1971. Changes in saccadic eye movements produced by cerebellar cortical lesions. Exp. Neurol. **32:** 123–132.
26. RITCHIE, L. 1976. Effects of cerebellar lesions on saccadic eye movements. J. Neurophysiol. **39:** 1246–1256.
27. WESTHEIMER, G. & S. BLAIR. 1974. Functional organization of primate oculomotor system revealed by cerebellectomy. Exp. Brain Res. **21:** 463–472.
28. ABRAMSON, A. & L. LISKER. 1968. Voice timing: Cross-language experiments in identification and discrimination. Paper presented at the meetings of the Acoustical Society of America, Ottawa, Ont., Canada.
29. IVRY, R. & H. S. GOPAL. Speech production and perception in patients with cerebellar lesions. *In* Attention and Performance, Vol. XIV, D. Meyer and S. Kornblum, Eds. Lawrence Erlbaum. Hillsdale, N.J. In press.
30. LIBERMAN, A. & I. MATTINGLY. 1985. The motor theory of speech perception revised. Cognition **21:** 1–36.
31. LISKER, L. 1975. Is it VOT or a first-formant transition detector? J. Acoust. Soc. Am. **56:** 1547–1551.
32. STEVENS, K. N. & D. H. KLATT. 1974. Role of formant transitions in the voiced-voiceless distinction for stops. J. Acoust. Soc. Am. **55:** 653–659.
33. IVRY, R. & P. LEBBY. Hemispheric differences in auditory perception are similar to those found in visual perception. Psychol. Sci. In press.

34. DARLEY, F., A. ARONSON & J. BROWN. 1969. Differential diagnostic patterns of dysarthria. J. Speech Hear. Res. **12:** 246–269.
35. ITO, M. 1984. The Cerebellum and Neural Control. Raven Press. New York.
36. YEO, C. H. 1991. Cerebellum and classical conditioning of motor responses. Ann. N.Y. Acad. Sci. **627:** 292–304.
37. THOMPSON, R. F. 1990. Neural mechanisms of classical conditioning in mammals. Philos. Trans. R. Soc. Ser. B **329:** 161–170.
38. STEINMETZ, J. E., D. G. LAVOND & R. F. THOMPSON. 1989. Classical conditioning in rabbits using pontine nucleus stimulation as a conditioned stimulus and inferior olive stimulation as an unconditioned stimulus. Synapse **3:** 225–233.
39. LAVOND, D. G., J. S. LINCOLN, D. A. MCCORMICK & R. F. THOMPSON. 1984. Effect of bilateral lesions of the dentate and interpositus nuclei on conditioning of heart-rate and nictitating membrane/eyelid responses in the rabbit. Brain Res. **305:** 323–330.
40. WICKENS, D. D., A. F. NIELD, D. S. TUBER & C. WICKENS. Strength, latency, and form of conditioned skeletal and automatic responses as functions of CS-UCS intervals. J. Exp. Psychol. **80:** 165–170.
41. LOGUE, S. F., P. D. MILLER & J. E. STEINMETZ. 1991. A signalled bar-pressing preparation for study of the neural bases of appetitive and aversive learning in the rat. Neurosci. Abstr. **17:** 660.

Control of Binocular Eye Movements in Normals and Dyslexics[a]

GUNNAR LENNERSTRAND,[b] JAN YGGE,[b]
AND CHRISTER JACOBSSON[c]

[b]Department of Ophthalmology
Karolinska Institute
Huddinge University Hospital
S-141 86 Huddinge Sweden

[c]Department of Applied Education
University of Växjö
S-351 95 Växjö, Sweden

INTRODUCTION

The importance of visual defects and abnormalities of binocular vision in dyslexia has been a subject of much dispute. In recent years the evidence for a neurobiological basis and possibly also a specific genetic defect has become stronger,[1-4] and the interest has therefore been focused less on ocular deviation and strabismus and more on perceptual abnormalities manifested in testing of visual and ocular motor function. For a more complete coverage of this field the reader is directed to recent reviews.[5-7]

In this paper we examine the possibility of a deficiency in the binocular control mechanisms as a contributing factor in dyslexia. There are reports of a mismatch in dyslexia between the "transient" and "sustained" channels of vision,[8,9] due to a weakness in the transient channel. This may also influence the motor control of binocular vision and tentatively lead to abnormal saccadic eye movements. It has been shown that saccadic latencies (i.e., reaction times) in dyslexic subjects are different from those of normal readers of the same age.[10] It has been suggested that deficiencies in the dynamic vergence control during binocular fixation and disturbances in the sense of direction manifested as an instability of ocular dominance, could contribute at least to some forms of dyslexia.[11] Some of these ideas have been tested in a population-based investigation, presently being conducted in the Kronoberg county of Sweden. The purpose of the study is to develop and evaluate methods for diagnosis and remediation of dyslexia by an interdisciplinary approach. As a part of the study, visual and oculomotor functions have been determined within the framework of a thorough general ophthalmological and orthoptic examination when the children were in grade three.[12,13] We here describe the findings relevant to binocular control, including some preliminary results from binocular recordings of eye movements obtained both during reading and with nonreading targets. Previous studies of eye movements in reading with high precision IR-technique have mainly been done monocularly. We have used a system that allowed dc-recordings of eye movements in the two eyes simultaneously, with the aim to analyze the synchrony

---

[a]This study was supported by grants from the Swedish Ministry of Social Affairs, the Bank of Sweden Tercentenary Foundation, the Swedish Research Council of Social Sciences, and the Sigvard & Marianne Bernadotte Research Foundation for Children Eye Care.

of eye movements and the control of alignment between the two eyes during non-reading and reading eye movements.

MATERIAL AND METHODS

The Study Group

The whole population of children attending the second grade (n = 2167) in Kronoberg county participated in the initial selection of subjects for the dyslexic and the control group. All the children were tested with regard to word decoding and reading comprehension, and with a nonverbal test for cognitive skills. Based on the outcome of these tests and on the teachers reports of the reading ability of the children, the poorest readers and control pupils in the same class matched for age, sex, and cognitive ability were selected. The number of matched pairs was 86.

Ophthalmological and Orthoptic Evaluation

A full examination was performed, but here only part of it is reported. The testing was done at a mean age of 9 years and 5 months. The sensory tests included monocular and binocular Snellen visual acuity for distance and near, monocular contrast sensitivity determined for near with the Vistech test,[14] stereoscopic vision with the TNO test, and ocular dominance testing with a synoptophore according to the method described by Dunlop, later modified by Stein and Fowler.[15] To ensure that the measurements of ocular dominance were performed in the same way as in the studies by Stein and coworkers,[15] our orthoptists were trained with the English group.

The motor tests included determination of ocular alignment with the cover tests. Measurements of vergence movements were done with prisms and with a synoptophore. Determination of vergence end-point with the synoptophore was done both subjectively with diplopia observations and objectively with recording of eye movements, using the infrared reflexion technique as developed in the Ober-2 system (Permobil AB, S-861 00 Timrå, Sweden). The Ober-2 system was also used for measuring pursuit movements in following/tracking of moving targets displayed on a computer screen and for recording eye movements and fixations during reading of text on paper.

RESULTS

Sensory Functions

Monocular Tests

Visual acuity with best correction for distance and near was significantly lower in dyslexics than in normal readers. Of the normal readers 94 percent had a distance acuity of 1.0 (20/20) or better, but only 83 percent of the dyslexics. For near acuity the corresponding numbers were 99 percent and 87 percent, respectively. Further details are shown in TABLE 1.

TABLE 1. Visual Acuity for Distance and Near, Best Eye

Visual Acuity	Dyslexics, No. (%)	Controls, No. (%)
Distance		
<1.0	15 (17.4)	5 (5.8)
1.0	62 (72.1)	60 (69.8)
>1.0	9 (10.5)	21 (24.4)
$p = 0.0017$, Wilcoxon–Mann–Whitney ($Z = 3.136$)		
Near		
<1.0	11 (12.8)	1 (1.2)
1.0	75 (87.2)	85 (98.8)
$p = 0.00029$, Wilcoxon–Mann–Whitney ($Z = 2.99$)		

Contrast sensitivity was lower in the dyslexic group than in controls, in the low (1.5–3 cycles per degree) as well as in the high spatial frequency range (18 cycles per degree), but not for medium spatial frequencies. These differences were statistically significant (Wilcoxon–Mann–Whitney test).

Binocular Tests

Stereopsis was normal (60 seconds of arc or better) in 57 dyslexics and 56 normal readers. Defects of stereoscopic vision was seen mainly in children with strabismus.

Ocular dominance and its stability. We found no difference in the stability of ocular dominance between dyslexics and normal readers (TABLE 2), if stability was defined as dominance of one eye at least 8 times out of 10 tests.[16] A strong left dominance, with all 10 trials favoring this eye, was much more common than a strong right dominance in both groups of children (TABLE 2). A statistical analysis (Fisher's exact test) showed no significant difference between stable and unstable ocular dominance in either group.

TABLE 2. The Results of the Ocular Dominance Test

Ocular Dominance	Dyslexics ($n = 81$)	Controls ($n = 81$)
Stable	38	45
Unstable	43	36
Strong LE dominance	17	16
Strong RE dominance	1	6

Note: LE = left eye; RE = right eye.

Ocular Motor Functions

Without Reading

Heterotropia and heterophoria were established with the cover test. Only the results of testing for proximate fixation are presented here since they relate more to the reading situation than the testing for distance. Heterotropia was found in 7 dyslexics and in 3 controls. Heterophoria was seen in 53 dyslexics and 63 control children. The distribution between esophoria and exophoria, and the magnitude of the deviations were not statistically different between groups. However, it can be noted that esophoria at near was more common in the controls than in dyslexics, while exophoria was equally common in both groups.

Vergence fusional range, measured at close range, were not different between groups when the values were corrected for the amount of latent strabismus, as seen in TABLE 3. The vergence movements were also tested with the synoptophore, and the child had to indicate when fusion was disrupted by the appearance of diplopia. Simultaneous recordings of eye movements with the Ober-2 equipment confirmed that vergence movements were interrupted at this moment (FIG. 1). Using a small fixation object subtending 2.5 degrees the mean divergence value for dyslexics was 4.1 degrees (S.D. = 1.24) and for controls 4.0 degrees (S.D. = 0.96). The convergence values for the same object size were 12.5 (S.D. = 7.86) degrees for dyslexics and 11.7 (S.D. = 7.87) for controls. The differences between groups were not statistically significant.

Pursuit movements during binocular viewing were elicited by asking the child to fixate a small target on the computer screen, moving from left to right at a speed of 7.5 degrees per second for 3.5 seconds. A typical recording is shown in FIG. 2. Dyslexics showed significantly larger saccadic components, irrespective of the direction of the saccade, that is, not only in the direction of target movement (catch-up saccades), but also backup saccades in the reversed direction (backup saccades).

During Reading

The children were reading texts adapted to their reading level with both eyes open, either in the ordinary right-to-left direction or with the text upside down. FIGURE 3 illustrates eye movements recorded binocularly during reading in the ordinary direction with the Ober-2 system in a control and a dyslexic pupil. So far our

TABLE 3. Vergence Fusion Capacities for Near Fixation

	Vergence Fusion in Prism Diopters [mean (S.D.)]		
	Dyslexics	Controls	Significance[a]
Convergence	26.5 (6.8)	26.3 (7.2)	$p = 0.75$
Divergence	10.5 (2.9)	10.2 (3.2)	$p = 0.44$
Total (con+div)	37.0 (7.1)	36.6 (7.3)	$p = 0.63$

[a] Student's t-test.

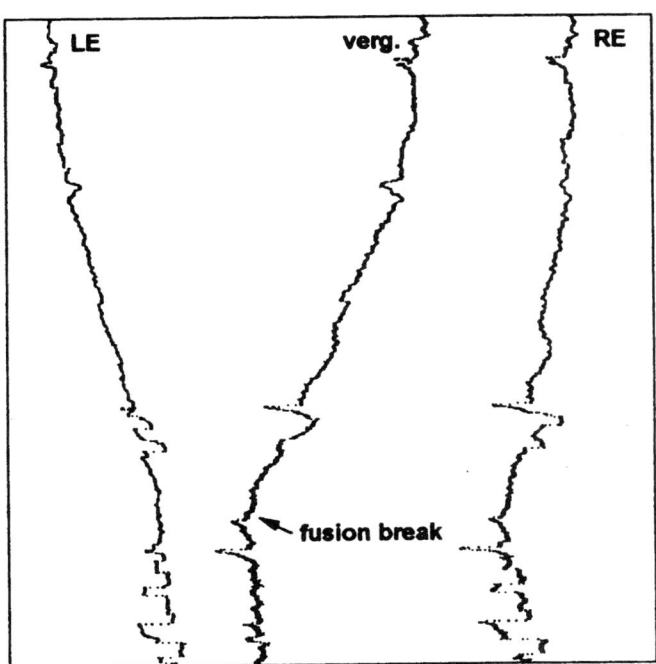

FIGURE 1. Binocular vergence eye movement during synoptophore investigation. The recordings were done with the Ober-2 infrared corneal reflection technique with a sampling frequency of 100 Hz. (*Key:* RE, right eye; LE, left eye; verg., vergence trace (RE–LE).) Note the vergence trace where the leftward deflection of the curve indicates a convergence. Fusion break indicates the point where the subject experienced diplopia. Time span in this picture is about 26 s.

eye movement analysis has been focused on the binocular coordination in the pulse of the saccade.

A *comparison of simultaneous saccades* in the two eyes revealed that the movements were not always of the same amplitude, and an index of the asymmetry was calculated (by dividing the standard deviation of the ratios of saccadic amplitudes of the two eyes, with the mean ratio). As seen in TABLE 4 the asymmetry index was significantly higher in dyslexics than in controls when the children were reading in the ordinary direction. In upside-down reading the asymmetry index increased significantly for the controls but remained the same for the dyslexics. However, the index was still larger in dyslexics than in controls. The index did not change if reading was done with one eye occluded in either group (TABLE 4).

The differences between groups for normal reading direction remained unchanged independent of the complexity of the reading material. However, the intragroup variations were quite considerable, and the index could therefore not be used as a marker to identify the dyslexics by their eye-movement performance during reading.

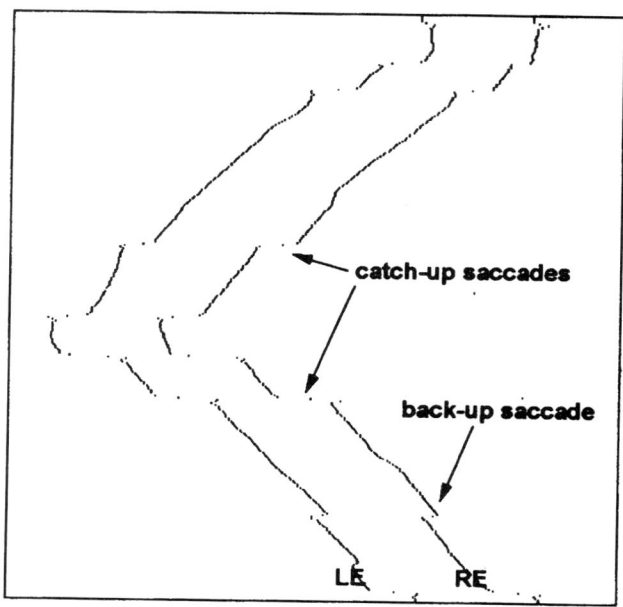

FIGURE 2. Smooth pursuit movement during tracking of an object moving with a velocity of 7.5 degrees/s, recorded with the Ober-2 technique. Note the occurrence of both catch-up and backup saccades. (*Key:* RE, right eye; LE, left eye.)

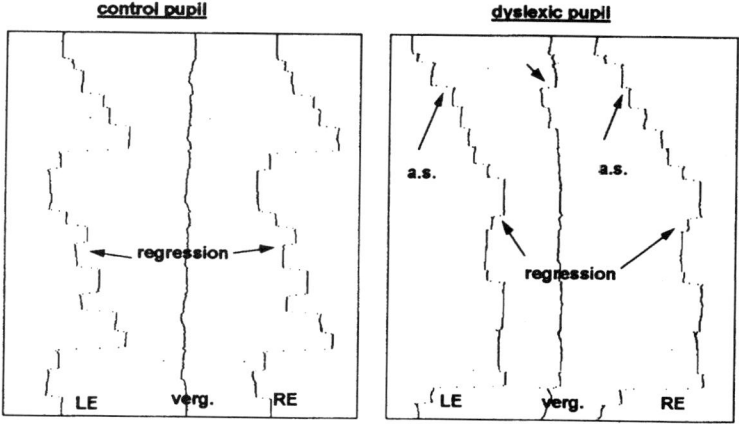

FIGURE 3. Eye movements during reading in a control (**left**) and a dyslexic (**right**) pupil. Note in both figure parts the occurrence of regressions and in the **right-hand** figure also the asymmetric saccades (a.s.) in the right and left eyes. The *arrowhead* indicates the vergence shift due to the asymmetric saccade. Time span of both pictures is about 5 s. (*Key:* RE, right eye; LE, left eye; verg., vergence trace (RE–LE).)

TABLE 4. Asymmetry Index in Dyslexics and Controls

	Binocular Reading		Monocular Reading	
	Normal Direction	Upside Down	Right Eye	Left Eye
Dyslexics	21	20	18	20
Controls	11	17	14	13
Significance[a]	$p < 0.001$	$p < 0.05$	$p < 0.001$	$p < 0.001$

[a]Student's t-test.

DISCUSSION

The reduction in visual acuity that we found in dyslexics has not previously been reported. This may be due to the fact that we have used well-defined groups of dyslexics and matched controls, and that we have tested for higher acuity values than has been done previously. However, reduced visual acuity was seen in only a few dyslexics, and furthermore we do not think that this difference could influence the development of reading skills. It is known that the acuity needed for letter recognition is about 20/200. All children in this study had considerably higher visual acuity. However, the acuity results may indicate differences in visual function, possibly related to performance in the two subsystems of vision, that is, the "transient" and the "sustained" channels.[17]

In our population of children we have further shown that the ability to discriminate contrast is somewhat lower in dyslexics than in controls for both the high and low spatial frequencies. The high-frequency decrease corresponded to the reduction in visual acuity, and could represent a sustained channel abnormality that has not been demonstrated before. The low-frequency defect, however, has already been demonstrated by others and is supposed to indicate reduced activity in the transient visual channel of dyslexics.[8,9] Research is being performed in different laboratories to further explore the possibilities of remediation in dyslexia by means of contrast enhancement.

With regard to the control of binocular coordination, we found no differences between dyslexics and controls in static functions such as size and type of latent strabismus, or in the amount of prism fusion capacity and stereoscopic acuity. Similar findings have been reported by others.[18–20] We also measured the range of fusion vergence movements with subjective and objective methods, but at the velocities and fixation target sizes that we used, there were no differences between the groups. These findings are in contradiction to those of Stein and coworkers.[11] Further we could not see any differences in the ocular dominance pattern determined with the synoptophore as claimed by Stein et al.,[16] because the distribution between children with stable, and unstable dominance was the same in both dyslexics and controls.

With high-precision eye movement recordings from both eyes during reading, we noted differences in the control of saccadic eye movements between dyslexic children and the matched controls. The symmetry of the saccades in the two eyes was poorer in the dyslexics than in the controls. An asymmetry index was created that allowed comparison between the two groups in different reading conditions. Reading of texts at different levels of complexity or monocularly instead of binocularly did not affect the asymmetry index. Reading with the text upside down reduced the saccadic symmetry in normal readers but not in dyslexics. It is possible that the variations noted between dyslexics and normal readers in the control of saccades during reading are related to differences between groups in the timing and sequencing of saccadic movements. Normally saccadic movements are produced in two states of attention: an engaged stage during fixation and a disengaged stage in casual looking around. In the engaged stage, saccades are inhibited; in the disengaged stage, saccades can be produced with extremely short latencies. Reading requires switching between the two stages: the engaged stage during fixation of one part of the text, and the disengaged stage in refixation on the next part. It has been shown in studies of the ability to fixate and of the reaction times in visually guided saccades that dyslexics have difficulties in remaining in the engaged stage, and that they very easily slip over into the disengaged stage.[10] The conclusion of these studies is that dyslexia involves insufficient control over the attentional system, which in turn leads to insufficient control over saccadic eye movements in reading.

The asymmetries in reading saccades that we have found could be interpreted in the same terms, and it could be suggested that the larger asymmetries in dyslexics are signs of the saccadic system working more in the disengaged state, while the normal readers show better coordination of the saccades in the two eyes as a sign of an engaged state of saccadic control. When the normal readers are presented with the text upside down, they revert into the disengaged state and show poorer coordination of saccades. The dyslexics remain in the disengaged state and their saccadic asymmetries are not changed.

REFERENCES

1. DUANE, D. 1989. Neurobiological correlates of learning disorders. J. Am. Acad. Child Adolesc. Psychiatry **28**: 314–318.
2. VON EULER, C., I. LUNDBERG & G. LENNERSTRAND. 1989. Brain and Reading. Structural and Functional Anomalies in Developmental Dyslexia with Special Reference to Hemispheric Interactions, Memory Functions, Linguistic Processing and Visual Analysis in Reading. Mamillan. London.
3. WHYTE, J. 1989. Dyslexia: Current research issues. Irish J. Psychol. **10**: 465–677.
4. PENNINGTON, B. Reading Disabilities; Genetic and Neurological Influences. Kluwer. Dordrecht, the Netherlands.
5. BEAUCHAMP, B. 1990. Visual correlates of dyslexia and related learning disabilities. Pediatr. Ann. **19**: 334–341.
6. EVANS, B. J. W. & N. DRASDO. 1990. Review of ophthalmic factors in dyslexia. Ophthal. Physiol. Opt. **10**: 123–132.
7. LENNERSTRAND, G. & J. YGGE. 1992. Dyslexia; Ophthalmological aspects 1991. Acta Ophthalmol. **70**: 3–13.
8. BREITMEYER, B. G. 1989. A visually based deficit in specific reading disability. Irish J. Psychol. **10**: 534–541.
9. LOVEGROVE, W. 1989. The visual deficit hypothesis: Nature, theory and treatment. *In* Current Perspectives in Learning Disabilities, N. Singh and I. Beale Eds. Springer-Verlag. Berlin/New York.
10. FISCHER, B. & H. WEBER. 1990. Saccadic reaction times of dyslexic and age-matched normal subjects. Perception **19**: 805–818.
11. STEIN, J. F. 1989. Visuospatial perception and reading problems. Irish J. Psychol. **10**: 521–533.
12. YGGE, J., G. LENNERSTRAND, I. AXELSSON & A. RYDBERG. 1992. Visual functions in a Swedish population of dyslexic and normally reading children. Acta Ophthalmol. In press.

13. YGGE, J., G. LENNERSTRAND, A. RYDBERG, S. WIJECOON & B. M. PETTERSSON. 1992. Oculomotor functions in a Swedish population of dyslexic and normally reading children. Acta Ophthalmol. In press.
14. GINSBURG, A. P. 1984. A new contrast sensitivity vision test chart. Am. J. Optom. Physiol. Opt. **61:** 403–407.
15. STEIN, J. F. & M. S. FOWLER. 1982. Diagnosis of dyslexia by means of a new indicator of eye dominance. Br. J. Ophthalmol. **66:** 332–336.
16. STEIN, J. F., P. RIDELL & M. S. FOWLER. 1986. The Dunlop test and reading in primary school children. Br. J. Ophthalmol. **70:** 317–320.
17. LIVINGSTONE, M. & D. HUBEL. 1988. Segregation of form, color, movement and depth: Anatomy, physiology and perception. Science **240:** 740–749.
18. NORN, M. S., E. RINDZIUNSKI & H. SKYDSGAARD. 1969. Ophthalmological and orthoptic examination of dyslexics. Acta Ophthalmol. **47:** 147–160.
19. BLIKA, A. 1982. Ophthalmological findings in pupils of a primary school with particular reference to reading difficulties. Acta Ophthalmol. **60:** 927–934.
20. AASVED, H. 1987. Ophthalmological status of school children with dyslexia. Eye **1:** 61–68.

Language Functions Related to Prefrontal Cortical Activity: Neurolinguistic Implications[a]

DAVID H. INGVAR

Department of Clinical Neurophysiology
University Hospital
S-221 85, Lund, Sweden

INTRODUCTION

Brain imaging techniques were first applied in 1972 to study language functions with the intra-arterial (IA) regional cerebral blood flow (rCBF) 133 xenon clearance method.[1,2] This initial study was followed by a number of 133 xenon rCBF investigations on speech functions; 133 xenon inhalation and intravenous single photon emission computerized tomography (SPECT) techniques have also been utilized.[3-13] In addition, several studies have used brain imaging with positron emission tomography (PET) to localize cortical and deeper rCBF and metabolic changes with a high degree of spatial and temporal resolution during language perception and production.[14-18] Recently, sophisticated rapid magnetic resonance imaging (MRI) methods have been introduced to localize frontal activations by language tests.[19]

Already in the first imaging study[1] some fundamental—and at the time new—observations were made. They have later been amply confirmed and indeed extended by subsequent investigations with the high-resolution techniques referred to earlier. First, language production (automatic speech) gave *bilateral*, to some extent symmetrical, rCBF augmentations dominating in premotor and lower rolandic regions, as well as in the upper temporal area (cf. especially references 3, 7-9). A selective involvement during automatic speech of Broca's and Wernicke's areas in the left hemisphere was not as predominant as one would have thought.

A second early, and likewise important observation was that widespread *frontal and prefrontal* structures are activated in almost all types of tests of language perception and production. This finding was related to a number of rCBF studies in our laboratory in which nonfocal bifrontal activity was shown during several forms of cognitive effort.[5-7,20] We have interpreted the bifrontal activation by language and cognitive tests in the light of current concepts on the functions of the prefrontal cortex. Several treatises and monographs from the last decades have stressed that the most important function of prefrontal cortical structures is to handle the temporal (serial, sequential) organization of behavior and cognition.[21-26] The evidence presented below strongly suggests that language should also be included among functions represented prefrontally.

In an earlier review[21] the serial aspects of language were discussed in the light of the prefrontal rCBF activation by language tests. This discussion is continued in the present paper in which rCBF patterns during *silent (inner) speech* are considered

---

[a]The author was supported by the Swedish Medical Research Council (project B 88-00084-24c), by the Wallenberg Foundation, and by the Swedish Bank Trecentenary Foundation in Stockholm.

especially, and related to recent language studies with PET and SPECT. Admittedly, the main emphasis here is given to our rCBF results obtained by relatively low-resolution 133 xenon techniques, by which cerebral activity changes cannot be ascribed to limited cortical areas. Hence, the discussion mainly concerns general nonfocal, especially prefrontal, rCBF effects, which are believed to be of great importance.

METHODS

The results from our laboratory, which are the main object of the present paper, are based upon measurements of rCBF with the IA 133 xenon clearance technique,[2,27] as well as on 133 xenon inhalation[5] and on intravenous (IV) 133 xenon injections.[28] While we have previously used two-dimensional methods, we have lately applied three-dimensional ones (SPECT[29]). For technical details the reader is referred to the descriptions of the original method. The rCBF results were treated statistically with methods described elsewhere.[7,9]

Two-dimensional 133 xenon rCBF measurements with IA, IV, or inhalation techniques, are beset by important limitations. Their temporal and spatial resolution are relatively low. They emphasize blood flow changes in outer superficial parts of the hemispheres. This appears to be the main explanation for differences between our two-dimensional rCBF landscapes and, on the other hand, results from three-dimensional SPECT and PET studies. The two-dimensional rCBF images thus mainly depict general, often nonfocal, flow changes in superficial cortical structures, that is, gyri facing the "outer" hemisphere surface. Such changes thus form the main basis for the ensuing discussion.

GENERAL FINDINGS

Speaking aloud (automatic enumeration of numbers, weekdays, etc.) showed bilateral, almost symmetrical cortical rCBF activity, predominating in the upper and lower rolandic, as well as in the upper temporal regions.[1,3,7,9,10] This pattern can mainly be explained by the important sensory–motor and auditory feedback caused by audible articulation.[1,3,7] As shown in a detailed statistical analysis, however, there were some, in part focal, asymmetries of which a few right-sided ones appeared related to prosodic voice control.[7,9]

Automatic speech, with its low semantic content, also activated to a limited extent prefrontal structures in part related to the supplementary motor area (SMA region), or the so-called upper speech cortex of Penfield. However, other forms of aloud speech (e.g., word fluency test) with a greater semantic content involving cognitive effort, showed clear-cut activity of prefrontal structures, mainly mesially and dominating on the left side.[12]

Speech Perception

Imaging studies in subjects perceiving simple words showed bilateral, upper temporal activity that was dominatant on the left side.[30] Word perception also showed diffuse and bilateral frontal/prefrontal activity, often dominating in a lower left-sided, prefrontal, Broca-related area. Similar and other forms of prefrontal activations during speech perception, as well as indeed a number of temporal and postcentral activity foci, have been observed in subjects listening to verbal instructions in psychological testing.[5,6,10,20]

Reading aloud showed clear-cut activity in "appropriate" centers for visual perception, auditory feedback, sensory–motor rolandic areas for articulation, as well as in the upper and lower prefrontal regions. *Reading silently* showed the same pattern, including prefrontal activity, but without flow increase in regions for mouth/tongue/larynx, etc., motor control and without temporal auditory feedback effects.[31]

Distinct prefrontal activity in various patterns have also been encountered in PET studies of speech perception, especially when semantic aspects were involved. Some of these prefrontal activations appeared less focal than those pertaining to the sensory (auditory/visual) input and the motor output.[10,15–18,26,32]

To summarize the studies quoted, it is possible to recognize that bilateral prefrontal activations in varying patterns and intensity form a common denominator during both speech perception and speech production (cf. references 21 and 23). Indeed, high-resolution PET techniques have confirmed and elaborated substantially this principal result originally obtained some 20 years ago by low-resolution two-dimensional rCBF methods. With PET greatly circumscribed, activity peaks can be shown during visual and auditory language perception in and around the occipital visual and temporal auditory areas, respectively.[17] Circumscribed prefrontal activity has also been demonstrated during audible speech with PET subtraction techniques.[15,17,32] According to these studies some similar prefrontal foci were also related to the semantic content of the words produced or perceived. This interpretation is supported in a general way by a recent SPECT study with factor analysis of rCBF measurements.[11]

Silent Speech

In order to "free" cortical speech landscapes from the important sensory–motor and auditory feedback effects, we have recently completed a two-dimensional intravenous 133 xenon study, comparing the rCBF landscapes during aloud and silent speech in 30 right-handed normals.[8,9] The test used was counting aloud and silently (101, 102, 103...). This simple test permitted reasonably satisfactory control of the performance in both situations. This study forms a part of several others we have made on rCBF changes during various forms of ideation, including, for example, motor ideation of handwriting and tennis movements (see reference 33 for a summary).

In the silent speech series there was one outstanding finding. *Counting aloud* confirmed that voluntary overt speech shows marked bilateral, somewhat asymmetrical activity of the rolandic/temporal regions as previously described.[7] Aloud counting showed only limited nonsignificant activity prefrontally. *Counting silently*, on the other hand, showed a completely different pattern. There were highly significant asymmetrical prefrontal activations. Postcentrally on the *right* side there were no significant rCBF changes. On the *left* side, however, moderately significant activity was recorded that involved the lower and middle rolandic areas, as well as the upper temporal and lower parietal region. This left-sided change suggested that silent speech activated cortical regions related to the classic speech centers, especially to Wernicke's area in the dominant hemisphere.[8,9]

The study of silent speech confirmed in principle earlier observations of ours on motor ideation (hand clenching performed or imagined). The actual movement showed a circumscribed upper *rolandic* sensory–motor activity of the hand area. Motor ideation of the same movement gave an almost exclusive *prefrontal* rCBF increase.[33,34] In short, our ideation studies have revealed a prefrontal localization of "programs" for movements and speech.[21]

THE CEREBELLUM

Following the introduction of three-dimensional SPECT measurements of rCBF in our laboratory, we noted a cerebellar activation in several studies of motor ideation.[33] During speech ideation (silent speech) some cerebellar asymmetries were also noted.[13] Cerebellar activity has also been recorded with PET during overt speech production.[17] These new findings show clearly that the cerebellum is involved in language mechanisms. The cerebellar activation during silent speech signals a most interesting cerebellar participation in abstract ideation, perhaps in cognition in general.[13] Future research will most certainly reveal further details of the cerebellar language effects, their localization and extent, as well as their relation to the temporal organization of language perception and production.

DISCUSSION

It is now some twenty years following the first demonstration that cognitive effort augments rCBF in prefrontal areas.[20] A wealth of subsequent studies, especially by Risberg and his collaborators,[5,6] have amply confirmed that frontal/prefrontal activation forms an integral part of augmented cognitive activity during psychological testing. In most cases, such tests include verbal instructions or performance. In view of the solid experimental and clinical evidence that the prefrontal cortex handles the temporal organization of behavior and cognition,[22,23] it appears "logical" that a clear-cut prefrontal component can be discerned in several of the language studies discussed here.

It should be stressed that prefrontal activation was not only seen in actual speech performance, that is, during language production (output), it was also clearly demonstrated in *language perception* (input) of simple words and sentences. This observation has wide implications as suggested previously.[21] It signals that "efferent" (precentral, prefrontal) cortical structures participate in "afferent" speech perception. Indeed, there has long been indirect evidence for this, that is, that simple and complex neuronal speech motor programs, "housed" in prefrontal regions, are used as templates in identification of words and sentences during language perception.[23,26] Such a general theory forms a basic component of the so-called *motor theory of speech perception* developed early by A. M. Liberman.[35]

Our general interpretation is then that the neuronal action programs for speech are localized in the prefrontal cortex—like other sequentially organized action programs for simple or complex movements. These programs are, as it appears from the brain imaging studies, used both in language perception and production.[21,23]

Several clinical observations support this interpretation. In the acute phase, prefrontal traumatic and vascular brain lesions may, as is well known, disturb the language programs and completely block all forms of speech production leading to aphasia and/or mutism. It is also an established fact that patients with aphasia of the

Broca type, in addition to the well-known "expressive" difficulties may show reduced capacity of language perception (cf. references 21, 26). Organic dementia with a prefrontal rCBF reduction may also cause reduced speech production and speech comprehension.[6] Finally, patients with schizophrenia with their many peculiar "aserial" types of speech disturbances often show a *"hypofrontal"* rCBF pattern indicating reduced prefrontal activity that cannot be activated by verbal cognitive tasks.[21,23,40] When the symptoms of psychosis subside, the prefrontal activation by verbal tasks returns.[12]

Some two-dimensional rCBF studies,[5,6,9,11] as well as several high-resolution PET and SPECT studies, demonstrate activation of circumscribed regions prefrontally during language tests, which probably represent functional subunits subserving speech.[16,17,26,32] There is evidence that such subunits on the left side participate in expressing and interpreting the semantic content of verbal messages.[5,6,12] Dorsolateral left-sided prefrontal regions may also contribute to "working memory" mechanisms that must be a prerequisite for language production and interpretation.[25] Right-sided prefrontal subunits appear to be involved in well-learned, more global attentional aspects of language, as well as in mechanisms controlling prosody.[36] Finally, emotional and "value"-related aspects of language may involve the mesial cingulate prefrontal cortex[16,32] (cf. references 26, 37).

It can be emphasized here that the semantic content of a verbal message has an important inherent temporal organization. It is in the final serial sequences of phonemes, morphemes, words, and sentences that the meaning, the semantic content of spoken or written messages is conveyed. Hence, it appears logical that prefrontal cortical structures known to control the temporal organization of behavior and cognition, should also be involved so clearly in the production and interpretation of semantically meaningful verbal messages.

Several of the interpretations given earlier are supported by the study of silent speech.[8,9] When counting aloud one is constantly "re-minded" of what to say by auditory and sensory–motor feedback of the well-known series of numbers to be articulated. Such automatic speech apparently does not need but limited prefrontal activity. However, silent counting requires the programming of a strict inner prefrontal serially and temporally organized "score" to be read off silently in one's mind. But, apparently, silent speech also to some extent activates regions related to classic speech centers in the dominant hemisphere, housing speech motor programs in lower rolandic regions, as well as lexicon functions related to Wernicke's area. As mentioned before, the cerebellum is also activated by silent speech.[13]

A COMMENT ON DYSLEXIA

The interpretation given of prefrontal participation both in language *production* and language *perception* warrants a comment on dyslexia. There is evidence that dyslectics lack the normal upper temporal activation when identifying rhyming words.[38] This finding suggests strongly that the deficient phonemic and linguistic awareness in dyslexia is related to a defect on the *input* side of the cortical language mechanisms. Indeed, in the upper temporal region and elsewhere, in clearly precentral/prefrontal parts of the cortex, pathoanatomical neuronal abnormalities have been found in autopsied patients with dyslexia.[39] The evidence given previously shows that prefrontal *(output)* cortical language mechanisms also participate in auditory and visual verbal perception. Therefore, the role of deficient prefrontal structures in dyslexia should also be considered.

CONCLUDING REMARKS

Brain imaging in language research has revealed a number of new features of brain mechanisms involved in language perception and production. There is a *bilateral* involvement of cortical fields during speech perception and performance. Another new finding is the participation of *prefrontal* structures both in language perception and production. Both in two- and three-dimensional 133 xenon, as well as in PET rCBF studies, prefrontal subunits have been demonstrated. On the left side they appear to subserve semantic functions and ("working") memory mechanisms.[16,17,25] On the right side the prefrontal subunits may be involved in attentional and prosodic control mechanisms.[6, 36]

Modern high-resolution brain imaging will, it seems, rather shortly reveal further details about the complex *"parallel distributed neurocognitive networks"*[26] that underlie the language functions of the brain. There is every reason to believe that this research will be of immense importance not only for language research but also for the understanding of human cognition in general.

ACKNOWLEDGMENTS

I would like to thank Jarl Risberg, Ph.D., and Erik Ryding, M.D., for providing valuable criticism and advice.

REFERENCES

1. INGVAR, D. H. & M. S. SCHWARTZ. 1974. Blood flow patterns induced in the dominant hemisphere by speech and reading. Brain **97**: 273–288.
2. LASSEN, N. A. & D. H. INGVAR. 1961. The blood flow of the cerebral cortex determined by radioactive Krypton 85. Experientia **17**: 42–43.
3. LARSEN, B., E. SKINHÜOJ & N. A. LASSEN. 1978. Variation in regional cortical blood flow in the right and left hemispheres during automatic speech. Brain **101**: 193–209.
4. ROLAND, P. E., E. SKINHÖJ & N. A. LASSEN. 1981. Focal activations of human cerebral cortex during auditory discrimination. J. Neurophysiol. **45**: 1139–1151.
5. RISBERG, J. 1980. Regional cerebral blood flow measurements by 133-Xe inhalation: Methodology and applications in neuropsychology and psychiatry. Brain Lang. **9**: 9–34.
6. ———. 1986. Regional cerebral blood flow. *In* Experimental Techniques in Human Neuropsychology, H. J. Hannay, Ed.: 514–543. Oxford Univ. Press. Oxford, England.
7. RYDING, E., B. BRÄDVIK & D. H. INGVAR. 1987. Changes of cerebral regional blood flow measured simultaneously in the right and left hemisphere during automatic speech and humming. Brain **110**: 1345–1358.
8. ——— 1989. Silent speech activates circumscribed speech centers selectively in the dominant hemisphere. J. CBF. Met. Suppl. 1 **9**: 317.
9. ———. 1992. Silent speech activates frontal cortical regions asymmetrically, as well as speech related areas in the dominant hemisphere. In press.
10. FRIBERG, L. & N. A. LASSEN. 1991. Language and the cerebral hemispheres: Impact of stimulus relevance and absence of lateralized activation response as revealed by rCBF studies. *In* Brain Work and Mental Activity, N. A. Lassen, D. H. Ingvar, M. E. Raichle, and L. Friberg, Eds.: 294–308. Munksgaard. Copenhagen.
11. MCLAUGHLIN, T., B. STEINBERG, D. CHRISTENSEN, I. LAW, A. PARVING & L. FRIBERG. 1992. Potential language and attentional networks revealed through factor analysis of rCBF data measured with SPECT. J. CBF Met. **12**: 535–545.

12. WARKENTIN, S., J. RISBERG, A. MADER, S. KARLSON & E. GRAAE. 1991. Cortical activity during speech production. Neuropsychiat. Neuropsychol. Behav. Neurol. **4:** 305–316.
13. DECETY, J., H. SJÖHOLM, E. RYDING, G. STENBERG & D. H. INGVAR. 1990. The cerebellum participates in mental activity: Tomographic measurements of regional cerebral blood flow. Brain Res. **535:** 313–317.
14. METTER, E. J., C. G. WASTERLAIN, D. E. KUHL, W. R. HANSON & M. E. PHELPS. 1981. 18-FDG-positron emission computed tomography in a study of aphasia. Annu. Neurol. **10:** 173–183.
15. MAZZIOTTA, J. C., M. E. PHELPS & E. HALGREN. 1983. Local cerebral glucose metabolic response to audiovisual stimulation and deprivation: Studies in human subjects with positron CT. Human Neurobiol. **2:** 1–13.
16. PETERSEN, S. E., P. T. FOX, M. I. POSNER, M. A. MINTUN & M. E. RAICHLE. 1988. Positron emission tomographic studies of the cortical anatomy of single word processing. Nature **331:** 585–589.
17. RAICHLE, M. E. 1991. Studies of the processing of single words in normal human subjects with PET. In Brain Work and Mental Activity. N. A. Lassen, D. H. Ingvar, M. E. Raichle, and L. Friberg, Eds.: 315–321. Munksgaard. Copenhagen.
18. HEISS, W. D., G. PAWLIK, G. R. FINK, M. GROND, K. HERHOLZ & J. KESSLER. 1991. Metabolic activation of the brain by speech and visual recognition. In Brain Work and Mental Activity, N. A. Lassen, D. H. Ingvar, M. E. Raichle, and L. Friberg, Eds.: 335–343. Munksgaard. Copenhagen.
19. BLAMIRE, A. M., G. MCCARTHY, R. GRUETTER, D. L. ROTHMAN, Z. RATTNER, F. HYDER & R. G. SHULMAN. 1992. Echoplanar imaging of the left interior frontal lobe during word generation. Social Magnetic Resonance in Medicine. 11th Annual Science Meeting, Aug. 8–14, Berlin, Germany.
20. RISBERG, J. & D. H. INGVAR. 1973. Patterns of activation in the grey matter of the dominant hemisphere during memorization and reasoning. Brain **96:** 737–756.
21. INGVAR, D. H. 1983. Serial aspects of language and speech related to prefrontal cortical activity. A selective review. Human Neurobiol. **2:** 177–189.
22. FUSTER, J. 1989. The Prefrontal Cortex. Anatomy, Physiology, and Neuropsychology of the Frontal Lobes, 2nd ed. Raven Press. New York.
23. INGVAR, D. H. 1985. "Memory of the future": An essay on the temporal organization of conscious awareness. Human Neurobiol. **4:** 127–136.
24. STUSS, B. T. & D. F. BENSON. 1986. The Frontal Lobes. Raven Press. New York.
25. GOLDMAN-RAKIC, P. S. 1988. Topography of cognition. Parallel distributed networks in primate association cortex. Annu. Rev. Neurosci. **14:** 137–156.
26. MESULAM, M.-M. 1990. Large-scale neurocognitive networks and distributed processes for attention, language, and memory. Annu. Neurol. **28:** 597–613.
27. LASSEN, N. A., K. HOEDT-RASMUSSEN, S. C. SÖRENSEN, E. SKINHÖJ, S. CRONQVIST, B. BODFORSS & D. H. INGVAR. 1963. Regional cerebral blood flow in man determined by Krypton-85. Neurology **13:** 719–727.
28. RYDING, E. 1986. Measurement of cerebral blood flow by intravenous administration of 133 xenon. Theory, technique and clinical applications, Ph.D. Thesis, Univ. of Lund, Lund, Sweden.
29. STOKELEY, E. M., E. SVEINSDOTTIR, N. A. LASSEN & P. ROMMER. 1980. A single photodynamic computer-assisted tomograph (DCAT) for imaging brain function in multiple cross-sections. J. Comput. Assisted Tomogr. **4:** 142–148.
30. NISHISAWA, Y., T. SKYHÖJ-OLESEN, B. LARSEN & N. A. LASSEN. 1982. Left-right cortical asymmetries of regional cerebral blood flow during listening to words. J. Neurophysiol. **48:** 458–466.
31. LASSEN, N. A., D. H. INGVAR & E. SKINHÖJ. 1978. Brain function and blood flow. Sci. Am. **239:** 62–71.
32. POSNER, M. I., S. E. PETERSEN, P. T. FOX & M. E. RAICHLE. 1988. Localization of cognitive functions in the human brain. Science **240:** 1627–1631.
33. DECETY, J. & D. H. INGVAR. 1990. Brain structures participating in mental simulation of motor behaviour: A neuropsychological interpretation. Acta Psychol. **73:** 13–34.

34. INGVAR, D. H. & L. PHILIPSON. 1977. Distribution of cerebral blood flow in the dominant hemisphere during motor ideation and motor performance. Annu. Neurol. **2:** 230–237.
35. LIBERMAN, A. M., F. S. COOPER, D. R. SHANKWEITER & M. STUDDERT-KENNEDY. 1967. Perception of the speech code. Psychol. Rev. **74:** 431–461.
36. BRÄDVIK, B., C. DRAVINS, S. HOLTÅS, I. ROSÉN, E. RYDING & D. H. INGVAR. 1991. Disturbances of speech prosody following right hemisphere infarcts. Acta Neurol. Scand. **84:** 114–126.
37. LURIA, A. R. 1977. Higher Cortical Functions in Man, 2nd ed. Basic Books. New York.
38. RUMSEY, J. M., P. ANDREASON, A. J. ZAMETKIN, T. AQUINO, A. C. KING, S. D. HAMBURGER, A. PIKUS, J. L. RAPOPORT & R. M. COHEN. 1992. Failure to activate the left temporoparietal cortex in dyslexia. Arch. Neurol. **49:** 527–532.
39. GALABURDA, A. M., G. F. SHERMAN, G. D. ROSEN, F. ABOITIZ & N. GESCHWIND. 1985. Developmental dyslexia. Four consecutive patients with cortical anomalies. Annu. Neurol. **81:** 222–233.
40. INGVAR, D. H. 1980. Abnormalities of activity distribution in the brain of schizophrenics. A neurophysiological interpretation. *In* Perspectives in Schizophrenia Research, D. Baxter and Melneshuk, Eds.: 73–98. Raven Press. New York.

Developmental Speech Perception: Implications for Models of Language Impairment

PATRICIA K. KUHL

Department of Speech and Hearing Sciences and
Virginia Merrill Bloedel Hearing Research Center
University of Washington, WJ-10
Seattle, Washington 98195

INTRODUCTION

This book focuses on the neural and psychological substrates that underpin language processing, with an aim toward understanding impairments evidenced by dyslexic and dysphasic individuals. Clinical evaluation[1] and research studies[2–4] suggest that dyslexic and dysphasic individuals have impairments in the perception of rapidly changing information, and in phonetic and phonological processing. Understanding these processes in normal and impaired individuals is thus of interest. The present paper contributes to this endeavor by describing recent studies on normal infants' abilities to perceive speech and by providing a model of developmental speech perception incorporating these data. The data and theory provide a framework for speculation about the nature of phonetic and phonological processing deficits in language-impaired individuals.

INFANTS' PERCEPTION OF SPEECH

There is a great deal of evidence supporting the view that at the beginning of life infants are exquisitely prepared to perceive human speech. Research studies have demonstrated that young infants are born with an ability to discern differences between the phonetic units used in the world's languages (for recent reviews, see references 5 and 6). This ability exists in the absence of experience with the sounds—infants perform in this way for foreign-language sounds they have never heard. Moreover, infants' abilities are not limited to the perception of fine differences between speech sounds. They are also excellent "categorizers." Infants can perceive a similarity among discriminably different speech sounds that belong to the same phonetic category (for review, see reference 7). Infants' abilities to perceptually group stimuli—to perceive speech-sound constancies—is enormously important. The lack of an ability to categorize phonetically is one of the bottlenecks preventing speech recognition by machine. Finally, infants show an ability to recognize the coherence between speech presented visually and auditorially.[8–11] They recognize that a wide-open mouth "goes with" the auditorially presented /a/ vowel, while retracted lips "go with" the vowel /i/. In short, speech is a biologically important stimulus for infants, and they appear well prepared to perceive it.

Recent studies in my laboratory focus on a different aspect of infants' perception of speech. The new work highlights *learning*—the change in infants' abilities that comes about as a function of language experience. Our studies that show that by 6 months of age infants' perception of speech is altered by exposure to a specific language.[12] These data have led to the formation of a theory of the development of speech perception called the Native Language Magnet (NLM) Theory.[13,14]

NLM theory is based on the notion that infants' initial perceptual abilities provide a rough division of stimuli into phonetic categories. To these abilities that are present at birth, NLM adds a powerful component that relies on linguistic input. According to the theory, language input results in the formation of stored representations of native-language phonetic categories. These phonetic category representations highlight the best exemplars, or "prototypes," of the category. Our studies have shown that prototypes function in a unique way: they act like perceptual magnets. Prototypes perceptually attract nearby members of the category, and this provides internal structure to the category (FIG. 1). The prototypes' magnet effect, as laid out in NLM, offers an explanation for infants' perception of native- and foreign-language speech perception, as well as second-language learning. It also provides a framework for examining the nature of speech representational systems in language-disordered populations.

Thus, NLM has two components, one focusing on infants' "built-in" abilities, and the other on infants' sensitivity to linguistic experience. Two behavioral phenomena reflect these two components: infants' demonstration of enhanced discriminability near the boundaries that separate phonetic categories[15–17] reflects the built-in component, and infants' demonstration of phonetic prototype effects reflects the learned component.[18,19,12] Infants' abilities to partition acoustic stimuli into categories is initially "language-general." It is exhibited for phonetic units the infant has never heard, and thus does not depend on linguistic experience.[20] This enhanced discrimination at phonetic boundaries is also demonstrated by nonhuman animals that have no prior experience with speech[21] (see reference 22 for review). I will argue here that infants' demonstration of enhanced discriminability near phonetic boundaries reflects an innate ability to partition into gross categories the acoustic events underlying speech, but that this ability is attributable to infants' *general* auditory perceptual processing mechanisms. I will also show, however, that infants' perception of phonetic prototypes is, by 6 months of life, both "language specific" and unique to humans.

Category Boundaries and Language Experience

Tests of categorical perception (CP) on adults by Liberman and his colleagues at Haskins Laboratories showed that adults' abilities to discriminate between speech stimuli located on a continuum between two phonetic categories is not equivalent across the continuum[23] (see reference 24 for review). Adults' discrimination abilities are enhanced in the region of the phonetic boundary, the location of the division between speech categories. Tests of CP use a series of computer-generated speech sounds that are created by altering some acoustic variable in small steps. On one end of the series the sounds are identified as one syllable, such as the syllable /ba/, while sounds on the other end are identified as /pa/ (FIG. 2). When listeners are tested in a discrimination task to see whether they can hear the difference between two adjacent /ba/'s (or/pa/'s) in the series, stimuli drawn from opposite sides of the phonetic boundary are more easily discriminated than stimuli falling on one side of

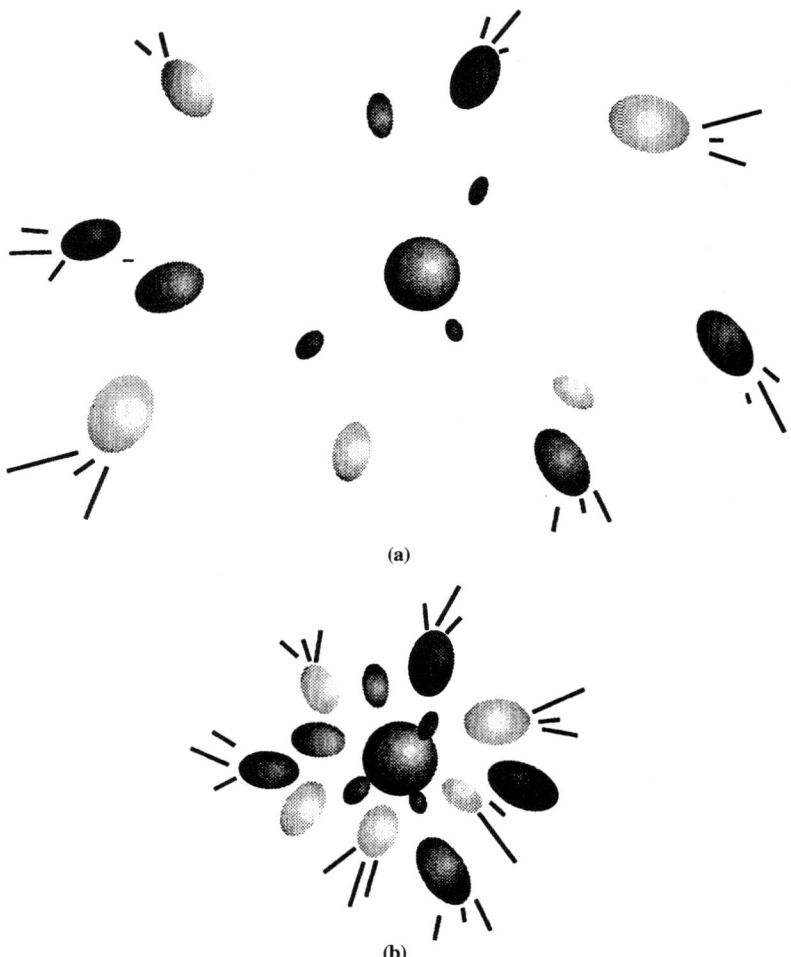

FIGURE 1. The *perceptual magnet effect*. Stimuli surrounding a phonetic prototype (a) are perceptually drawn toward the prototype (b), thereby shrinking the perceived distance between the prototype and other members of the category.

the boundary, even though the physical difference in the two cases is the same. Tests on infants revealed the effect as well, both for consonants[15–17] and for vowels.[25] Moreover, young infants demonstrated the phenomenon not only for the sounds of their own native language, but also for sounds from foreign languages that they had never heard.[20] Thus, infants' initial discrimination abilities are independent of linguistic experience.

Studies in my laboratory have also revealed, however, that the boundary phenomenon is not unique to human listeners. Enhanced discriminability in the region of the

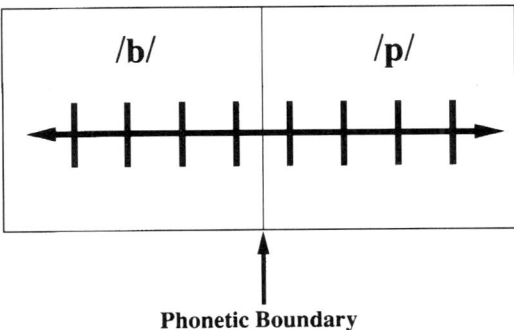

FIGURE 2. Classic categorical discrimination: For both adults and infants discriminability is enhanced in the region of the phonetic boundary between /ba/ and /pa/.

phonetic boundary is displayed by nonhuman animals[21,26] (see reference 27 for review). I have elsewhere argued that the tendency to partition sounds into gross categories on the basis of certain acoustic features is one that is deeply embedded in our phylogenetic history, and one that played a role in the selection of candidates for a phonetic inventory.[22,28] The view developed here is that boundary effects are not due to innate mechanisms that prespecify all of the potential phonetic units used in speech. Rather, NLM holds that perceptual boundaries result from the general auditory processing mechanism and the fact that in the evolution of speech existing auditory abilities were exploited in the selection of linguistically contrastive sounds.[28]

Research on the boundary phenomenon shows that it is modified by linguistic experience. For example, when Japanese listeners are tested on a series of sounds that range from /ra/ to /la/, a distinction that is not phonemic in Japenese, they do not show enhanced discrimination at the phonetic boundary between the two sounds. In contrast, American listeners do show a boundary effect for the /ra–la/ stimuli.[29] American listeners do not show enhanced discrimination at the phonetic boundary between the Spanish prevoiced and voiceless unaspirated sounds.[30] These examples illustrate that by adulthood we are "language-specific" listeners. Our abilities to hear differences between sounds have been restricted as a result of exposure to our native language and the alterations in our perceptual systems that result from this experience. Infants, on the other hand, are born "Citizens of the World"—their built-in discriminative abilities suffice for the acquisition of any language. The question is: When, how, and why do our initial "language-general" abilities become "language-specific"?

Category Centers and Language Experience

Category recognition studies done in my laboratory with 6-month-old infants have demonstrated that infants recognize *phonetic constancies.* Even though the members of phonetic categories differ greatly from a physical standpoint, infants detect their similarities. They can perceptually sort vowels into categories, such as the categories /a/ versus /i/, /a/ versus / ɔ /, and /a/ versus /ae/, when the categories are composed of sounds produced by many different people (for review, see reference 7). Infants also demonstrate the ability to perceive categories based on the initial or the final consonant of sets of syllables, such as those beginning with /s/ as opposed to /sh/,[31] or /m/ versus /n/.[32] Finally, infants detected category membership based on a featural distinction separating nasals and stops.[33] These data suggest that infants possess an ability to perceive a kind of constancy for speech sounds.[7]

The boundary effect, which examines infants' *discrimination* abilities, cannot fully explain infants' *categorization* abilities. Phonetic categorization requires more than simple discrimination. Infants recognize categories composed of stimuli that are discriminably different from one another. Thus, the perception of stimulus differences is not the key issue. The central problem is *similarity:* infants display an ability to perceive similarity among discriminably different stimuli.

This work in my laboratory on infants' categorization abilities led to the work on phonetic prototypes. Our work suggested that infants' abilities to categorize were enhanced when they were trained with good instances of phonetic categories.[18,19] Our focus on the prototypes of speech categories was thus based on the assumption that prototypes exemplify the *centers* of speech categories, optimum stimuli that may be used as referents in the categorization process, and the belief that prototypes tap listeners' mental representations for speech categories.

Phonetic Prototypes and Their Function in Perception

Previous studies supported the idea that certain speech stimuli had privileged status when compared against other stimuli.[34-37] The approach we adopted was to ask adult listeners to rate the category goodness of individual exemplars from a phonetic category. Stimuli that were rated as the best exemplars, or prototypes, were then examined further in tests that compared the perception of prototypes to the perception of nonprototypes from the same category.

We used vowels in the initial tests,[18,19] and have now undertaken a set of studies involving consonants.[38] To conduct the vowel tests, many instances of the vowel /i/ were computer synthesized and then rated. The findings showed that adults' ratings were very consistent. There was a particular location in the /i/ vowel space that produced better ratings. As one moved away from that "hotspot," the ratings became consistently worse.[18,19]

Two /i/ vowels were selected from the set. One was the vowel given the highest average category goodness rating; it was designated the prototype (P) /i/. The second one was an /i/ that had been given a relatively poor average rating; it was designated the nonprototype (NP) /i/. Both P and NP were always rated as /i/ vowels by listeners. The poor /i/ was simply judged to be produced less well. Variants of P and of NP were created by manipulating the first and second formants of the two vowels. The 32 variants formed four rings around each vowel [FIG. 3(a)]. Each ring was a controlled distance from the center stimulus (for further details, see reference 19).

These stimuli were used to test the hypothesis that category goodness (typicality) has an effect on speech perception. A discrimination test was used to test the degree of perceptual similarity between each variant and its referent (P or NP). Adults, 6-month-old infants, and rhesus macaques were tested in a discrimination task that was virtually identical for the three groups of subjects.[19] The question was: Is the

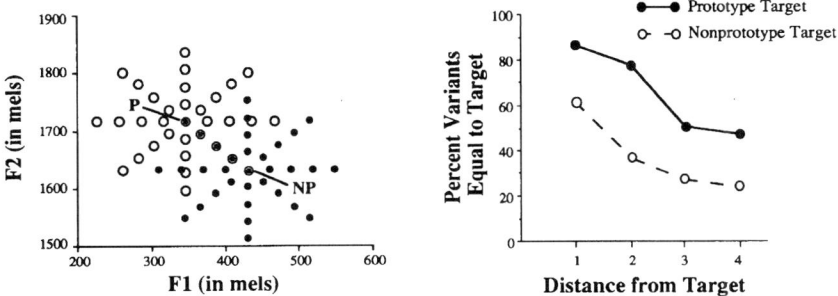

FIGURE 3. (a) The prototype /i/ (P) and its 32 variants *(open circles)* and the nonprototype /i/ (NP) and its 32 variants *(closed circles).* (b) Results showing that the prototype is equated to its variants more often than is the case for the nonprototype, and thus that it exhibits a stronger perceptual magnet effect.

prototype perceived as more similar to its variants than is the case for the nonprototype?

Human adults and infants showed the same pattern of results, that shown in FIGURE 3(b). The plot shows the percentage of variants on the four rings that were equated to the P or NP. As shown, the prototype produced a stronger magnet effect. A greater number of variants were equated to the prototype than to the nonprototype, even though distance was controlled in the two sets of stimuli. The results suggested that the prototype perceptually assimilates or attracts surrounding stimuli to a greater extent than is the case for the nonprototype. The prototype appears to draw other stimuli toward it, effectively reducing the perceptual distance between the prototype and surrounding stimuli. This behavioral result led to the simile I have developed to describe the prototype's effect on perception: The prototype functions like a perceptual *magnet* (FIG. 1).

Monkeys demonstrated a strikingly different pattern of response. They exhibited no magnet effect.[19] Monkeys treated the variants surrounding the prototype and the nonprototype in exactly the same way. In both cases, variants were discriminated from the target at a particular distance from the target. These results are interesting because they reveal a dissociation between humans and monkeys in a test of phonetic perception, unlike the case of categorical perception.[6,28] Thus, the perceptual magnet effect differs in significant ways from the phenomenon of categorical perception.

Linguistic Experience and the Magnet Effect: A Cross-Language Study

The results on 6-month-old infants showing that they demonstrated the magnet effect raised interesting questions: What makes a particular vowel a prototype? And regarding development, how might the prototype get into the mind of the baby?

Two different possibilities were entertained regarding the developmental question, and each made a prediction about the nature of the magnet effect. The first answer regarding development is that phonetic prototypes are part of infants' biological endowment for language. An alternative is that prototypes depend on linguistic input. The two models make different predictions about infants' perception of vowels from a foreign language. The first hypothesis—that vowel prototypes are innately

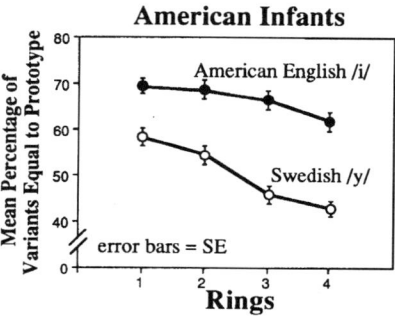 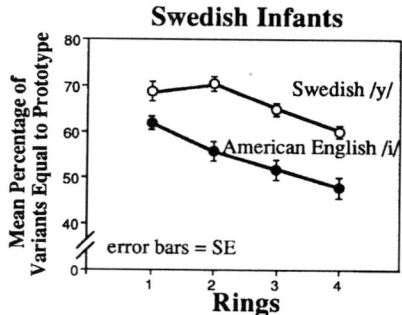

FIGURE 4. American (a) and Swedish (b) 6-month-old infants were tested on two vowel prototypes, American English /i/ and Swedish /y/. Infants from both countries equated variants to their native-language vowel prototype more often than for the foreign-language vowel prototype. Both groups produced a stronger magnet effect for their native-language phonetic prototype.

"fixed"—predicts that the prototype's magnet effect would exist for vowels of all languages, even ones that the infant has never heard. The second hypothesis predicts that the magnet effect would exist only for vowels in the infant's own language.

An international research team examined the two hypotheses in a cross-language test. Infants from United States and Sweden were tested on two vowel prototypes, the American English vowel /i/ used in our previous tests and the Swedish vowel /y/.[12] The Swedish /y/ prototype was synthesized and then modified to create 32 additional variants in the same way as previously described. In both countries, tests on adult native speakers revealed that the foreign vowel was perceived as a non-prototype (see 12 for details).

Careful controls were adopted for the cross-language infant test. We moved the entire laboratory (computer, loudspeaker, cables, reinforcers, everything used to conduct the experiment), and three trained experimenters, from Seattle to Stockholm. Except for the critical variable, the language experience of the 6-month-old infants who were tested, the methods and procedures used to conduct the study in the two countries were identical. The question was: Would the magnet effect be exhibited universally for both prototypes by infants, or would 6-month-olds from the two countries show the effect only for the native-language prototypes?

The results demonstrated that infants from both countries showed a significantly stronger magnet effect for their native-language prototype (FIG. 4), confirming the hypothesis that linguistic experience in the first half-year of life alters phonetic perception. American infants demonstrated a significantly stronger magnet effect for the American English /i/ prototype when compared to the Swedish /y/ prototype. Swedish infants demonstrated a significantly stronger magnet effect for the Swedish /y/ when compared to the American English /i/ prototype. This is the youngest age at which language input has been shown to alter infants' phonetic perception.

MAGNET EFFECTS AND SPEECH REPRESENTATION

The findings revealed that by 6 months of age, infants' perception of the sounds of their native language differs from their perception of the sounds of a foreign language. Native-language prototypes exhibit the magnet effect, while foreign sounds are treated as nonprototypes in the native language. This result allows the inference that infants have had sufficient listening experience with the ambient language to alter some aspect of the speech representational systems of the young child. How do we explain the magnet effect? What is the mechanism that underlies it?

Theories of Categorization and Representation

There are two views concerning the form that category representations might take. My NLM model is not substantially affected by this debate about the type of representation; my data can easily be accommodated by either form of representation. However, it is worth noting that the data from experiments on infants' formation of categories outside the domain of speech lend some support to an abstract summary view (typically called the *prototype* view, where the term prototype refers to some summary statistic of a set of stimuli instead of referring simply to an "ideal exemplar").

The prototype view of categorization derives from Rosch and her colleagues.[39] Prototype theory asserts that people calculate and store some sort of summary statistic that characterizes a category as a whole. As people experience new items from a category, a generalization about those items as a group is formed, such as an average of all the experienced exemplars. Category decisions are made by comparing newly encountered items to this summary representation.

Recently, an alternative to prototype theory has been described that can also account for typicality effects.[40,41] According to the "exemplar-based" models of categorization, classification can be accounted for by the storage and retrieval of individual exemplars. Exemplar theories maintain that newly encountered items act as retrieval cues to access stored individual exemplars from a category. Since the most representative stimuli (prototypes) are similar to a large number of individual exemplars, they are more likely to be accessed quickly; thus, the exemplar model offers an explanation for the results of studies showing the superior or more efficient recognition of prototypic items from a category.

Data on infants' category representations come from experiments on faces and dot patterns. For example, Strauss[42] presented 10-month-old infants with a number of schematic faces varying in length, width, and amount of separation between the eyes, during the familiarization phase of an habituation experiment. After familiarization, infants treated the average face, a face that they had not actually seen during the experiment, as more familiar than either the most frequently presented face or a novel face that was not the average. This result suggests that infants summarized the faces that they were exposed to in the form of an average of all the faces they experienced.

Research on the perception of dot patterns suggests a similar conclusion. Bomba and Siqueland[43] tested 3- and 4-month-old infants' abilities to represent dot patterns. Infants were shown distorted dot patterns that were generated from a symmetrical form (triangle, square, or diamond). After familiarization of the patterns from a single category, infants treated the prototype of that category as more familiar than a previously unseen prototype of another category or an experienced exemplar.

The work on infants' perception of visual stimuli demonstrates infants' capacity to form representations based on experience. Work on phonetic prototypes' in infants using similar designs is now underway, and will be helpful in understanding the form that infants' speech representations take and infants' abilities to retain speech information in long-term memory. At the present time we do not take a position on whether the prototype abstraction view or the exemplar-based view offers the best description of infants' stored representations for speech. The magnet effect in infants could be accommodated by either form of representation. The type of long-term memory and representation involved in the speech case also fits together with recent work demonstrating long-term memory for human body movements.[44] The parallels between infant speech perception and the representation of faces and human action are quite interesting.[45,46]

A THEORY OF DEVELOPMENT

The studies described here suggest a new theory of the development of speech perception, called the *Native Language Magnet (NLM) Theory* of developmental speech perception. The theory accounts for the early period of speech perception covering roughly the first year of life, prior to the time that infants acquire word meaning and contrastive phonology. The theory holds that infants' early representations of speech information constitute the beginnings of language-specific speech perception and play a critical role in infants' perception of native and foreign-language sounds.

What is Given by Nature and What is Gained by Experience?

The results of the studies on phonetic prototypes led to the formulation of a new theory of developmental speech perception, the NLM theory.[13,14] NLM accounts for the early period of speech perception covering roughly the first year of life, prior to the time that infants acquire word meaning and contrastive phonology. The theory holds that infants come into the world with language-relevant abilities that are innate and attributable to general mechanisms of auditory perception. Some of the characteristics of this basic innate mechanism were uncovered in our studies with animals described earlier (for review, see reference 22); they are also suggested by studies of infants' perception of nonspeech (e.g., reference 47). To this innate component, the model adds a powerful component that derives from linguistic experience. The model holds that by 6 months of age infants develop stored representations of speech information, based on their perception of ambient language input. These initial representations constitute the beginnings of language-specific speech perception and play a critical role in infants' perception of native- and foreign-language sounds.

NLM holds that what is given by nature is the ability to partition the sound stream into gross categories separated by natural boundaries, as is schematically illustrated in FIGURE 5. These boundaries, shown here as divisions in a two-formant vowel space, convey the fact that infants are born with a capacity to resolve the acoustic differences between sounds. This allows infants to separate phonetic units into rough categories that conform to those of language. The boundaries do not indicate an absolute failure to detect within-category distinctions nor perfect success in the discrimination of between-category contrasts. The boundaries simply reflect infants' better discrimination for between- as opposed to within-category contrasts as discovered in tests of consonants and vowels with infants. This separation of phonetic units into rough categories would also be displayed by nonhuman animals.[22] If the model is correct, the boundaries do not derive from a specialized speech-specific

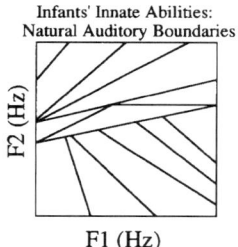

FIGURE 5. At birth infants perceptually partition the acoustic space underlying phonetic distinctions in a language-general way.

mechanism. These are results produced by the general auditory processing mechanism. According to the view presented here, infants' speech processing abilities are thus not initially the result of a language-specific speech module, though they may eventually become organized in this way (for a development of this view, see references 48 and 49).

Given that the acoustic space is initially divided by natural boundaries, boundaries that are also shared by certain nonhuman animals, what is acquired in human ontogeny? Based on the data gathered in the perceptual magnet studies reported here, we can now say that by 6 months of age infants have something more than the basic boundaries they were born with. By 6 months of age infants demonstrate perceptual magnet effects that are language specific. This is illustrated in the plots shown in FIGURE 6. Here I schematically portray magnet effects demonstrated by 6-month-old infants being raised in Sweden, America, and Japan. The graphs are not meant to be precise with regard to the locations of vowel magnets. They convey in conceptual terms the idea that linguistic experience in the three different cultures has resulted in magnets that differ in number and location for infants growing up listening to the three different languages.

Where do these perceptual magnets come from? They are the result of infants' perception and representation of language input. Infants are exposed to human speech from the first moments of postnatal life (even before birth, see reference 50). The ambient speech heard by infants is typically restricted to a single language and

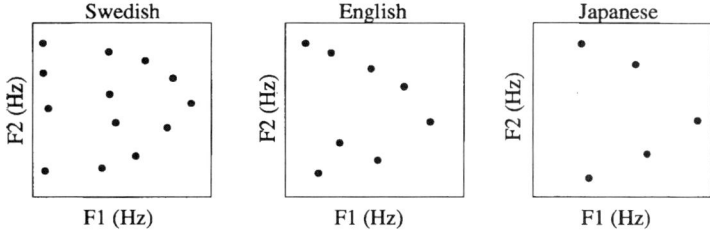

FIGURE 6. By 6 months of age, infants reared in different linguistic environments show an effect of language experience. They have acquired language-specific magnets that reflect the ambient language input.

reflects distributional properties that are characteristic of that particular language. For example, in the case of the three languages shown here—Swedish, English, and Japanese—the distributional properties of vowels produced by native speakers would be expected to differ considerably. According to the model, infants begin to form memory representations of the ambient language input, representations that reflect these distributional properties. NLM thus does not hold that there is a single identical version of each vowel represented in all individuals: there is no one /i/ vowel, for example. An individuals' representation of /i/ reflects /i/ vowels spoken by native speakers of a particular dialect and a particular language. Note that if language input to the child is to play this role, then detailed attention needs to be directed toward describing it (for a current description of work on the vowels contained in Motherese, see references 13 and 51). Note also the importance of infants' innately given perceptual boundaries in this scheme: infants perceptual boundaries delimit the space incorporated by an individual magnet. Infants' organization of language input is thus appropriately constrained so that magnets reflect a single category rather than the entire vowel space. Thus, magnets are formed because infants are prepared to respond to linguistic input (for a discussion of the potential physiological underpinnings of infants' receptivity, see reference 14). Magnets are a natural result of infants' coding of the input of native-language speakers.

According to NLM, native-language speech perception comes about in the absence of word acquisition and linguistic contrast. Previous research indicated that infants' perception of foreign-language contrasts changed near the end of the first year. Studies by Werker and her colleagues[52–54] show that 10- to 12-month-old infants fail to discriminate certain foreign-language contrasts, ones that they discriminated earlier in life. The fact that the language-general pattern of perception appeared to give way to a language-specific pattern near the end of the first year, coinciding with infants' production and comprehension of first words, led to a number of hypotheses,[55] one of which was that the change in phonetic perception reflected infants' acquisition of word meaning and their understanding of contrastive phonology.

The data and theory presented here support a different view. NLM suggests that early language input results in infants' development of native-language phonetic *representations*, and that this process precedes word acquisition and the understanding of contrastive phonology. NLM holds that infants' native-language speech representations alter phonetic perception, causing subsequent change in their perception of foreign-language contrasts. If the theory is correct, the infant does not have to acquire words or contrast in order to display language-specific phonetic perception.

NLM theory thus provides an account of infants' development of native-language speech perception, which then explains their perception of foreign-language sounds. The theory holds that acquisition of native-language magnets subsequently alters the perception of differences in phonetic space. Magnets attract surrounding category members. This will cause certain perceptual distinctions to be minimized (those near the magnets themselves), while others are maximized (those sounds that are not near a native-language magnet). The effects of magnet acquisition on the boundaries that divide the underlying phonetic space are shown in the schematic diagrams of FIGURE 7. In essence, magnets cause certain boundaries to functionally disappear as the perceptual system is reconfigured to incorporate a languages' particular magnet placement.

Magnet theory accounts for Werker's discovery that infants aged 10–12 months fail to discriminate foreign-language contrasts that they once discriminated. After the

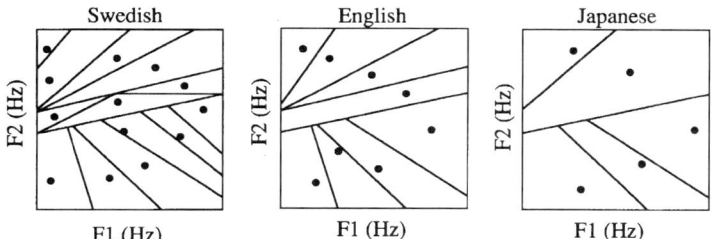

FIGURE 7. Language-specific magnets cause certain phonetic boundaries to disappear for each group of infants.

language-specific magnets are in place, and have reorganized the underlying perceptual space, infants will fail to discriminate sounds that they earlier discriminated. The developing magnet pulls sounds that were once discriminable toward a single magnet, making them no longer discriminable. On this account, magnet effects occur first, before the failure to discriminate; they will developmentally *precede* and underlie infants' failure to discriminate foreign-language contrasts. As discussed by Werker and Polka,[56] the new data gathered on vowel perception is interpretable when viewed in this way. NLM thus offers a *mechanism* that explains the reorganization Werker postulated in infants' phonetic perception.

The NLM theory also helps explain the results of studies on adults' perception of sounds from a foreign language. These studies show that not all foreign-language contrasts are difficult to discriminate. Foreign-language units that are similar to a native-language category are difficult to perceive as different from the native-language sound; sounds that are not similar to a native-language category are relatively easy to discriminate.[57] The case of /r–l/ discrimination by native speakers of Japanese provides the canonical example of a difficult foreign-language contrast.[29,58,59] I would suggest that foreign contrasts are made difficult to discriminate by the fact that a prototype of a native-language category attracts both foreign-language sounds. The difficulty in discriminating two foreign-language sounds depends on their proximity to a native-language magnet. The nearer they are, the more difficult to discriminate. NLM thus provides a model that is compatible with Best's[60] levels of relative difficulty in discriminating various foreign-language contrasts.

Finally, NLM theory applies to adults' acquisition of a second language. The model holds that the native-language categories of the listener interfere with the ability to perceive certain phonetic distinctions in the new language. The proximity principle again holds: the nearer a new sound is to a native-language magnet, the more it will be assimilated by it, making the new sound indistinguishable from the native-language sound. Phonologists have argued that the phonetic categories of ones' native language form some sort of "sieve" through which the phonetic units of the newly acquired language must pass.[61] NLM provides a potential mechanism by which this could come about.

Two additional points need to be made. First, we cannot as yet specify the state of the initial mechanism with regard to the magnet effect. We do not know whether magnet effects are present at birth for at least some vowels or whether they develop with exposure to a particular language. We are at present testing very young infants with various prototype and nonprototype stimuli. These studies should reveal whether or not infants initially show a magnet effect for all prototypes in the absence of language experience, or whether magnet effects are initially absent and develop with language experience. In either case, by 6 months of age infants' phonetic perception has been altered by language experience. A second point that has not been made is that NLM, as described here, has focused on the perceptual aspects of speech representations. In fact, the model holds that infants' speech representations are "polymodal" very early on (for further discussion, see reference 14).

In summary, in the studies reviewed here we have shown that linguistic experience has an effect prior to the time that infants utter or understand their first words. Infants' abilities to learn by simply listening to the ambient language suggests a powerful linguistic representational system that responds automatically given proper input. Nature's initial structuring in the form of natural boundaries, combined with the role experience plays in defining the centers of phonetic categories, provides infants with a strong foundation for higher language processes. The Native Language Magnet model describes how innate abilities interact with infants' early experience to produce a language-specific pattern of speech perception, and explains the available facts in infant speech perception.

IMPLICATIONS FOR LANGUAGE IMPAIRMENT

What does this view offer to the study of language disorders and dyslexia? One contribution is to focus on the effects of early perceptual predispositions and early learning on the phonetic representations that are formed. The working hypothesis that stems from the work of Tallal,[2] Galaburda and Livingstone,[3] and Llinás[4] is that dyslexic and other language-impaired individuals do not perceive rapidly changing information, particularly rapidly changing speech information, in the same way that nonimpaired individuals do. Tallal's early work generated the hypothesis that temporal processing of rapid information was impaired, regardless of whether the information was speech or nonspeech.

Impairments in the ability to process speech input could have two deleterious effects on an impaired individual. First, impaired individuals' perceptual boundaries could be different. I know of no studies that specifically test dyslexic individuals on the perception of stimuli from a phonetic continuum. One can speculate that, for example, the location of the phonetic boundary on a continuum that ranges from /ba/ to /wa/, one that relies on the rate of change of frequency information (e.g., reference 62), could be substantially altered in impaired individuals. Second, the phonetic representations formed by these individuals could well be very different from those formed by nonimpaired individuals who heard the same input. This difference would be due to the abnormal processing of language input. Thus, temporal processing deficits could result in the formation of aberrant representations, prototypes that are not like those of normal individuals.

This is not to say that language-impaired individuals lack the ability to extract from ambient language experience the relevant data to construct representations. It simply highlights the fact that their processing deficits could result in representations that are not normal. This has implications for treatment. Perhaps, for example, dyslexics might benefit from "stretched" speech, speech that has been altered so as to expand the rapid temporal events in speech (see reference 63). Stretched speech may match the dyslexic's representations better than speech presented at normal rates. With future research aimed at assessing the perceptual representations of language-impaired individuals, we might look forward to treatments that target specific problems encountered by these individuals.

REFERENCES

1. DENCKLA, M. B. 1992 A neurologists's overview of dyslexia. This volume.
2. TALLAL, P. 1992. Neural basis of temporal perceptual motor processing: Implications for speech and reading. This volume.
3. GALABURDA, A. M. & M. LIVINGSTONE. 1992. Neuropathological evidence a defect in developmental dyslexia. This volume.
4. LLINÁS, R. R. 1992. Cerebellar involvement in temporal sensory-motor processing: Relevance for speech, reading and writing. This volume.
5. EIMAS, P. D., J. L. MILLER & P. W. JUSCZYK. 1987. On infant speech perception and the acquisition of language. In Categorical Perception: The Groundwork of Cognition, S. Harnad, Ed.: 161–195. Cambridge Univ. Press. New York.
6. KUHL, P. K. 1987. Perception of speech and sound in early infancy. In Handbook of Infant Perception, Vol. 2, From Perception to Cognition, P. Salapatek and L. Cohen, Eds.: 275–382. Academic Press. New York.
7. ———. 1985. Categorization of speech by infants. In Neonate Cognition: Beyond the Blooming, Buzzing Confusion, J. Mehler and R. Fox, Eds.: 231–262. Erlbaum. Hillsdale, N.J.
8. KUHL, P. K. & A. N. MELTZOFF. 1982. The bimodal perception of speech in infancy. Science 218: 1138–1141.
9. ———. 1984. The intermodal representation of speech in infants. Infant Behav. Dev. 7:361–381.
10. ———. 1988. Speech as an intermodal object of perception. In Perceptual Development in Infancy: The Minnesota Symposia on Child Psychology, Vol. 20, A. Yonas, Ed.: 235–266. Erlbaum. Hillsdale, N.J.
11. MACKAIN, K., M. STUDDERT-KENNEDY, S. SPIEKER & D. STERN. 1983. Infant intermodal speech perception is a left-hemisphere function. Science 219: 1347–1349.
12. KUHL, P. K., K. A. WILLIAMS, F. LACERDA, K. N. STEVENS & B. LINDBLOM. 1992. Linguistic experience alters phonetic perception in infants by 6 months of age. Science 255: 606–608.
13. KUHL, P. K. 1992. Infants' perception and representation of speech: Development of a new theory. In The Proceedings of the International Conference on Spoken Language Processing. J. Ohala, T. Nearey, B. Derwing, M. Hodge, and G. Wiebe, Eds.: 449–456. Univ. of Alberta Press. Edmonton, Alta., Canada.
14. ———. 1993. Innate predispositions and the effects of experience in speech perception: The native-language magnet theory. In Developmental Neurocognition: Speech and Face Processing in the First Year of Life, B. de Boysson-Bardies, S. de Schonen, P. Jusczyk, P. MacNeilage, and J. Morton, Eds. Kluwer. Dordrecht, the Netherlands.
15. EIMAS, P. D., E. R. SIQUELAND, P. JUSCZYK & J. VIGORITO. 1971. Speech perception in infants. Science 171: 303–306.
16. EIMAS, P. D. 1974. Auditory and linguistic processing of cues for place of articulation by infants. Percept. Psychophys. 16: 513–521.
17. ———. 1975. Auditory and phonetic coding of the cues for speech: Discrimination of the /r-l/ distinction by young infants. Percept. Psychophys. 18: 341–347.
18. GRIESER, D. & P. K. KUHL. 1989. Categorization of speech by infants: Support for speech-sound prototypes. Devel. Psych. 25: 577–588.
19. KUHL, P. K. 1991. Human adults and human infants show a "perceptual magnet effect" for the prototypes of speech categories, monkeys do not. Percept. Psychophys. 50: 93–107.
20. STREETER, L. A. 1976. Language perception of 2-month-old infants shows effects of both innate mechanisms and experience. Nature 259: 39–41.

21. KUHL, P. K. & J. D. MILLER. 1975. Speech perception by the chinchilla: Voiced-voiceless distinction in alveolar plosive consonants. Science **190**: 69–72.
22. KUHL, P. K. 1987. The special-mechanisms debate in speech research: Categorization tests on animals and infants. *In* Categorical Perception: The Groundwork of Cognition, S. Harnad, Ed.: 355–386. Cambridge Univ. Press. New York.
23. LIBERMAN, A. M., F. S. COOPER, D. P. SHANKWEILER & M. STUDDERT-KENNEDY. 1967. Perception of the speech code. Psych. Rev. **74**: 431–461.
24. REPP, B. 1984. Categorical perception: Issues, methods, findings. *In* Speech and Language, Vol. 10. Advances in Basic Research and Practice, N. J. Lass, Ed.: 243–335. Academic Press. New York.
25. SWOBODA, P. J., J. KASS, P. A. MORSE & L. A. LEAVITT. 1978. Memory factors in vowel discrimination of normal and at-risk infants. Child Devel. **49**: 332–339.
26. KUHL, P. K. & J. D. MILLER. 1978. Speech perception by the chinchilla: Identification functions for synthetic VOT stimuli. J. Acoust. Soc. Am. **63**: 905–917.
27. KUHL, P. K. 1986. Theoretical contributions of tests on animals to the special-mechanisms debate in speech. Exp. Biol. **45**: 233–265.
28. ———. 1988. Auditory perception and the evolution of speech. Hum. Evol. **3**: 19–43.
29. MIYAWAKI, K., W. STRANGE, R. VERBRUGGE, A. M. LIBERMAN, J. J. JENKINS & O. FUJIMURA. 1975. An effect of linguistic experience: The discrimination of [r] and [l] by native speakers of Japanese and English. Percept. Psychophys. **18**: 331–340.
30. ABRAMSON, A. S. & L. LISKER. 1970. Discriminability along the voicing continuum: Cross-language tests. *In* Proceedings of the Sixth International Congress of Phonetic Sciences Prague 1967. Academia. Prague.
31. KUHL, P. K. 1980. Perceptual constancy for speech-sound categories in early infancy. *In* Child Phonology, Vol. 2, Perception, G. H. Yeni-Komshian, J. F. Kavanagh, and C. A. Ferguson, Eds.: 41–66. Academic Press. New York.
32. HILLENBRAND, J. 1983. Perceptual organization of speech sounds by infants. J. Speech Hear. Res. **26**: 268–282.
33. ———. 1984. Speech perception by infants: Categorization based on nasal consonant place of articulation. J. Acoust. Soc. Am. **75**: 1613–1622.
34. MILLER, J. L., C. M. CONNINE, T. M. SCHERMER & K. R. KLUENDER. 1983. A possible auditory basis for internal structure of phonetic categories. J. Acoust. Soc. Am. **73**: 2124–2133.
35. MILLER, J. L. & L. E. VOLAITIS. 1989. Effect of speaking rate on the perceptual structure of a phonetic category. Percept. Psychophys. **46**: 505–512.
36. SAMUEL, A. G. 1982. Phonetic prototypes. Percept. Psychophys. **31**: 307–314.
37. VOLAITIS, L. E. & J. L. MILLER. 1992. Phonetic prototypes: Influence of place of articulation and speaking rate on the internal structure of voicing categories. J. Acoust. Soc. Am. **92**: 723–735.
38. DAVIS, K. & P. K. KUHL. 1992. Best exemplars of English velar stops: A first report. *In* The Proceedings of the International Conference on Spoken Language Processing, J. Ohala, T. Nearey, B. Derwing, M. Hodge, and G. Wiebe, Eds.: 495–498. Univ. of Alberta Press. Edmonton, Alta., Canada.
39. MERVIS, C. B. & E. ROSCH. 1981. Categorization of natural objects. Annu. Rev. Psych. **32**: 89–115.
40. MEDIN, D. L. & L. W. BARSALOU. 1987. Categorization processes and categorical perception. *In* Categorical Perception: The Groundwork of Cognition, S. Harnad, Ed.: 455–490. Cambridge Univ. Press. New York.
41. NOSOFSKY, R. M. 1988. Exemplar-based accounts of relations between classification, recognition, and typicality. J. Exp. Psych.: Learn., Mem., Cognition. **14**: 700–708.
42. STRAUSS, M. S. 1979. Abstraction of prototypical information by adults and 10-month-old infants. J. Exp. Psych.: Hum. Learn. Mem. **5**: 618–632.
43. BOMBA, P. C. & E. R. SIQUELAND. 1983. The nature and structure of infant form categories. J. Exp. Child Psych. **35**: 294–328.
44. MELTZOFF, A. N. 1990. Towards a developmental cognitive science: The implications of cross-modal matching and imitation for the development of representation and memory

in infancy. *In* The Development and Neural Bases of Higher Cognitive Functions, A. Diamond, Ed. Ann. N.Y. Acad. Sci. **608:** 1–31.
45. MELTZOFF, A. N. & P. K. KUHL. 1989. Infants' perception of faces and speech sounds: Challenges to developmental theory. *In* Challenges to Developmental Paradigms: Implications for Theory, Assessment and Treatment, P. R. Zelazo & R. Barr, Eds.: 67–91. Erlbaum. Hillsdale, N.J.
46. MELTZOFF, A. N., P. K. KUHL & M. K. MOORE. 1991. Perception, representation, and the control of action in newborns and young infants: Toward a new synthesis. *In* Newborn Attention: Biological Constraints and the Influence of Experience, M. J. S. Weiss & P. R. Zelazo, Eds.: 377–411. Ablex. Norwood, N.J.
47. JUSCZYK, P. W., D. B. PISONI, M. A. REED, A. FERNALD & M. MYERS. 1983. Infants' discrimination of the duration of a rapid spectrum change in nonspeech signals. Science **222:** 175–177.
48. LIBERMAN, A. M. 1992. In speech perception time is not what is seems. This volume.
49. LIBERMAN, A. M. & I. G. MATTINGLY. 1985. The motor theory of speech perception revised. Cognition **21:** 1–36.
50. LECANUET, J. 1993. Fetal responsiveness to voice and speech. *In* Developmental Neurocognition: Speech and Face Processing in the First Year of Life, B. de Boysson-Bardies, S. De Schonen, P. Jusczyk, P. MacNeilage, and J. Morton, Eds. Kluwer. Dordrecht, the Netherlands.
51. MOON, S. J. & B. LINDBLOM. 1989. Formant undershoot in clear and citation-form speech: A second report. Quarterly Progress and Status Report **1:** 121–123. Stockholm: KTH Speech Transmission Laboratory.
52. WERKER, J. F. & R. C. TEES. 1984. Cross-language speech perception: Evidence for perceptual reorganization during the first year of life. Infant Behav. Devel. **72:** 49–63.
53. WERKER, J. F. & C. E. LALONDE. 1988. Cross-language speech perception: Initial capabilities and developmental change. Devel. Psych. **24:** 672–683.
54. WERKER, J. F. & PEGG. 1992. Infant speech perception and phonological acquisition. *In* Phonological Development, C. A. Ferguson, L. Menn & C. Stoel-Gammon, Eds. York Press. Timonium, Md.
55. WERKER, J. F. 1993. The ontogeny and developmental significance of language specific phonetic perception. *In* Developmental Neurocognition: Speech and Face Processing in the First Year of Life, B. de Boysson-Bardies *et al.*, Eds. Kluwer. Dordrecht, the Netherlands.
56. WERKER, J. & L. POLKA. Developmental changes in speech perception: New challenges and new directions. J. Phonetics. In press.
57. BEST, C. T., G. W. MCROBERTS & N. M. SITHOLE. 1988. Examination of perceptual reorganization for nonnative speech contrasts: Zulu click discrimination by English-speaking adults and infants. J. Exp. Psych.: Hum. Percept. Perform. **14:** 345–360.
58. LOGAN, J. S., S. E. LIVELY & D. B. PISONI. 1991. Training Japanese listeners to identify English /r/ and /l/: A first report. J. Acoust. Soc. Am. **89:** 874–886.
59. STRANGE, W. & S. DITTMANN. 1984. Effects of discrimination training on the perception of /r-l/ by Japanese adults learning English. Percept. Psychophys. **36:** 131–145.
60. BEST, C. T. 1993. Language-specific developmental changes in non-native speech perception: A window on early phonological development. *In* Developmental Neurocognition: Speech and Face Processing in the First Year of Life, B. de Boysson-Bardies, S. de Schonen, P. Jusczyk, P. MacNeilage, and J. Morton, Eds. Kluwer. Dordrecht, the Netherlands.
61. TRUBETZKOY, N. S. 1939/1969. Principles of phonology. [Originally published in German (Grundzüge der Phonologie) as *Travgaux du cercle linguistique de Prague 7*. Transl. C. A. M. Baltaxe], Univ. of California. Berkeley.
62. MILLER, J. L. & A. M. LIBERMAN. 1979. Some effects of later-occurring information on the perception of stop consonant and semivowel. Percept. Psychophys. **25:** 457–465.
63. MEHLER, J., N. SEBASTIAN, G. ALTMANN, E. DUPOUX, A. CHRISTOPHE & C. PALLIER. 1992. Understanding compressed sentences: The role of rhythm and meaning. This volume.

In Speech Perception, Time Is Not What It Seems

ALVIN M. LIBERMAN

Haskins Laboratories
270 Crown Street
New Haven, Connecticut 06511-6695

The subject of this symposium and the titles of some if its papers imply a belief that general principles of temporal processing can enlighten us about language behavior and the ills that attend it, whether in speech or in writing–reading. To determine just how well-founded that belief is, we must, I think, resolve two issues. One concerns the relation between the two kinds of language behavior we are trying to understand, the other looks in a different direction, at the relation of speech, the more basic of these behaviors, to the nonlinguistic modalities where the roots of that understanding are presumed to lie.

The salient fact about the relation of speech to writing–reading is the vast difference in the underlying biology. Speech is a product of biological evolution, having emerged with us as the most important of our species-specific characteristics. Writing systems, on the other hand, are recently developed artifacts, part discovery, part invention. In the case of an alphabet, the momentous discovery was that human beings had, for untold thousands of years, been speaking phonologically. Quite without knowing it, they had all been using a marvelously generative scheme for producing an indefinitely large number of meaningful words by variously combining and permuting a small number of meaningless segments. Once that was understood, it remained only to invent the idea that if each of the meaningless segments were to be represented, however arbitrarily, by a distinctive optical shape, than all could write and read, provided only that they knew the language and could manage to become consciously aware of the internal phonological structure of its words.

Seen this way, an alphabetic transcription is an accurate account of species-specific behavior, hence an early achievement of ethological science. Accordingly, one might characterize the relation of speech to writing–reading by a simple equation: the speaker–listener is to the writer–reader as an ordinary human being is to an ethologist.

What, then, is biologically distinct about the species-specific behavior that an alphabetic transcription is an ethological account of? In short, what evolved? Not why, or when, or by what progression from earlier-existing states. Only what.

I mean, in due course, to suggest that what evolved were processes that are specific to speech, hence part of the larger specialization for language and not likely, therefore, to be properly understood by reference to putatively comparable processes in nonlinguistic modalities. Touching more particularly on the point of this symposium, I will say that the evolution of these speech-specific processes was itself guided largely by requirements of temporal processing, which is our subject, then quickly add that these requirements were special, having been imposed by the special nature of phonologic communication.

But first I must take account of the opposite view, which is that the processes we are here concerned with are not specific to speech, that language simply appropriated, for phonological purposes, motor and auditory mechanisms of a very general sort.

(For representative examples of this view, see Crowder and Morton,[1] Fujisaki and Kawashima,[2] Oden and Massaro,[3] Samuel,[4] Miller,[5] Stevens,[6] Cutting and Rosner,[7] Hillenbrand,[8] Diehl and Kluender,[9] Lindblom[10]). Borrowing a word that Fodor[11] used to characterize a much broader version of this view, I will call it "horizontal," in contrast to my view, which is appropriately called "vertical." By any name, however, the horizontal view is the more conventional and also the more congenial to the purpose of this symposium. It rests on four assumptions that compare neatly with four facts about writing–reading.

The first assumption is that the ultimate constituents of language are sounds. Obvious though this may seem, it is, nevertheless, only an assumption, and, as I will argue, quite wrong. However, its counterpart in writing–reading is a hard fact: the constituents of an alphabet are optical shapes and nothing else.

The second assumption is that the constituent sounds are produced by articulatory maneuvers and motor control processes that are not specific to speech, but are, rather, of some quite general sort. As for its counterpart in writing, we know that the movements the writer makes cannot be specific biological adaptations to language, if only because writing was not part of linguistic evolution.

The third assumption is companion to the second. Just as the production of speech sounds is managed by processes of a general nonlinguistic sort, so too is their perception. According to the horizontalists, perception of speech is no different from perception of other sounds. All are governed by the same general processes of hearing, processes that evoke in a common perceptual register a common set of auditory primitives: pitch, loudness, timbre, and the like. The representations evoked by a stop consonant and a squeaking door are made of the same perceptual stuff; they differ only in the relative values assigned to the primitives they share. This assumption that perception of speech sounds is generally auditory corresponds to the fact that perception of alphabetic characters is generally visual.

We come, then, to the fourth assumption, which is made necessary by the second and third. For if the motor and perceptual representations are not themselves distinctly linguistic, they must be made so, and that can be dome only by a cognitive translation. Accordingly, horizontalists say explicitly that, after experiencing the purely auditory percept that was evoked by the acoustic signal, the listener connects it to language by giving it a phonologic name or otherwise associating it with a phonologic unit. Thus, perceiving speech is, to the horizontalist, a matter of experiencing something auditory and calling it something linguistic. For speech perception, this proves to be a very troubling, if necessary, assumption, but for reading it is an indisputable fact; the purely visual percepts evoked by the letters of the alphabet do require to be translated into units of the language. Indeed, as I mean to emphasize later, it is just the need for this translation that distinguishes reading from speech perception.

Thus, the first shortcoming of the horizontal view is that everything it assumes about speech is a fact about writing–reading, so the horizontal view cannot rationalize the profound biological difference between the two kinds of behavior that are the objects of our concern. But if a theory of speech cannot cope with a fact about language as basic and obvious as the difference in a naturalness between its spoken and written forms, then there must be something profoundly wrong with it.

Other shortcomings go deeper. Perhaps the deepest has to do with the most basic requirement that a communication system must meet, which is simply that sender and receiver be bound by a common understanding about what counts: what counts for the sender must count for the receiver. Though this requirement does not commonly figure in the evaluation of theories of language, Ignatius Mattingly and I have thought it important enough to deserve a name, so we have called it the "requirement for parity," and we have challenged theories to explain how it was established as language developed in the history of our species and as it develops anew in each child. [12–14]

To see the point most clearly, consider parity in the case of writing–reading. If someone draws a "B" and a squiggle, all who are literate in the Roman alphabet understand that the one has linguistic significance and the other does not. Moreover, all know what the particular linguistic significance of the "B" is. Thus, parity exists, so all can use this signal for communication. As for the origin of parity in this case, it is to be found in an agreement, arrived at by those who presided over the development of the Roman alphabet, that invested a select set of optical shapes with linguistic significance by arbitrarily assigning each one to a phonological segment.

But, surely, we cannot make a similar statement about speech. People did not simply agree that "da" would count but a snapping of the fingers would not. Neither was it an agreement that determined what "da" would count for. Yet, as we have seen, the horizontal view allows no alternative, since it assumes that the motor and perceptual representations of speech are connected to language, and to each other, only because speaker and listener choose to call them by the same phonologic names or somehow connect them to the same phonologic units. Indeed, the harder one looks at the parity question from the horizontal point of view, the more one is forced to the unacceptable conclusion that phonology must have been an invention, a new and better mode of communication devised by human beings who were smart enough to appreciate the generative advantages of the phonological principle and creative enough to have seen how to exploit it, given the resources of the vocal tract and the ear.

Having said that speech as seen on the horizontal view would not plausibly meet the parity requirement, which is imposed on all forms of communication, I turn now to requirements that are specific to phonology. There are two. The first, which must be met if phonology is to serve its generative function, is that the segments of the phonological structure be commutable—that is, that they be discrete, invariant, and categorical. The second, which is only slightly less obvious, has to do with rate and, accordingly, with the subject of this symposium: temporal processing. The point is that if all utterances are to be formed by variously stringing together an exiguous set of segments, then, inevitably, the strings must run to considerable lengths. Moreover, these segments must be organized into words, the words into phrases, and the phrases into sentences. There is, then, a need for rapid production and perception of the segments.

But discrete, invariant, and categorical sounds would require correspondingly discrete, invariant, and categorical gestures, so, on the horizontal view, communication could be managed only at unacceptably slow rates. To know how slow, one has only to consider writing, even cursive writing, where it is similarly necessary that the optical shapes be discrete, invariant, and categorical. So, if the ultimate constituents of speech were sounds, speaking would be like writing: it would not be possible to say "bag," but only "b" "a" "g." And to say "b" "a" "g" is not to speak but to spell.

I should add that the problem is fundamentally insoluble on the horizontal strategy, for if Nature had tried to avoid the limitations on rate by endowing her human creatures with acoustic devices specifically adapted to producing a rapid-fire string of sounds, she would have defeated the ear. The point is that, as I speak to you now, I am producing phonological segments at a rate that averages about 10 per second and, for short stretches, reaches 20 or more. If each of those were a discrete sound, rates that high would seriously strain the temporal resolving power of the ear and its ability to place the segments in their proper temporal order. Thus, phonological communication would be impossible.

The foregoing arguments of plausibility are about just those shortcomings of the horizontal view that are most relevant to the purpose of this symposium. They reduce to the consequences of the most general assumption of this view, which is that there is, at the level of action and perception, no such thing as a distinctly and specifically linguistic mode. Thus, the question, "What evolved?", that I earlier asked gets from the horizontal view the simple answer, "No more in speech than in writing–reading." Since that answer flies in the face of the most obvious fact about the relation between these two behaviors, I find the view that supplies it a poor guide to the understanding we seek.

I turn, then, to the view that I think more likely to be helpful, the view that I earlier referred to as "vertical." (For general accounts, see Liberman and Mattingly,[15] Mattingly and Liberman,[16] Mattingly and Liberman,[17] Liberman and Mattingly.[18]) The first assumption of this view is that nature managed the rate problem by defining the constituents of language, not as sounds, but as gestures. Thus, the constituent we write as "b" is a closing of the vocal tract at the lips; "m" is a closing at the lips and an opening at the velum; and so on. Putting aside admittedly difficult questions about exactly how these gestures are to be characterized, we see nonetheless clearly the great advantage of the gestural strategy, which is that it permits coarticulation. Given phonologic segments that are instantiated as more or less abstract motor units, and given successive segments that are realized at the periphery by independent articulators such as the lips for "ba" and the tongue for "a," the speaker says, not "b" "a," but "ba." At all events, coarticulation is characteristic of all languages, and it is, without question, the necessary condition for the rapid rates of phonologic communication that are, in fact, achieved.

The second assumption of the vertical view is that the articulatory movements and their controls were not lying conveniently to hand, just waiting to be used by language. They are, rather, the products of evolution. Consider, for example, that the movements we make when we speak are a distinct set, different from those we make with the same organs when we chew, swallow, move food around in the mouth, lick our lips, or worry a sore tooth with the tip of the tongue. Phonologic gestures serve a linguistic function and no other. Presumably, they were selected in evolution largely because of the ease with which they lent themselves to being coarticulated. As for their controls, they must be specialized, too. Is there another motor system in which the kinematics are managed by, and perfectly preserve information about, strings of temporally ordered motor units that are discrete, invariant, and categorical?

Of course, the organs that are used in speech are also controlled by motor systems that have nothing to do with speech, and these must certainly affect speech as well. Indeed, they will often take precedence over speech, as in breathing, coughing, or gagging. And, surely, the phonological specialization has much in common with other motor systems—for example, the need to control degrees of freedom—but, as I said earlier, it also has to manage the rapid production of strings of discrete, invariant, and categorical motor units, and that task seems peculiar to phonological communication. So, somewhere upstream from the final common paths, there must be a specialization for that special phonological task. Just where that "somewhere" is can only be determined empirically.

The third assumption of the vertical view takes account of the perceptual consequences of coarticulation. These are happy consequences from the standpoint of rate of communication, since coarticulation folds into a single piece of sound information about several phonologic segments, and so, by achieving parallel transmission, considerably relaxes the constraint on rate imposed by the temporal resolving power of the ear. Therefore, listeners can perceive phonologic structures as fast as the coarticulating speaker can produce them. But this comes at the cost of a considerable and specifically linguistic complication in the relation between acoustic signal and phonologic message. Thus, as all speech researchers know, the acoustic signal for each particular phonologic segment is different, often grossly, depending on the segments with which it is coarticulated. For some segments, the signal also varies as a function of rate of articulation and condition of linguistic stress. What remains constant is only some representation of the articulatory gesture. One is led, then, to suppose that the phonologic component of the language specialization has two complementary processes: one for computing the articulatory movements from the more abstract specification of the gestures, as in the second assumption just given, the other for automatically analyzing the acoustic signal in such a way as to recover the coarticulated gestures that caused it.

As in speech production, so, too, in speech perception, we recognize that the most peripheral structures and functions are shared with processes that are not linguistic, and it must, again, be an empirical matter to determine where the division into phonologic and nonphonologic occurs. What is clear, I think, is that it does not occur at a point where a preliminary auditory representation is cognitively translated into something phonologic, for there is no such preliminary auditory representation.

There is no need, then, on the vertical view, as there was on its horizontal opposite, for a fourth assumption about a cognitive translation into language because the motor and perceptual representations of speech are, by their nature, already linguistic, hence perfectly appropriate for further processing by the other components of the language system. Indeed, it is exactly this that is the primary biological difference between speech and writing–reading.

As for parity, we see, on the vertical view, that it is the very essence of the system, for what evolved was nothing less than a communicative modality, including the specifically phonological gestures that are integral parts of it. Accordingly, these gestures form a natural class, so their representations are set apart, biologically, from all others by their membership in that class, not by having phonologic names assigned to them. Speaker and listener can communicate in a perfectly natural way, as writer and reader cannot, because the speaker sends and the listener receives exactly the same specifically phonologic gestures; there is no need to connect a generally motor representation that underlies production to a generally auditory representation that underlies perception by means of an agreement that arbitrarily makes them comparable.

The vertical view also allows us to understand exactly what it is that the would-be reader must learn that experience with speech will not have taught him. Consider that a speaker does not have to know how to spell a word in order to produce it. Indeed, he does not even have to know that it has a spelling. He has simply to think of the word; the phonological specialization spells it for him, automatically selecting and coordinating the relevant gestures. The listener is in similar case, for to perceive a word, he need not puzzle out the complex relation between acoustic signal and the string of segments it conveys, or even be in any way aware of how very complex that relation is. Rather, he need only listen, relying on the automatic processes of phonology to parse the signal into its segments and arrange them in the proper temporal order. Speaker and listener lack awareness of these processes of production and perception, because the governing mechanisms are modular, hence insulated from consciousness. Of course, these modular processes do make their representations available to consciousness; indeed, if they did not, then alphabetic writing and reading would be impossible. But, as we have seen, these representations, being immediately phonologic, do not require the translation that would put them at the focus of attention. Taking all this into account, we understand why experience with speech, no matter how extensive, is not likely to produce the awareness of phonological structure that the would-be reader needs if he is to understand the phonologic principle, and so be able to connect the alphabetic transcription to the language it indexes.[19]

Like writing–reading, speech must, of course, be learned, but, unlike writing–reading, it need not be taught. The language module does, of course, depend on the phonologic environment for its proper development and calibration, and in this respect is no different, in principle, from such modules as those that are, for example, responsible for stereoscopic vision and sound localization.[20] But this kind of learning is precognitive, which is to say that it requires little more than the appropriate stimulation from the environment. Given the phonologic environment in which it finds itself, the language module will adapt without cognitive effort on the part of the child. Reading an alphabetic script, on the other hand, requires a cognitive, conscious understanding of the facts of phonological structure. Thus, we see how reading and writing are intellectual achievements in a way that the development of speech is not.

Now, at last, I redeem the promise of my title by describing the results of two kinds of experiments that show how very special are the perceptual consequences of the flow of time in the speech signal. The first has to do with the fact that speech perception requires the listener to respond to resonances that move rapidly up or down in center frequency. In the case of stop consonants, for example, the critically important resonances complete excursions as large as 500 Hz in about 50 ms. On the horizontal view, one might suppose that tracking these rapid changes is an auditory process that produces a correspondingly auditory representation and that this representation can be used as a base for obtaining psychophysical data relevant to the processes of speech perception. That matters are not so straightforward is shown by the results of experiments on a phenomenon, called *duplex perception,* in which a speech pattern is divided into two discordant or discontinuous parts, with the result that one of the parts is simultaneously perceived as two distinct events, one phonetic, the other not.[17,18,21–23] For example, a rapid movement up or down in center frequency that can be made responsible for the perceived difference between "da" and "ga" will be perceived as a nonspeech chirp (which is what it sounds like in isolation) and, at the same time, be responsible for the phonologic distinction. A duplex percept of this kind provides a unique opportunity to measure the listener's ability to discriminate tokens of the same rapidly changing resonance (in the same acoustic context) when, on the one side of the duplex percept, the resonance is producing the nonspeech chirp, and when, on the other, it is, at the same time, evoking the phonologic segment. The finding is that the discrimination functions obtained with these simultaneously available percepts are very different, both in shape and in level. Apparently, responding to rapidly changing resonances when they cue a phonologic segment does not depend on the same processes that underlie perception of these same resonances when, failing to engage the language module, they are perceived as acoustic events.[24] Hence, generalizing psychophysical results from the auditory to the phonologic modalities is, at best, a chancy thing.

The second relevant observation is more directly about the processing of temporal order. It pertains to the fact that, as Gunnar Fant pointed out many years ago, there is no direct correspondence in segmentation between the acoustic signal and the perceived phonetic message.[25] Since then, dozens of experiments have justified two important generalizations about temporal order in speech: (1) the articulation of a phonological segment typically has acoustic consequences that cover a wide span of the signal and overlap quite thoroughly with the acoustic consequences of the articulation of other segments in the string; and (2) the speech-perceiving system is sensitive to all these consequences, no matter how widely distributed, overlapped, or acoustically heterogeneous. In the contrast between the words "slit" and "split," for example, the acoustic information that has been shown to contribute to the perception of "p," the second segment in the string of five, includes at least the following: the duration, spectral shaping, and amplitude contour at offset of the band-limited noise at the beginning of the syllable; the duration of the interval of silence following the noise; the presence of a transient burst of sound following the silence; the onset frequencies of the three important resonances following the burst; the trajectories of the resonances following their onsets; the duration of those trajectories; and the duration (and possibly the amplitude envelope) of the voiced portion of the syllable (see Repp,[26] and the further references therein). That the perceptual mechanism somehow converges this information onto a phonetic percept that is perfectly unitary and properly positioned in the temporal order bespeaks a special process that is adapted to a special circumstance.

To summarize: Speech rests on a biologically coherent mechanism, adapted in evolution to the special requirements of phonologic communication, including especially the need for rapid production and perception of a small set of empty and commutable segments. I think it the better part of wisdom to take account of the special characteristics of this evolutionary product as we try to understand how it manages, nevertheless, to share organs and neural processes with nonlinguistic modalities. As for reading and writing, they surely connect to the biologically primary processes of language, but only after a cognitive translation that establishes the connection. There must, of course, be temporal processes that serve the visual aspects of reading, all of which occur before the translation, and also other temporal processes that are part of the translation itself, but it seems unlikely that these bear any relation to the temporal processes of speech.

REFERENCES

1. CROWDER, R. G. & J. MORTON. 1969. Pre-categorical acoustic storage (PAS). Percept. Psychophys. **5**: 365–373.
2. FUJISAKI, M. & T. KAWASHIMA. 1970. Some experiments on speech perception and a model for the perceptual mechanism. Annu. Rep. Eng. Res. Inst. (Faculty of Electrical Engineering, University of Tokyo) **29**: 207–214.
3. ODEN, G. C. & D. W. MASSARO. 1978. Integration of featural information in speech perception. Psychol. Rev. **85**: 172–191.
4. SAMUEL, A. G. 1977. The effect of discrimination training on speech perception: Noncategorical perception. Percep. Psychophys. **22**: 321–330.
5. MILLER, J. D. 1977. Perception of speech sounds in animals: Evidence for speech processing by mammalian auditory mechanisms. *In* Recognition of Complex Acoustic Signals. Life Sciences Research Report 5, T. H. Bullock, Ed.: 49. Dahlem Konferenzen. Berlin.
6. STEVENS, K. N. 1975. The potential role of property detectors in the perception of consonants. *In* Auditory Analysis and Perception of Speech, G. Fant and M. A. Tatham, Eds. Academic Press. New York
7. CUTTING, J. E. & B. S. ROSNER. 1974. Categories and boundaries in speech and music. Percept. Psychophys. **16**: 564–570

8. HILLENBRAND, J. 1984. Perception of sine-wave analogs of voice onset time stimuli. J. Acoust. Soc. Am. **75**: 231–240
9. DIEHL, R. & K. KLUENDER. 1989. On the objects of speech perception. Ecol. Psychol. **1**: 121–144.
10. LINDBOLM, B. 1991. The status of phonetic gestures. *In* Modularity and the Motor Theory of Speech Perception, I. G. Mattingly and M. Studdert-Kennedy, Eds. Erlbaum. Hillsdale, N.J.
11. FODOR, J. 1983. The Modularity of Mind. MIT Press. Cambridge, Mass.
12. MATTINGLY, I. G. & A. M. LIBERMAN. 1990. Speech and other auditory modules. *In* Signal and Sense: Local and Global Order in Perceptual Maps, G. M. Edelman, W. E. Gall, and W. M. Cowan, Eds. Wiley. New York.
13. LIBERMAN, A. M. & I. G. MATTINGLY. 1989. A specialization for speech perception. Science **243**: 489–494.
14. LIBERMAN, A. M. The relation of speech to reading and writing. *In* Orthography, Phonology, Morphology, and Meaning, R. Frost and L Katz, Eds. North-Holland. Amsterdam, the Netherlands.
15. LIBERMAN, A. M. & I. G. MATTINGLY. 1985. The motor theory of speech perception revised. Cognition **21**:1–36.
16. MATTINGLY, I. G. & A. M. LIBERMAN. 1988. Specialized perceiving systems for speech and other biologically significant sounds. *In* Functions of the Auditory System, G. M. Edelman, W. E. Gall, and W. M. Cowan, Eds.: 775–793. Wiley. New York.
17. ———1990. Speech and other auditory modules. *In* Signal and Sense: Local and Global Order in Perceptual Maps, G. M. Edelman, W. E. Gall, and W. M. Cowan, Eds. Wiley. New York.
18. LIBERMAN, A. M. & I. G. MATTINGLY. 1989. A specialization for speech perception. Science **243**: 489–494
19. LIBERMAN, I. Y. 1973. Segmentation of the spoken word. Bull. Orton Soc. **23**: 65–77.
20. LIBERMAN, A. M. 1992. Plausibility, parsimony, and theories of speech. *In* Analytic Approaches to Human Cognition, J. Alegria, D. Holender, J. Junca de Morais, and M. Radeau, Eds.: 25–40. Elsevier. Amsterdam, the Netherlands.
21. RAND, T. S. 1974. Dichotic release from masking for speech. J. Acoust. Soc. Am. **55**: 678–680.
22. BENTIN, S. & V. A. MANN. 1990. Masking and stimulus intensity effects on duplex perception: A confirmation of the dissociation between speech and nonspeech modes. J. Acoust. Soc. Am. **88**(1): 64–74.
23. WHALEN, D. H. & A. M. LIBERMAN. 1987. Speech perception takes precedence over nonspeech perception. Science **23**: 169–171.
24. MANN, V. A. & A. M. LIBERMAN. 1983. Some differences between phonetic and auditory modes of perception. Cognition **14**: 211–235
25. FANT, C. G. M. 1962. Descriptive analysis of the acoustic aspects of speech. Logos **5**: 3–17.
26. REPP, B. H. 1985. Perceptual coherence of speech: Stability of silence-cued stop consonants. J. Exp. Psychol.: Human Percept. Perform. **11**(6): 799–813.

Understanding Compressed Sentences: The Role of Rhythm and Meaning[a]

JACQUES MEHLER,[b, c] NURIA SEBASTIAN,[d]
GERRY ALTMANN,[e] EMMANUEL DUPOUX,[f, c]
ANNE CHRISTOPHE,[c] AND CHRISTOPHE PALLIER[c]

[c]LSCP, CNRS-EHESS
54 Boulevard Raspail
75006 Paris, France

[d]Facultat de Psicologia
Universitat de Barcelona
Campus de Pedralbes
08028 Barcelona, Spain

[e]Department of Experimental Psychology
University of Sussex
Brighton BN1 9OG, England

[f]France Telecom
6, Place D'Alleray
75015 Paris, France

INTRODUCTION

The language user can recognize words uttered by different speakers, even when they vary their intonation and speaking rate. In this paper we focus on the user's ability to recognize word forms regardless of whether they are spoken fast or slow. Indeed, speech rate is highly variable in natural context. For example, a word uttered in isolation may be twice as long as the same word uttered in the middle of a sentence. However, regardless of the mode in which a word is pronounced, the two resulting acoustic signals activate the same lexical representation. That people have this ability suggests that speech must be coded in a time-invariant fashion.

Psychologists are quite familiar with the study of perceptual invariance for the visual domain.[1,2] When it comes to speech, however, the study of perceptual invariance, in particular that of time, has generated less interest, and we are thus still unable to explain how the acoustic/phonetic processors solve this problem. Cognitive scientists who work in the area of speech recognition generally assume that subjects use their lexical knowledge to normalize the signal. Undeniably, lexical processing does intervene at some level, but we believe that normalization of the signal is a necessary part of prelexical processing, that is, it has to take place prior to the intervention of lexical lookup routines.

---

[a]This research was supported by grants from the Centre National pour des Etudes de Telecommunication (Convention No. 00 790 92 45 DIT), from the HFSP program "Contrasting Language Phonologies Project," the Spanish Ministerio de Educacion y Ciencia: DGICYT CE 90-008, and from the 1991/1992 Actions Intégrées Franco-Espagnoles.

[b]To whom correspondence should be addressed.

Indeed, automatic speech recognition systems tend to be effective when the lexicon contains a small number of items. However, they are quite poor when the lexicon contains a large number of entries. Thus, pattern matching to a small set of items might be exempt from the usual problems that arise from changes in time and rate. That, however, is not the general case. Mehler, Dupoux, and Segui[3] have argued that the problem of time invariance has to be placed in the context of language acquisition rather than exclusively within the context of speech processing in adults. Indeed, if time invariance can only be attained through pattern matching of forms stored in the lexicon, it becomes difficult, if not outright impossible, to explain how children can acquire the lexicon of their maternal language to start with. To acquire a lexicon, the many different acoustical renderings of a given word must be placed within one and the same category, presumably one that is allowed by the phonology of the language. If we apply this point of view, infants must first use the input to adjust their invariant prelexical representation so that it fits the language in the environment. Once this task has been solved, they can begin to acquire the word forms used in their language. The only alternative proposal we can imagine would roughly claim that infants or young children have perfect and unlimited memories and that, initially, they represent a huge constellation of acoustical forms, indeed, all the speech signals they have ever been exposed to. At first no organization of these acoustic forms occurs. Later, as the child hears an acoustic signal, and according to some metric or another, he links or assimilates it to the most similar entry already in the constellation. Only when the lexical category itself has become established (one wonders how) does the child recognize new versions of the old entry. Of course, for such a mechanism to work one would have to explain how all the acoustic signals that stimulate the child from this massively unstructured memory space come to be grouped into word forms.

Given all we know about neonates and their abilities, cognitive science should get rid of models that are as unrealistic as the one just described. The proposal sketched at the end of the preceding paragraph should thus not be taken too seriously. Indeed, there are studies suggesting that an intermediary representation between the acoustic signal and the lexicon exists that is already functional in infants who have not yet mastered the lexicon.[4,5] This intermediary code is computed after the speech signal is stripped from variations due to speaker identity, rate of speech, illocutionary force, etc.[6] There is little one can say now about the nature of this intermediary code. Possibly, this representation reflects, in part, universal properties of our endowment and in part language-specific properties that arise when a brain like ours is put into contact with a linguistic environment. While all languages rely on segmental as well as prosodic information, some languages may pay closer attention to the distribution of stress, and others to syllable structure. Regardless of how languages reduce the diversity in the signal into a relevant invariant code, it seems ill-advised to deny the existence of such a code. For our purpose what appears essential is the fact that signals are normalized in order to map the speech signal onto an invariant code.

In this paper we present some exploratory studies to establish how time invariance is achieved when listening to sentences that have very different rates of speech. Although we have carried out a number of experiments in different languages, countries, and teams, all make use of the *speech compression technique* rather than of the fast or slow rates of naturally articulated speech. We grant that our studies are limited because we do not yet understand how the time invariance processes that apply for compressed speech can be extrapolated to unaltered speech. However, there is an advantage to the use of compressed speech: namely, in normal circumstances temporal normalization occurs instantaneously and effortlessly, and is therefore difficult to study. The use of speech rates much faster than what can be naturally produced may push the system to its limit, and allow us to observe the time course of normalization.

PERCEPTION OF COMPRESSED SENTENCES

The digitization of speech makes it possible to resynthesize the signal with a different duration while leaving most other parameters of the signal unaltered. Thus, it is possible to take a sentence spoken at a normal rate and reproduce it with half the duration leaving the timbre of the voice and the spectral features relatively intact. The speech compression algorithm we used is based on the pitch synchronous overlap and add (PSOLA) technique;[7] roughly speaking, it takes adjacent pitch periods (in the case of voiced portions) and averages them smoothly; for unvoiced segments the algorithm picks out an arbitrary time window to do the averaging. It is enough to say that this method allows one to double the number of words that are pronounced in a given unit of time with only rare instances of any significant decrement in perceptual performance. Speech compression has furnished psycholinguists with a practical tool to inspect speech perception from a novel vantage point.

The identity of speech segments, if guessing is ruled out, must be computed on the basis of acoustical cues. Many are, however, time dependent. How does the perceptual apparatus overcome these huge variations in speaking rates to pull out the appropriate segments? Miller[8,9] has identified two mechanisms: one, that evaluates speaking rate on the basis of local indices (for instance, syllable duration), and the other that determines segment identity on the basis of both the instantaneous acoustic cues that characterize segments and the speaking rate established by the former mechanism. Miller synthesizes a syllable that comprises a vowel preceded by a /b/ or a /w/ consonant just by changing the transition's slopes. When one measures real speech it becomes apparent, however, that these slopes vary with the rate of speech. Conversely, when subjects listen to an ambiguous syllable, either /ba/ or /wa/, the perceived phonetic identity will be influenced by the duration of the whole syllable, and also, to a lesser extent, by the rate of the preceding context. Miller's studies suggest that speech rate is used to determine the segmental identity of the signal. Moreover, Miller and Eimas[10] have shown that the intercategory boundary depends on speech rate in the same way for adults and infants. This last result suggests that the mechanisms for extracting time invariance are rather primitive and low level. We turn to complementary studies that were carried out using the speech compression algorithm, which makes it possible to present continuous speech rather than just isolated syllables.

A team of investigators from different countries and different linguistic communities, namely, Altmann (English), Dupoux, Christophe, and Pallier (French), Sebastian (Spanish and Catalan), Myagishima (Japanese, personal communication), observed an interesting phenomenon that was at the origin of these compression studies. When naive subjects listen to sentences compressed to 50 percent of their initial duration, they find the first sentences difficult to understand, although the ones that follow become easier and often as natural as the uncompressed sentences themselves. This evolution suggests that subjects *adapt* to altered speaking rates. What are the mechanism and the processes that make such an adaptation possible? In this paper we present studies that explore the perception of compressed speech.

TABLE 1. Percentage of Recalled Open-class Words in Function of Adaptation Condition

Adaptation Rate (%)	French	English
Nothing	61	23
100	61	21
50	86	44
40	89	27

We use different compression rates and adaptation sentences in the same or in a different language than the test sentences.

In order to experimentally investigate adaptation to high compression rates, we conducted two parallel and complementary experiments, one in French and one in English, in Paris and at Sussex University, respectively. We asked subjects to listen to and transcribe one by one, five sentences compressed to 40 percent (of their initial duration). There were two experimental conditions and two control conditions. In the experimental ones, subjects had previously heard a set of ten different compressed sentences at either 40 percent or 50 percent. In the two control groups, subjects either did not receive adaptation sentences or they heard them with their original duration (100 percent). The English and French sentences were translations of each other, and the overall length in number of syllables was matched across languages. Words with similar relative frequencies were selected in both languages. The material was recorded by the same English–French female bilingual who was very fluent in both languages. The subjects' performance was assessed on the basis of the number of items[g] they reported for each test sentence. All groups listened to the same five test sentences so that any differences in performance must be attributed to the conditions leading up to the test sentences.

The results of the French and English experiment are presented in TABLE 1. First and foremost, notice that the performance of the control groups is very different in the two languages. The two French control groups transcribed correctly over 60 percent of the open-class words, while the two English control groups transcribed roughly 20 percent of the open-class words. It is unclear why performance by these control groups differs so dramatically. We cannot affirm that the testing conditions and the ambient noise were identical in the two laboratories. Neither can we maintain that the bilingual speaker was entirely comparable in the two languages; indeed, the original rate of the English sentences was slightly faster than that of the French sentences. It is also possible that the languages in question and the materials had contrasting effects. At any rate, we believe that the two experiments should be considered separately and that a direct comparison of the two should only be subject to extreme caution.

The performance of the French subjects was alike whether they heard the test sentences without any prior context or after hearing ten uncompressed sentences. However, their performance improved significantly after they had heard compressed sentences, regardless of whether these were compressed to 40 percent, the same rate as the test sentences, or to 50 percent. This result corroborates our subjective

---

[g]Three different scores were considered: the number of words, the number of open-class words, and the number of syllables. No significant effects emerge by scoring one way rather than another.

impression that the ability to perceive compressed speech improves by shear exposure to high rates of speech. The fact that the absence of context yielded similar performances to those obtained with the context of natural sentences is interesting. It suggests that the improvement we measured in the other two conditions is not just a general improvement in doing this kind of a task, such as improving one's transcription skills or getting better at recovering materials stored in immediate memory. Instead, the improvement has to come from more perceptual levels.

The results of the English experiment parallel the results of the French study with the exception of one condition. Indeed, although there was an improvement for the group that got the sentences compressed at 50 percent, there was no sign of improvement for the group that listened to the sentences at 40 percent, namely, the same rate as the test sentences. These contrasting results are, at first glance, rather antiintuitive. Indeed, why should subjects' performance only improve when they listen to compressed sentences, but at a compression rate that differs from that in the test sentences and not otherwise? One hypothesis that comes to mind is that subjects will adapt, if and only if they can "handle" the context sentences. Indeed, the overall performance on the test sentences hinges, up to a certain point, on how the compressed sentences are initially perceived. If subjects can pay attention to the context sentences and understand many of the words in them, adaptation arises. Presumably when the context sentences were compressed to 50 percent subjects can "handle" the stimuli like normal speech and their performance improves. This, apparently, was not so when the context sentences were compressed to 40 percent. Other studies will tell whether this interpretation is satisfactory or not.

Sebastian carried out experiments in Spanish and Catalan using a similar design, but reducing the number of groups to one experimental (adaptation at 36 percent) and one control (no adaptation sentences). In her case, the test sentences were compressed at 36 percent of their original duration. She found a significantly improved performance for subjects who were adapted with sentences compressed to the same rate as the test sentences (see TABLE 2). Moreover, despite the fact that the test sentences were compressed to nearly a third of their original duration, the performance of the control group is better than 50 percent. As we suggested earlier, with compression rates that allow the controls a performance close to 50 percent adaptation, the presentation of compressed sentences usually improves perception.

So far, the experiments reported before suggest that the adaptation to compressed speech, which is easy to observe informally, is also rather easy to corroborate in the laboratory. Out of four different experiments, we failed to find improvement in intelligibility of compressed speech in only one experiment, the one in which the subjects' initial performance was very low. What we need to address next is the kind of mechanism that subjects use in order to improve their performance. How long does it take for adaptation to set in? What aspect of the adapting stimuli is necessary to obtain improved perception? Dupoux and Green[11] have gathered some data that specifically explores these issues.

TABLE 2. Percentage of Recalled Open-class Words in Function of Adaptation Condition

Adaptation Rate (%)	Spanish	Catalan
Nothing	67	62
36	92	79

Dupoux and Green[11] carried out an experiment to determine the time course of adaptation. To this end, they presented the same five sentences in different serial positions in lists of 20 sentences. This allowed them to examine the performance on a given sentence when it was preceded by fifteen, ten, five, or no compressed sentences. Their study discloses that the more compressed sentences one hears the better one becomes at reporting a given sentence. This slow growing improvement requires ten or more sentences to reach asymptote.

The preceding results mesh badly with the intuitive observations outside of the laboratory. Indeed, naive subjects feel that one or two sentences are sufficient for them to tune into high rates of compression. Dupoux and Green show that this phenomenological experience is unfounded and that adaptation is, in all likelihood, a slow process by which subjects learn to adjust their perceptual processes to the new rates. Such a slow pace could reflect a rather central learning strategy (subjects learn to guess more efficiently). But a slow process is not necessarily a postperceptual or strategic process. An analogy that one could use at this point is a situation where subjects wear distorting optical prisms. Indeed, after a more or less prolonged time of complete clumsiness, subjects who wear these tend to adapt, in the sense that they become able to reach out and grasp objects in their surroundings without making errors they initially could not avoid making. If the prisms are removed, subjects make errors in the reverse direction to what they did when the prisms were first worm. This process may take days or even weeks to reach its peak, yet it is doubtlessly a low-level process, not a central nor a strategic one.

The prism analogy has of course its limitation since when a subject has adapted to compressed speech it is not the case that he or she cannot process normal uncompressed speech anymore. Dupoux and Green have gathered some data showing that if subjects are presented with normal speech after having adapted to compressed speech, they do not go back to their original unadapted performance level when they are again presented with compressed speech. Indeed, subjects tend to keep the same performance level they had before switching to normal speech. So maybe the more correct analogy would be the situation that arises when one is faced for the first time with a very heavy foreign accent. As with the prism, adaptation may take some time, but unlike with the prism, one may retain understanding for this particular signal through an extended period of time. Incidentally, subjects who adapt to very fast rates tend to report that when they go back to normal rates of speech they hear it as being far too slow. Attempts to establish an objective measure of these subjective reports have been so far unsuccessful. Obviously, more work is required before the mechanisms of adaptation can be fully understood.

Be that as it may, we can ask a slightly different question: How similar do the relevant parameters in the induction and test sentences have to be in order for adaptation to arise? One way to study this situation is to explore whether the meaning and the rhythm of the induction sentences have to be processed and represented for adaptation to arise.

Recent studies have suggested that prelexical representations are language specific. In particular, Cutler et al.,[12,13] Sebastian et al.,[14] and Otake et al.[15] have claimed that speakers of French, English, Spanish, Catalan, and Japanese use language-specific processing routines. Indeed, Cutler et al. have shown that native speakers of French are faster when they have to respond to the first syllable in a word (PA in PAlace or PAL in PALmier) as compared to cases in which the target is either one segment longer or one segment shorter than the first syllable. Speakers of English, in contrast, show no such effect regardless of whether they have to listen to English or French stimuli. Similar differences have been found with speakers of

Japanese who make mora-based responses that the English or French speakers do not. The speakers of Spanish use either the syllable or a demisyllable, depending on the speed of their response.

Different languages use different timing units to represent the speech signal. If so, could the commonality of timing units be one of the factors that determines whether there is adaptation or not? For adaptation to arise, must the timing units in the induction and test sentences resemble one another? Would speakers of French find a Spanish context more useful for adapting to fast rates of speech than English? Would speakers of Spanish benefit from Catalan because both are syllable-timed languages? Obviously, to answer such questions, we have to control for how familiar subjects are with the induction language. Indeed, whether subjects understand or not the context language may have a vast effect on performance. Suppose subjects listened to Jabberwocky-like sentences, or, for that matter, to a text by Derrida. Would they show signs of adapting to faster rates? If they did, one would have the demonstration that understanding the sentences is unnecessary for adaptation to arise. If they do not, we would have to conclude that the process of understanding is an essential component for adaptation to take place.

CROSS-LINGUISTIC COMPRESSION STUDIES

As we argued earlier, adapting to compressed speech is a phenomenon that takes time to reach asymptote and seems, at least in part, located on the level of prelexical representations. To establish whether this is the case, one needs to evaluate the improvement in one language after subjects listen to induction sentences in either the same or in a different language. Subjects may benefit from prior stimulation, regardless of the induction language. If so, one might conclude that speech normalization to very fast speech uses universal representations. Alternatively, subjects may be able to benefit from the induction sentences only if they are related to the test sentences. If this were the case one might argue that adaptation rests on processing structures that are language specific. If so, we might be able to isolate natural language families in terms of the prelexical units they employ. Maybe all the languages that use the same prelexical units might promote adaptation, regardless of whether subjects understand the language or not.

Below we present studies on two kinds of populations, monolingual subjects of different linguistic communities and bilingual subjects.

Monolingual Subjects

The studies reported in the first part of this section were carried out using French and English monolingual subjects who were tested in Paris and at Sussex University. The experimental design is quite similar to the one presented earlier, namely, subjects of the experimental groups are tested on five compressed sentences after having been habituated on ten induction sentences. Subjects have to write down all they can recall about the test sentences, while they simply have to listen attentively to the induction sentences. All subjects were students between 20 and 25 years old.

The results for the French subjects were quite unequivocal. The subjects who listened to English compressed induction sentences performed like the control group who heard the compressed test sentences without any induction context. Likewise, subjects who heard the induction sentences at a natural rate performed as poorly as the controls, who, as we know, only heard the test sentences. These results suggest that French subjects do not improve their ability to perceive compressed French sentences by being exposed to compressed English sentences.

Similarly, English subjects tested in the converse situation did not improve their performance when presented with compressed French sentences. Unfortunately, the interpretation of these results is clouded by the fact that as we mentioned before, English subjects did not improve their performances in the condition where they were presented with compressed English. To understand what is really going on, another study with controls who have higher base performance rates would be needed in order to ascertain that the obtained pattern of results is truly genuine.

The picture can be extended, however, by considering a similar experiment conducted by Sebastian and described as follows. She showed that Spanish subjects, adapted to compressed Catalan sentences, perform significantly better on compressed Spanish sentences than the control group, which received the test sentences without having been subjected to the compressed context. Last but not least, Miyagishima (personal communication) showed that French monolingual subjects do not improve their performance on five compressed French sentences, as compared with a control group, after listening to compressed Japanese. Thus, there is no benefit when the French are habituated to either Japanese or English (if one wants to be lenient and draw this conclusion from the previously reported experiment), but there are benefits when the Spanish subjects are habituated to Catalan.

The tentative results just reported are compatible with, at least, the following two interpretations: (1) *Adaptation takes place at the prelexical level.* We know that French does not rely upon the same prelexical representations as Japanese or English,[9,12] and the failure to observe adaptation when one of these two languages is used as context might be attributed to the fact that the adaptation process or mechanism is determined by the prelexical representations. The Spanish results would then suggest that Spanish and Catalan rely on similar prelexical representations. (2) *Adaptation depends on understanding the words.* Spanish and Catalan have many words that derive from the same roots; at any rate, many more than French and English or Japanese. This last interpretation might seem unlikely, however, since Sebastian reported that Spanish monolinguals were generally unable to identify more than six words out of the ten test sentences.

What interpretation (2) suggests is that understanding the adaptation sentences is essential for habituation to take place. If so, bilingual subjects should benefit from the compressed context sentences even when they are in a different language than the test sentence, providing they understand both languages.

Studies of Compression with Bilingual Subjects

In a series of studies, English–French bilingual subjects were tested with a design that is similar to the one used with monolingual subjects. As in the study with monolingual subjects, we failed to observe any substantive improvement on English test sentences regardless of whether the subjects had been tested in a cross-language condition or not. Subjects, of course, understood both languages perfectly well. This result confirms that regardless of comprehension, habituating to French or English does not help subjects to report sentences in English. Likewise, when subjects have to process French test sentences, adapting to English context sentences does not help at all. Insofar as we can see, these observations could have arisen for one of two reasons. First, when one adapts to a language one uses the phonological representation of that language to draw generalizations. If the representations of context and test languages do not coincide, there will be no savings when one is habituated to one and tested in the other. Second, for adaptation to arise, one has to be able to cope with the context sentences as if they were speech, namely, at rates that put the controls at more or less 50 percent correct. The English sentences, however, were hardly comprehensible even by monolingual native speakers of English. Thus, we cannot choose between these two alternatives until a new study becomes available.

Spanish and Catalan, as opposed to English and French, have quite similar phonologies. Indeed, as we pointed out earlier, both languages are, at a first approximation, syllable-timed languages; moreover we know from a previous study that the control groups perform rather well on both types of stimuli.

The Spanish–Catalan bilingual study that was run by Sebastian provides unambiguous evidence of improved performance on test sentences regardless of whether the bilingual subjects were presented with habituation sentences in one language or the other. This result suggests that both Spanish and Catalan rely on rather similar phonological representations, at any rate, at the level of description that is relevant to understand performance in this task. Alternatively, it could be that understanding language is an essential part of the process of rate adaptation. It should be recalled, however, that the monolingual Spanish subjects who listen to Catalan induction sentences also improve their performance on the test sentences. These subjects did not have any understanding of spoken Catalan. Even though the roots of many of the open-class items might have been similar, the subjects were unable, as was mentioned before, to understand these roots when they received a Catalan pronunciation. Yet, the monolingual adaptation data look very similar to the bilingual data presented earlier, suggesting that full understanding may not be a prerequisite for adaptation to compressed speech. Still, as we stated before, several essential studies are necessary before we have a better understanding of the processes that underlie the adaptation to fast rates.

CONCLUSION

The series of studies previously presented all have a common aim, namely, to establish how the human brain processes the speech signal and frees itself of potential misinterpretations, incomprehension, and other major obstacles. These studies represent a small set of the future studies that will be necessary to understand how the human brain computes time invariance from the speech signal. Even to draw preliminary conclusions we will need more data than are currently available.

Yet these studies have, by and large, demonstrated that the language user adapts to exceptionally high compression rates. This result concurs with the incidental observations mostly carried out in the open. It is difficult to state that listening to compressed speech engages exactly the same kinds of processes that one encounters when listening to speakers who use very rapid rates. However, barring such a reservation, it still is the case that subjects report hearing a sentence that is spoken with recognizable timbre, but only very, very rapidly. Indeed, subjects do not report hearing distorted or artificial sounding speech for large ranges of compression. Thus, one can speculate that the language user has little if any difficulty in processing speech, even when its temporal properties are entirely novel. How the brain manages to make the necessary computations is what the preceding experiments have tried to clarify.

From the results reported, it appears that subjects slowly learn to cope with compressed speech at relatively high rates. It was shown that to become asymptotic subjects may require up to ten sentences of practice. Furthermore, it appears that the induction sentences need not be comprehensible to subjects in order for the adaptation or learning to be effective. If comprehension is not an essential ingredient for learning, what other parameters are essential? We explored whether or not the language phonology of the induction sentences and of the test sentences have to be closely related to observe improved performances. Unfortunately, the results so far available are insufficient to settle the issue. Experiments in progress should clarify the critical case of English versus French. Indeed, if language phonology matters, a syllable-based language like French should not help speakers to adapt to a stress-based language like English. So far we have tested several groups, but the outcome of these studies remains uninterpretable because the control groups in the different languages perform very differently. Conversely we should predict that French and Spanish should adapt each other, since they both are syllable-based languages.

Thus, it may be the case that the technique allows us to define families of languages sharing processing strategies: any pair of languages drawn from the same family should adapt each other, but not languages of disjoint families. If this turns out to be the case, the study of speech compression would become one of the central methods for establishing the representations on which subjects rely when they process speech. Only more studies will uncover whether or not this is the case.

ACKNOWLEDGMENTS

We thank the CNET who provided the speech compression software package which allowed us to prepare our stimuli in comparable ways across the different studies reported here.

REFERENCES

1. HELMHOLTZ, H. 1921. Schriften zur Erkenntnistheorie. Julius Springer. Berlin.
2. BORING, E. G. 1942. Sensation and Perception in the History of Psychology. Appleton. New York.
3. MEHLER, J., E. DUPOUX & J. SEGUI. 1990. Constraining models of lexical access: The onset of word recognition. *In* Cognitive Models of Speech Processing: Psycholinguistic and Computational Perspectives, G. Altmann, Ed. MIT Press. Cambridge, Mass.
4. BIJELJAC-BABIC, R., J. BERTONCINI & J. MEHLER. How do four-day-old infants categorize multisyllabic utterances? Dev. Psychol. In press.
5. BERTONCINI, J. & J. MEHLER. 1981. Syllables as units in infant speech perception. Infant Behav. Dev. **4:** 247–260.
6. KUHL, P. 1983. Perception of auditory equivalence classes for speech in early infancy. Infant Behav. Dev. **6:** 263–285.
7. CHARPENTIER, F. J. & M. G. STELLA. 1986. Diphone synthesis using an overlap-add technique for speech waveforms concatenation. Proceedings of the IEEE International Conference ASSP, Tokyo: 2015–2018.
8. MILLER, J. L. 1981. Effects of speaking rate on segmental distinctions. *In* Perspectives on the Study of Speech, P. D. Eimas and J. Miller, Eds. Erlbaum. Hillsdale, N.J.
9. ———. 1985. Rate-dependent processing in speech perception. *In* Progress in the Psychology of Language, A. Ellis, Ed. Erlbaum. London.
10. MILLER, J. L. & P. EIMAS. 1983. Studies in the categorisation of speech by infants. Cognition. **16:** 135–165.
11. DUPOUX, E. & K. GREEN. Adaptation to compressed sentences. In preparation.

12. CUTLER, A., J. MEHLER, D. NORRIS & J. SEGUI. 1983. A language specific comprehension strategy. Nature **304:** 159–160.
13. ———. 1986. The syllable's differing role in the segmentation of French and English. J. Mem. Lang. **25:** 385–400.
14. SEBASTIAN, N., E. DUPOUX, J. SEGUI & J. MEHLER. 1992. Contrasting syllabic effects in Catalan and Spanish. J. Mem. Lang. **31:** 18–32.
15. OTAKE, T., G. HATANO, A. CUTLER & J. MEHLER. Mora or syllable? Speech segmentation in Japanese. Submitted for publication in J. Mem. Lang.

Timing in Speech Production with Special Reference to Word Form Encoding

WILLEM J. M. LEVELT

Max Planck Institute for Psycholinguistics
Nijmegen, The Netherlands

INTRODUCTION

The ability to speak is probably our most complex cognitive–motor skill. It is, moreover, a uniquely human and a universal skill. In speaking, myriad processes involving a wide range of cerebral structures cooperate in the generation of a temporally organized structure, an articulatory pattern that has overt speech as its physical–acoustic effect.

The temporal organization of speech is multileveled. There are, on the one hand, the relatively slow strategic processes involved in planning the speech act. When we speak, our attention is almost fully dedicated to *what* we say. *How* we say it largely takes care of itself. Words, for instance, are produced at a speed of about 2 per second, but so-called anacruses are possible of up to 7 words per second. At this rate we retrieve lexical items from a mental lexicon that contains thousands, and probably tens of thousands of items. In fluent speech our average syllabic rate is about 3 per second, whereas individual speech sounds come as fast as 10 to 15 phonemes per second. And normally, all this happens without any attentional control.

These high-speech automatic processes are, moreover, surprisingly error proof in normals. Estimates of the rate of lexical selection errors range around one per thousand, whereas phonemic errors are even rarer. What are the mechanisms that subserve this perfect, multilevel timing in speech production?

In the following I will discuss some recent research in our laboratory that is concerned with the time course of spoken word production at three levels of processing, as depicted in FIGURE 1. The first one concerns lexical selection, the second one phonological encoding and syllabification, and the third one phonetic encoding, in particular the retrieval of syllabic gestural scores.

LEXICAL SELECTION

How do we select the appropriate words for the concepts that we want to express? Ardie Roelofs[1] proposed an activation spreading model for this process. FIGURE 2 presents a fragment of the lexical network.

Lexical items are represented at three levels. An item's meaning is specified at the conceptual level by way of a network of labeled relations. The concept of sheep, for instance, is represented by a conceptual node SHEEP, which entertains an *isa* relation to ANIMAL, etc. The next level is a syntactic stratum. Each lexical concept (such as SHEEP) connects to a so-called *lemma* node at this stratum. Its network

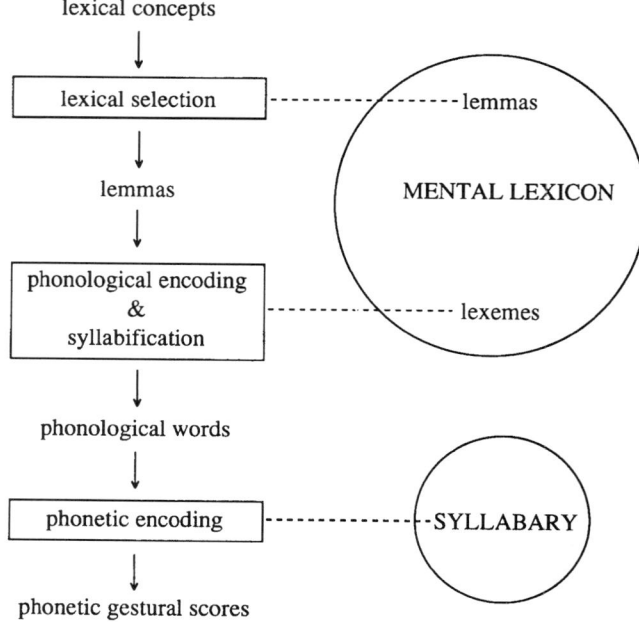

FIGURE 1. Producing words in speech production. Three levels of processing.

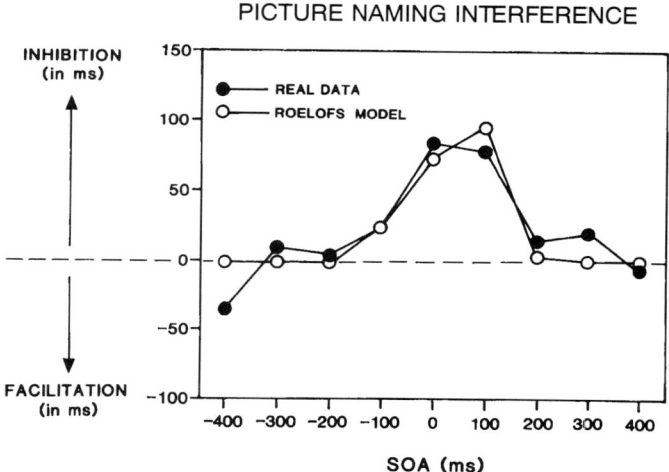

FIGURE 2. Fragment of lexical network. *Arrows* represent types of connections, not the flow of information. (From Bock and Levelt.[2] Reproduced by permission.)

LEVELT: TIMING IN SPEECH PRODUCTION

connections at this level represent the item's syntactic properties (for instance that *sheep* is a noun or that French *mouton* has male gender). Finally, there is the lexeme or sound form stratum. Here the item is represented by a *lexeme* node, which in turn connects to segmental and other sound form nodes that specify the item's phonological properties (see below). Each lemma node connects to one lexeme node. But in case of homonyms two different lemma nodes project onto the same lexeme node (see below).

The network has a simple activation spreading regime, which runs in discrete time steps (see Roelofs' original publication for details).

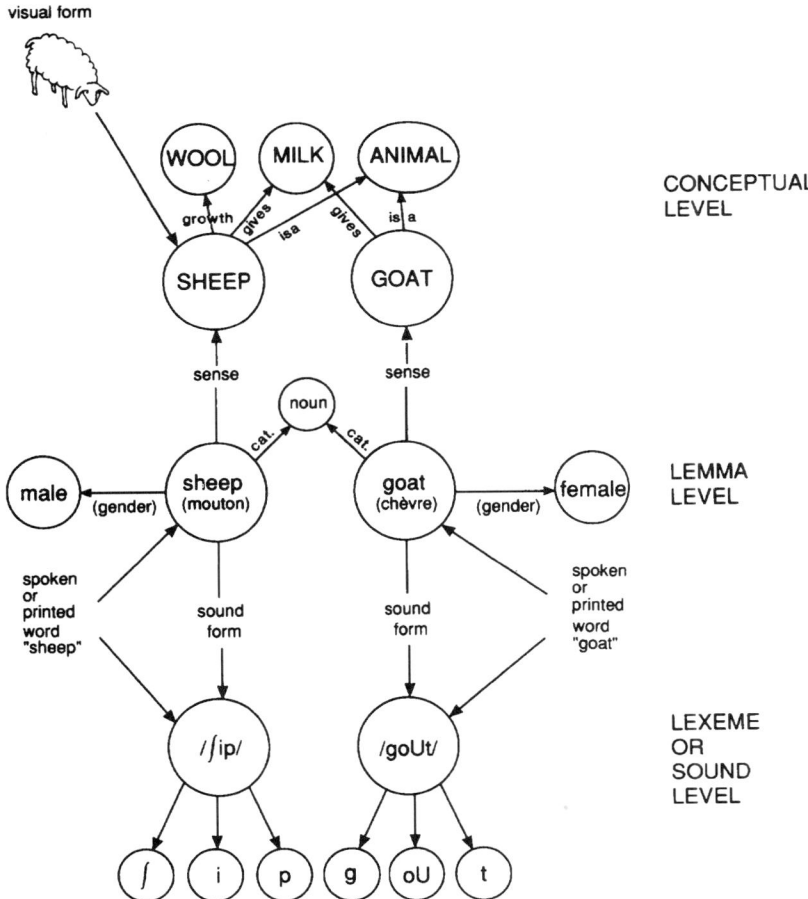

FIGURE 3. Picture naming latency differences for semantically related vs. unrelated primes at nine different SOAs and model simulations. (After Roelofs.[1] Reproduced by permission.)

Roelofs defined lexical selection as the selection of an appropriate lemma node. The time course of lexical selection (for instance, in picture naming) is predicted from a simple probabilistic rule. The probability that a particular lemma is selected during time interval i is the ratio of its activation to the sum activation of all active lemmas (the Luce ratio).

The probabilistic character of the rule creates the possibility of explaining errors of lexical selection, such as *nephew* for *uncle*. Given the rule, there is always a small probability that a nontarget item will be selected, such as *goat* instead of *sheep*. When the concept node SHEEP is active, some of its activation will spread to the semantically related concept GOAT, and down to its lemma node *goat*. Hence, errors of selection will often be semantic in character.

But Roelofs tested his (computer-implemented) model by way of reaction time experiments. The basic procedure was to do a picture naming experiment, and to measure the subjects' naming latencies. This process was interfered with by presenting visual prime words that the subject had to ignore. The visual prime could be semantically related to the target word (for instance, "goat" when the picture was one of a sheep), or it could be unrelated. The prime word could be presented at various moments, either before, simultaneous with, or after picture onset (i.e., at different stimulus onset asynchronies or SOAs). The model gave precise predictions for the effect of different types of prime word at different SOAs, and they were surprisingly well confirmed by the experimental data. In addition, the model could account for the major data sets in the literature. FIGURE 3 presents the classic data obtained by Glaser and Düngelhoff[2] and the model's excellent fit.

As soon as a lemma has been selected, it sends its activation down to its lexeme node.

PHONOLOGICAL ENCODING

In phonological encoding we generate the phonological form of an utterance, in particular its segmental and prosodic structure. Central to phonological encoding is the construction of successive syllables, the basic units of articulation. In connected speech syllabification often straddles word boundaries. When we say *Peter gave it*, we contract *gave* and *it* to form a single so-called "phonological word" /geI-vIt/. Here, the syllable boundary ignores the word boundary.

FIGURE 4 diagrams some of the main processes involved in phonological encoding. After a lemma (such as *gave* or *it*) is selected, its lexeme is activated (here FIG. 4 connects to FIG. 3), and two kinds of phonological information become available. The first one is the word's segmental composition, roughly the string of phonemes it consists of. The second one is the word's metrical or foot structure; this is the word's syllabicity (the number of syllables the word contains), and the word's stress pattern over these syllables.

The metrical patterns of successive words will be grouped into (larger) phonological words. And, finally, the "spelled out" string of segments will be associated to a phonological word's metrical frame. This process of association provides, one by one, the successive syllables of which the phonological word is composed.

I now discuss some aspects of the five processes depicted in FIGURE 4, beginning with lexeme activation, and ending with syllabification.

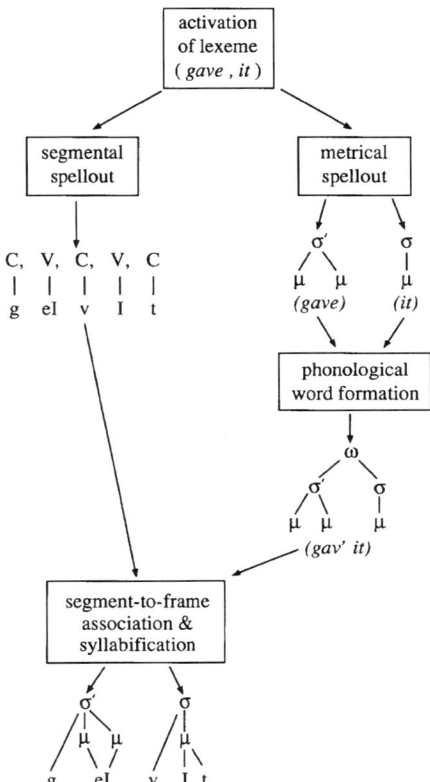

FIGURE 4. Processes involved in the phonological encoding of words.

Lexeme Activation

The proximal cause for a lexeme's activation is the *selection* of its lemma (see FIG. 2). Levelt *et al.*[4] showed experimentally that a merely *activated* lemma does not send its activation to its lexeme node. This state of affairs is different from what one would expect on the basis of existing connectionist and cascading accounts of lexical access, where activation spreads uninterruptedly throughout the lexical network. The mechanism of phonological encoding is apparently carefully sealed from the competitive storms in lexical selection; it has to deal only with the eventual winner, the selected target word.

Another important aspect of lexeme activation is that it is the seat of the word frequency effect in production. Since Oldfield and Wingfield's seminal paper,[5] it is known that in picture naming it takes longer to access low-frequency names than high-frequency names. Wingfield[6] showed that this is not due to recognizing the depicted objects; the effect is of lexical origin. Jörg Jescheniak and I (in preparation) replicated both findings and then asked ourselves whether the locus of the effect is at the lemma level or at the lexeme level.

In order to test whether it is at the lemma level, we gave our (Dutch) subjects a gender decision task. They were presented with pictures, and on the appearance of each picture they had to push one of two push buttons, corresponding to the gender of the picture's name (is it a *het* or a *de* word?). Gender is a property of lemmas (see FIG. 2). If lemma thresholds are frequency sensitive, then the same frequency effect as in naming should appear in this task. But it did not. After acquainting themselves with stimuli and task, gender decision showed no effect of word frequency, whereas the frequency effect in naming appears fully fledged for the same pictures, and cannot even be eradicated by repeated presentations of the pictures.

That the effect is indeed due to accessing the word's sound form could be shown in an experiment where subjects were asked to name the low-frequent item of a homonym pair. For instance, they would name the animal *bee,* where there is a high-frequent homophone *be.* Our network theory has different lemma nodes for these two items (one is a noun, the other a verb). But they project onto one and the same lexeme node, /bi/. Therefore *bee* should behave like a high-frequent item rather than like a low-frequent one, and that is what we found.

The conclusion here is that a lexeme's threshold activation, that is, the activation needed for releasing its phonological information, is frequency dependent. In normal speech, the release of this information is occasionally (but rarely) blocked, leading to the much studied "tip-of-the-tongue" phenomenon (see Levelt[7] and Brown[8] for reviews). The same mechanism is involved in the pathological case of anomia.

Segmental Spellout

Since the beginning of speech error research it has been known that a word's segments can be independently affected or displaced in spontaneous speech. A spoonerism such as *With this wing I thee red,* shows that a word's phonological form does not become available as an indivisible template. Rather, phonemes are independently released and positioned into some independently generated metrical word or syllable frame (Shattuck-Hufnagel[9]). But speech errors do not tell us whether a word's segments are simultaneously, or rather successively released. What is the timing of segmental spellout?

Following up on initial findings by Antje Meyer[10, 11] that suggested successive spellout of segments, Meyer and Schriefers[12] used the priming technique to measure the time course of phonological spellout. In a picture naming task they presented their subjects with prime words that were phonologically related to the picture's name or with unrelated control words. For instance, the picture could be one of a cigar (Dutch name: *sigaar,* pronounced [si-xa:r]). The prime word could be *citroen* ([si-tru:n], which shares the first syllable of the target (begin-related prime). Or it could be *bulgaar* ([būl-xa:r]), which shares the second syllable of the target (end-related prime). As a control prime, a phonologically unrelated word was used, such as *boutique.*

The prime could be presented such that its related syllables ([si] and [xa:r], respectively, for begin- and end-related primes) began at either 300 or 150 ms before the picture, simultaneously with the picture, or 150 ms after picture onset. The subjects were instructed to ignore the prime and to name the picture as soon as it appeared. Naming latencies were measured.

The central finding was this: At SOA = −300 ms neither of the two primes had any significant effect on the naming latencies (as compared to the controls). The begin-related primes, however, began facilitating the response at SOA = −150 ms, where end-related primes were still without effect. The facilitatory effect of end-related primes began 150 ms later, at SOA = 0. This shows that a word is not phonologically encoded as a whole, but incrementally from beginning to end. Antje Meyer and Herbert Schriefers[12] could show that the same holds for monosyllabic words.

Linda Wheeldon and I (in preparation) obtained rather precise data on the time course of phonological spellout by way of a quite different technique. We replaced the usual picture naming task by a *translation* task. Here (Dutch) subjects were given a list of English–Dutch translation equivalents, for instance *hitch-hiker–lifter*. Since all subjects knew (some) English, each word's translation was easily memorized. As soon as this was the case, we introduced the experimental task. The subject was given a phoneme target, for instance /f/, and instructed to push a yes button every time the Dutch translation of a new English word on the screen contained that target. Hence, the subject pushed the yes button shortly after the word *hitch-hiker* was presented on the screen; this is because *lifter* contains an /f/. And, of course, we measured the response latencies. Notice that subjects did not utter the Dutch translation words; they only performed their phoneme monitoring.

It is likely that this task directly measures the timing of segmental spellout. If a word like *lifter* is spelled out "from left to right," then its consonantal phonemes /l/, /f/, /t/, and /r/ will become available one after another, and this should affect the monitoring latencies. When /l/ is the target phoneme, monitoring should be relatively fast, and it should be increasingly slower when /f/, /t/, and /r/ are the target phonemes.

The experiment was run over 20 items, all with CVCCVC structure like *lifter*, where each of the consonants involved could be a target. The results confirmed the expectations. The monitoring latency was 1178 ms on average for the first consonant (i.e., for /l/ in *lifter*), 1233 ms for the second consonant (i.e., for /f/), 1289 ms for the third consonant (/t/ in the example), and 1302 ms for the final consonant (/r/ in *lifter*). We are confident that the subjects are not monitoring their internal speech in this experiment. The results are essentially the same when subjects are given a concurrent counting aloud task during the experiment.

It is interesting to consider the size of these significant increases. The first and third consonant are exactly one syllable apart, their latency difference is 111 ms. The second and fourth consonant are also one syllable apart, their latency difference is 69 ms. The average duration of a spoken syllable is about 250 to 350 ms. Apparently, the speed of spelling out is two or three times as fast as the speed of articulation.

It is an important question what it is that is spelled out. The segments are probably not fully specified. Stemberger[13] argued this point on the basis of speech errors such as *in your really gruffy—scruffy clothes*. In *scruffy* the second segment (/k/) is probably unspecified for voicing. It will acquire the correct feature (−voiced) at a later stage in the process (see below); in English +voiced is impossible in the context s–r. But in the error, where /s/ is lost, the context (−r) is insufficient to provide the feature specification, and it may then happen that the underspecified segment surfaces as /g/ instead of /k/. It is fully in line with modern phonology (cf. Archangeli[14]) to suppose that a word's segments are stored and spelled out in underspecified form.

It is, in fact, better to reverse terminology here. It is not so much segments that are spelled out, but small sets of feature specifications. The second segment of *scruffy*, for instance, is probably only specified as +velar, no more. Segmental spellout, then, is the retrieval of these minimal feature specifications for successive "timing slots."[a]

Metrical Spellout

When speakers are in a tip-of-the-tongue state, they can often report on the number of syllables and the stress pattern of the trouble word. This suggests that metrical spellout can proceed independently of segmental spellout. In Levelt,[15] I proposed that (for English) the metrical spellout of a word consists of the number of syllables, their weights, and stress pattern. For the word *neglect* it would be

$$[\sigma \quad \sigma'] \\ | \quad /\backslash \\ \mu \quad \mu \quad \mu$$

where the first syllable is light (one μ) and the second one is heavy (two μ) and accented.

If metrical structure is independently represented, it should be possible to prime its spellout, independent of the word's segmental composition. Paul Meyer and I (in preparation) could show that this is indeed the case. In one experiment we used the priming procedure that Antje Meyer and Herbert Schriefers[12] had used (see above). The subjects had to name pictures that all had two-syllable names. For half of the pictures the name had iambic meter (such as [si-xa:r], similar to *cigar* in English); for the other half, the meter was trochaic (such as [moU:tər], like *motor* in English). For each picture subjects heard a disyllabic prime word that they had to ignore. The prime word could be presented at different SOAs, but here I will ignore that variable. The experimental variable was whether the prime word corresponded in meter to the target word, and we measured subjects' naming latencies.

The results of this experiment were clear. We obtained a highly significant 58-ms facilitation effect when the prime had the same meter as the target, but this occurred under one condition only: the first segment of prime and target had to be identical. For instance, *saloon* is a better prime for *cigar* than is *salmon*, but *balloon* and *ballot* are equally ineffective. This effect had been predicted by Paul Meyer. If segmental and metrical spellout run in parallel, as is suggested in FIGURE 4, priming metrical spellout will only be effective if it is the slowest of the two processes. In the effective condition segmental spellout is given a head start; segmental spellout is facilitated by the word-initial identity of prime and target.

These findings could be replicated by using the translation task as experimental procedure (see above). Here the subjects produced the Dutch translation of an English word on the screen, while they heard an acoustic metrical prime that they had to ignore.

Together, these results form the first reported experimental evidence for the independent generation of a word's metrical form.

---

[a]The timing slots are probably also specified as C (consonantal) or V (vocalic or sonorant), as indicated in FIGURE 4. A word can namely be primed by another word of the same CV-composition, as Paul Meyer and I (in preparation) could recently show.

Phonological Word Formation

Any utterance has a multilevel prosodic structure. At the top level there are intonational phrases, defined by a characteristic pitch contour. Intonational phrases consist of phonological phrases. These are metrical phrases that have lexical heads-of-phrase as their final elements (as in *The committee / had considered / that the students / might have needed / personal computers /*). In their turn, phonological phrases consist of phonological words. In the example, the phonological phrase *might have needed* consists of two phonological words, *might've* and *needed*. At all three levels metrical planning is sensitive to syntax (see Levelt[7] for a review). Here I will only consider the formation of phonological words.

A major process in phonological word formation is *encliticization*. Here a light lexical element is attached to a preceding head word, like in *might've*, or *gav'it*. This process is sensitive to syntax. Encliticization is blocked when there is a major syntactic boundary between the two elements (one cannot cliticize *it* to *gave* in *What Peter gave, it should be stressed, is irrelevant*). But though phonological word formation depends on syntax and on the metrical composition of the lexical elements involved, it is independent of the segmental composition of these elements. Hence, one can characterize phonological word formation as a purely metrical process. The formation of *gav'it*, for instance, can be formally represented as

$$
\begin{array}{ccc}
\text{gave} & \text{it} & \text{gav'it} \\
[\sigma'] & + \quad [\sigma] & \rightarrow \quad [\sigma' \ \sigma] \\
/\backslash & | & /\backslash \ | \\
\mu \ \mu & \mu & \mu \ \mu \ \mu
\end{array}
\tag{1}
$$

Although the rules of cliticization and phonological word formation are rather well-understood (see, for instance, Nespor and Vogel[16]), literally nothing is known about the implementation of these rules in the *process* of phonological word formation as it develops over time.

Segment-to-Frame Association and Syllabification

The final stage of phonological encoding consists of associating the string of spelled-out segments to the phonological word's metrical frame. Above I mentioned Paul Meyer's finding that for metrical priming to appear, segmental spellout should be given a head start. This indicates that metrical spellout is relatively fast. Normally, the metrical frame is already there to absorb successive segments as they are spelled out. Levelt[15] proposed that segments are, one by one, attached to the metrical frame, going "from left to right," so to say. The following rules of attachment (for English) were proposed in that paper (still excluding the diphthong rule):

(i) A vowel only associates to μ; a diphthong to $\mu\mu$.
(ii) The default association of a consonant is to σ. A consonant associates to μ if and only if any of the following conditions hold:

—the next element is lower in sonority;
—there is no σ to associate to;
—associating to σ would leave a μ without an associated element.

(In addition there is the general convention that attachment to σ can only occur to the left of a syllable's morae).

For the rationale of these rules I refer the reader to the original paper. Here I will, by way of example, apply the rules to the generation of the phonological word *gav'it*. The spelled-out segments /g/, /eI/, /v/, /I/, and /t/ are successively attached to the right-hand structure in (1). The first segment, /g/, is a consonant and has to attach to σ, according to rule (ii). The second segment is the diphthong /eI/, which attaches to μμ, according to rule (i). The third segment is /v/. According to rule (ii) it must associate to σ, but that can only be done to the left of a syllable's morae. Hence, the association has to go to the next σ, inducing a syllable break. The fourth segment /I/ attaches to μ according to rule (i). And the fifth segment /t/ will attach to the same μ because the second condition under rule (ii) holds. The final result is

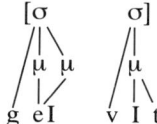

It is important to notice that syllabification takes place "on the fly" as successive segments are attached to the metrical frame. Different from what standard terminology in phonology suggest, there is no *resyllabification*. It is not the case that a word's segmental syllable composition is stored, retrieved, and subsequently changed (resyllabified) as phonological words are formed. That would be a wasteful process. Rather, the independent spellout of segmental and metrical information makes it possible that phonological word formation runs on metrical information only. Syllabification then comes "for free" at the later stage of segment-to-frame association.

The eventual output of phonological encoding is a metrically structured string of phonological syllables. If, as I suggested earlier, phonological segments are underspecified, then these phonological syllables are underspecified as well. How, then, does the speaker compute the full phonetic form of each syllable? This brings us, finally, to phonetic encoding (see FIG. 1).

PHONETIC ENCODING

Phonetic encoding involves the production of what Browman and Goldstein[17] have called a *gestural score*. A gestural score is a specification of the gestural "tasks" that have to be performed over time by the various articulatory subsystems in order to produce the target utterance. According to Browman and Goldstein there are five subsystems whose gestures can be independently controlled. Hence there are five "tiers" in a gestural score. They are the glottal and the velar system, and three tiers in the oral system.

TABLE 1 represents the tasks that can be specified for each of these subsystems. At the lips tier, for instance, the task is two-dimensional. Lips can be instructed to protrude, and they can be instructed to open or close.

Normally, a word's articulatory gesture results from performing tasks at different tiers simultaneously. But a task underspecifies the gesture. Take, for instance, the task of closing the lips. It can be realized in infinitely many ways. One can move the

TABLE 1. Gestural Tasks on Articulatory Tiers

Tier	Task Variables
Glottal	Aperture
Velar	Amount of closure
Oral—Tongue body	Place and amount of constriction
—Tongue tip	Place and amount of constriction
—Lips	Protrusion and aperture

upper lip, the lower lip, the jaw, or all three of them to different degrees. Which combination will be used by the speaker depends on myriad circumstances, such as the starting position of the articulators or arbitrary physical contingencies (e.g., having a pipe in the mouth).

How the articulatory system factually executes a particular gestural task is a fascinating problem in coordinative structures theory (Saltzman and Kelso[18]), but it is not the topic of phonetic encoding. Our problem is "merely": Where do gestural scores come from? There are two approaches here, which are not mutually exclusive, I believe, but rather complementary.

The first one is the direct route. The idea is that a word's phonological specification is already an abstract rendering of its gestural score. The features in successive timing slots are essentially specifications of phonological tasks; for instance, that there should be velar closure at some early moment in the word *scruffy*. A sophisticated rendering of this direct route can be found in the work by Browman and Goldstein.[17]

Here I would like to argue for a more indirect route. I suppose that speakers have access to a *mental syllabary*. This is a repository of phonetic programs or gestural scores for the syllables in the speaker's language. As phonological syllables are generated one after another (see above), they will function as access codes to the syllabary. Each of them will trigger the retrieval of the corresponding gestural score, which in turn will be executed by the articulatory system.

One argument for the existence of a syllabary is that syllables are real units of articulation; within-syllable phonetic coherence is much larger than between-syllable coherence. Moreover, most syllables are highly overused units of articulation. It would be wasteful to fully program them time and again.

The syllabary theory is, of course, more attractive for languages such as Chinese and Japanese, where the number of syllables is no more than a few hundred, than for English, which has some 6,000–7,000 different syllable patterns. But even for English the amount is not excessive; the number of words the speaker has in store is very much larger.

An obvious advantage of the syllabary theory is that phonological underspecification becomes an almost trivial problem. There is no need to "complete" the specifications of successive segments in a word. The only condition that has to be satisfied in the syllabary is that each phonological syllable (consisting of underspecified segments) corresponds to one and only one gestural score. That score, then, is fully specified in the syllabary.

One nontrivial prediction from the syllabary theory is that there should be a frequency effect. Just as low-frequent words are harder to access than high-frequent ones (see above), low-frequent syllables should be harder to access than high-

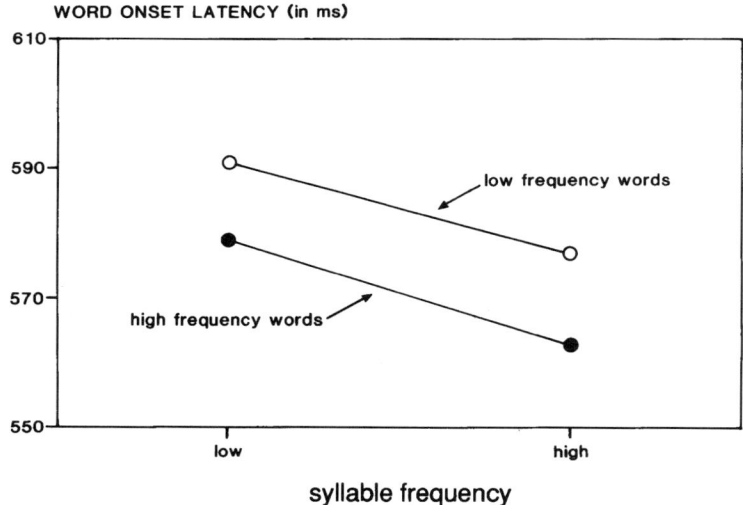

FIGURE 5. Naming latencies for high- and low-frequency words consisting of high- or low-frequency syllables.

frequent ones. Moreover, these two effects should be independent, because lexicon and syllabary are independent stores.

In order to test this theory, Linda Wheeldon and I (in preparation) had people produce two-syllable words (in response to abstract visual patterns that they had learned to associate with these words). We used four types of words. There were low-frequent words consisting of low-frequent syllables (such as *lantern*), low-frequent words consisting of high-frequent syllables (such as *litter*), high-frequent words that consisted of low-frequent syllables (such as *language*), and high-frequent words consisting of high-frequent syllables (such as *lady*). The response latencies obtained are presented in FIGURE 5. The results are as predicted; there is both a word and a syllable frequency effect, and the two effects are independent (or additive). Although these findings are open to alternative explanations, they do invite further exploration of the syllabary notion.

CONCLUSION

The present paper outlined some of the major steps involved in spoken word production. I reviewed a research program that analyzes each step by experimental procedures specifically affecting or tapping into its time course. As the partitioning of this complex system becomes more transparent, further questions can be profitably raised. Among them are issues in language and speech pathology, such as the origins of disturbances of lexical selection, anomias, and disorders of timing in word formation. Also one can, with some confidence, begin to relate various component processes in the model to specialized cerebral structures by making use of brain scanning imagery in combination with experimental procedures of the sort described in this paper.

But it will still be a major step to the analysis of larger stretches of connected speech. Response latencies in normal picture naming are around 600 ms. But we speak at a rate of two to three words per second. Clearly, there is substantial overlap in accessing successive words. It is still largely an enigma how this parallel lexical processing is organized in the brain.

REFERENCES

1. ROELOFS, A. 1992. Cognition **42**: 107–142.
2. GLASER, W. R. & F.-J. DÜNGELHOFF. 1984. J. Exp. Psychol. **10**: 640–654.
3. BOCK, J. K. & W. J. M. LEVELT. 1993. Language production: Grammatical encoding. *In* Handbook of Psycholinguistics, M. Gernsbacher, Ed. Academic Press. New York.
4. LEVELT, W. J. M., H. SCHRIEFERS, D. VORBERG, A. S. MEYER, T. PECHMANN & J. HAVINGA. 1991. Psych. Rev. **98**: 122–142.
5. OLDFIELD, R. C. & A. WINGFIELD, 1965. Q. J. Exp. Psychol. **17**: 273–281.
6. WINGFIELD, A. 1968. Am. J. Psychol. **81**: 226–234.
7. LEVELT, W. J. M. 1989. Speaking: From Intention to Articulation. MIT Press. Cambridge, Mass.
8. BROWN, A. S. 1991. Psychol. Bull. **109**: 204–223.
9. SHATTUCK-HUFNAGEL, S. Speech errors as evidence for a serial order mechanism in sentence production. *In* Sentence Processing: Psycholinguistic Studies Presented to Merrill Garrett; W. E. Cooper and E. C. T. Walker, Eds.: 295–346. Erlbaum. Hillsdale, N.J.
10. MEYER, A. S. 1990. J. Mem. Lang. **29**: 524–545.
11. ———. 1991. J. Mem. Lang. **30**: 69–89.
12. MEYER, A. S. & H. SCHRIEFERS. 1991. J. Exp. Psychol.: LMG **17**: 1146–1160.
13. STEMBERGER, J. P. 1982. Lingua **56**: 43–65.
14. ARCHANGELI, D. 1988. Phonology **5**: 183–207.
15. LEVELT, W. J. M. 1992. Cognition **42**: 1–22.
16. NESPOR, M. & I. VOGEL. 1986. Prosodic Phonology. Foris. Dordrecht, the Netherlands.
17. BROWMAN, C. P. & L. GOLDSTEIN. 1991. Gestural structures: Distinctiveness, phonological processes, and historical change. *In* Modularity and the Motor Theory of Speech Perception, I. G. Mattingly and M. Studdert-Kennedy, Eds.: 313–338. Erlbaum. Hillsdale, N.J.
18. SALTZMAN, E. & J. A. S. KELSO. 1987. Psychol. Rev. **94**: 84–106.

Phonological Skills and Learning to Read

USHA GOSWAMI

Department of Experimental Psychology
University of Cambridge
Downing St.
Cambridge CB2 3EB, England

INTRODUCTION

One of the success stories in research in developmental psychology over the last decade has been the establishment of a relationship between phonological skills and learning to read. A child's ability to isolate and manipulate the constituent sounds of spoken words at preschool has been shown to have a direct relationship to that child's later progress in reading and spelling. Children with reading difficulties have been shown to have specific problems in phonological tasks, problems that are not only more marked than those of their peers, but also more marked than those of younger children who have attained similar levels of word reading. Moreover, training children's phonological skills has been shown to have a beneficial effect on their reading development. So the connection between phonological skills and reading is now well-established.

The question that my research has tried to address is how exactly the phonological skills that are known to be available to preschoolers might relate to the strategies that they adopt once they are faced with the task of decoding printed words. The focus of this research has been on the kinds of analogies that children make between spelling patterns as they are learning to read. For example, a child who learns to read one word, such as "beak," might be able to work out that words with similar spelling patterns, such as "peak," "weak," and "speak," are likely to have similar pronunciations to "beak" (they will rhyme). However, a child who learns to read a word like "beak" might make other kinds of analogies, too. Words like "bean," "bead," and "beat" share a spelling sequence with "beak" at the beginning, and so these words, too, will share an analogous pronunciation with "beak." Yet although both kinds of words share a spelling unit with "beak" of equivalent size (3 letters, 2 phonemes), the analogy between "beak" and "peak" seems somehow more salient than the analogy between "beak" and "bean." Quite why this should be the case is one of the issues that will be addressed in this paper.

TRADITIONAL MODELS OF READING DEVELOPMENT

The Sequence of Stages of Reading

Surprisingly, traditional models of reading development treat the use of analogy as a fairly sophisticated strategy, one that can only be expected to emerge in the final stages of learning to read. These models of reading development are stage models.[1,2] Such models agree that children pass through at least three rather different stages as they learn to read. The first stage is a *logographic* one. During this initial stage, children learn associations between pronunciations and whole words. The spelling sequences making up these words remain fairly unanalyzed, and are retained more as holistic patterns. The term "logographic" is the key to understanding the nature of reading at this stage. As adult readers, we can all "read" logographs like £ or lb. However, we do not analyze the relationship between components of these patterns and their associated sounds. Children in the first stage of learning to read are said to be in a similar position.

The second stage in the development of reading according to these models is an *alphabetic* one. During the alphabetic stage, children learn associations between different alphabetic letters and their sounds, and accordingly apply this knowledge to their reading. For example, a child who knows the sounds for the letters C, A, and P will be able to pronounce the written word "cap." This child can build up the pronunciation of the word by blending together its constituent sounds. Similarly, a child who knows the sounds for the letters C, I, M, and E may mispronounce the nonsense word "cime" by giving it a hard C (saying "kime").[2]

Clearly, therefore, a reliance on letter-sound rules can lead a child to make errors. In fact, for many irregular words, such as "light" and "people," the use of letter-sound rules will lead the child very far indeed from an accurate pronunciation. The irregularity of English orthography at the letter-sound level is a widely acknowledged drawback of the use of "phonics" programs for teaching reading. However, the use of an alphabetic strategy does provide children with a method for attacking unknown words.

The final stage proposed by these models of learning to read is an *orthographic* one. During the orthographic stage of learning to read, children are thought to become able to use larger spelling sequences in words as a basis for pronouncing new words. For example, a child might recognize that spelling units like "-ight" and "-tion" have consistent pronunciations in different words ("light," "might," "fight," "station," "lotion," "mention"). The orthographic stage thus sees the emergence of the use of orthographic analogies in reading. Children become able to read new words on the basis of known words. Children are also thought to pick up knowledge of higher level orthographic rules at this stage, such as the "Rule of E." Such "rule learning" could also arise as a process of analogical reasoning, as children might notice that an E at the end of different written words consistently lengthens the vowel ("time," "lame," "home"). Of course, this is a rather different kind of analogy from the use of shared spelling sequences in words to predict pronunciation, and it is the use of these kinds of analogies between shared spelling patterns in words that are discussed here.

The Orthographic Analogy Stage

Why were orthographic analogies (using "light" as a basis for reading "fight") thought to be relatively sophisticated developmentally? The answer lies in some research conducted by Marsh and his colleagues,[2] who studied children's use of analogies to read nonsense words. The nonsense words that they devised were ingenious ones, as they all had at least two possible pronunciations. One pronunciation could be arrived at by the use of letter-sound rules, whereas the other depended on the use of analogy. Two examples are the nonsense words "puscle" and "biety." If children use letter-sound correspondence rules as a basis for reading these words, then they would produce pronunciations like "puskle" and "beety." However, if they read them on the basis of analogies to the real words "muscle" and "piety," then their pronunciations would rhyme with these real words. Marsh *et al.* found that whereas younger children tended to pronounce these nonsense words by using letter-sound correspondence rules, older children would use analogies. The youngest children read very few nonsense words by analogy, producing rhyming pronunciations for only 14 percent of the words at age 7, and 34 percent at age 10.

On the basis of these nonsense word studies, it was concluded that orthographic analogies were characteristic of fairly sophisticated readers. This tied in with the idea that analogy was a late-emerging reasoning strategy anyway. Piagetian theory suggested that analogical reasoning was only available in early adolescence.[3] So the finding that younger readers apparently preferred to rely on grapheme-phoneme conversion rules when reading new words aloud was not seen as surprising.

However, Marsh *et al.*'s studies had an important flaw, which was that they did not control for the children's knowledge of the analogous real words on which the nonsense word pronunciations had to be based. If a 7-year-old child does not have the word "muscle" in her reading vocabulary, then she is unlikely to use an analogy when trying to read the nonsense word "puscle," even if she has an analogy strategy available. Because more recent developmental research suggests that analogical reasoning is available to children as young as 3 years of age,[4] the apparently late emergence of analogies in reading could well be an artifact of vocabulary knowledge.

To try and study children's use of orthographic analogies in more depth, I thus decided to carry out some experiments in which the basis for an analogy was available to the child in the form of a "clue" word. These "clue" word studies showed up some very interesting differences in the kind of analogies between spelling patterns that the children were willing to make. Furthermore, these differences in analogizing turned out to be intimately connected to the level of the children's phonological skills, which in turn suggested that phonological and orthographic knowledge were interacting from the very beginning of learning to read. The interactive model of reading development that can be proposed on the basis of these analogy experiments stands in marked contrast to the developmental changes in reading strategy proposed by stage models.

THE USE OF ORTHOGRAPHIC ANALOGIES IN READING

The Clue Word Studies

In order to provide a proper test of children's ability to use analogies in reading, then, it is important to be sure that they know the real words that are meant to provide a basis for the analogy. In the clue word studies that I carried out, the analogous base words were explicitly taught to the children prior to the analogy test in the form of "clue" words. The clue words were printed on cards in large type, and each clue word remained in front of the child throughout an experimental trial. The experimental trials consisted of the presentation of various analogous and nonanalogous test words, also printed on cards, that the child was required to read. Prior knowledge of these words had been checked in a pretest, and re-presentation of the words with the clue word was scored as an "analogy" test.

In the first clue word studies, children aged from 5 to 7 years were tested with both real words and nonsense words.[5,6] The analogous test words shared either a beginning spelling sequence with the clue word (e.g., *"beak"*–"bean," "bead," "beat"; *"hark"*–"hard," "harm," "harp") or an end spelling sequence (e.g., *"beak"*–"peak," "weak," "speak"; *"hark"*–"dark," "bark," "lark"). The nonanalogous words shared either some spelling-sound correspondences with the clue words ("Common Letter words," e.g., *"beak"*–"bank," "bask") or had quite different spelling patterns ("Control words," e.g., *"beak"*–"rain," "tail"). The Control words were actually analogous words for clue words used in different experimental trials (e.g., "rain," "tail"–*"rail"*). My prediction was that the Control words should only be read correctly when they were acting as analogous words. It was also predicted that the analogous words should be read more accurately than the Common Letter words when the clue word was available.

Both of these predictions turned out to be correct. All of the children read more analogous words correctly than either Common Letter or Control words at analogy test, whether the analogous words were real words or nonsense words (e.g., *"beak"*–"beal," "neak"). The analogy effect did not vary with reading level, as even children who were in the very earliest phases of learning to read (they did not yet score on a standardized test of reading) were able to make some analogies. So analogy does not seem to be a reading strategy that is characteristic of sophisticated readers. Instead, it seems to be a strategy that is available from the very beginning of reading development.

The possibility that analogy is a strategy that children actually bring with them to the reading task is obviously a very different proposition to the idea that analogy emerges only in the final stages of reading. However, it could be objected that the analogy effect found in these studies was simply an artifact of the clue word design. In the clue word task, the children only saw two words on a given trial, the clue word and the test word, and this could have encouraged a "spurious" use of analogy that would not be found in "normal" classroom reading.

Now "normal" classroom reading usually involves story books. Children usually come across unknown words that they need to decode when they are reading passages of prose. So there is a simple way to examine this objection to the apparently early use of analogy, and that is to embed the test words in passages of prose. The clue words can be taught as part of the title of each story, and the test words can be hidden in the story itself. Experiments using this prose technique found that the analogy effect remained robust.[6] Children made approximately the same number of analogies when reading the stories as they did in the clue word task. So analogies may be ubiquitous in "normal" reading.

One consistent difference did emerge in children's use of analogies in the clue word studies, however. This difference was a qualitative one. The children consistently made more analogies between shared-spelling sequences at the ends of words ("beak"–"peak") than between shared spelling sequences at the beginning of words ("beak"–"bean"). This "End" effect was found for both real words and nonsense words, and with both younger and older readers. In fact, the children who were not yet scoring on a standardized test of reading *only* made analogies between spelling sequences at the ends of words. This End effect in analogizing led me to think more about phonological skills.

Phonological Knowledge and Orthographic Analogies

A child who uses a shared-spelling sequence at the end of two words as a basis for an analogy about pronunciation is predicting that the two words will have rhyming pronunciations. Words that are spelled the same at the end usually (although not always) rhyme with each other, and so such a child would be quite correct in predicting that "peak" should rhyme with "beak," or that "dark" should rhyme with "bark." A child who is trying to make an analogy about the pronunciation of shared spelling sequences at the beginnings of words has a more difficult task. Although we popularly refer to the similarity between words that begin with the same sound as "alliteration," alliteration really refers to the very first sound in the word. "Beak" and "bean" are linked via alliteration, but so are "beak" and "bowl," and "beak" and "bite," even though the latter pairs of words are quite different in sound. So there is no culturally recognized sound category for describing the similarity between "beak" and "bean."

This difference between the sound categories that correspond to spelling patterns at the beginnings and ends of words is recognized by linguistic theory. Some linguistic theories of syllable structure propose that syllables are not simply linear strings of phonemes.[7] Instead, there is a level of structure intermediate between the syllable and the phoneme, which is called the *onset* and the *rime*. Onsets in spoken words correspond to any consonants at the beginning of the written word, while rimes correspond to the vowel and any subsequent consonants. So while the spoken word "clap" can be thought of as made up of four phonemes, /k/, /l/, /ə/, and /p/, it can also be thought of as consisting of two subsyllabic units, the onset (corresponding to "cl-") and the rime (corresponding to "-ap").

Onsets and rimes are particularly interesting with respect to phonological development, as there is now a lot of evidence to suggest that whereas onset–rime knowledge develops prior to learning to read, phonemic knowledge develops as a consequence of reading. Most of this evidence concerns traditional rhyme. Children as young as 3 years of age can recognize and produce rhyming words in experimental tasks, and even younger children produce rhymes spontaneously in the context of language games or early babbling.[8-11] Furthermore, research has shown that rhyming skills measured prior to beginning school, when children are 4 and 5 years old, is a significant predictor of the same children's reading and spelling progress at 8 and 9 years.[12] The possibility that this relationship is a causal one is supported both by training studies and by the study of backward readers. Training children who have poor phonological skills in rhyming notably improves their progress in reading and spelling,[12] whereas the rhyming skills of backward readers are significantly worse than those of younger children reading at the same level.[13-15] So there is a lot of evidence to link rhyming skill to reading progress.

There is also a lot of evidence that knowledge about phonemes develops later than knowledge about onsets and rimes.[16] Onset–rime judgments are considerably easier than phonemic ones until children begin learning to read.[17] Once reading is taught, however, a spurt in phonemic knowledge occurs,[18] and this spurt is found in other scripts, too.[19] Furthermore, illiterate adults find phonemic judgments very difficult,[20] and there is also evidence that spelling knowledge changes a child's phonemic awareness.[21,22] So knowledge about onsets and rimes appears to develop prior to knowledge about phonemes.

It thus seems apparent that the phonological awareness of children who have yet to learn to read is somewhat different in nature from that of children who are already reading. Prereaders have phonological awareness of syllables, onsets, and rimes. They do not know much about phonemes. Readers very quickly develop an awareness of phonemes, reaching ceiling on certain phonemic tasks within a very short space of time.[17] Readers can segment a word like "clap" into its four phonemic units, whereas a prereader is more likely to segment it into two phonological units, the onset (corresponding to the spelling sequence "cl-") and the rime (corresponding to the spelling sequence "-ap").

If we now relate this evidence about phonological development to children's orthographic analogies, we can see a connection emerging. We already know that children are more likely to make analogies between spelling sequences at the ends of words ("beak"–"peak") than between spelling sequences at the beginnings of words ("beak"–"bean"). A possible explanation for this difference is that it reflects phonological knowledge. End analogies ("beak"–"peak") are rime analogies. The child is making a prediction about pronunciation that involves a recognizable phonological unit, the rime. Beginning analogies ("beak"–"bean") do not involve a phonological unit that is familiar to beginning readers. Beginning analogies are based on a spelling sequence that corresponds to the onset-and-part-of-the-rime. As such, they may well be more difficult analogies for beginning readers to use.

Onset–Rime Knowledge and Orthographic Analogies

It is possible, therefore, that a child's phonological knowledge has a very specific effect on how that child initially learns about the orthography. If children are aware of onset–rime units prior to learning to read, then these may be the phonological units that they expect the orthography to represent. Even if their expectations are not this specific, they may find it relatively easy to learn orthographic correspondences for onsets and rimes in the initial phases of reading, because these correspondences reflect their phonological knowledge. Connections between individual alphabetic letters and their sounds should be more difficult to learn, as these correspondences require phonemic knowledge. So the most natural way into reading may be to learn how sequences of alphabetic letters correspond to onsets and rimes. This idea about initial reading would certainly explain the End analogy effect, but so far, it is just a hypothesis.

One way of testing this "phonological status" hypothesis (that the phonological status of a spelling unit influences how easily it is learned) is to manipulate the predictions that it makes about transfer. A neat way of doing this would be to try and reverse the End analogy effect. If it is Beginning analogies that correspond to natural phonological units rather than End analogies, then the hypothesis would predict that Beginning analogies should be more frequent than End analogies in early reading. This prediction can be tested experimentally by studying the transfer of consonant clusters. A consonant cluster at the beginning of a word corresponds to the onset. We have already seen this for the "cl-" in "clap," and the same is true of the "tr-" in "trim" or the "fl-" in "flan." Consonant clusters at the ends of words, however, correspond to part of the rime. The consonant cluster "-sk" in "desk" or the consonant cluster "-ft" in "loft" are good examples.

If orthographic analogies partly reflect phonological knowledge, then a simple prediction follows. Children who learn clue words with initial consonant clusters like "trim" should make analogies to new words sharing the same initial consonant clusters, like "trap" and "trot." Children who learn clue words with end consonant clusters, however, like "desk," should not make analogies to new words sharing the same consonant clusters, like "risk" and "husk." The relevant clue word experiment confirmed that this was the case. Six-year-old children who learned clue words like "trim" improved in reading words like "trap" and "tred" at analogy test, whereas when they learned clue words like "desk," they did not improve in reading words like "risk" and "mask." In this experiment, the Beginning–End effect in analogizing was completely reversed. So the phonological status of a spelling unit indeed affects transfer in reading.

Correlational Studies

If orthographic analogies are linked to phonological knowledge, than another prediction follows as well. Children who have better onset–rime knowledge should make more analogies. If a child's phonological knowledge feeds directly into that child's approach to reading, then children with good onset–rime skills should be more likely to make connections between shared spelling sequences in words that reflect onsets and rimes than children with poor onset–rime skills. Variations in onset–rime knowledge should correspond to variations in the use of orthographic analogies.

This prediction was tested in two different studies, both of which contrasted rime analogies ("beak"–"peak") with analogies between the onset-and-part-of-the-rime ("beak"–"bean"). In the first study,[23] I measured the number of analogies that children made in the clue word task, and then looked at how these were related to two different measures of phonological skill. The first was an onset–rime measure, Bradley and Bryant's oddity task. The second was a phoneme measure. For this, I used Content et al.'s phoneme deletion task,[24] in which two puppets are speaking a secret language. One puppet (the experimenter's) always says whole words, and the other puppet (the child's) always repeats them with a sound missing. This sound is either the first sound ("bean"–"ean") or the last sound ("bean"–"bea") in the word. The children in the study were also given a measure of verbal skills [the British Picture Vocabulary Scales (BPVS)], and a measure of memory (the WISC digit span subtest).

As would be expected, simple correlations showed that all of the phonological measures were related to the reading measure, which was Beginning or End analogies. However, verbal skills were also significantly related to analogizing, in contrast to memory skills and reading age. In order to examine the specific relationship between onset–rime skills and orthographic analogies, I used multiple regression equations. In these equations, the variance accounted for by verbal skills (BPVS) and phonemic knowledge (the deletion measure) was controlled before the contribution of the onset–rime measure (the oddity task) was calculated. The equations showed a very consistent set of results. Performance in the different oddity tasks was significantly related to rime analogies even after controlling for verbal skills and phonemic knowledge, but not to beginning ("beak"–"bean") analogies. So the relationship between onset–rime skills and rime analogies seemed to be a specific one. This relationship was especially strong for the rhyme oddity measure. Rhyme oddity accounted for 20 percent of the variance in rime analogies even after controlling for verbal skills and phoneme deletion (initial sound measure).

Further support for the specificity of the relationship between rhyme and analogy came from a second set of multiple regression equations, in which the entry of the two phonological variables was reversed. If oddity (rhyme) performance was entered before the phoneme deletion measures, then no significant relationship remained between phonemic knowledge and analogies. So the relationship between rhyme and rime analogies does not arise from individual differences in phonological awareness *per se*. It seems to be specific to the level of phonological skill that is being measured.

These results were replicated in a larger study in which more phonological measures were taken, and in which a larger range of reading ability was sampled.[25]

In this second study, the phonological measures included syllable and phoneme segmentation measures, as well as a test of nonsense word reading (phonological recoding). The study again showed a specific relationship between the onset–rime (oddity) measures and rime analogies. No relationship between the syllable or phoneme measures and rime analogies remained after controlling for reading ability and nonsense word reading, whereas the relationship between rhyme oddity and rime analogies did remain significant after these controls. For Beginning analogies ("beak"–"bean") it was a phonemic measure (consonant deletion) that retained a significant relationship with analogy after reading ability and nonsense word reading were controlled, and the oddity measures that did not. This latter finding is consistent with the idea that Beginning analogies require more complex phonological skills than rime analogies (and in particular, some knowledge about phonemes).

Phonological Priming

We thus have at least two pieces of evidence for the idea that onset–rime knowledge feeds directly into learning to read via the use of onset–rime analogies. First, children make more analogies between spelling units of equal length when these spelling units correspond to onsets and rimes. Analogies between words like "beak" and "peak" are more frequent than analogies between "beak" and "bean," and analogies between words like "trim" and "trot" are more frequent than analogies between "desk" and "risk." Second, children's onset–rime awareness is directly linked to the number of analogies that they make. Children with better onset–rime skills make more analogies. However, if it is true that these onset–rime analogies are really based on spelling units (that is, that they are truly orthographic in nature), then we can make another prediction as well. Children should restrict their use of rime analogies to words that share spelling sequences. They should not simply make analogies to *any* word that shares a rhyming sound with the clue word.

The prediction about shared orthography is an important one for ruling out a "phonological priming" explanation of children's analogies in reading. If children who learn to read a word like "beak" go on to read "peak" because of some kind of rhyme-based priming, then there would be no grounds for arguing that they were analyzing spelling patterns at all. The way to rule out a phonological priming argument is to compare children's analogies to rhyming words that either share orthography or do not. Children should use a word like "head" as a basis for an analogy to a word like "bread" because of the shared orthographic unit. They should not use their knowledge of a word like "head" as a basis for an analogy to a rhyming word with a completely different spelling pattern, such as "said."

This "phonological priming" explanation of the analogy effect was examined in a clue-word experiment that compared transfer between words that shared both a spelling sequence and a rhyming sound ("head"–"bread," "bone"–"cone"), and words that shared a rhyme only ("head"–"said," "bone"–"moan").[26] The results of the experiment supported the orthographic interpretation of analogy. The children (6-year-olds) made significantly more analogies to test words like "bread" that shared a spelling pattern with the clue word, than to phonological priming control words like "said," that did not. So children do seem to be thinking about the relationship between consistent spelling patterns and consistent sounds when they use analogies in reading. This orthographic effect came out even more strongly in a prose version of the task, in which the test words were embedded in simple stories ("real reading").

THE ROLE OF ANALOGY IN READING DEVELOPMENT

An Orthographic Analogy Model of Reading Development

Given the evidence considered so far, what conclusions can we draw about the role of analogy in reading development? Some conclusions are obvious. First of all, analogy is available from the very beginning of learning to read. It is not a developmentally sophisticated strategy characteristic of children in the final stages of learning to read, but a strategy that children bring with them to the reading task. Second, the analogies that children make are closely connected to the phonological status of the spelling sequences on which they are based. Children are more likely to use analogies between spelling sequences that reflect either rimes ("beak"–"peak") or onsets ("trim"–"trot") than between spelling sequences of equal length that require segmentation of the rime ("beak"–"bean," "desk"–"risk"). Third, children's use of analogy is specifically connected to their phonological skills. Children who have better onset–rime skills make more analogies.

These facts, however, have quite far-reaching implications for theories of reading development. Not only do they question the assumption that an analogy strategy is only used in the final stages of learning to read, they actually question the whole notion of the appropriateness of developmental stage models of reading. A major implication of the clue word studies is that phonological and orthographic knowledge *interact* from the very beginning of learning to read.

One way of thinking about this interactive process is to realize that young children do not come to the task of decoding written words without any useful knowledge at all (see also Stuart and Coltheart[27]). In fact, they have a lot of knowledge about language, not only in terms of its meaning, but also in terms of its sound. This phonological knowledge is involved in their analysis of written words from very early in the reading process. As children begin to understand the relationship between phonology and orthography, their phonological knowledge in its turn becomes more refined. Children start out with phonological knowledge at the level of syllables, onsets, and rimes, and via reading itself they gain more and more knowledge about phonemes.

This interactive process suggests an alternative model of reading development, which we can call an analogy model of reading.[28] When children first learn to recognize written words (or at least, single-syllable words, which are those most frequently encountered in their reading books), they associate the spelling sequences representing those words with two sounds, the onset and the rime (see also Wimmer and Goswami[29]). So they code a simple word like "bug" in terms of two phonological units, the onset, corresponding to "b-," and the rime, corresponding to "-ug." As children develop better phonemic skills, the nature of this "phonological underpinning" will change, enabling the children to represent other phonological units in the word, such as those that correspond to the onset–vowel unit ("bu-"), and those that correspond to the individual alphabetic letters U and G (the phonemes).

An analogy model of reading would predict that these changes in the nature of the phonological underpinning of words will be reflected in changes in transfer. Children in the earliest phases of learning to read, who code written words in terms of the two phonological units of the onset and the rime, should only transfer pronunciations to words that share entire rimes with the word that they know. If these children can read "bug," then they should show transfer (make analogies) to words such as "rug" and "dug." Children who are more advanced in reading and who learn to read a word like "bug" should be able to transfer pronunciations for other spelling units in this word as well. Their more refined phonological underpinning should enable transfer between onset–vowel units ("bug"–"bud"), and between single phonemes ("bug"–"cup") too.

Testing an Orthographic Analogy Model of Reading Development

The analogy model of reading suggested here is consistent with the experimental evidence discussed so far in this paper. Children at the very beginning of learning to read (those who do not yet score on standardized tests of reading) do restrict their use of analogy to rime analogies. The early clue-word studies showed that these children used analogies from "beak" to read words like "peak," but not to read words like "bean" (onset–vowel words). Children who are a bit further in their reading use other analogies, such as onset–vowel analogies ("beak"–"bean"), as well. However, the model has not yet been tested directly. If children in the initial phases of reading development really do code spelling patterns in terms of onset–rime units, then they should have very little knowledge of the individual phonemes making up the onsets and the rimes in these words.

One way of testing this idea about how words are initially phonologically underpinned by children is to study transfer between vowel sounds in words. Vowels provide a good test of the theory because they are always part of the rime. According to the analogy model, children should initially code vowel sounds in terms of the sound of the entire rime of the word, and should have no knowledge of vowel pronunciation independently of this rime unit. Knowledge about the sounds of vowels in isolation should only arise gradually, as children learn more about the connections between orthography and phonology via being taught to read. So the transfer of vowel sounds should be restricted initially to transfer of the entire rime unit. Later, however, children should become able to make connections between the sounds of individual vowels in different words, irrespective of whether the entire rime is shared or not, and to make analogies about vowel sounds as isolated units.

This prediction can be tested quite easily within the clue-word paradigm. In the initial phases of reading, children who are taught a pronunciation for a clue word like "beak" would not be expected to use this word as a basis for an analogy to a word like "heap," which shares a vowel grapheme. Similarly, children who are taught a pronunciation for a clue word like "bug" would not be expected to use this word as a basis for an analogy to "cup." Once children have begun learning to read, however, analogies should extend beyond shared letters corresponding to the rime unit. Analogies between shared vowels should start emerging as well. The early clue-word experiments did control for shared phonemes in words (e.g., "beak"–"bank"), but not for shared vowels. In order to test the analogy model of reading development, a new set of clue-word studies was therefore carried out, this time focusing specifically on vowel analogies.

The ideal way to examine whether a more refined phonological underpinning of words develops with reading experience would be to use the same clue and test words with children of different reading levels. If the clue and test words remain constant, but the kinds of analogies that children make vary with reading level, then we would have firm grounds for concluding that the nature of the phonological underpinning of the words was changing with reading development. However, since children become able to read more and more words as their reading develops, these experimental controls are not possible in the real world. Clue and test words that are appropriate for 5-year-old readers are inappropriate for 7-year-old readers, who can probably read many words that 5-year-olds cannot. The approach taken here was thus to use different clue and test words with children of different reading levels, examining the *same* contrasts within each word set. The spelling sequences manipulated in each experiment were shared-vowel-only (e.g., "bug"–"cup," "beak"–"heap," "trim"–"skid," "wink"–"tick"), shared rime (e.g., "bug"–"rug," "beak"–"peak," "wink"–"pink"), and shared onset–vowel unit (e.g., "bug"–"bud," "beak"–"bean," "trim"–"trip").

Three experiments were conducted altogether, involving 5- to 7-year-old children at three different reading levels (averaging 6 years, 5 months; 6 years, 10 months; and 7 years, 6 months, respectively).[28] In each experiment, the children were pretested on the words being used, and transfer from the clue word was then measured in an analogy test. The results were in line with the hypothesis. The youngest readers only made analogies between spelling patterns representing the rimes of the clue and the test words. Children who learned clue words like "bug" only made analogies to test words like "rug," and showed no transfer to the onset–vowel ("bug"–"bud") or shared-vowel-only words ("bug"–"cup"). Slightly older readers made analogies between both rimes ("beak"–"peak") and onset–vowel units ("beak"–"bean"), replicating the results of previous studies. These children also made analogies to the shared-vowel-only words ("beak"–"heap"), suggesting that they had fairly well-developed phonemic knowledge. So knowledge about phonemes may develop very quickly once children are learning to read, as suggested by the evidence on phonological development.[18]

The oldest readers tested also made analogies between both rimes ("wink"–"pink") in words and shared onset–vowel units ("trim"–"trip"). However, these children did not make analogies to the shared-vowel-only test words ("trim"–"skid," "wink"–"tick"). So the vowel transfer found in the previous study was not maintained. This result can either be taken to show that the phonological underpinning of the vowel as an isolated unit (phoneme) may not be well-established until later in reading development, or that children need a certain amount of graphemic overlap in order to use analogies to read new words. The shared-vowel grapheme in "beak" and "heap" represents 50 percent of the spelling pattern of each word, a quite noticeable graphemic overlap. In contrast, the shared-vowel grapheme in "trim" and "skid" represents only 25 percent of the spelling pattern of each word, a much less salient graphemic similarity. If children vary their use of analogies with the amount of graphemic overlap between words, then this would account for the lack of vowel transfer found in this study. It would also be a rather sensible way to constrain the use of analogies in reading. Analogies between single letters in words may often be misleading in terms of pronunciation, especially when the shared letters are vowels (e.g., "cost"–"cold," "mint"–"mild").

In general, then, the idea that a more refined phonological underpinning of words develops with increasing reading experience was supported by these studies on vowel transfer. The proposal that phonological and orthographic knowledge interact from the beginning of learning to read thus seems to be correct. Children come to the reading task with phonological knowledge about onsets and rimes, and this affects their initial analysis of the printed letter string. Learning to read then affects their phonological analyses, and they soon become aware of single phonemes in words as well. This phonemic knowledge then feeds back into the kinds of connections that they make between shared spelling patterns when they are reading (analogies). So the same interactive process underlies reading development from the very beginning of learning to read. Rather than using qualitatively different strategies as reading develops, children use the same basic strategy all the way through. They try to link their phonological knowledge to consistent patterns in the orthography, but they do this at different levels as they become better readers. Phonological and orthographic knowledge affect each other throughout learning to read.

ORTHOGRAPHIC ANALOGIES AND DYSLEXIA

Implications of the Orthographic Analogy Model

This interactive model of reading development has clear implications for children with reading difficulties, who are known to have poor phonological skills. For them, the interaction between phonological and orthographic knowledge cannot get off the ground, as they lack the phonological skills required to initiate this process. In particular, these children are unlikely to be able to use orthographic analogies as a way into reading, since they have such poor rhyming skills.[13,14] Backward readers are not only worse at producing or at recognizing rhymes than their age mates, they are also significantly impaired in their recognition and production of rhyme when compared to younger children reading at the same level as them (the stringent "reading level" match experimental design[30]). This difficulty in rhyming will cause obvious difficulties in using orthographic analogies. Even if backward readers have the cognitive ability to use analogies, which they probably do, they lack the phonological knowledge necessary to use similarities in spelling patterns as a basis for making predictions about shared sound. They simply cannot hear the shared sounds reliably in the first place.

The obvious consequence of the absence of this phonological knowledge is that backward readers may develop recognition units for words that either lack any phonological underpinning, or that have an incomplete or an inadequate phonological underpinning. Dyslexic children may be able to recognize individual words in reading, but they will not necessarily be able to use their knowledge of the pronunciation of these words as a basis for transfer. Since the pronunciation of the words is not represented in a way that allows access to their constituent phonological subunits, backward readers may not be able to utilize shared spelling sequences in words, even if they can see their orthographic similarity. This inability to use analogy would stem directly from a deficit in onset–rime knowledge, with a consequent deficit in the ability to establish any phonological underpinning for words that *are* recognized. Without adequate phonological underpinning, there is no basis for analogy.

The Use of Analogies by Dyslexic Children

Although this latter idea is purely speculative, it is consistent with what we know about the reading skills of dyslexic children. These children are thought to learn to read words by a process of holistic recognition,[31] relying heavily on their visual memories to pronounce known words. If this view is correct, it would mean that dyslexic children establish direct recognition units for words that lack phonological underpinning. We also know that dyslexic children do not spontaneously connect shared spelling patterns in words in the way required for analogy. Lovett and her group have studied the use of orthographic analogies in dyslexic children by giving them lists of analogous words to read. For example, they taught a group of dyslexic 8-year-olds to read a list of words like "beak" and "part."[32] The children were then given a transfer list of analogous words to read, like "peak" and "cart." Absolutely no transfer was found to these new words, even though the children did remember the spelling patterns of the words in the original training list. So the children were not making analogies.

As noted previously, this failure to use analogies may be a direct consequence of poor phonological skills, and so the proper way to test the hypothesis just outlined would be to train dyslexic children in rhyme, and then to see whether they could begin making analogies. Although no one has studied this connection directly, at least two types of evidence are consistent with this proposal. The first comes from the effect of rhyme training on reading in nondyslexic children, and the second comes from the design of instructional programs to teach reading by analogy in the classroom.

A study in which children with poor phonological skills were trained in rhyme was carried out by Bradley and Bryant.[12] They gave one group of the children (none of whom were diagnosed as dyslexic) rhyme training over a period of two years, using a concrete version of the oddity task based on pictures. The children were given a set of pictures such as a hat, a cat, a bat, and a pig, and they had to categorize them by rhyme. Another group of the children learned to categorize the same pictures semantically, using categories such as "farm animals." This "semantic control" group received an equal amount of individual attention from the experimenters with the same stimuli, but learned a different kind of categorization. Finally, half of the children who received the rhyme training spent the second year of the study learning how to represent the rhyming words with plastic letters. For example, for the rhyming category "cat," "hat," and "bat," the child would learn that to make "cat" into "hat," the plastic letters representing the rime (AT) did not change. The only letter that was removed was the onset (C), which was replaced by another one (H). So the training in sound categories was supplemented by orthographic training in onset and rime, too.

When the children's reading and spelling progress was measured two years later, it was the group that had received training with both rhyme and plastic letters that was significantly ahead of the semantic control group in reading. The children who had received rhyme training alone also showed reading benefits, but were not significantly ahead of this control group. So helping children to categorize words on the basis of rhyme and then teaching them about the connection between rhyme and orthographic categories had the greatest effects on reading. It can be argued that this training procedure was effectively teaching the analogy process to the children.

A study of analogy instruction in the classroom that supports the important role of rhyme was carried out by White and Cunningham.[33] They designed an analogy training program to be used by classroom teachers, and then tested it over two consecutive years in the Hawaii school district. Their subject population comprised children from minority and low-socioeconomic-status groups, who often experience difficulties in learning to read. The analogy instruction began with instruction about rhyme, which was accompanied by the learning of a series of analogy base words representing common spelling patterns, such as "look." The words that had been learned were put up on a "word wall" in the classroom, color-coded by vowel. After 3 to 4 months of rhyme work, explicit teaching about "word families" began. Children learned about a small group of families at a time, such as the "nine," the "mat," and the "job" families. The teacher would present a new word from one family, such as "spine," and the children would have to decide how to pronounce this word, and which family it belonged to. Similar instruction was also given in spelling.

The analogy training lasted for an entire year, after which White and Cunningham compared the reading progress of the children in these "analogy" classrooms to the progress of the children in the "control" classrooms. A clear advantage in reading development for the children taught by analogy was found, and this advantage was significant in measures of both decoding and comprehension. These results were replicated in a similar study conducted a year later. Since the rhyme training formed a significant part of the teaching program, and preceded the training about orthography (word families), it is at least plausible to argue that this study shows that rhyme training forms an important part of learning to use analogies in reading. Short-term training studies that have looked at the benefits of analogy training in the classroom also support this claim. Training studies that have included word family training have generally found an effect of analogy instruction,[34] whereas training studies that have omitted such training have not.[35]

CONCLUSION

The orthographic analogy research can be used as a basis for proposing a model of reading development that is rather different from the currently popular stage models of reading. An interactive analogy model of reading development provides a plausible account of why phonological skills are important for learning to read. According to the model, early phonological (onset–rime) skills feed into reading via analogies, and as orthographic knowledge develops, phonological knowledge in turn becomes more refined. In particular, phonemic knowledge will develop, partly as a consequence of learning to read, and partly as a result of beginning to spell.

An interactive model can also explain why backward readers have difficulties in making progress in reading. Dyslexic children have poor phonological skills, and so the interactive process of applying phonological knowledge to understand the orthography will be severely hampered. In particular, an initial inability to code spelling patterns in terms of phonological units like onsets and rimes, and thus use orthographic analogies to build up knowledge about the orthography, would go some way toward explaining the difficulties experienced by dyslexic children. The popular view of the reading skills that dyslexic children do acquire is that they are based on visual recognition. Dyslexic children may establish visual recognition units for words, but these recognition units will lack adequate phonological underpinning (onsets and rimes), and thus provide an inadequate basis for transfer.

REFERENCES

1. FRITH, U. 1985. Beneath the surface of developmental dyslexia. *In* Surface Dyslexia, K. Patterson, M. Coltheart, and J. Marshall. Eds. Academic Press. Cambridge.
2. MARSH, G., M. P. FRIEDMAN, V. WELCH & P. DESBERG. 1981. A cognitive-developmental approach to reading acquisition. *In* Reading Research: Advances in Theory and Practice, Vol. 3, G. E. MacKinnon and T. G. Waller, Eds.: 199–221. Academic Press, New York.
3. PIAGET, J., J. MONTANGERO & J. BILLETER. 1977. Les correlats. *In* L'Abstraction Reflechissante, J. Piaget, Ed. Presses Univ. de France. Paris.
4. GOSWAMI, U. & A. L. BROWN. 1989. Melting chocolate and melting snowmen: Analogical reasoning and causal relations. Cognition 35: 69–95.

5. GOSWAMI, U. 1986. Children's use of analogy in learning to read: A developmental study. J. Exp. Child Psychol. **42:** 73–83.
6. ———. 1988. Orthographic analogies and reading development. Q. J. Exp. Psychol. **40A:** 239–268.
7. TREIMAN, R. 1988. The internal structure of the syllable. *In* Linguistic Structure in Language Processing, G. Carlson and M. Tanenhaus, Eds. Kluger. Dordrecht, the Netherlands.
8. CHUKOVSKY, K. 1963. From Two to Five. Univ. of California Press. Berkeley.
9. LENEL, J. C. & J. H. CANTOR. 1981. Rhyme recognition and phonemic perception in young children. J. Psychol. Res. **10:** 57–68.
10. MACLEAN, M., P. E. BRYANT & L. BRADLEY. 1987. Rhymes, nursery rhymes and reading in early childhood. Merrill-Palmer Q. **33:** 255–282.
11. OPIE, I. & P. OPIE. 1987. The Lore and Language of Schoolchildren. Oxford Univ. Press. Oxford.
12. BRADLEY, L. & P. E. BRYANT. 1983. Categorising sounds and learning to read: A causal connection. Nature **310:** 419–421.
13. ———. 1978. Difficulties in auditory organisation as a possible cause of reading backwardness. Nature **271:** 746–747.
14. HOLLIGAN, C. & R. S. JOHNSTON. 1988. The use of phonological information by good and poor readers in memory and reading tasks. Mem. Cognition **16:** 522–532.
15. OLSON, R. K., B. J. DAVIDSON, R. KLIEGL & G. FOLTZ. 1985. Individual and developmental differences in reading disability. *In* Reading Research: Advances in Theory and Practice, Vol. 4, G. E. MacKinnon and T. G. Waller, Eds.: 1–64. Academic Press. New York.
16. GOSWAMI, U. & P. E. BRYANT. 1990. Phonological Skills and Learning to Read. Erlbaum. Hillsdale, N.J.
17. TREIMAN, R. & A. ZUKOWSKI. 1991. Levels of phonological awareness. *In* Phonological Processes in Literacy, S. Brady and D. Shankweiler, Eds. Erlbaum. Hillsdale, N.J.
18. LIBERMAN, I. Y., D. SHANKWEILER, F. W. FISCHER & B. CARTER. 1974. Explicit syllable and phoneme segmentation in the young child. J. Exp. Child Psychol. **18:** 201–212.
19. COSSU, G., D. SHANKWEILER, I. Y. LIBERMAN, G. TOLA & L. KATZ. 1987. Awareness of phonological segments and reading ability in Italian children. Haskins Labs Status Rep. on Speech Research, Vol. SR-91.
20. MORAIS, J., L. CARY, J. ALEGRIA & P. BERTELSON. 1979. Does awareness of speech as a sequence of phones arise spontaneously? Cognition **7:** 323–331.
21. EHRI, L. C. & L. S. WILCE. 1980. The influence of orthography on readers' conceptualisation of the phonemic structure of words. Appl. Psychol. **1:** 371–385.
22. TUNMER, W. E. & A. R. NESDALE. 1985. Phonemic segmentation skill and beginning reading. J. Ed. Psych. **77:** 417–527.
23. GOSWAMI, U. 1990. A special link between rhyming skills and the use of orthographic analogies by beginning readers. J. Child Psychol. Psychiatr. **31:** 301–311.
24. CONTENT, A., J. MORAIS, J. ALEGRIA & P. BERTELSON. 1982. Accelerating the development of phonetic segmentation skills in kindergarteners. Cahiers Psychol. Cognition **2:** 259–269.
25. GOSWAMI, U. & F. MEAD. 1992. Onset and rime awareness and analogies in reading. Reading Res. Q. **27**(2): 152–162.
26. GOSWAMI, U. 1990. Phonological priming and orthographic analogies in reading. J. Exp. Child Psychol. **49:** 323–340.
27. STUART, M. & M. COLTHEART. 1988. Does reading develop in a sequence of stages? Cognition **30:** 139–181.
28. GOSWAMI, U. 1992. Towards an orthographic analogy model of reading development: Decoding vowel graphemes in beginning reading. Submitted for publication in J. Exp. Child Psychol.
29. WIMMER, H. & U. GOSWAMI. 1992. The influence of orthographic consistency on reading development: Word recognition in English and German children. Submitted for publication in Cognition.

30. BRYANT, P. E. & U. GOSWAMI. 1986. The strengths and weaknesses of the reading level design: Comment on Backman, Mamen and Ferguson. Psychol. Bull. **100:** 101–103.
31. SNOWLING, M. 1987. Dyslexia: A Cognitive Developmental Perspective. Blackwell. Oxford.
32. LOVETT, M. W., M. J. RANSBY, N. HARDWICK, M. S. JOHNS & S. A. DONALDSON. 1989. Can dyslexia be treated? Treatment-specific and generalised treatment effects in dyslexic children's response to remediation. Brain Lang. **37:** 90–121.
33. WHITE, T. G. & P. M. CUNNINGHAM. 1990. Teaching disadvantaged students to decode by analogy. Paper presented at the Annual Meeting of the American Educational Research Association, Boston, Mass., April.
34. PETERSON, M. E. & L. P. HAINES. 1992. Orthographic analogy training with kindergarten children: Effects on analogy use, phonemic segmentation, and letter-sound knowledge. J. Reading Behav. **24:** 109–127.
35. BRUCK, M. & R. TREIMAN. 1992. Learning to pronounce words: The limitations of analogies. Reading Res. Q. **27**(4): 374–389.

An Operant Conditioning Paradigm for Assessing Auditory Temporal Processing in 6- to 9-Month-Old Infants

APRIL ANN BENASICH AND PAULA TALLAL

Center for Molecular and Behavioral Neurosciences
Rutgers University
197 University Avenue
Newark, New Jersey 07102

Specific language impairment (SLI) in children, also referred to as developmental dysphasia, is characterized by a relatively specific failure of normal language functions in the absence of such factors as deafness, mental retardation, motor disability, childhood schizophrenia, or infantile autism. Highly significant and persistent deficits have been shown in the ability of children with language disorders, specifically SLI, to process rapidly changing nonverbal auditory stimuli. SLI children have been shown to be selectively impaired in their ability to both perceive and produce those speech sounds that are characterized by brief or rapidly changing temporal cues in their acoustic spectra. The degree of temporal processing deficit has also proved to be highly correlated with the degree of language comprehension deficits over a broad age range of SLI individuals (4–24 years).

These findings suggest that auditory temporal processing deficits might serve as a behavioral "marker" of language impairment and could be useful in early identification of language impairment. However, procedures for testing specific temporal auditory processing deficits have currently only been developed for use with children over the age of 4 years. We have developed an infant operant conditioning paradigm that facilitates assessment of auditory temporal processing in the first year of life.

Auditory temporal processing thresholds of 16 infants from 6 to 9 months of age were examined using the infant auditory temporal processing paradigm.[1] Infants from 6 to 9 months of age were recruited from local obstetric and pediatric practices. All infants were full-term, had uneventful pre- and perinatal circumstances, Apgar scores of 9 or 10, and birthweights above 2500 grams. Twelve were first born, three were second born, and one was a third child. Nine were boys and 7 were girls. Mean age at testing was 6.9 (1.6) months. There was no history of hearing dysfunction, no recent occurrences of otitis media, and no family history of congenital hearing loss, speech, or language disorder.

Infants had to learn to discriminate between two auditory tone sequences and associate each auditory stimulus with a directional response. They anticipated which of two toys would be illuminated and set in motion by looking at the correct place. The experiment consisted of three phases: a *shaping* phase, an *association* phase, and a *variable interstimulus interval (ISI) test* phase. During the shaping and association phases the tone pair that comprised each stimulus was separated by a 500-ms ISI; in the variable ISI test phase the ISI within each stimulus varied between 8 and 300 ms. Trial-by-trial sessions for two infants completing the ATP variable ISI test phase are presented in FIGURES 1 and 2.

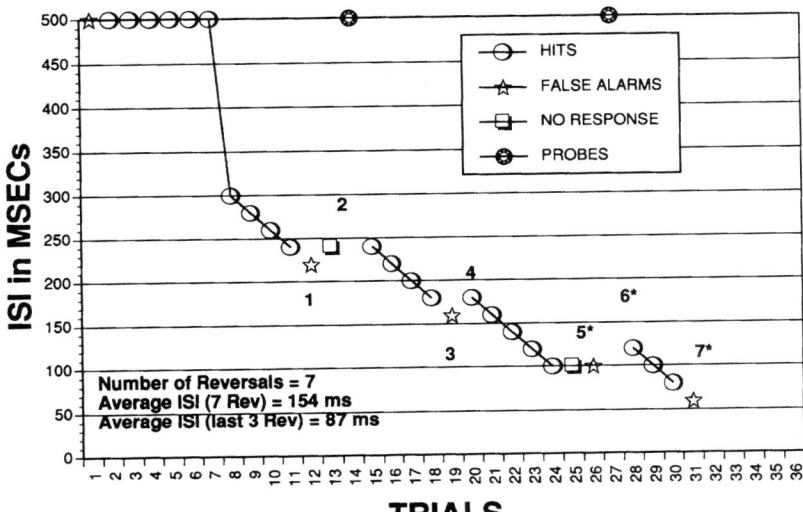

FIGURE 1. Trial-by-trial record from a 26-week-old infant.

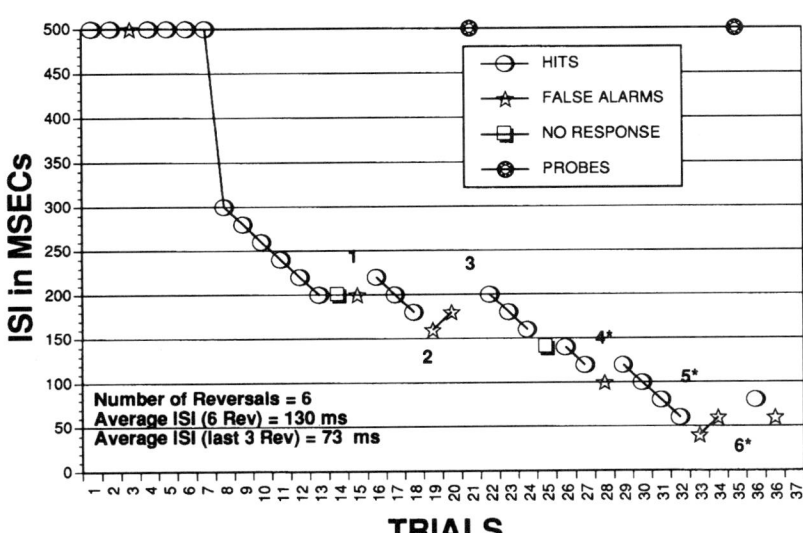

FIGURE 2. Trial-by-trial record from a 30-week-old infant.

The mean auditory temporal processing (ATP) threshold for all completed test sessions after a minimum of six reversals was 107 ms, and the standard deviation was 49 ms ($N = 9$). The mean ATP threshold for the last three reversals was 69 ms, and the standard deviation was 24 ms ($N = 9$). Latencies for false alarms were significantly longer than latencies for hits for infants completing the association and variable ISI test phases, as well as for infants who failed to complete the variable ISI test phase. The mean latency for hits was 1.24 s (SD = 0.5; $N = 9$), and the mean latency for false alarms was 2.35 s (SD = 0.8; $N = 9$), a significant difference (paired $t(8) = 5.36$, p (1-tailed) = 0.0003). Mean latencies for uncompleted test sessions was 1.67 s (SD = 0.4; $N = 3$) for hits and 3.44 s (SD = 0.6; $N = 3$) for false alarms, also a significant difference (paired $t(2) = 16.14$, p (1-tailed) = 0.002).

Thus, infants from 6 to 9 months of age learned to discriminate between two auditory tone sequences and associate each auditory stimulus with a directional response. The feasibility of using an infant operant conditioning paradigm to assess early auditory temporal processing was demonstrated, although based on a small sample. Auditory temporal processing thresholds were in the same range (56 to 76 ms at 500 Hz) reported by Werner *et al.*[2] for a similar task assessing gap detection thresholds, in a broad-band noise, for 3 to 12 month olds.

Our ultimate goal is the development of an assessment instrument that can be used in the first year of life, in conjunction with existing perceptual–cognitive paradigms, that would elucidate the developmental course of temporal processing abilities and their relationship to early speech perception and language development.

REFERENCES

1. BENASICH, A. A. & P. TALLAL. 1992. An infant operant conditioning paradigm to assess auditory temporal processing in infants. Paper presented at the International Conference on Infancy Studies, Miami, Fla., May.
2. WERNER, L. A., G. C. MAREAN, C. F. HALPIN, N. B. SPETNER & J. M. GILLENWATER. 1992. Infant auditory temporal acuity: Gap detection. Child Devel. **63**: 260–272.

Successive Information Processing Strategies: WISC-R Sequential Scores and Reading

HADASSAH WEITZMAN BENNETT

Jewish Board Family and Children Services
25 Amberson Avenue
Yonkers, New York 10705
and
David Yellin College
Jerusalem, Israel

INTRODUCTION

Current thinking and research validate the appropriateness of the many-faceted, dynamic neuropsychologically based information processing theory of Luria/Das *et al.*[1] as a conceptual model for understanding the complex higher cognitive skill of reading. While Leong,[2] Das,[3] and others related simultaneous and successive strategies to reading, successive processes have been marked as being a primary factor. This paper attempts to strengthen that notion.

SUBJECTS

Subjects were drawn from the second grade population in a large, urban, multi-ethnic middle socioeconomic population. Thirty poor readers were randomly drawn from those children who scored one standard deviation (SD) or more below the district mean on the Stanford Reading Test, Form B. Thirty skilled readers were randomly chosen from those who scored one SD or more above the mean.

PROCEDURE

Previously defined simultaneously and successive tests were administered in random order to all subjects. Individual and group mean scores of the poor and skilled readers were compared. To explore the sequential-linguistic link, the groups were compared on the Bannatyne "sequential" (digit span, coding arithmetic) subtests of the WISC-R and on the picture arrangement subtest of the WISC-R.

RESULTS

As expected, the skilled readers were more proficient on the Bannatyne sequential subtests of the WISC-R. A 2 (reading skill) × 2 (processing strategy) ANOVA with repeated measures of the second factor showed significant main effects for reading and for processing and for an interaction of the two. Tukey *post hoc* comparisons found successive processing to be the primary discriminator. A 2 (reading skill) × 7 (test) ANOVA with repeated measures of the second factor showed significant main effects for reading and for test and for the interaction between them. Tukey *post hoc* comparisons revealed one/simultaneous test (Ravens) and three successive tests (social, recall, free recall, and visual short-term memory) to be significant discriminators between the two groups of readers (see FIG. 1). Finally, the two reading groups scored in the predicted fashion on the picture arrangement subtest, and a positive correlation (0.25) was found between the students' scores on this subtest and on the successive strategy tests (FIG. 2).

DISCUSSION

The link between successive processing and reading has been demonstrated by Leong.[4] Other researchers have also linked reading to language, phonological processing, working memory, automaticity, and efficient control. These other factors are all components of the Luria Das Model, and therefore bolster the goodness of fit of this model for the analysis of reading.

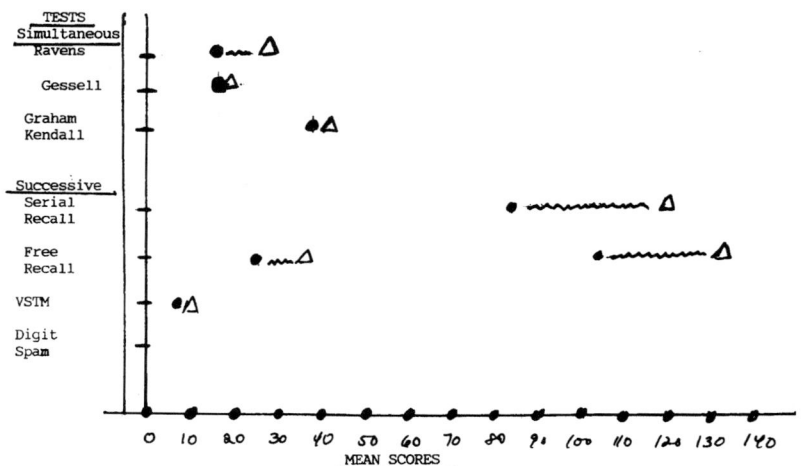

FIGURE 1. Simultaneous and successive tests. (*Key:* ● = poor readers; Δ = skilled readers; ~~~ = significant differences; F (Geisser Greenhouse df = 1, 58) = 13.72, $p < 0.01$; Tukey *post hoc* HSD comparisons $\alpha = 0.05$.)

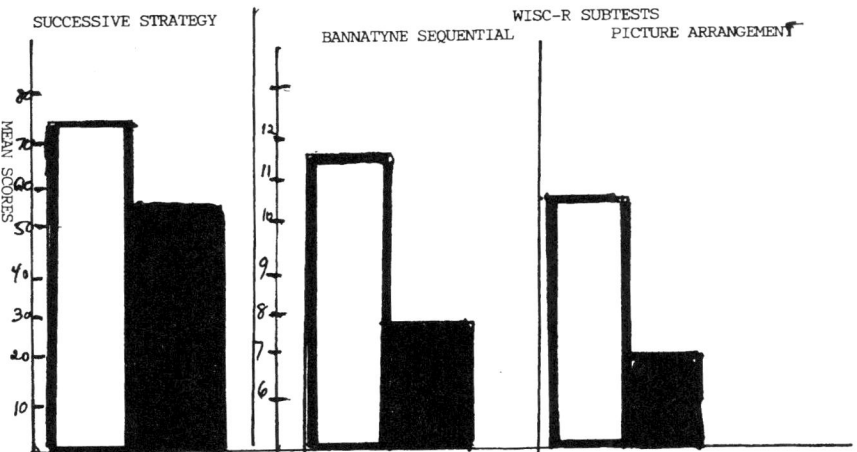

FIGURE 2. Skilled and poor readers' performance. (*Key:* ▫ = skilled; ■ = poor.)

REFERENCES

1. DAS, J. P., J. KIRBY & R. F. JARMAN. 1979. Simultaneous and Successive Cognitive Processes. Academic Press. New York.
2. LEONG, C. K. 1980. Cognitive patterns of "retarded" and below-average readers. Contemp. Educ. Psychol. **5:** 101–117.
3. DAS, J. P. 1984. Simultaneous and successive processing in children with reading disabilities. Top. Lang. Disord. **4:** 34–47.
4. LEONG, C. K. & S. S. SHEH. 1982. Knowing about language—Some evidence from readers. Ann. Dyslexia **32:** 149–161.

Effects of Naming Speed Differences on Fluency of Reading after Practice

PATRICIA GREIG BOWERS AND ALLISON KENNEDY

Department of Psychology
University of Waterloo
Waterloo N2L 3G1, Canada

Dyslexic children read nonwords poorly and recognize familiar words slowly. Ehri[1] suggests that the phonological weakness that impairs nonword decoding also impedes the formation of sufficiently precise and complete word representations, resulting in slow word retrieval. Less exposure to print is also associated with slower and less accurate performance on tests of orthographic skill.[2] Are phonemic insensitivity and less print exposure the basic sources of the dyslexic's slow reading speed? We argue that an additional source of the halting reading style of dyslexics is indexed by slow naming of the simplest symbols, reflecting an underlying dysfunction in automatic processes dependent upon precise timing of subprocesses, and affecting orthographic codes.[3] The hypothesis that speed of naming simple digits is a marker for a process independent of phonemic sensitivity that affects both lexical access speed and facility in forming orthographic codes, was investigated in two studies.

A longitudinal sample of 37 children selected in grade 2 as poor and average readers, reread passages at a level of difficulty appropriate to each child, in grades 2, 3, and 4. Phoneme deletion assessed by a modified Auditory Analysis Test[4] (e.g., "Say block ... without the /b/") and continuous-list digit naming speed (e.g., 1 5 8 2 4 3, repeated eight times) were consistently related to speed and errors on reading a passage for the first and fourth times. However, hierarchical regression analyses revealed that after controlling for Woodcock Reading Mastery Test (WRMT): Word Identification, only digit-naming speed contributed significant unique variance to reading speed. Controlling for speed of first reading, digit-naming speed predicted speed of the fourth reading to a small but significant extent. In grades 3 and 4, a curvilinear relationship between the fourth time reading and naming speed is apparent, with the relationship stronger in the slower readers (see TABLE 1).

In a second experiment, 35 grade 2 and 39 grade 3 readers practiced a total of 18 easy regular and exception words and nonwords (e.g., not, one, dep) ten times. They were presented in isolation on a computer in random order, and latency to correct vocal response was measured. Recognizing a word or nonword as fast as a simple digit, or unitizing retrieval, was assessed for three levels of WRMT reader skill. Good readers showed greater unitization than average or poor readers. Even after ten practices, poor readers failed to unitize any items, replicating Ehri and Wilce.[5] In grade 2, naming speed but not phoneme deletion predicted significant unique variance in latency for exception words and nonwords at trial 10, controlling for latency at trial 1 and general language ability (TABLE 2). When digit-naming speed is entered at step 3 before phoneme deletion at step 4, phoneme deletion accounted for only 2 percent of unique variance in nonword latency. Neither naming speed nor phoneme deletion contributed unique variance to speed at trial 10 in grade 3. Perhaps the orthographic patterns were too simple to reveal effects in older children.

TABLE 1. Hierarchical Regressions Predicting Text Speed on First and Fourth Reading

		Grade 2		Grade 3		Grade 4	
		1st Reading	4th Reading	1st Reading	4th Reading	1st Reading	4th Reading
Section A		Words/min	Words/min	Words/min	Words/min	Words/min	Words/min
Variable	Step	R^2 change	R^2 change	R^2 change	R^2 change	R^2 change	R^2 change
Word identity	1	0.50^a	0.54^a	0.34^a	0.26^b	0.48^a	0.38^a
Phoneme deletion	2	0.00	0.01	0.00	0.00	0.02	0.02
Digit naming	3	0.16^a	0.20^a	0.22^a	0.40^a	0.15^a	0.14^b
Section B							
Variable	Step						
1st words/min	1		0.90^a		0.85^a		0.62^a
Digit naming	2		0.014^c		0.05^a		0.017
Digit squared[d]	3		0.01		0.04^a		0.075^b

[a] $p < 0.001$.
[b] $p < 0.01$.
[c] $p < 0.05$.
[d] Digit squared: Digit naming speed score squared, representing the curvilinear component.

Both studies provide evidence that "slow namers" not only read more slowly but also benefit less from each practice of words or text. We suggest that slow naming speed indexes a process independent of phonemic sensitivity that moderates the effect of reading exposure on the formation of subword and word orthographic patterns. Phoneme deletion, although correlating with reading skill, did not predict significant fluency gains after practice. Dyslexic readers are apt to have two partially independent cognitive dysfunctions.

TABLE 2. Hierarchical Regression Predicting Latency at Trial 10 for Accurate Item Naming in Grade 2

		Regular Words	Exception Words	Nonwords
Variable	Step	R^2 change	R^2 change	R^2 change
Oral language[a]	1	—	—	—
Trial 1 latency	2	0.59^b	0.21^c	0.15^c
Phoneme deletion	3	0.01	−0.02	0.08
Digit naming	4	0.00	0.14^c	0.08^c

[a] Oral language was measured by Peabody Picture Vocabulary Test—Revised.
[b] $p < 0.01$.
[c] $p < 0.05$.

REFERENCES

1. EHRI, L. C. 1992. Reconceptualizing the development of sight word reading and its relationship to recoding. *In* Reading Acquisition, P. B. Gough, L. C. Ehri, and R. Trieman, Eds. Erlbaum. Hillsdale, N.J.
2. CUNNINGHAM, A. E. & K. E. STANOVICH. 1990. Assessing print exposure and orthographic processing skill in children: A quick measure of reading experience. J. Educ. Psychol. **82:** 733–740.
3. BOWERS, P. G. & M. WOLF. Theoretical links between naming speed, precise timing mechanisms and orthographic skill in dyslexia. Reading Writ. In press.
4. ROSNER, J. & D. P. SIMON. 1971. The auditory analysis test: An initial report. J. Learn. Disabilities **4:** 1–15.
5. EHRI, L. C. & L. S. WILCE. 1983. Development of word identification speed in skilled and less skilled beginning readers. J. Educ. Psychol. **75:** 3–18.

Short-circuiting Phonological Limitations in Dyslexia: The Beneficial Effect of Accelerated Reading Pace

ZVIA BREZNITZ
School of Education
University of Haifa
Haifa 31905, Israel

Both dyslexic and normal beginning readers rely heavily on phonological processing when reading. Normal beginning readers have not yet established an orthographic lexicon, while dyslexics appear unable to bypass the phonological route due to impaired phonological skills. As dyslexics seem to possess normally functioning orthographic skills, it is suggested that encouragement of greater reliance on the unimpaired orthographic route, as opposed to training of phonological skills, may improve their reading performance.

Studies carried out by the present author found that the acceleration of reading rate increases the decoding and comprehension scores of beginning readers, particularly in poor readers (see reference 1 for a review). This finding led to the hypothesis that dyslexics might enjoy a similar benefit. This study compares the effect of reading rate acceleration on the reading performance of dyslexics and matched-pair normally achieving beginning readers. It also examines the effect of auditory intervention, which is assumed to reduce the level of phonological route involvement in reading.

METHOD

Subjects included 52 dyslexics (mean age 9.2 years) and 52 matched-pair normally achieving first-grade readers (mean age 6.7 years). All subjects read six forms of a reading comprehension test, with and without auditory interference, under three reading rate conditions: (1) at their own natural self-paced reading rate, (2) at a faster reading rate based on the highest reading rate achieved per letter in the self-paced condition, and (3) again at their own self-paced reading rate, in order to eliminate a possible warm-up effect. So as not to monopolize all attention, a familiar Hebrew children's tune was chosen as an auditory distractor. Measures were reading time, comprehension, and oral reading errors. Reading errors were coded according to four categories; substitution, repetition, deletion, and addition.

RESULTS

The following results were achieved:

1. forced acceleration of dyslexics' reading rate increased reading performance
2. dyslexics' errors pattern differed from their matched controls in both the self- and fast-paced reading rate conditions

3. control subjects profited from usage of the phonological route, while its partial blockage reduced their reading effectiveness
4. partial blockage of the dyslexics' phonological route, by way of auditory interference, improved their reading performance.

CONCLUSION

Forced fast pace helps both groups of subjects, but for different reasons. Whereas control subjects, who are at the acquisition stage of reading, appear to make better use of the auditory channel if prompted to read faster, for dyslexics, the advantage may be due to a greater reliance on the orthographic channel. This interpretation is in line with the differential errors pattern exhibited by the two groups. Furthermore, the impact of the partial blockage of the auditory channel is dramatically different in both groups. Thus, *the manipulation that was found to reduce reading effectiveness of controls enhanced comprehension of dyslexics.*

REFERENCES

1. BREZNITZ, Z. 1991. The beneficial effect of accelerating reading rate on dyslexic readers' reading comprehension. *In* Dyslexia: Integrating Theory and Practice, M. Snowling and M. Thompson, Eds. Whurr. London.

Language and Memory in Children with Combined Complex-Partial Epilepsy and Reading Disorder

MELINDA BROMAN

Division of Pediatric Neurology
SUNY Health Science Center
Box 118
450 Clarkson Avenue
Brooklyn, New York 11203

The present study examined the neuropsychological pattern that characterized a group of seven children ages 6 to 16 with combined severe reading disorder (RD) defined as a significant discrepancy {one standard deviation (SD) unit or more} between the IQ and standardized reading score persisting for two or more years despite reading remediation, and complex-partial epilepsy (CPE). The office neurological exam was normal except for soft signs in all cases. In six cases, the etiology of the epilepsy was unknown; in the seventh, the presumed etiology was herpes encephalitis. A breakdown of the sample showing the locus of seizure activity is shown in TABLE 1.

All subjects received a battery of neuropsychological tests. The resulting data are presented according to the range and median performance for the seven cases in TABLE 2. In the case of language and memory data, average performance for the group is expressed in terms of median SD units from the normative mean.

Pictured-object naming and rapid automatized naming (RAN) emerged as consistent, significant impairments related to RD/CPE. All but one case showed a specific, severe difficulty with the task of memorizing a series of words. None of the

TABLE 1. Regional Focus (i) of Epileptic Activity According to EEG and Clinical Findings

Patient ID/Age	Epileptiform Discharge Focus (i)	Slow Wave Focus (i)	Side of Initial Motor Seizures	Automatisms
M.G. 6:11	RP	—	R or L	No
S.F 10:7	LT–P+RP	—	R or L	No
E.G. 10:10	LT–P	—	—	Yes
C.W. 12:12	(1)LT, (2)RF	(1)LT, (2)RT	G(akinetic)	Yes
T.K. 14:8	L+RT	—	R or G	No
M.J. 15:4	LT+RF	—	G	Yes
G.S. 17:5	(1)LT, (2)LP	RT	R or G	Yes

Note: EEG findings are from a single recording or separate recordings, indicated by numbers (1) and (2).
Key: R = right; L = left; T = temporal; P = parietal: F = frontal; G = generalized.

TABLE 2. Neuropsychological Test Findings

	Range	Average (Median)
WISC-R		
Verbal IQ	65–103	77
Performance IQ	73–102	87
Full-Scale IQ	68–95	82
Raven CPMT	81–114	88
WRAT-R		
Reading	<46–76	59
Spelling	49–79	61
Arithmetic	55–98	75
Expressive Language		
Rapid Automatized Naming (RAN)	−1 to −3 SDs<M	−3 SD
Boston Naming Test (BNT)	−2 to −3 SDs<M	−3 SD
Semantic fluency	−2 SD to +1.3 SD	−1 SD
Phonemic fluency	−3 SD to +2 SD	−2 SD
Repetition	−3 SD to +1.5 SD	−1 SD
Receptive Language		
Token test	−3 SD to +1.5 SD	Average
Binet absurdities	−3 SD to Average	−1.5 SD
Menyuk sentences	−3 SD to Average	−3/Average (bimodal)
Language Cognition/Acquisition		
WISC-R Information and Vocabulary	−3 to +1.6 SD	−2 SD
Peabody Picture Vocabulary Test (PPVT-R)	Z = 42 to 91	77
WISC-R Similarities and Comprehension	−2.3 to +1.6 SD	−1.3 SD
Memory—Verbal		
Digit Span	−3 SD to +0.3 SD	−1.3 SD
Rey Auditory Verbal Learning Test	−3 SD to Average	−3 SD
Prose Passage	−3 SD to +1 SD	Average
Wechsler Memory Scale (WMS) Paired-Associate Learning	−3 SD to Average	−1 SD
Memory—Visual		
Benton Visual Retention Test (BVRT-R)—Multiple choice	−0.5 to +1.5 SD	+1 SD
Revised BVRT	−3 SD to +1.3 SD	−1.3/+1.3 (bimodal)
WMS Visual Reproduction	−3 SD to +2 SD	+1 SD

six idiopathic cases demonstrated a significant generalized (i.e., across modalities) memory deficit, nor even a generalized memory deficit within the verbal modality. The disorders of rapid name retrieval and naming accuracy are among the strongest predictors of RD found in many studies of dyslexic children without neurological impairments.[1] The lack of association of a generalized verbal memory impairment and the association of naming impairments replicate the chief finding of a clinical neuropsychological study[2] of adult patients with temporal lobe epilepsy (TLE).

Stores and Hart[3] reported an association between focal epilepsy, including CPE, and impairments of oral reading. The present data indicate an overlapping neuropsychological deficit pattern between the two disorders. The increased incidence of dyslexia in CPE could be due to the presence of microscopic structural anomalies in functional language zones in the temporal and parietal lobes. Autopsy studies indicate that a common pathological basis would not be unexpected [for example, focal cortical dysplasias: Galaburda et al.[4] (dyslexia); Goldring[5] (focal seizures)].

REFERENCES

1. DENCKLA, M. B., R. G. RUDEL & M. BROMAN. 1981. Tests that discriminate between dyslexic and other learning-disabled boys. Brain Lang. **13:** 118–129.
2. MAYEUX, R., J. BRANDT, J. ROSEN & D. F. BENSON. 1980. Interictal memory and language impairment in temporal lobe epilepsy. Neurology **30:** 120–125.
3. STORES, G. & J. HART. 1976. Reading skills of children with generalized or focal epilepsy attending ordinary school. Dev. Med. Child Neurol. **18:** 705–716.
4. GALABURDA, A., G. SHERMAN, G. ROSEN, F. ABOITZ & N. GESCHWIND. 1985. Developmental dyslexia: Four consecutive patients with cortical anomalies. Ann. Neurol. **18:** 222–233.
5. GOLDRING, S. 1987. Pediatric epilepsy surgery. Epilepsia Suppl. 1 **28:** S82–S102.

Magnocellular Visual Deficits Affect Temporal Processing of Dyslexics

CHRIS CHASE[a] AND ANNETTE R. JENNER[b]

[a]*School of Communication and Cognitive Science*
Hampshire College
Amherst, Massachusetts 01002

[b]*Department of Neurobiology*
Harvard Medical School
220 Longwood Avenue
Boston, Massachusetts 02115

INTRODUCTION

A recent study[1] of five dyslexic brains found neurological abnormalities in a part of the visual system called the *lateral geniculate nucleus* (LGN). About 25 percent of the magnocells were smaller than normal, and cell locations were disorganized. Other parts of the LGN were normal. Livingstone *et al.*[1] speculated that smaller magnocells would have smaller axons and that these abnormalities may affect the speed with which information is processed in the magnocellular pathway.

This experiment compared the visual processing speed in the magno- and parvocellular channels of seven dyslexic adults and controls using flicker fusion threshold tasks. Five different stimuli (see FIG. 1) were tested in an effort to selectively activate the magno- and parvocellular channels.[2] Four tasks (one, two, four, and five) were selected that were expected to activate the magnocellular channel; the third task alternated between equiluminant red and green squares to measure the color fusion threshold (a unique parvocellular function). Dyslexics were hypothesized to have lower luminance flicker thresholds on the magnocellular tasks but to have normal threshold on the parvocellular task.

METHOD

Fifteen subjects were recruited from local colleges and a residential private school that specialized in working with dyslexic high school students. The seven dyslexic subjects were diagnosed through professional testing as having a reading disability and all had an educational history of reading and writing problems. Eight controls had normal educational histories and did not exhibit any current reading or writing difficulties. Subjects' ages ranged from seventeen to twenty-two.

A random, two stair procedure was used to determine the flicker fusion threshold for the six different pairs of stimuli just described. The stimuli were presented spatiotemporally so that the fused image resulted in an overlapped composited image, as shown in the far right column of FIGURE 1. For the red and green color displays the contrast was set to be equiluminant for each subject using another random two stair-step procedure to determine a luminance intensity at which the flicker vanished. For the shape discrimination and apparent motion tasks, subjects were asked to notice a point at which the display appeared to no longer flicker and

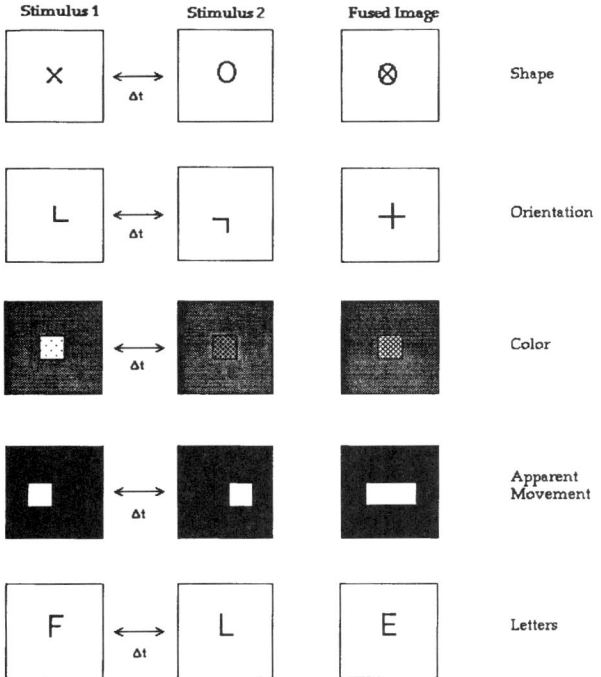

FIGURE 1. Experimental stimuli. The first two columns present examples of the stimuli used in the five tasks. The last column is an example of the fused image. For the apparent movement stimuli, the *white foreground square* was presented on a black background with a slight overlap between the two to present the appearance of a moving box at rapid flicker rates. Display luminance measured 0.67 cd/m^2 using an Minola LS-100 photometer. In the third task the *equiluminant colored squares* were presented with a grey background (11.51 cd/m^2). *Black figures* on white background were used in the other three tasks (87.13 cd/m^2).

make a yes or no judgment. For the color fusion task, subjects were asked to judge when the square change from a red/green alternation to a single brown or yellow appearance. The threshold value of eight response reversals were recorded, and task averages were computed for each subject.

All stimuli were presented on a NEC Multisync color monitor using Microexperimental Lab (MEL) software, subtending a visual angle of 0.56° at a viewing distance of 30 cm, which was maintained throughout the experiment with a chin rest. The stimuli that presented characteristics of color and apparent movement were twice as large and subtended 1.12°. Testing occurred in a dark room (0.011 cd/m^2 measured on a white sheet of paper along side the computer screen); subjects dark adapted for five minutes, during which instructions were given and informed consent was obtained.

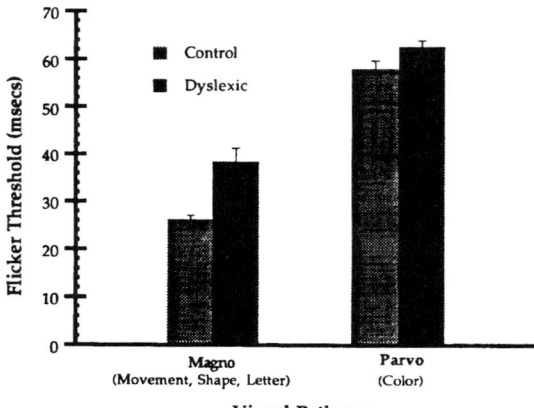

FIGURE 2. Flicker fusion thresholds of dyslexics and controls for magno- and parvocellular tasks.

RESULTS

Flicker thresholds on the color fusion task (parvocellular channel) were compared to the average performance on three magnocellular tasks that involved perceptions of shape and movement (one, four, and five). Task two was eliminated from the data analysis due to technical difficulties with the display. The 2 × 2 (group × visual channel) analysis of variance revealed main effects for group, $F(1, 12) = 21.97$, $p = 0.0005$, and channel, $F(1, 12) = 244.84$, $p < 0.0001$, as well as an interaction, $F(1, 12) = 4.60$, $p = 0.05$. Flicker rates for magnocellular tasks were faster than parvocellular tasks (31.9 Hz versus 16.7 Hz, respectively). The dyslexic group had higher fusion thresholds that control only for the magnocellular tasks; their magno flicker fusion averaged 26.1 Hz compared to 38.4 for controls (see FIG. 2).

DISCUSSION

These results provide further support for the hypothesis that dyslexics have slower visual processing speed for certain types of perceptual tasks. Compared to controls, the dyslexics had significantly lower flicker fusion rates for the perception of shape and movement, but were comparable on color fusion. The fact that the tasks involving shape perception and movement had similar high flicker thresholds lends support to the claim that they were being processed by the magno system, whereas the lower color fusion threshold reflected processing by the slower parvo channel.

These findings are consistent with other studies that have reported dyslexics to have low flicker fusion thresholds.[3,4] However, these results provide additional evidence that visual-processing speed impairment of dyslexics is specific to tasks involving the magnocellular channel. Results also are consistent with the anatomical and neurophysiological data of Livingstone et al.,[1] providing converging support for the idea that smaller magnocells produce a functional processing speed deficit.

The results of this experiment should be viewed cautiously. The number of dyslexic subjects is small, and the numbers and types of perceptual displays are not necessarily representative of the domain of magno and parvo tasks. In particular, only one parvo display was employed. Replication with additional subjects and a broader variety of magno and parvo displays would strengthen these conclusions.

REFERENCES

1. LIVINGSTON, M. S., G. D. ROSEN, F. W. DRISLANE & A. M. GALABURDA. 1991. Proc. Natl. Acad. Sci. U.S.A. **88:** 7943–7947.
2. LIVINGSTON, M. S. & D. H. HUBEL. 1987. J. Neurosci. **7:** 3416–3468.
3. DiLOLLO, V., D. HANSON & J. S. McINTYRE. 1983. J. Exp. Psych. Hum. Percept. Perform. **9(6):** 923–935.
4. WILLIAMS, M. C. & K. LECLUYSE. 1991. J. Am. Optom. Assoc. **61(2):** 111–123.

Flicker Contrast Sensitivity and the Dunlop Test in Reading-disabled Children[a]

PIERS CORNELISSEN,[b] ALEXANDRA MASON,[b]
SUE FOWLER,[c] AND JOHN STEIN[b]

[b]Physiology Department
Oxford University
Parks Road
Oxford OX1 3PT, England

[c]Orthopic Department
Royal Berks Hospital
Reading, Berkshire, England

Up to 3–10 percent of school children have particular difficulty learning to read.[1] Given that fluent reading demands rapid integration of both visual and linguistic information, it is plausible that problems with either visual or language processing could contribute to these children's difficulties. As regards language processing, there is convincing evidence that poor phonological awareness contributes to reading failure in many children.[2,3] However, the question whether visual problems contribute to reading failure remains unresolved.

Two kinds of experiment have suggested that children with reading disability (RD) process visual information differently when they are compared with normal children of the same age. In the first kind, Lovegrove et al.[4] have shown that many RD children show reduced contrast sensitivity for flickering grating stimuli (>5 Hz), and for low spatial frequency static stimuli (<1.5 cycles/degree) (for a review, see reference 4). These findings have been interpreted as evidence for reduced efficiency of the "transient" visual system, which normally responds best to low spatial, high temporal frequencies. Indeed, using measures of type I visible persistence, which is thought to depend on transient system function, Lovegrove et al.[5] have found that as many as 75 percent of RD children fall into a "weak transient system" category.

In the second experimental approach, the stability of binocular visual direction sense has been measured in RD children using the Dunlop Test (DT). Stein et al.[6] found that as many as 65 percent of 9–11-year-old RD children may experience unstable visual direction sense, as revealed by failure in the DT. By comparison, only 20 percent of unselected primary school children of the same age fail the DT (for a review, see reference 6). However, until now there has been no suggestion that these two phenomena might be associated in reading disability, so we investigated this possibility by measuring flicker contrast sensitivity in two experiments.

In experiment one, we measured the flicker contrast sensitivity of 12 RD children who passed the DT, 12 RD children who failed the DT, and 12 normal, control children (mean ages 9:3). Subjects viewed sinusoidal gratings (0.5, 1.5, 3.0, and 6.0 cycles/degree) that were displayed on a VDU (Joyce screen) and were modulated in counterphase at 20 Hz. The circular grating patches subtended 8° at the retina, were

---

[a]This work was supported by the Wellcome Trust and the Science and Engineering Research Council.

presented for 1000 ms, and had a mean luminance of 3.5 cd/m². FIGURE 1 shows mean contrast sensitivity plotted against spatial frequency, where sensitivity is the reciprocal of threshold. From FIGURE 1 it can be seen that, on average, all RD children were less sensitive to flicker than normals at all spatial frequencies (about 0.25 log units). But RD children who failed the DT were significantly less sensitive to the flickering gratings than those who passed it (about 0.15 log units). Analysis of variance showed that both main effects of spatial frequency and group (i.e., normals, RDs who passed the DT, and RDs who failed the DT) were significant ($F_{3,138} = 73.8, p < 0.0005$, and $F_{2,138} = 53.6, p < 0.0005$, respectively). No significant interaction between spatial frequency and group was found ($F_{6,132} = 0.17, p > 0.9$). Finally, Scheffe's multiple comparison technique confirmed that the mean contrast sensitivity of each of the three groups was significantly different from the other two, where each comparison exceeded the critical values $\alpha = 0.001$ and $F_{2,138} = 7.27$.

We wanted to be sure that these findings could not be attributed to systematic differences in age, reading ability, or IQ. Therefore in experiment two we compared the flicker contrast sensitivities of 15 children who passed the DT with 15 children who failed the DT. But this time both groups were matched as closely as possible for age, reading age, and IQ (group means 9:0, 7:11, and 112, respectively). FIGURE 2 shows that despite these more stringent controls, DT failure was still significantly correlated with reduced flicker contrast sensitivity (about 0.14 log units) at all spatial frequencies. Analysis of variance confirmed this effect ($F_{3,115} = 48.9, p < 0.0005$ and $F_{1,115} = 18.1, p < 0.0005$, for spatial frequency and DT, respectively).

Together these results suggest that flicker contrast sensitivity and DT performance are linked in RD children. Furthermore, they support the idea that abnormal visual processing could affect how children read.

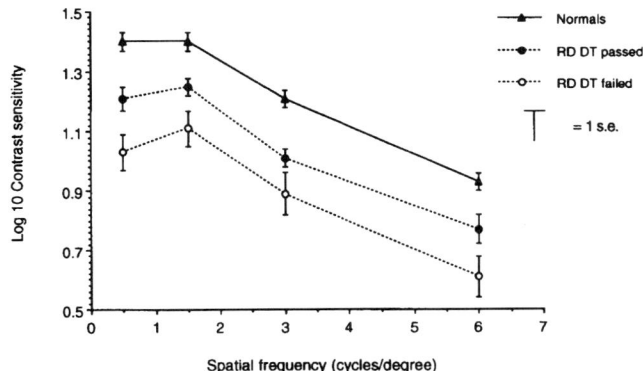

FIGURE 1.

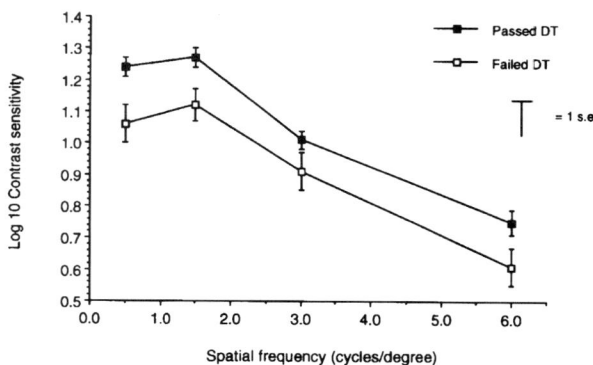

FIGURE 2.

REFERENCES

1. RUTTER, M. & W. YULE. 1975. The concept of specific reading retardation. J. Child Psychol. Psychiatry **16:** 181–197.
2. BRADLEY, L. & P. BRYANT. 1978. Difficulties in auditory organization as a possible cause of reading backwardness. Nature **301:** 419–421.
3. WAGNER, R. & J. TORGESON. 1987. The nature of phonological processing and its causal role in the acquisition of reading skills. Psychol. Bull. **101:** 192–212.
4. LOVEGROVE, W. J., R. P. GARZIA & S. B. NICHOLSON. 1990. Experimental evidence for a transient system deficit in specific reading disability. J. Am. Optom. Assoc. **61**(2): 137–145.
5. LOVEGROVE, W. J., F. MARTIN & W. SLAGHUIS. 1986. A theoretical and experimental case for a visual deficit in specific reading difficulty. Cognitive Neuropsychol. **3**(2): 225–267.
6. STEIN, J. F. 1991. "Visuospatial sense, hemispheric assymetry and dyslexia." *In* Vision and Visual Dysfunction, Vol. 13, Vision and Visual Dyslexia, J. F. Stein, Ed. Macmillan. London.

Alertness: Vigilance and Wakefulness in Developmental Disorders of Reading and Attention

DRAKE D. DUANE

Institute for Developmental Behavioral Neurology
Arizona State University
10250 North 92nd Street
Scottsdale, Arizona 85258

Wakefulness in adults is associated with stable ocular pupil size that may be quickly assessed quantitatively by pupillometry.[1] Some developmental disorders are speculated to be associated with disordered vigilance.[2] We have previously shown in a large pool of developmentally disabled students of elementary through college age a high frequency of pupillary instability.[3] This study investigates the relationship between attention/reading disorder, daytime wakefulness, and behavioral as well as physiologic measures of vigilance.

Fifty children (41M/9F) between 10 and 15 years of age (mean 12; SD 1.84) met DSM-III-R diagnosis of attention deficit hyperactivity disorder (ADHD) and/or developmental disorder of reading (RD). In addition to psychometric evaluation, a routine EEG supplemented by computer-assisted topographic mapping and auditory N-100/P-300 evoked potential studies (Bio-logic Systems Corp., Mundelein, Illinois), all subjects underwent quantitative measurements of pupil size and stability utilizing monocular pupillometer (Micromeasurements, Farmington, Connecticut). Subjects were initially drug free. After three minutes of dark adaptation, a 10-minute recording was performed between noon and 4:00 P.M.

Moderate or severe pupillary instability assessed semiquantitatively was observed in 11 of 32 ADHD only (34 percent), 8 of 15 ADHD + RD (53 percent), and 1 of 3 RD only (33 percent). Daytime drowsiness, despite adequate nocturnal rest, correlated moderately with cognitive impairment on the Letter Cancellation Task and prolonged N-100/P-300 latency.

The N-100/P-300 latencies in the 50 patients diagnosed as ADHD and/or RD were contrasted with 20 control subjects between ages 9 and 15 years of age (mean 12; SD 1.9) without personal or family history of developmental disorder. Study subjects displayed significantly longer P-300 latency (mean = 329.6 ms; SD = 32.96; Mann-Whitney U $P < 0.001$) compared to the controls (mean = 292.3 ms; SD = 14.13). Additionally, these patients displayed longer N-100 latency (mean = 108.8 ms; SD = 24.60; Mann-Whitney U $P < 0.001$) compared to the control group (mean = 87.0 ms; SD = 8.35). Among the study subjects, the most common alteration was a prolonged (>320 ms) P-300 latency, which was observed in 31, followed by prolonged (>100 ms) N-100 latency, noted in 25 of the 50 subjects.

Baseline cognitive and pupillary observations were contrasted with cognitive performance and pupillary stability following protocol acute dosages of alerting compounds. Improved wakefulness marked by improved pupillary stability was commonly but not invariably associated with improved cognitive performance. This paradigm permits accurate prediction of clinical response to pharmacologic intervention.

Overall, these studies suggest that a common feature of developmental disorders of attention is cognitive impairment of vigilance with which there is a not uncommon correlate of impaired alertness and a common correlate of prolonged physiologic latency. These observations are consistent with the conference theme of disordered temporal processing in developmental disorders.

ACKNOWLEDGMENT

Statistical analysis performed by Cary Chivalier, Ph.D.

REFERENCES

1. Yoss, R. E., N. J. Moyer & K. N. Ogle. 1969. The pupillogram and narcolepsy: A method to measure decreased levels of wakefulness. Neurology **19:** 921–928.
2. Weinberg, W. A. & R. A. Brumback. 1990. Primary disorder of vigilance: A novel explanation of inattentiveness, daydreaming, boredom, restlessness and sleepiness. J. Pediatr. **116:** 720–725.
3. Duane, D. D. & L. Y. Epcar-Zigler. 1991. Pupillometry, sleepiness and vigilance in developmental disorders. Neurology, Suppl. 1 **41:** 236.

Dyslexia: A Study of Preserved and Impaired Visuospatial and Phonological Functions

G. F. EDEN,[a,c] J. F. STEIN,[a] M. H. WOOD,[b]
AND F. B. WOOD[b]

[a]*University Laboratory of Physiology*
Parks Road
Oxford OX1 3PT, England

[b]*Section of Neuropsychology*
Bowman Gray School of Medicine
Winston-Salem, North Carolina 27157-1043

In a preliminary study[1] we showed for a small sample of children, that oculomotor and visuospatial as successfully as phonological tests differentiate reading-disabled from normal children. We now present results from a larger sample of children that confirm our previous findings. We compared the phonological and visuospatial abilities of the following groups of children (mean age 11.3 years), selected from a larger epidemiological sample of normal ($n = 485$) and poor reading ($n = 295$) children from the Bowman Gray Learning Disability Project: Normal (N) children ($n = 39$): selected from those in the normal sample, whose reading ability at the fifth grade level was between 85 and 115 on the Woodcock-Johnson standardized score and whose IQs on the WISC was between 85 and 115; reading-disabled (RD) children ($n = 26$): selected from the poor reading sample; whose reading ability was below 85 on the Woodcock-Johnson standardized score, but whose IQs were normal (85–115); backward readers (BR): also selected from the poor reading sample, but whose reading was below 85, and whose IQs on the WISC were also below 85 ($n = 12$). The N and RD groups were compared to see whether phonological and visuospatial tests could be used to discriminate between them. The BR's abilities were also compared with those of the RDs to determine whether differences in phonological and visual processing differentiate RDs from the BRs. The remaining children that did not meet any of the just stated three criteria ($n = 16$) were normal readers. They were included in order to extend the range of reading and IQ levels, providing a more representative population to correlate the visual with the phonological tests. In the tests for phonemic awareness mean scores of the RD groups were significantly worse than those of the Ns. This was true for the Test of Auditory Analysis Skills (third and fifth grade), Pig Latin correct score (fifth grade), and the Lindamood test of phonemic awareness in third grade, but not for fifth grade. The BRs performed significantly worse than the RDs on all three tests. Further, the RDs performed poorly in rapid naming in the third grade. They needed more time for Automized Rapid Naming of numbers and letters than the Ns. The RDs also had a significantly lower score for the Boston Naming Test at third grade and semantic (but not linguistic) Verbal Fluency at fifth grade. The BRs performed slightly better than the RDs in some of these tests, but not significantly. We found no significant

[c]To whom correspondence should be addressed.

TABLE 1. Means (and SE), Compared by Two-tailed t-test: Normals, Reading-Disabled, and Backward Readers on Temporal and Spatial Dots, Fixation Tasks, and Eye-Movement Recordings

VISUAL TESTS	5th Grade	
means and t-test of:	Normals Reading Disabled	Reading Disabled Backward Readers
DOTS		
Temporal Dots Number of correct answers (out of 12)	••• $p<0.0015$ N: n=39 5.18 (0.39) RD: n=26 3.35 (0.35)	ns BR: n=12 4.33 (0.58)
Spatial Dots Number of correct answers (out of 12)	• $p<0.0773$ N: n=39 6.26 (0.41) RD: n=26 5.15 (0.46)	ns BR: n=12 5.50 (0.70)
INDIRECT FIXATION		
Dot Localisation /Fixation Points scored correct	•• $p<0.0168$ N: n=39 240.00 (6.7) RD: n=26 223.15 (6.2)	ns BR: n=12 210.67 (22.99)
Vertical Tracking Number of errors (out of 18)	•• $p<0.0337$ N: n=38 1.03 (0.19) RD: n=26 1.85 (0.36)	ns BR: n=12 1.42 (0.31)
Completion Time (minutes)	ns N: n=38 1.79 (0.20) RD: n=26 2.27 (0.22)	ns BR: n=12 1.85 (0.21)
DIRECT FIXATION		
Fixation measured in degrees left eye	•• $p<0.0244$ N: n=38 0.66 (0.07) RD: n=25 1.12 (0.22)	ns BR: n=12 0.58 (0.09)
Divergence measured in degrees under synoptophore both eyes together	••• $p<0.0036$ N: n=38 6.71 (0.82) RD: n=26 3.44 (0.51)	ns BR: n=12 5.04 (1.45)

TABLE 2. The Means (and SE) Compared by Two-tailed t Test: Normals, Reading-Disabled, and Backward Readers on the Benton Judgement of Lines

Judgement of Lines means and t-tests of:	3rd Grade		5th Grade	
	Normals Reading Disabled	Reading Disabled Backward Readers	Normals Reading Disabled	Reading Disabled Backward Readers
JL Score	*** $p<0.0029$	ns	** $p<0.0127$	* $p<0.0597$
	N: n=39 10.92 (0.91)		N: n=39 14.69 (0.49)	
	RD: n=26 6.27 (1.23)	BR: n=12 4.58 (1.14)	RD: n=24 12.62 (0.63)	BR: n=12 10.09 (1.23)
Left vs. right Performance				
JL Left	** $p<0.0190$	ns	*** $p<0.0035$	ns
	N: n=39 72.67 (3.52)		N: n=39 86.49 (1.59)	
	RD: n=26 58.31 (5.06)	BR: n=12 53.41 (4.46)	RD: n=23 79.56 (2.53)	BR: n=12 71.08 (4.72)
JL Right	*	ns	ns	* $p<0.0643$
	N: n=39 71.16 (3.75)		N: n=38 82.81 (1.79)	
	RD: n=26 59.04 (5.14)	BR: n=12 51.92 (4.56)	RD: n=25 77.10 (3.09)	BR: n=12 65.28 (6.24)
Numbers of Reversals	ns	ns	** $p>0.0057$	ns
	N: n=38 5.49 (0.76)		N: n=38 0.03 (0.03)	
	RD: n=25 7.07 (1.48)	BR n=12 4.00 (1.13)	RD: n=25 1.28 (0.54)	BR n=12 1.67 (1.14)
Reversals				
Reversals at: affecting performance at:	3rd Grade		5th Grade	
	3rd Grade	5th Grade	3rd Grade	5th Grade
Left and right Performance:				
JL Left	ns	ns	ns	*** $p<0.0015$
JL Right	ns	* $p>0.0960$	ns	ns

Note: Overall test performance, left-versus-right performance, and tendency of right–left reversal in reporting the line segments and its influence on final score are shown.

differences between the N and RD groups for Verbal Memory, tested by the Prose Recall story and Rey Auditory Verbal Learning in third and fifth grades.

In a variety of visual tests (tested in fifth grade) RDs performed significantly worse than Ns (TABLE 1)—counting of rapidly repeated dots on a computer screen (Temporal Dots)—and were less severely impaired when the same number of dots were displayed simultaneously (Spatial Dots). Tasks requiring stable fixation were performed worse by RDs than Ns. These included the ability to judge visual direction when fixating a small dot on the computer screen, and control of their eye movements during vertical tracking of lines. Eye-movement recording confirmed larger fixation instability in RD subjects and lower amplitudes of divergent and, to a lesser degree, convergent eye movements. Depth perception (measured by the TNO test) was also reduced in the RD group. Unlike in the phonological tests, BRs were never significantly worse than RDs on any of the visual tests; indeed, some performed better.

We propose that while the verbal deficits are most likely to be attributed to left-hemisphere dysfunction, right-hemisphere impairment may be responsible for the visual impairments in these RD subjects. This theory is supported by our finding mild left neglect in the RDs. Not only did RDs show inferior performance on the Benton Judgement of Lines, but their performance was significantly worse on the left side compared to normals. Further, RDs had a higher tendency for right–left reversal when reporting orientation of line segments (TABLE 2). This suggests that RDs may use a right-to-left scanning strategy. However, this strategy was not associated with Attention Deficit Disorder (assessed using the Herjanic DICA), a condition that has been shown to affect other aspects of cognitive ability.[2] Further, RDs showed selective distortion of the left perceptual field when drawing clocks and geometric shapes such as the Rey Figure. Correlations for the entire sample between verbal ability and visual tests showed significant shared variance between the three tests of phonemic awareness and those examining fixation control (dot localization and vertical tracking), left neglect, as well as the temporal and spatial dot task.

These results therefore support the hypothesis that children with reading problems often suffer both phonological and visuospatial problems.[3]

REFERENCES

1. EDEN, G. F., J. F. STEIN & F. B. WOOD. 1992. Visuospatial ability and language processing in reading disabled and normal children. *In* Facets of Dyslexia and Its Remediation. Studies in Visual Information Processing, S. F. Wright and R. Groner, Eds. North-Holland/Elsevier. Amsterdam, the Netherlands.
2. FELTON, R. H. & F. B. WOOD. 1989. Cognitive deficits in reading disability and attention deficit disorder. J. Learn. Disabilities **22**: 3–13.
3. STEIN, J. F. & M. S. FOWLER. 1989. Disordered right hemisphere function in dyslexic children. *In* Brain and Reading, C. von Euler, I. Lundberg, and G. Lennerstrand, Eds.: 139–158. Macmillan. London.

Auditory and Visual Temporal Processing in Dyslexic and Normal Readers

MARY E. FARMER AND RAYMOND KLEIN

Dalhousie University
Halifax, Nova Scotia
Canada B3H 4J1

It has been suggested[1] that the phonological difficulties evidenced by many developmental dyslexics may be symptomatic of an underlying temporal processing deficit for any sounds that must be processed in rapid succession. Evidence from studies involving visual stimuli[2] suggests the possible existence of a temporal processing deficit in dyslexics in the visual modality. The current study investigated the possibility that temporal processing deficits in both the auditory and visual modalities coexist in severely reading disabled adolescents. Tasks were devised to assess ability at making judgments of numerosity, temporal order, and pattern sequence matching, using rapid presentation of stimuli, in both modalities. A visual task employing simultaneous presentation of pattern stimuli was included. It was hypothesized that the dyslexics would be impaired relative to the age-matched controls on the auditory and visual tasks involving sequential presentation, but not on the visual task involving simultaneous presentation. It was also hypothesized that scores

TABLE 1. Scores (and Standard Deviations) for Each Group on the Word Attack, Phonemic Awareness, and Auditory and Visual Tasks

	DYS	AM	RM	F
WATT	20.60 (8.31)	33.10 (4.84)	23.85 (8.08)	16.00[a]
ODD	14.70 (3.50)	16.95 (2.37)	16.60 (1.88)	4.12[b]
RHYM	17.00 (5.32)	22.90 (7.15)	18.15 (3.76)	6.27[a]
AUDAN	12.45 (4.93)	17.10 (4.50)	13.90 (3.48)	6.04[a]
CFUS (ISI in ms)	6.50 (5.52)	2.95 (2.21)	3.90 (3.78)	4.08[b]
ATOJ (% correct) (mean for all ISIs)[c]	80.37 (21.90)	96.55 (6.26)	87.05 (13.44)	7.27[a]
TONESEQ (% correct) (mean for all ISIs)[c]	88.17 (12.83)	92.30 (9.32)	87.99 (10.86)	2.11
FFUS (ISI in ms)	43.50 (8.13)	38.50 (13.49)	38.00 (8.34)	1.75
VTOJ (% correct) (mean for all ISIs)[c]	93.25 (11.10)	96.55 (6.55)	88.08 (17.17)	3.61[b]
MATSEQ (% correct) (mean for all ISIs)[c]	89.00 (13.58)	96.09 (6.81)	84.59 (14.35)	7.51[a]
MATSIM (% correct) (mean for both durations)[c]	91.38 (12.31)	96.63 (5.90)	92.25 (8.52)	3.63[b]

[a] $p < 0.01$.
[b] $p < 0.05$.
[c] Accuracy increased for all groups as ISI (or duration) increased. There was no significant ISI by group interaction.

TABLE 2. Correlation Matrix for the 10 Selected Task Variables for all Groups Combined

	READLEV	WATT	PHONAWAR	CISI	ATOJD	TSD	FISI	VTOJD	MATSEQD	MATSIMD
READLEV	1.000	0.739[a]	0.453[a]	-0.304[a]	0.444[a]	0.210	-0.073	0.325[a]	0.340[a]	0.032
WATT	0.739[a]	1.000	0.587[a]	-0.321[a]	0.483[a]	0.206	-0.174	0.355[a]	0.474[a]	0.023
PHONAWAR	0.453[a]	0.587[a]	1.000	-0.336[a]	0.378[a]	0.339[a]	-0.175	0.292[b]	0.433[a]	0.136
CISI	-0.304[a]	-0.321[a]	-0.336[a]	1.000	-0.155	0.045	0.221[b]	-0.027	-0.395[a]	-0.055
ATOJD	0.444[a]	0.483[a]	0.378[a]	-0.155	1.000	0.368[a]	-0.087	0.281[b]	0.399[a]	0.028
TSD	0.210	0.206	0.339[a]	0.045	0.368[a]	1.000	0.026	0.211	0.207	0.014
FISI	-0.073	-0.174	-0.175	0.221[b]	-0.087	0.026	1.000	-0.035	-0.053	-0.191
VTOJD	0.325[a]	0.355[a]	0.292[b]	-0.027	0.281[b]	0.211	-0.035	1.000	0.313[a]	-0.132
MATSEQD	0.340[a]	0.474[a]	0.433[a]	-0.395[a]	0.399[a]	0.207	-0.053	0.313[a]	1.000	0.345[a]
MATSIMD	0.032	0.023	0.136	-0.055	0.028	0.014	-0.191	-0.132	0.345[a]	1.000

[a] $p < 0.01$.
[b] $p < 0.05$.

on the visual and auditory tasks would be significantly correlated with each other and with scores on reading and phonemic awareness tasks.

Subjects were 20 dyslexic students (DYS), 20 age-matched normal readers (AM), individually matched for age and intelligence level, and 20 younger normal readers (RM), individually matched for reading level and intelligence. Mean ages of the DYS, AM, and RM groups were 14.07 (1.01), 14.10 (0.98), and 8.8 (1.37) years, respectively. Median single-word reading level for the DYS, AM, and RM groups, respectively, was 3B, 8E, and 3B (grade equivalent, measured by the Wide Range Achievement Test—Revised). Three auditory tasks were administered: a click fusion task (CFUS) to measure the interstimulus interval (ISI) required to perceptually segregate two clicks; a temporal order judgment task (ATOJ) with two high/low tones, and ISIs of 40, 120, and 360 ms; and a tone sequence matching task (TONESEQ), with two sets of four high/low tones and ISIs of 40, 120, and 360 ms. Analogous visual tasks used light flashes (FFUS), two meaningless symbols (VTOJ) with ISIs of 50, 100, and 250 ms, and two sets of four light flashes sequentially presented in a matrix (MATSEQ), with ISIs of 50, 100, and 250 ms. A further task, similar to the last, presented each of two sets of light flash patterns simultaneously (MATSIM), with durations of 100 and 400 ms.

Results for the three groups on all tasks are given in TABLE 1. A composite variable (PHONAWAR) was derived for the phonemic awareness tasks for use in a correlation matrix, along with scores representing the two reading tasks, the three auditory tasks, and the four visual tasks. This correlation matrix is shown for all groups combined in TABLE 2.

The results of this study provide qualified support for Tallal's hypothesis[1] of a temporal processing deficit in dyslexics for any rapidly presented auditory stimuli. Dyslexics required longer ISIs to perceptually segregate clicks, and were less accurate at perceiving the order of a pair of tones. They were not less accurate at making same/different judgments for sequences of tones, however. We speculate that the dyslexics may have been processing the sequences holistically (as rhythmic patterns) rather than sequentially. Support for a visual temporal processing deficit was equivocal. Dyslexics did not need longer ISIs to perceptually segregate two flashes. However, the range of ISIs may have been too broad, and the steps too gross, to capture subtle differences. Dyslexics were not less accurate at ordering two symbols. However, the trend was toward impairment. The finding that the dyslexics were impaired on the simultaneously presented pattern matching task was unexpected. However, the high correlation between MATSIMD and MATSEQD for the dyslexics ($r = 0.697, p < 0.01$) and the lack of any significant correlation for the other two groups, indicates that the dyslexics were using similar strategies for these two tasks. The possibility of a developmental resolution of a visual temporal processing deficit, at an earlier stage than that of an auditory deficit, must be considered.

REFERENCES

1. TALLAL, P. 1984. Temporal or phonetic processing deficit in dyslexia? That is the question. Appl. Psycholinguist. **5:** 167–169.
2. DILOLLO, V., D. HANSON & J. S. MCINTYRE. 1983. Initial stages of visual information processing in dyslexia. J. Exp. Psychol.: Hum. Percept. Perform. **9:** 923–935.

Event-related Potentials and Dyslexia

A. J. FAWCETT,[a] A. K. CHATTOPADHYAY,[b]
R. H. KANDLER,[b] J. A. JARRATT,[b]
R. I. NICOLSON,[a] AND M. PROCTOR[a]

[a]*Department of Psychology*
Post Office Box 603
University of Sheffield
Sheffield S10 2 UR
United Kingdom

[b]*Royal Hallamshire Hospital*
Sheffield S10 2 JF
United Kingdom

Developmental dyslexia is conventionally defined as "a disorder in children who, despite conventional classroom experience, fail to attain the language skills of reading, writing and spelling commensurate with their intellectual abilities." There is evidence that dyslexic children are slow in a number of language-related tasks.[1] Recently, however, speed deficits have been discovered[2] even in selective choice reaction time (SCRT) to one of two pure tones (the subject had one response key only, and had to press it only on hearing the low tone). By contrast, the dyslexic children performed at normal levels on a simple reaction time (SRT) task to the target tone. The authors suggested that dyslexic children showed speed deficits from two sources—slowness of access to the lexicon together with general slowness of stimulus categorization—but the evidence was necessarily indirect.

In principle, event-related potentials (ERP) offer the potential for identifying whether this slowing is attributable entirely to stimulus categorization problems, or whether there is some response selection component. In ERP research, a set of electrodes is attached to selected points on the subject's skull, and the electrical activity following some external event (presentation of a stimulus) is then monitored. SCRTs have been extensively studied using ERPs, and there is a robust finding that in these types of task the ERP trace shows a broad, positive component, peaking around 300 ms, and this peak is known as the P300 (or alternatively as P3). Both the origin and the functional role of the P300 remain active research frontiers.[3] There has been extensive research on the antecedent conditions for the P300. Although the P300 amplitude has been most researched, the P300 latency is of more direct relevance here, in that the latency is thought to provide an index of stimulus classification speed uncontaminated by response selection factors.[4]

Eleven subjects, 6 dyslexic and 5 control, were selected from our older panels of dyslexic and control 16-year-old children, and participated in the experiment with full, informed consent. They were paid for participation. All children had an IQ of 90 or above, and had no known emotional or neurological problems. The dyslexic children had been clinically diagnosed as dyslexic several years previously, and all had a reading age of at least 18 months lower than their chronological age, whereas the controls were all reading at or around their age. Furthermore, availability of their SRT and SCRT allowed us to match the groups on SRT. Mean data for the dyslexics and controls were 15.6 versus 15.5 years chronological age; 111 versus 107 for IQ (WISC-R); 12.3 versus 15.0 reading age (Schonell); 23.8 versus 25.0 SRT (cs); and 42.5 versus 27.8 SCRT (cs).

The experiments were conducted using a Nicolet Pathfinder II system that was programmed to deliver binaural pure tone stimuli in an "oddball" SCRT paradigm. Subjects were requested to respond only to the rare tone (4000 Hz) and not to the frequent tone (1000 Hz). Potentials recorded within 750 ms after stimulation were averaged separately for the frequent and rare tones. Samples contaminated by excessive artifact were automatically rejected. To ensure reproducibility, two consecutive series comprising 20 percent rare and 80 percent frequent tones, presented in a pseudorandom sequence, were averaged until 100 artifact-free samples had been collected. In one dyslexic subject it was impossible to generate artifact-free data, and the results were excluded from the analysis. Recordings were made using Ag/AgCl electrodes. Skin–electrode impedances were less than 5 kohm. Potentials were recorded from Cz (10–20 system) referred to linked mastoids. An earth was located at Fpz. Subjects reclined in a comfortable chair, with their eyes closed. They were asked to tap with their forefinger on hearing the rare tone. Recording and analysis were carried out by clinicians who were unaware of the subjects' diagnoses. An experimenter who knew the children was present in a support role.

Latencies to the N1 and P2 peaks were measured for the frequent tones, and to the N2 and P3 (P300) peaks for the rare tones. The amplitude differences between these peaks were also measured, namely N1–P2 and N2–P3. FIGURE 1 shows representative traces for a dyslexic and a control subject. The individual latency data are plotted in FIGURE 2. The clinicians attempted to separate the groups on the basis of the individual data. By ranking the P3 (rare) latencies, all ten subjects were correctly assigned between the two categories. Ranking of amplitudes did not provide a separation between the groups. Mann-Whitney statistical analysis revealed two significant differences between the groups, namely that the dyslexic group had significantly longer N2 (rare) and P3 (rare) latencies [$z = 2.19, p < 0.05$ and $z = 2.61, p < 0.01$, respectively]. Student's t-test carried out on the latency measurements gave similar results [$t(8) = 2.48, p < 0.05$ and $t(8) = 5.59, p < 0.001$, respectively]. Correlations between ERP components and the prior SRT and SCRT data were then determined. Of particular interest was the high correlation with dyslexia of the P300

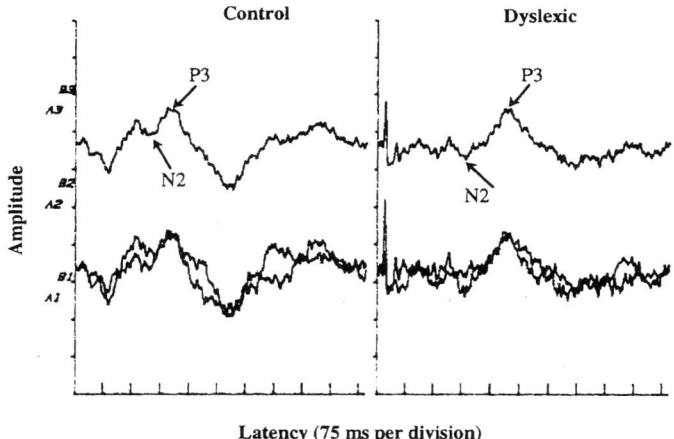

FIGURE 1. ERP traces for a control child and a dyslexic child for the rare stimulus.

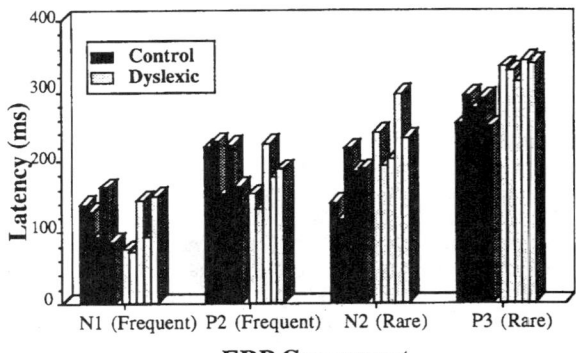

FIGURE 2. Individual latency data.

(rare) latency ($r = 0.89$). Several ERP measures correlated moderately highly with SCRT latency, but not SRT latency, with the P300 (rare) having correlations of 0.69, −0.34, respectively.

Before considering the interpretation of the results, it is important to attempt to relate them to the large and variable extant literature on ERPs and dyslexia. Surprisingly, there appear to be few other direct investigations of P300 latency in the dyslexia literature. Researchers have focused on topics such as the cortical distributions of ERPs and dyslexia;[5] the amplitude of the P300,[6] or its latency in linguistically based tasks.[7] The only directly comparable study,[8] using an auditory oddball paradigm, found significantly slower P300 latency in the dyslexic group and lower amplitudes (though only significantly lower for the Pz electrode). The present study therefore replicates and extends these findings.

In summary, the group of dyslexic children showed a temporal processing speed deficit compared with same-age controls in P300 latency in selective choice reaction to auditory tones. The differences between the groups were sufficient to allow a differential diagnosis purely on the basis of the ERP data. Furthermore, the latencies correlated highly with selective choice reaction latencies obtained in earlier experimentation. The data provide convergent evidence that the deficit is not attributable to motor response selection or execution, and appears to be linked to the need to make a discrimination between stimuli. This is particularly significant in that it provides further evidence that dyslexic children have a deficit in response categorization even for nonlinguistic stimuli.

REFERENCES

1. DENCKLA, M. B. & R. G. RUDEL. 1976. Rapid 'Automatized naming (R.A.N.). Dyslexia differentiated from other learning disabilities. Neuropsychologia **14:** 471–479.
2. NICOLSON, R. I. & A. J. FAWCETT. 1992. Reaction times and dyslexia. Q. J. Exp. Psychol.: Hum. Exp. Psychol. In press.
3. WOODWARD, S. H., W. S. BROWN, J. T. MARSH & M. E. DAWSON. 1991. Probing the time-course of the auditory oddball P3 with secondary reaction time. Psychophysiology **28:** 609–618.

4. COLES, M. G. H., G. GRATTON & M. FABIANI. 1990. Event-related brain potentials. *In* Principles of Psychophysiology: Physical, Social and Inferential Elements, J. T. Cacioppo and L. G. Tassinary, Eds. Cambridge Univ. Press. Cambridge, England.
5. DUFFY, F. & G. MCANULTY. 1990. Neurophysiological heterogeneity and the definition of dyslexia: Preliminary evidence for plasticity. Neuropsychology **28**: 555–571.
6. KLORMAN, R. 1991. Cognitive event-related potentials in attention deficit disorder. J. Learn. Disabilities **24**: 130–140.
7. TAYLOR, M. J. & N. K. KEENAN. 1990. Event-related potentials to visual and language stimuli in normal and dyslexic children. Psychophysiology **27**: 318–327.
8. ALONSO, T. O., M. NAVARRO & E. V. ABAD. 1990. P300 component of the auditory event-related potentials and dyslexia. Funct. Neurol. **5**: 333–338.

Left Hemisphere Specialization for Auditory Temporal Processing in Rats[a]

ROSLYN HOLLY FITCH, CHRISTINE P. BROWN,
AND PAULA TALLAL

Center for Molecular and Behavioral Neuroscience
Rutgers University
Newark, New Jersey 07102

The existence of asymmetry in the human brain is well established, particularly left hemisphere specialization for language processing. Reports of left hemisphere specialization for acoustic processing in nonhuman species have also accumulated. We have demonstrated a right ear advantage (REA) in male rats for the discrimination of 2-tone sequences. The current study was designed to (1) further assess the effects of repeated testing on this REA, and (2) assess the effect of "speeding up" stimulus presentation on the REA, based on studies that have shown a stronger REA in humans for consonants containing rapid formant transitions as compared to these same stimuli when extended by computer.

Three adult male rats were tested in an operant conditioning apparatus designed to allow shaping of subjects through a series of phases culminating in a Go/No-Go target identification task. Subjects were required to discriminate among four twotone sequences by pressing an illuminated button following presentation of their target (either a high–low or low–high tone sequence, with an interstimulus interval (ISI) of 250 ms) to get a water reward. Negative sequences included low–low, high–high, and the opposite mixed pair. The apparatus was custom designed to allow monoaural presentation of stimuli, with concurrent white noise presented to the contralateral ear. Subjects were tested for 18 sessions (one session per day), at which time the ISI between tones was shortened from 250 ms to 100 ms. Responses, ear of presentation, stimuli, and latencies to respond were recorded by computer.

Latencies to respond to target (hits) versus negative sequences (false alarms) were analyzed to assess auditory discrimination in the right versus left ear. Patterns of laterality and discrimination were assessed across days of testing, and before and after shortening of the ISI. Response latencies for the first 6 days (block 1) showed a near-significant REA, based on an interaction between response type (hits versus false alarms) and ear ($p<0.07$). This interaction has consistently been found to be highly significant for the first six days of testing in identical studies. Simple effects within the interaction showed that latencies to false alarms were significantly longer than for hits for the right ear ($p<0.009$) but *not* left ear. These four latency values were collapsed into a single laterality score for each subject for each block, with positive laterality scores signifying a REA (see FIG. 1). Analysis of laterality scores across blocks showed that laterality scores for block 1 were significantly higher than for block 3 ($p<0.05$), thus representing a decrease in the REA across the first 18 days (3 blocks) of testing. Laterality scores for block 5 were significantly higher than for block 3 ($p<0.05$), signifying a renewal in the REA after shortening of the ISI.

Discrimination scores were also calculated, and did not show any significant

[a]This research was supported in part by an award to one of the authors (R.H.F.) from the Rita Rudel Memorial Foundation, and by the National Institute on Deafness and other Communication Disorders Grant 1-RO3-DC1038 to two of the authors (P.T. and R.H.F.).

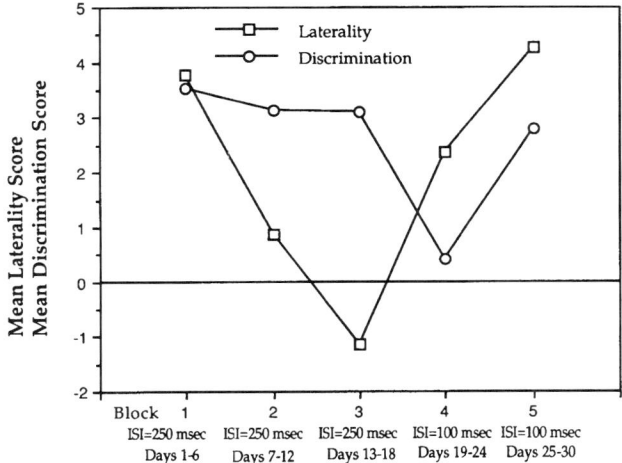

FIGURE 1. Laterality and discrimination as a function of day and ISI.

changes across blocks. The stability of overall discrimination level suggests that changes in the REA with repeated testing and reductions in the ISI cannot be attributed to changes in overall discrimination levels.

The current evidence of lateralization for auditory temporal processing in rats parallels mechanisms that have been demonstrated in humans. Combined results suggest the widespread cross-species existence of specialized mechanisms in the left hemisphere for processing auditory temporal information, which may in turn represent evolutionary precursors to lateralized mechanisms for speech perception in humans. The fact that the REA was reduced following repeated testing may reflect changes in the nature of the processing mechanisms underlying the task, and may parallel the effects of repeated dichotic testing with the same stimuli on humans. However, to our knowledge this has not been examined, since most REA scores are derived from a single dichotic listening session for humans. The fact that the REA was renewed by shortening the ISI emphasizes the interpretation that this REA is a reflection of lateralization for temporal processing mechanisms.

Differential Diagnosis between Learning-disabled and Dysphasic Children

J. FORTIN,[a,b] J. G. DUDLEY,[b] AND Y. JOANETTE[a,b]

[a]*Laboratoire Théophile-Alajouanine*
Centre de Recherche du Centre Hospitalier Côte-des-Neiges
4565 Chemin de la Reine-Marie
Montréal, Québec, Canada H3W 1W5

[b]*École d'orthophonie et d'audiologie*
Université de Montréal
C.P. 6128, Succursale A
Montréal, Québec, Canada H3C 3J7

INTRODUCTION

Two approaches have been proposed to classify subjects with developmental language and/or speech deficits. The first is based on different tasks to determine subgroups of children with reading impairment,[1] while the second is based on pre-established diagnostics to determine specific patterns of deficits.[2] The present study employs discriminant function analysis to identify patterns of verbal and nonverbal abilities in a population of children with developmental disorders divided into dysphasic, dyslexic, apraxic, and learning disabled, without major language disorder, subgroups.

METHODS

Subjects

One hundred and one native French speaking children, aged between six and twelve years, were selected if they were previously diagnosed by a multidisciplinary team as belonging to an identifiable subgroup (dysphasic, dyslexic, apraxic, or learning disabled), and if they were receiving specific educational treatment for their diagnostic categories. Children with low-performance I.Q. scores, who were unable to complete one or more tasks or who had more than one of the diagnostic categories, were excluded.

Material

All subjects were given a naming test, Franco-Quebecois adaptations of the Northwestern Syntax Screening Test (TSR) and of the fifth part of the Token Test (TJ-5), the Raven's Progressive Matrices, and a test of auditory perception (discrimination between /ba/ and /da/).

SUMMARY OF RESULTS

The dysphasic group made significantly more errors on the auditory perception task than did the learning-disabled and dyslexic groups. The learning-disabled group made fewer errors than all other groups. The apraxic children did not differ from the dysphasic and dyslexic groups. On the TSR, the dysphasic and apraxic groups had significantly lower scores than the other groups that did not differ between themselves. On the TJ-5, the dysphasic group had lower scores than all other groups. On the Raven's Matrices, the learning-disabled group had significantly higher scores than the other groups that did not differ between themselves. On the naming test (TDEN), the learning-disabled and dyslexic groups had the highest scores, and the apraxic and dysphasic groups had the lowest scores (TABLE 1). In the discriminant function analysis (TABLE 2), the token test (TJ-5) was removed and all other variables retained. Age was entered first to restrict age effect, and all other variables were then entered. The dysphasic and learning-disabled groups had the highest reclassification rate (100 percent and 98 percent). The dyslexic group had 77 percent, and the apraxic group 91 percent of correct reclassification.

CONCLUSION

These findings are in accordance with previous results in the literature.[2] The dyslexic group was the most difficult to identify. Future research should consider including other tests, such as the verbal visual scanning test proposed by Doehring,[3] in order to improve the reclassification of dyslexic subjects.

TABLE 1. Means, Standard Deviations, F and *Post Hoc* Results for Dysphasic, Learning-disabled, Dyslexic, and Apraxic Groups

		DYSP (Dysphasic)	LD (Learning Disabled)	DYSL (Dyslexic)	APR (Apraxic)	F	Post Hoc
Age (years)	$\bar{x}$	7.75	9.16	9.08	8.27	4.42	dysp < ld, dysl, apr
	SD	1.65	1.71	2.22	1.73		
TAP (test of auditory perception)	$\bar{x}$	12.91	3.76	8.77	11.55	19.89	dysp = apr dysp, apr > ld, dysl, dysl > ld
	SD	5.64	4.65	5.70	6.90		
TSR (test of receptive syntax)	$\bar{x}$	31.50	41.09	41.39	31.09	13.37	dysp = apr, ld = dysl, dysp, apr < ld, dysl
	SD	9.52	5.54	4.19	11.49		
TJ-5 (token test, part 5)	$\bar{x}$	59.06	80.53	77.08	75.82	12.34	dysp < ld, dysl, apr
	SD	18.39	14.41	15.22	11.63		
Raven Progressive Matrices	$\bar{x}$	20.41	25.98	20.85	18.36	8.97	ld > dysp, dysl, apr
	SD	5.41	5.52	7.44	5.87		
TDEN (naming test)	$\bar{x}$	40.94	47.64	47.46	37.46	8.14	dysp, apr < ld, dysl
	SD	8.83	7.73	6.86	6.15		

TABLE 2. Group Identification Using Discriminant Function Analysis of Selected Measures

Given by a Multidisciplinary Team	Identified by the Tests				
	Dysphasic	Learning Disabled	Dyslexic	Apraxic	Total
Dysphasic	32 100%				32
Learning Disabled	1 2%	44 98%			45
Dyslexic		3 23%	10 77%		13
Apraxic			1 9%	10 91%	11
Total	33	47	11	10	96% of correct re-classification

Variables: Age, auditory perception (TAP), test of receptive syntax (TSR), Raven Progressive Matrices, naming test (TDEN).

REFERENCES

1. DOEHRING, D. G. & I. M. HOSHKO. 1977. Classification of reading problems by the Q-factor analysis. Cortex 13: 281–292.
2. STARK, R. E. & P. TALLAL. 1988. Language, Speech, and Reading Disorders in Children: Neuropsychological Studies, R. J. McCauley, Ed. College-Hill Press. Boston, Mass.
3. DOEHRING, D. G. 1973. Patterns of Impairment in Specific Reading Disability: A Neuropsychological Investigation. Indiana Univ. Press. Bloomington, Ind.

Do Adult Dyslexics Show Low-level Visual Processing Deficits?

S. HAYDUK,[b] M. BRUCK,[a,b] AND P. CAVANAGH[c]

[b]Department of Psychology
McGill University
1205 Dr. Penfield Avenue
Montreal, Quebec H3A 1B1
Canada
[c]Department of Psychology
Harvard University
Cambridge, Massachusetts 02138

INTRODUCTION

Some researchers claim that a deficit in low-level visual processing is a major factor in the etiology of developmental dyslexia.[1,2] According to this view, these visual deficits are specific to the transient pathway of the visual system; sustained pathway processing is intact.

The following results provide support for this hypothesis. Dyslexic children show poorer pattern contrast sensitivity, and poorer flicker contrast sensitivity than normal readers. These processing deficits are most prominent for low spatial frequency and high temporal frequency stimuli, which are processed by the transient system. Disabled readers do not differ from normal readers in the oblique effect, in orientation tuning, and in spatial frequency tuning; these findings are indicative of normal sustained pathway functioning.

Previous research in this field has focused on the dyslexic child. The objective of the present study is to determine if the transient pathway deficits persist into adulthood.

METHOD

Subjects

There were 17 dyslexic subjects with childhood diagnoses of dyslexia. These subjects had normal childhood IQ scores, but significant childhood word recognition and spelling deficits. At the time of this study, these adults were between 18 and 31 years of age. As adults they continued to show performance decrements on standardized reading and spelling tests. There were 18 normal reading subjects matched with dyslexics for age, gender, and educational status. Group characteristics and standardized test scores are shown in TABLE 1.

---

[a]To whom correspondence should be addressed.

TABLE 1. Background Information on Subjects

	Normal Readers	Disabled Readers
Age (years)	24	24
Percent male subjects	71	68
Education (years post high school)	3.0	3.0
Standardized Test Scores		
WRMT Word Recognition (%)	64	13
WRMT Word Attack (%)	76	20
WRMT Read Comprehension (%)	85	47
WRAT Spelling (%)	78	11
PPVT-IQ	110	90
Culture Fair Test IQ	108	97

Stimuli

The stimuli consisted of sine wave gratings and sine wave annuli (rings). The luminance of alternate bars of the stimuli flickered in counterphase. The spatial frequency (high—33 Hz versus low—2 Hz), temporal frequency (high—12 cpd versus low—2 cpd), and placement (foveal versus peripheral) of the stimuli were varied. A yes/no detection task was used to measure the minimum amount of contrast required to perceive alternating bars in the stimuli (i.e., the contrast threshold) on 75 percent of the trials.

There were six conditions: (1) foveal placement control: low temporal frequency/low spatial frequency; (2) foveal placement sustained: low temporal frequency/high spatial frequency; (3) foveal placement transient: high temporal frequency/low spatial frequency; (4) peripheral placement control: low temporal frequency/low spatial frequency; (5) peripheral placement sustained: low temporal frequency/high spatial frequency; (6) peripheral placement transient: high temporal frequency/low spatial frequency.

Procedures

The stimuli were presented on a Macintosh computer. Each of the six conditions was presented separately in random order. Gratings were presented for foveal placement; annuli were presented for peripheral placement. On each trial the stimulus appeared at a selected level of contrast for 105 ms. Subjects indicated whether they detected the alternating bars.

Hypotheses

Both groups were expected to show higher contrast thresholds from foveal to peripheral vision. Dyslexics were predicted to show higher contrast thresholds than normal readers in the transient conditions only.

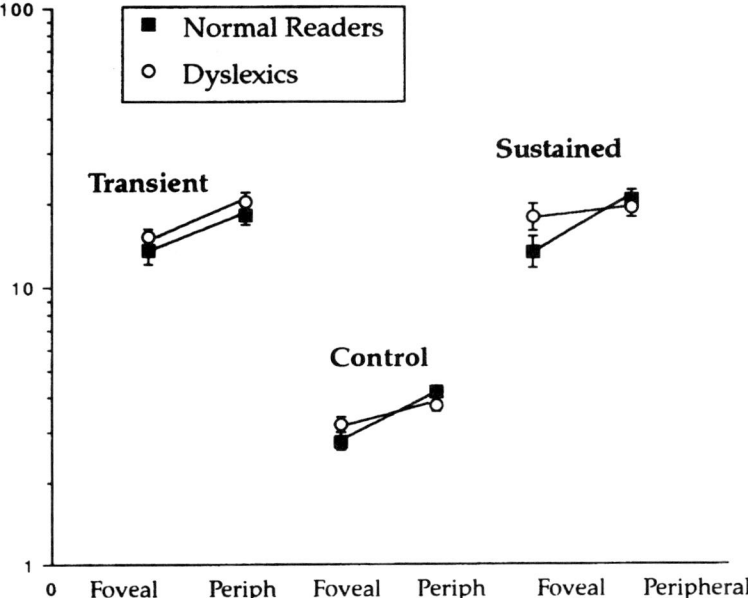

FIGURE 1. Contrast thresholds of normal readers and dyslexics.

RESULTS AND DISCUSSION

The results are presented in FIGURE 1. As predicted, both groups showed higher contrast thresholds in peripheral vision than foveal vision. The dyslexics' contrast thresholds were higher than those of control subjects for only one of six tasks (the foveal placement sustained condition); this is not consistent with any predictions of the model.

Thus, transient pathway deficits do not characterize adults with childhood diagnoses of dyslexia. The results suggest that either low-level transient deficits do not persist into adulthood or that previous work with dyslexic children reflects performance factors (e.g., vigilance, decision criteria) rather than early visual deficits.

REFERENCES

1. LOVEGROVE, W., R. GARZIA & S. NICHOLSON. 1990. Experimental evidence for a transient system deficit in specific reading disability. J. Am. Optometric Assoc. **61:** 137–146.
2. LOVEGROVE, W., R. MARTIN & W. SLAGHUIS. 1986. A theoretical and experimental case for a visual deficit in specific reading disability. Cognitive Neuropsychol. **3:** 225–267.

Visual Word Recognition in Developmental Dysgraphia: One Lexicon or Two?

JAMES M. HODGSON[a,b] AND GRETCHEN JOHNSON

Institute of Health Professions
Massachusetts General Hospital
Boston, Massachusetts 02114

INTRODUCTION

Abstract orthographic representations are often accorded two important roles in written language processing. In reading, they support "direct" visual word recognition, obviating the need for prelexical conversion of orthographic strings to phonological form. Among the kinds of evidence adduced in support of that role are demonstrations that spelling-sound regularity effects are limited to relatively uncommon words.[1] In spelling, orthographic representations provide the word-specific graphemic information that permits accurate production despite the complex relationship between sublexical phonological elements and graphemes found in deep orthographies like English. Though both of these phonology-independent lexical representations have been labeled "orthographic," it remains unclear whether they reside in separate input and output lexicons or are stored in a single central repository.[2]

Developmental dysgraphia is a condition in which individuals experience significant and persistent difficulty in developing normal spelling skills. Their lexical productions are replete with phonologically plausible errors (e.g., *curtious, preshious, museam*). This pattern of performance suggests specific difficulty in forming output orthographic representations, leading to an inordinate reliance on phonological recoding. The data reported here assess whether this profile of impaired orthographic processing with an unusual reliance on recoding is characteristic of their reading as well. Though the issue of one versus two orthographic lexicons is too complex to be adequately addressed by a single experiment of the sort reported here,[2] it is worth noting that, other things being equal, a single orthographic store model would expect relatively symmetrical impairments of function in orthographic reading and spelling.

METHODS AND RESULTS

A group of 24 educationally successful adult dysgraphics and an age- and education-matched control group participated in two speeded pronunciation tasks, one

---

[a]To whom correspondence should be addressed.
[b]Current address: Graduate Program in Communication Sciences and Disorders, MGH Institute of Health Professions, 101 Merrimac Street, Boston, Massachusetts 02114.

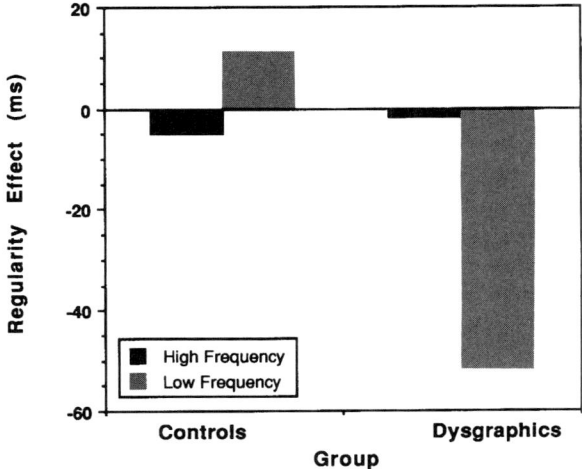

FIGURE 1. Regularity effects on naming latencies of dysgraphic and control subjects for high- and low-frequency words.

using words and the other, single-syllable pseudowords. Materials for the word naming task consisted of 144 one- and two-syllable words crossed for frequency and regularity. In a 2(Group) × 2(Regularity) × 2(Frequency) ANOVA, strong main effects of group and frequency were obtained [$F(1, 46) = 9.326, p = 0.004$; $F(1, 46) = 57.21, p < 0.001$]. Our primary interest lies in the interaction of the three factors [$F(1, 46) = 5.5, p = 0.023$]. Those data are presented in FIGURE 1. The control group produced the expected pattern: a small but significant regularity effect for low-frequency words, but no effect of regularity for high-frequency words [$F(1, 23) = 6.446, p = 0.018$]. The dysgraphic group also produced a marginally significant regularity by frequency interaction [$F(1, 23) = 3.961, p = 0.059$], but of an unexpected sort. Like the controls, they showed no effect of regularity for high-frequency words. For low-frequency words, however, there was a pronounced negative regularity effect.[c]

Could this negative effect of regularity for low-frequency words be due to a few subjects with seriously impaired phonological skills? FIGURE 2 represents a plot of individual regularity scores for low-frequency items against the number of pronunciation errors made in the pseudoword naming experiment. A multiple regression analysis in which the effects of age and education were controlled showed that phonological skill could explain only 1 percent of the variance in regularity effects [$r^2 = 0.01$; $F(2, 20) = 0.2148$, n.s.].

---

[c]Elimination of the one subject whose negative regularity effect for low-frequency items was extreme resulted in a smaller mean effect (−23.6 ms), but a slightly more robust one statistically [$F(1, 22) = 4.232, p = 0.052$].

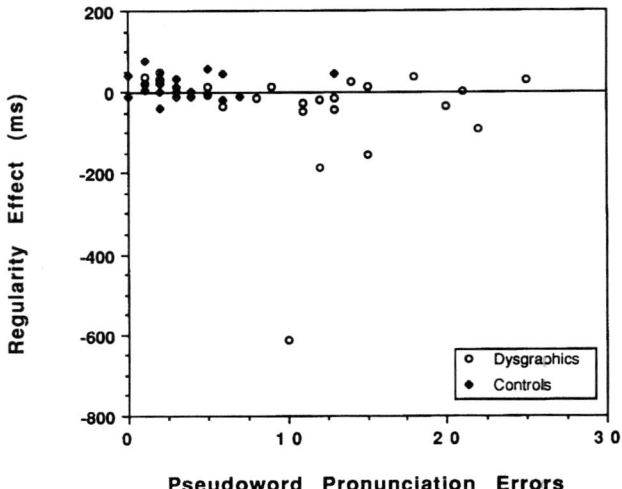

FIGURE 2. Regularity effects on naming latencies for dysgraphic and control subjects for low-frequency words as a function of pseudoword pronunciation accuracy.

CONCLUSIONS

These findings show clearly that the reading of developmental dysgraphics is quite different in character from their spelling. The absence of regularity effects for high-frequency words suggests that they are employing some form of frequency-sensitive input orthographic representation. The striking advantage for low-frequency exception over regular words suggests that phonological recoding plays a very small role in their reading. It may be that these words are recognized by means of some form of visually based representation that exploits the visual distinctiveness that correlates highly with exceptional spelling-sound correspondence.

REFERENCES

1. SEIDENBERG, M., G. WATERS, M. BARNES & M. TANENHAUS. 1984. J. Verbal Learn. Verbal Behav. **23**: 383–404.
2. COLTHEART, M. & E. FUNNELL. 1987. *In* Language Perception and Production: Relationships Between Listening and Speaking, Reading and Writing, A. Allport, D. Mackay, W. Prinz, and E. Sheerer, Eds. Academic Press. London.

Automaticity and Reading in Learning-disabled College Students

TERESA ANN HUTCHENS

Department of Educational and Counseling Psychology
University of Tennessee
Knoxville, Tennessee 37996-3400

INTRODUCTION

Speed of naming for rapidly presented serial stimuli, a measure of automatized processing, has been shown to discriminate learning-disabled (LD) and normal achievers.[1-3] Rapid automatized naming (RAN) and rapid alternating stimuli (RAS) are associated with speed of serial processing, tapping visual perception, and linguistic retrieval. The discriminability of RAN and RAS performance was examined in LD and normal college students. The impact of inhibition and attention assessed by a trigrams series was also examined.[4]

Subjects were undergraduate students (18–27 years, inclusive). The two groups ($N = 80$), the learning disabled, diagnosed at the college level, and the normal, demonstrating average achievement skills, were matched by age ($X = 21 - 10$), gender, and IQ ($\pm$ one $s_e m$). Intellectual functioning corresponded to the average to superior ranges for all subjects (PPVT-R, $\bar{X} = 105.55$). Each participant was tested individually on all tasks including expanded RAN, RAS, and trigrams measures.

Highly significant differences were found between the learning disabled and normal groups' response times for all RAN ($p < 0.01$) and RAS ($p < 0.001$) measures.

TABLE 1. Covariate-Adjusted Analyses of Group Differences

	Simple Difference Scores		Covariate-Adjusted (Co: Trigrams)	
	t Statistic[a]	p	t Statistic[a]	p
Rapid Automatized Naming Tasks				
Colors	4.72	0.0001[b]	2.91	0.0060[b]
Objects	5.66	0.0001[b]	4.65	0.0001[b]
Digits	4.62	0.0001[b]	3.62	0.0008[b]
Letters	4.70	0.0001[b]	3.65	0.0008[b]
Words	4.96	0.0001[b]	3.73	0.0006[b]
Rapid Alternating Stimulus Tasks				
Colors/Objects	4.34	0.0001[b]	2.90	0.0006[b]
Digits/Letters	6.15	0.0001[b]	5.22	0.0001[b]
Objects/Digits/Letters	5.32	0.0001[b]	4.12	0.0002[b]
Colors/Objects/Digits/Letters	5.70	0.0001[b]	4.35	0.0001[b]

[a]Matched records were analyzed as a single observation, with 40 matched pairs: df = 39.
[b]$p < 0.01$.

TABLE 2. Covariate-Adjusted Analyses of Group Differences on Reading Subtests of the Woodcock-Johnson Achievement Battery

	Simple Difference Scores		Covariate-Adjusted (Co: Trigrams)	
	t^a	p	t^a	p
Letter–Word recognition	−2.89	0.0062^b	−1.41	0.1670
Word attack	−2.79	0.0082	−1.21	0.2323
Passage comprehension	−0.91	0.3699	0.18	0.8550
Reading cluster	−2.96	0.0052	−1.35	0.1844

[a]Matched records were analyzed as a single observation, with 40 matched pairs: df = 39.
[b]$p < 0.01$.

Learning-disabled subjects consistently required a significantly longer time for serial naming of single- and cross-categorical stimuli than did their matched normals. Mean scores were also compared on the trigrams task (LD: $\bar{X}$(sd) = 22.65 (3.72); Normal: $\bar{X}$(sd) = 26.33 (3.35). A high level of statistical significance indicated relatively poorer performance of the LD group ($t = -4.29$, $p < 0.01$).

Significant differences on measures of reading skill (Reading Cluster, Woodcock-Johnson, Achievement) were also identified; however, when mean differences in RAN and RAS response times for the two groups were analyzed, results were no longer significant when the difference attributable to performance on trigrams was removed. Contrary to expectation, variance in speed of serial naming was not predictive of reading skill; regression equations were not significant. Differences between reading scores in LD and normal groups were explained by variability in the more attentional, inhibition task, trigrams, but not response speed in the naming paradigms. Results implicate broadly based processing deficits in the learning disabled, while specific deficits in reading may be more directly related to frontal lobe function.

REFERENCES

1. DENCKLA, M. B. 1972. Color naming defects in dyslexic boys. Cortex **8**: 164–176.
2. GESCHWIND, N. 1965. Disconnexion syndromes in animals and man. *In* Selected Papers on Language and the Brain, N. Geschwind, Ed. Reidel. Boston.
3. WOLF, M. 1986. Dyslexia, dysnomia, and lexical retrieval: A longitudinal investigation. Brain Lang. **28**: 154–168.
4. PASSLER, M. A., W. ISAAC & G. W. HYND. 1986. Neuropsychological development of behavior attributed to frontal lobe functioning in children. Dev. Neuropsychol. **1**: 349–370.

Naming and Gesture by Normal and Language-impaired Children: Evidence from a Modified Rapid Automatized Naming Test[a]

WILLIAM F. KATZ,[b,c] SUSAN CURTISS,[d]
AND PAULA TALLAL[e]

[c]Callier Center for Communication Disorders
University of Texas at Dallas
1966 Inwood Road
Dallas, Texas 75235-7298

[d]Department of Linguistics
University of California at Los Angeles
405 Hilgard Avenue
Los Angeles, California 90024-1543

[e]Center for Molecular and Behavioral Neuroscience
Rutgers University
Newark, New Jersey 07102

It is claimed that language- and reading-impaired children show interesting deficits in perceptual and motor development, particularly in processing rapid, sequentially presented information.[1-3] A task used to assess such deficits in reading-impaired children is the rapid automatized naming (RAN) test.[1] This test requires subjects to rapidly name symbols (e.g., letters, numbers, colors, objects) presented randomly in rows along a page. Relatively little research has investigated RAN performance by learning-impaired (LI) children. The present investigation examines whether deficits in rapid verbal processing characteristic of language- and reading-impaired children are deficits specific to rapid verbal behavior, or to rapid motor behavior in general.

A total of 67 LI and 54 age-matched control children were tested with the RAN and with a manual version of the RAN (RAN-manual), in which subjects were required to provide a nonverbal, pantomime response. Subjects also completed tests of rapid oral and manual sequencing skills, and standardized tests of reading ability. Each child was tested at 4, 6, and 8 years old.

The results (FIG. 1) show that LI children performed significantly poorer on both versions of the RAN in comparison with age-matched controls. Thus, for children tested at each of three ages, the RAN-manual test distinguished LI and learning-

---

[a]This research was funded by NS Grant 08176-01A1 to one of the authors (W.F.K.), by a grant, NINCDS-NS9, to another of the authors (P.T.), and by support from the MacArthur Foundation.
[b]To whom correspondence should be addressed.

TABLE 1. Pearson Product–Moment Correlations Comparing Oral, Motor, Manual, and Reading Tests with RAN-Verbal (V) and RAN-Manual (M) Speed of Performance

	Language Normal						Language Impaired					
	4 (n = 49)		6 (n = 53)		8 (n = 54)		4 (n = 37)		6 (n = 65)		8 (n = 66)	
Age in Years	V	M	V	M	V	M	V	M	V	M	V	M
Oral Motor												
Test type												
DDK single syllable	0.34	0.01	0.09	0.11	−0.13	0.01	0.36	0.15	0.21	0.14	0.03	0.20
DDK multiple syllable	0.31	−0.15	0.39[a]	0.16	0.21	−0.04	0.19	0.22	0.34[a]	0.10	0.29	0.11
Rapid word production	−0.02	−0.34	0.04	0.15	0.12	0.16	0.12	0.24	0.11	0.10	−0.02	0.23
Manual												
Finger opposition	0.23	0.06	0.15	0.13	0.31	−0.03	0.44[a]	0.52[b]	0.16	0.34[a]	−0.11	0.17
Coin-in-box	−0.05	0.06	0.15	0.24	0.13	0.09	0.34	0.57[b]	0.39[b]	0.31[a]	0.34[a]	0.33[a]
Reading												
Composite	—	—	0.36[a]	0.05	0.36[a]	0.08	—	—	0.36[a]	0.19	0.64[b]	0.32[a]

Note: DDK = Diadochokinesis.
[a] $p < 0.01$.
[b] $p < 0.005$.

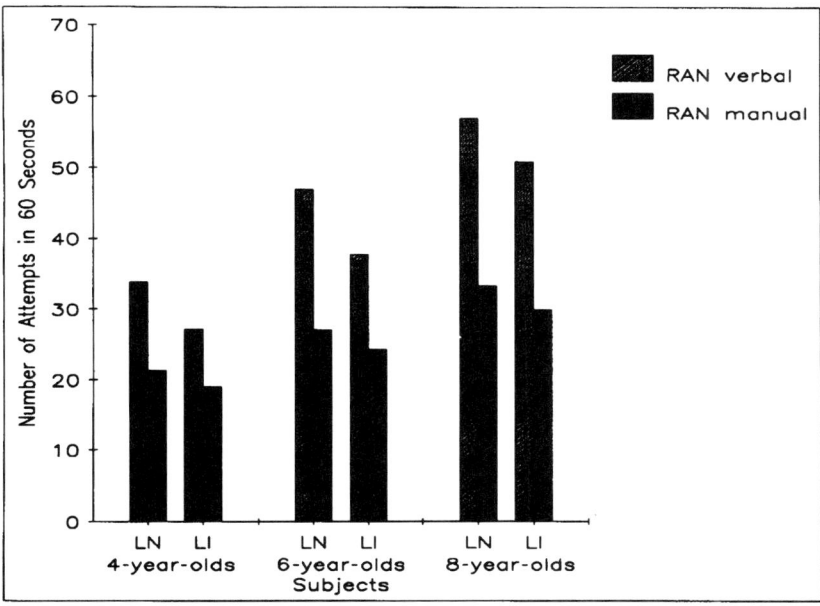

FIGURE 1. RAN-verbal and RAN-manual speed of performance. Data for language-normal (LN) and language-impaired (LI) children tested at ages 4, 6, and 8 years old.

normal (LN) performance as well as the RAN-verbal test. There was little relationship between RAN scores and tests of oral motor function (TABLE 1). However, a number of significant correlations were noted between RAN scores and tests of manual skills. Manual skills were significantly correlated with RAN scores for the LI children, but not for the LN children. Correlations between RAN scores and tests of reading ability were significant for normal and LI subjects, and were particularly high for 8-year-old LI children.

Although the present data must be considered preliminary, the results are consistent with the notion of a common deficit underlying both language impairment and developmental dyslexia; namely, impairment with rapid, serial behavior in timed identification (naming, pantomime) tasks. Additional experimentation should be conducted to clarify the exact processes (e.g., perceptual, phonological, memory-related, motoric) involved in this deficit.

REFERENCES

1. DENCKLA, M. B. & R. RUDEL. 1976. Rapid "automatized" naming (R.A.N.): Dyslexia differentiated from other learning disabilities. Neuropsychologia **14:** 471–479.

2. TALLAL, P., R. STARK & E. D. MELLITS. 1985. Identification of language-impaired children on the basis of rapid perception and production skills. Brain Lang. **25:** 314–322.
3. WOLFF, P., G. MICHEL & M. OVRUT. 1990. The timing of syllable repetitions in developmental dyslexia. J. Speech Hear. Res. **33:** 281–289.

An Investigation of Frontal Executive Dysfunction in Attention Deficit Disorder Subgroups

SARAH L. KEMP[a,b] AND URSULA KIRK[b]

[a]*Tulsa Developmental Pediatrics*
4520 South Harvard
Tulsa, Oklahoma 74135
and
University of Oklahoma College of Medicine
Tulsa, Oklahoma 74129

[b]*Teachers College*
Columbia University
New York, New York 10027

Children with attention deficit disorder (ADD) demonstrate problems that resemble frontal executive system dysfunction observed in adult frontal patients.[1] This study examined the hypothesis that performance on tests of frontal executive function (FEF) and posterior cortical dysfunction would distinguish 12-year-old males with medically diagnosed ADD from normal controls (NCs), and ADD subgroups from each other. Three groups of 20 subjects each were examined: ADD boys with no learning disability (ADDPure), ADD boys with reading and math disabilities (ADDRM), and NCs.. After one year's search, only ten boys could be located who met the criteria for the fourth experimental group, ADD with reading disability only (ADDR).

Discriminant analysis evaluated 33 variables and classified 94.29 percent of all subjects correctly as NC, ADDP, ADDR, and ADDRM on the basis of two functions: an Attention/Language function [Wilk's lambda (df 57) = 0.92, $p < 0.0001$], which explained 78 percent of the variance, and an Attention/Maintenance function [Wilk's lambda (df 36) = 0.32, $p < 0.002$], which explained 17 percent of the variance. With one exception, *The Boston Naming Test*,[2] performance on tests that loaded on these functions reflected FEF. Ninety percent of the ADDRs and the ADDRMS, 95 percent of the ADDPS, and 100 percent of NCs were correctly assigned to their predetermined groups (see FIG. 1 for the scatterplot).

Different patterns of performance distinguished NCs from ADDs, and ADD subgroups from each other. NCs were successful on all tests of FEF and posterior cortical function. ADDPs succeeded on the tests loading on the Automaticity/Language function, but were deficient on those loading on Attention/Maintenance: supraspan memory, accuracy in speeded addition, and shift/maintenance of set. In contrast, ADDRs succeeded on tests reflecting the Attention/Maintenance function, but were deficient on tests reflecting the Automaticity/Language function: solving word problems, rate of speeded math, linguistic fluency, and confrontation naming. ADDRMs' performance was deficient on tests across both functions. See TABLE 1 for standardized discriminant function coefficients for the selected variables. In addition, Univariate ANOVAs revealed that all ADDs were deficient in motor speed and that ADDRs were the most deficient. Although ADDRs were slower in accessing numbers, colors, and words than NCs, ADDRMs were slower only in accessing words.

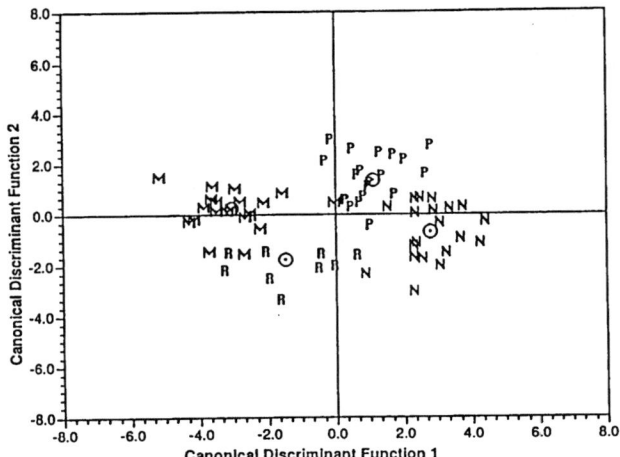

FIGURE 1. Scatter plot of normal controls, ADD pure, ADD reading disabled, and ADD reading and mathematics disabled with group centroids. (*Key*: N: normal control; P: ADD pure; R: ADD reading disabled; M: ADD reading and mathematics disabled; ◉: group centroid.

In conclusion, the results of this study indicate that ADD subgroups can be distinguished by different patterns of FEF deficits and that patterns of deficits may contribute differentially to their performance in school. Performance on these neuropsychological tests could provide a valuable clue to early identification of children with different types of ADD from among the 5–6 percent of children between ages 4 and 16 who are likely to be diagnosed as ADD each year.[3] Insight into the pattern

TABLE 1. Standardized Discriminant Function Coefficients of the Selected Variables

Standardized Canonical Discriminant Function Coefficients	
	Function 1
(P) Boston Naming total score	0.401
(F) Speeded addition aud–oral time	−0.905
(F) Speeded addition vis–written time	−0.302
(F) Lurian word problems—written correctly	0.764
(F) FAS—linguistic fluency—tot/3 min	−0.421
	Function 2
(F) WCST failure to maintain score	0.269
(F) Speeded addition aud–oral correct	0.337
(F) Rey A–V Learning combination (trials 1–5)	−1.422
(F) Trails B—time	0.900

Note: P = posterior test; F = frontal test.

of deficits exhibited by children, and in particular ADD subgroups, could lead to more effective interventions and compensatory methods for learning.

REFERENCES

1. LURIA, A. R. 1980. Higher Cortical Functions in Man. Basic Books. New York. (Original work published 1966).
2. KAPLAN, E., & H. GOODGLASS & S. WEINTRAUB. 1983. The Boston Naming Test, rev. ed. Boston University, Boston, Mass.
3. BARKLEY, R. A. 1990. Attention Deficit Disorder: A Handbook for Diagnosis and Treatment. Guilford Press. New York.

Deficits in Auditory Sequential Processing found for Both Gifted and Average IQ Reading-impaired Boys

R. HARTER KRAFT

Department of Applied Behavioral Sciences
Division of Human Development
University of California at Davis
Davis, California 95616

Identifying underlying processing deficits in the learning-disabled gifted has historically been one of the greatest challenges for educators and practitioners in the health sciences. Atypical laterality[1] and sequential processing deficits (e.g., reference 2) have been suggested as causes of these disabilities. The present study investigates these hypotheses by comparing the performances of age-matched elementary schoolchildren who were identified by their school psychologists as gifted-IQ[a] reading impaired,[b] average-IQ reading impaired, and gifted-IQ able readers on a battery of laterality, sequential processing, and cognitive tasks.

The results of within- and between-group comparisons of children's performances on the laterality measures do not support the atypical laterality hypothesis.[1] As reported in TABLE 1, the mean Edinburgh Inventory hand-preference score for all three groups indicated that most of the children were strongly right-handed. Children's mean performance for reporting back the dichotically presented verbal stimuli also indicated a robust right-ear advantage across groups: nonsense syllables $[t(100) = 9.58, p < 0.001]$ and digit stimuli $[t(100) = 6.16, p < 0.001]$. In addition, there were no significant between-group differences for any of the laterality tasks (see TABLE 1), nor did any of the laterally indices account for a significant proportion of variance when regressed on children's reading achievement scores.

There was support, however, for the sequential processing deficit hypothesis.[2] Compared to the gifted able readers, both reading-impaired groups demonstrated similar patterns on tests of sequential processing and short-term memory (see FIG. 1), which distinguished them from the patterns of performance found when these tasks were performed by gifted able readers. Specifically, both reading-impaired groups demonstrated a deficit in remembering and reproducing stimuli in the exact sequence heard, regardless of stimulus type, whether WISC digit span, $F(2,98) = 23.16, p < 0.001$) or "Morse code" sequences, $F(2,98) = 23.52, p < 0.001$. Regressing the digit span scores on the WRAT reading scores produced an R^2 of 0.358, $F(1,99) = 56.38, p < 0.001$. Regressing the auditory "Morse code" sequences produced an R^2 of 0.173, $F(1,99) = 20.68, p < 0.001$. When both of these scores were entered into the regression equation, the cumulative R^2 was 0.42 (i.e., accounted for 42

---

[a]Children were classified into IQ groups on the basis of their full-scale IQ scores on the WISC-R: gifted IQ = full-scale IQ scores > 130; average IQ = full-scale IQ scores between 90 and 110.

[b]Children were classified into reading groups on the basis of their Gray Oral Reading scores and their teachers' agreements with those classifications. Reading-impaired status was defined as reading at least 1.5 years below grade level. Reading-able status was defined as reading at or above grade level.

TABLE 1. Mean Age, Laterality, and Wide Range Achievement Scores[a] for Children Classified into IQ and Reading Ability Groups

Groups	n	Age	Laterality Scores[b]			Achievement z Scores			
			Hand	Eye	Syllables	Digits	Read	Spell	Math
Gifted-IQ able readers	40	9.31 (1.97)	0.71 (0.44)	0.60 (0.67)	0.15 (0.13)	0.08 (0.12)	1.00 (0.72)	0.77 (0.92)	0.40 (1.01)
Gifted-IQ impaired readers	21	9.35 (2.07)	0.77 (0.29)	0.24 (0.94)	0.15 (0.16)	0.07 (0.16)	−0.54 (0.42)	−0.37 (0.52)	0.25 (0.89)
Average-IQ impaired readers	40	9.69 (2.33)	0.76 (0.27)	0.35 (0.89)	0.15 (0.18)	0.08 (0.12)	−0.72 (0.50)	−0.58 (0.60)	−0.53 (0.93)

[a]Numbers in parentheses are the standard deviations.
[b]The formula used to compute each laterality score was $[(R - L)/(R + L)]$.

percent of the variance in the reading scores), demonstrating that a common component is shared among these three tasks. This significant relationship between digit span and reading achievement is consistent with findings from many other studies, as summarized by Naidoo.[3] Our findings are consistent also with Gould and Glencross's[2] conclusion that the underlying factor for this relationship is not verbal ability *per se,* because entering children's WISC-R verbal ability scores into the regression

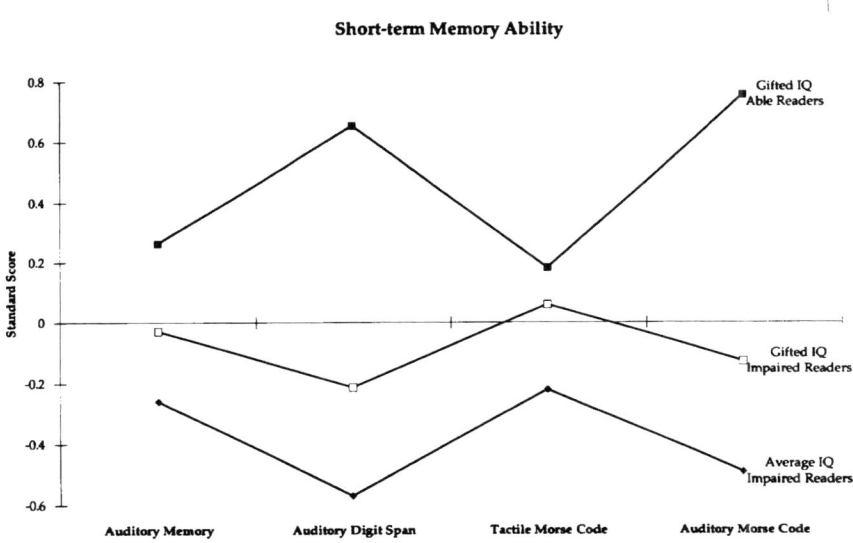

FIGURE 1. Graph illustrating children's mean performance on short-term memory tasks. The auditory memory task required that subjects remember and report back as many of the stimuli as possible, but the temporal order of the reproduction did not matter. The digit span and Morse code tasks require that the subject remember and reproduce the stimuli in either the exact order they were presented or backwards from the order in which they were presented.

equation with digit span produced an R^2 of 0.575, while the R^2 produced when entering the verbal ability scores alone produced an R^2 of 0.399. Thus digit span accounts for 17.6 percent of the variance in children's reading ability above and beyond their overall verbal ability.

The fact that the reading-impaired performed significantly better [t (60) = 2.55, p = 0.013] when asked to remember and report back auditorily presented digits in any order compared to being required to report the digits in the exact sequence heard suggests that the sequential processing component of these tasks was the significant factor rather than the short-term memory component *per se*. Regression analyses of the WRAT reading achievement scores provided further support for this conclusion. When entered into the equation alone, children's short-term memory scores for digits produced an 8 percent increase in R^2 [F (1,99) = 8.66, p < 0.005]. Adding digit span to the equation increased the cumulative R^2 to 0.36. Entering digit span alone in step one and then adding the short-term memory scores produced an R^2 of 0.36 in step one and step two. These results indicate that of the variance in children's reading achievement scores accounted for by their digit span scores, 8 percent represents a common short-term verbal memory component and 28 percent represents some other common components such as sequential processing. The fact that they did not show the same processing deficit when asked to remember and reproduce the tactilely presented "Morse code" stimuli further suggests that the specific underlying component reflected in these findings is an auditory temporal order and sequential processing deficit.

REFERENCES

1. GESCHWIND, N. & A. M. GALABRUDA. 1987. Cerebral Lateralization: Biological Mechanisms, Associations, and Pathology. MIT Press. Cambridge, Mass.
2. GOULD, J. H. & D. J. GLENCROSS. 1990. Do children with a specific reading disability have a general serial-ordering deficit? Neuropsychologia **28:** 271–278.
3. NAIDOO, S. 1978. The assessment of dyslexic children. *In* Dyslexia: An Appraisal of Current Knowledge, A. Franklin and S. Naidoo, Eds. Oxford Univ. Press. New York.

Toward Objective Measurements of Physical versus Mental Overload or Subjective Fatigue when Performing Sequential Eye Scanning and Reading Tasks

E. CHRISTINE KRIS

48 Garden Street
Cambridge, Massachusetts 02138

INTRODUCTION

Purposes and Methods

To differentiate between efficient versus problematic performance indicators on perceptual scanning tasks and reading, simultaneous vertical and horizontal binocular eye movement (EOG), bihemispheric brainwave (EEG), and cardiac (EKG) surface electrical recordings are made continuously during vestibular rotation and visual pursuit, as well as during self-initiated scanning eye motions during eye calibrations, sequential target tracking, picture recognition and naming, and word and sentence reading, to ascertain the *developmental learning level*, the *sensory and perceptual learning style*, that is, *sound-symbol* versus *visual pattern analytic-synthetic information processing*, leading to word and sentence decoding and encoding for meaning.

Performance efficiency is measured in terms of an ergonomic assessment of *work-load* (amount) and *mental-load* (difficulty) levels correlated to grade-level expectations.

Results

Combined EEG, EOG, and EKG provide continuous eye–brain, and heart interaction patterns that facilitate differential diagnoses of normal versus stressed and/or organic, pathological indicators of reading performance deficits with special reference to binocular oculomotor defocusing (attention gaps) versus oculomotor dysfunctions; regressions to correct versus inability to read and comprehend; scanning rate maintenance versus slowing of word and line reading; normal bihemispheric EEG recordings versus hypersynchronous, paradoxically slowed EEG discharges when mentally overloaded; and heart rate (EKG) irregularities during "stressed conditions." Case illustrations are provided.

METHODS OF RECORDING AND MEASUREMENT

Bidimensional, binocular EOGs using two pairs of nonpolarizable Ag/AgCl electrodes vertically and horizontally placed about each eye at one-half interpupillary distance, and bilateral, bipolar fronto-parietal and temporo-occipital EEG leads differentially input-coupled into a Beckman Type T 9-channel AC/DC portable electroencephalograph-oculograph with variable time constants, have been previously described. The EKG is recorded by means of two Beckman electrodes and a ground electrode, using the NASA "D" settings, with leads attached to the right shoulder, and below the heart at the left apex. More recently, a Cadwell-Schwarzer 14-channel fiber-optic, portable polygraphic recorder has been used with similar methods of electrode placement.

I. Comparison of simultaneously recorded binocular, bidimensional electrooculographic (EOG) eye scanning and bihemispheric bipolar electroencephalographic (EEG) response patterns during reading of mid-first, mid-second grade, and end of second grade paragraphs.

1. By a bright, normal first grade student;
2. By a 10-year-old dyslexic girl;
3. Comparison of EOG and EEG response patterns of the same 10-year-old girl during

    (a) Sequential encoding of the two lines of the Rey-Maze, showing slow and irregular eye scanning and normal, open-eye EEG traces.
    (b) EOG and EEG recording while decoding a two-line word sequence from a Gates grade 2.9 reading paragraph, showing that eye-scanning is irregular and unfocused eye-drift occurs while she attempted to decode a difficult word-sequence. During this episodic attention interruption the EEG presents paradoxical high-voltage hypersynchronized 5–7 c/s waves in the fronto-parietal bipolar derivations bilaterally, while 3 c/s slow waves appear in the right temporo-occipital bipolar derivation during the second half of the 6-s discharge.

        - We conclude that hypersynchronous high-voltage slow wave discharges represent a form of "paradoxical, light sleep-like withdrawal," similar to the paradoxical hypersynchronous high-voltage alphalike discharges in response to stimulation in organically depressed patients (see references 6, 7, and 12).
        - We further conclude that binocular oculomotor performance can be used as a telltale indicator of focused versus drifting attention in children and others who present with otherwise normal oculomotor functions; and that the reading rate (in numbers of seconds per graded line) and number of regressions for self-correction reflect decoding/encoding difficulties, while line-following problems reflect oculomotor problems. When EOG and EEG recordings are made simultaneously, it is possible to differentiate and correlate states of physical fatigue versus mental overload due to stimulus difficulty.

II. Simultaneous vertical and horizontal binocular EOG, and bihemispheric parieto-occipital EEG and heart-rate monitoring during slow reading for decoding and rereading for comprehension. (Subject: D. S. CA. 16 years, 8 months.)

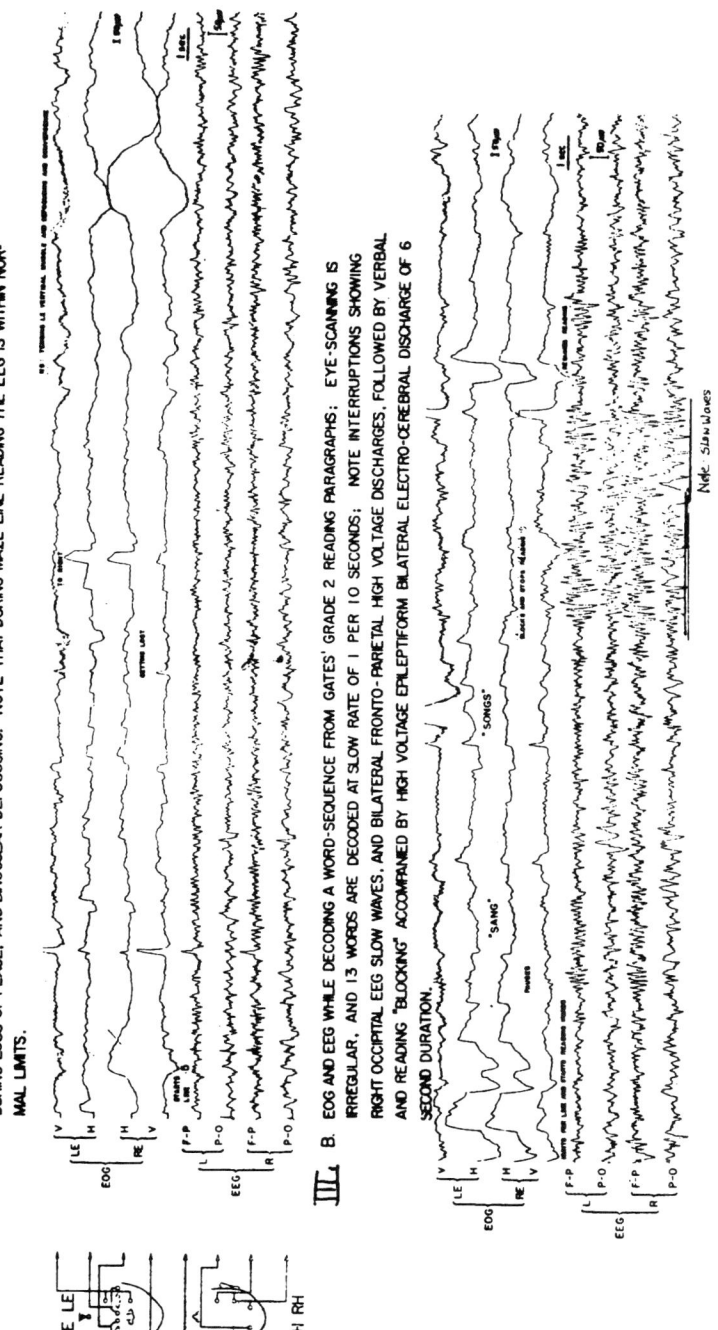

FIGURE 1. Simultaneous binocular, vertical, and horizontal eye-motion and bilateral EEG recordings showing continuous eye–brain interaction patterns of a 10-year-old dyslexic girl, while reading.

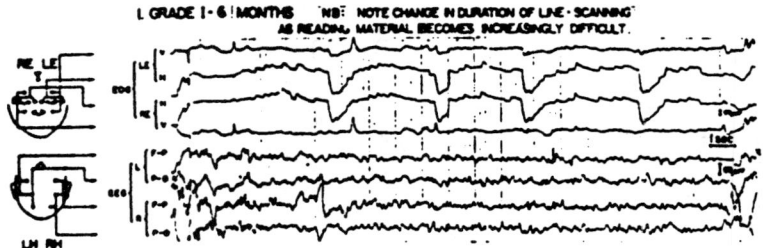
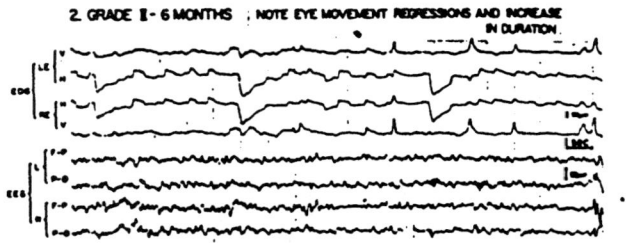
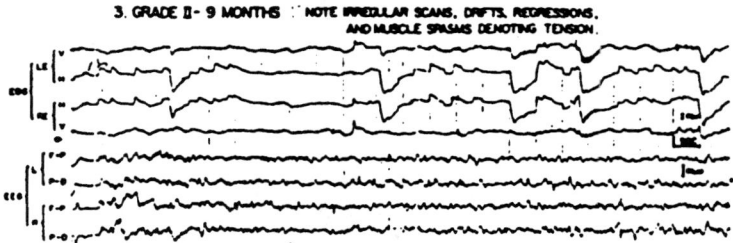

FIGURE 2. (a) Simultaneous binocular, vertical, and horizontal eye-motions and bilateral EEG recording of a 6-year-old boy of superior intelligence, showing eye scanning patterns during reading of Gates Gifted Paragraphs for Grade I—6 Months, Grade II—6 Months, Grade II—9 Months.

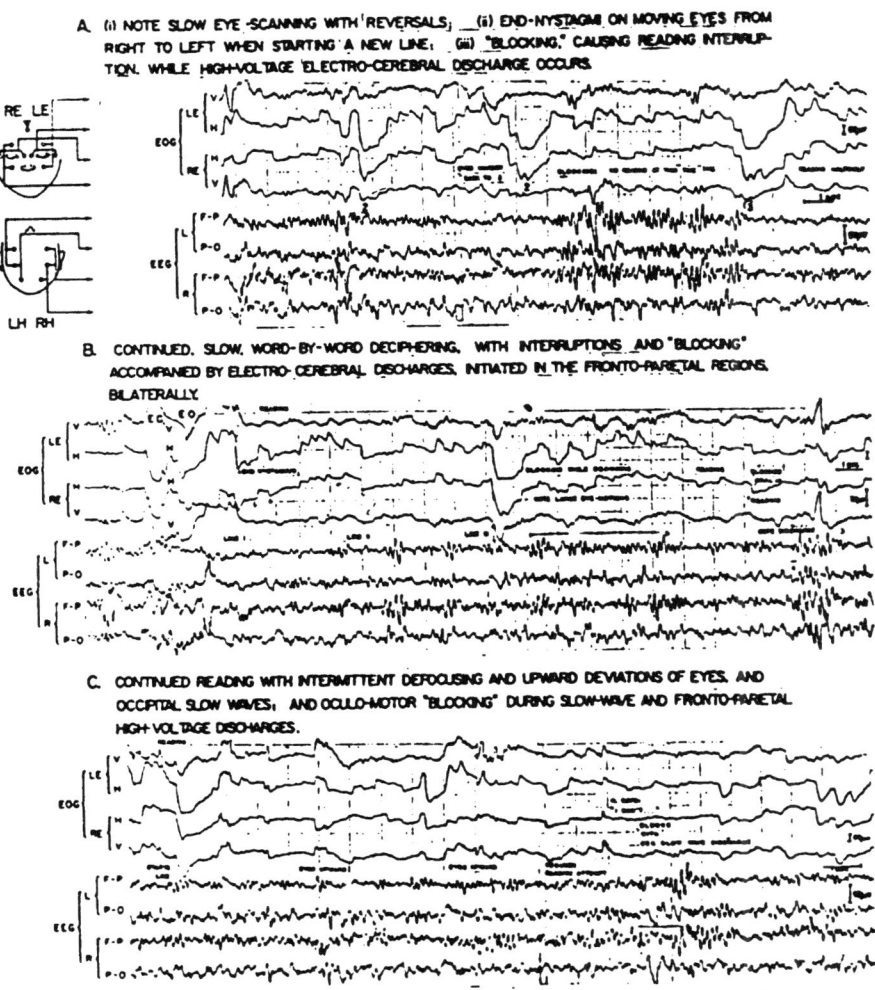

FIGURE 2. (b) Bidimensional binocular EOG and bilateral EEG recording, showing eye-motion and brain-wave activation during reading, in a 10-year-old developmental dyslexic girl.

D. S. was a right-handed, right-eye-sighting, underachieving, restless, irritable, and easily fatigued high school dropout of above average intelligence who was reluctant to be examined. No one had been able to help him before with reading and learning. He showed abnormalities in all three surface-electrical psychophysiological recordings during reading and vestibular rotation tests.

When first scanning 9 lines of a Spache Graded Reading Test, he used only his *right eye* during initial decoding, while the left eye drifted. When rereading the same text for encoding meaning, he used both eyes and scanned conjointly for 7 of the 9 lines. Then he blocked on a hard word, and presented midpoint fixation drift, and started to reread the entire paragraph, for better understanding. During the "blocking" episode, he presented high-voltage slowing in the left parieto-occipital EEG, which was generally abnormal due to irregular sharp-wave discharges. Also his cardiac record showed a flattened, irregular pattern, and he had three brief cardiac slowing episodes and one temporary cardiac arrest, from which he spontaneously recovered, during a 3-hour recording session. He was then treated both holistically and specifically, in a special hospital school environment.

III. Simultaneous bipolar, bihemispheric 6-channel EEG; heart-response pattern and rate analysis using the NASA "D" lead EKG settings; and binocular, bidimensional EOG 4-lead recording of eye-movements during reading. (*Note:* Slow reading, right eye intermittent drift, and cardiac arrhythmia.) (Subject: J. R. CA 12 years, 8 months, 11-17-1990.)

J. R. is a bright, normally intelligent, sensitive, motivated participant in school and social activities, but becomes easily physically fatigued and psychologically discouraged when school work, and especially reading tasks are too long and too hard. While placed in a seventh grade, he read fifth-grade-level texts and took from 5.5 to 7.5 seconds to read 5 word lines. He often lost his place and starting-point orientation, during binocular defocusing, which frequently occurred after left-hemisphere frequency changes and some EEG spiking in the left parietotemporal and occipital derivations. There was also occasional EEG flattening in these areas, followed by higher voltage beta-frequency sharp-wave discharges. Cardiac response-patterns were affected by stressful situations, such as mental overload during difficult reading tasks, and during the postrotation period after vestibular stimulation.

He presented with significant arrhythmias on inspiration–expiration, and with frequent premature heartbeats. His reading performance improved when he received new reading glasses and some line-following exercises that are helping him to overcome alternating visual suppression on binocular testing. He continues to suppress right-eye vision when his right eye drifts. A whole-line window was cut into a card that he could move over a given reading line, thereby reducing the confusing stimulus field of too many unfamiliar words and lines; he improved with tutoring and placement in a less competitive school. His cardiac condition was monitored by a pediatric cardiologist who recommended regular exercise such as noncompetitive running under supervision, and swimming. Recommendations were followed, and cardiac regulation has improved, as has cerebral blood-flow, which, in turn, lessened his tension states and EEG regulation, so that there are now longer periods of relaxed alpha states recorded. He continues to be monitored.

IV. Simultaneous monitoring of heart rate, horizontal binocular eye movements for left and right eye, and bihemispheric bipolar EEG, from left fronto-parietal and left temporo-occipital, and right fronto-parietal and right temporo-occipital derivations, are used to provide diagnostic indicators of correlated cardiac, oculomotor, and cerebral activation patterns during waking activities (reading) and during rest with eyes closed.

(a) Cardiac sensitivity is measured by heart rate changes, recorded by Beckman electrodes, using the NASA "D" leads. (*Note:* Heart rate increased to 96 beats/min while reading and 72 beats/min at rest.)
(b) Eye position and eye movement measurements during eye calibration, starting point search and location confusion (right for left), and poor oculomotor coordination and eye scanning while reading, necessitate following a pointer, and later her finger, to assist in line following.
(c) Studies of open-eyed and closed-eyed EEG response patterns. (*Note:* Extremely high-voltage discharges during the open-eyed place finding and reading tests in the right temporal, occipital area, while A is attempting to read "reading readiness words and phrases"; and high-voltage spike-wave discharges of focal epileptiform type when the eyes are closed and A is resting, in 1975 before being treated, and in 1977, after more than a year of anticonvulsant medication.

Subject A was an 8 year and 4 months old elementary school student when she first came to be examined at the M.I.N.D. Diagnostic Learning Center. She was extremely hyperactive, sadly depressed about her inability to learn in school, and sensitive about being in constant need of attention, structure, and support at home, among four other siblings.

She was treated neurologically, ophthalmologically, neuropsychologically, and psychoeducationally, and placed in a sheltered, small special education class in her own school district, where she began to thrive after one year of anticonvulsant medication trials (Clonapin yielded best results), and she was allowed to progress at her own pace. She is now a successfully integrated young adult, who is fully employed and enjoys being a contributor at home and in society.

CONCLUSIONS

It has become clear that the use of only single-system studies, that is, eye movements, brainwaves, or cardiac responsiveness mislead investigators in setting up paradigms for study and treatment, and hamper diagnosticians from arriving at appropriate diagnoses, treatment, and pedagogic remedial training.

Since individuals present with different areas of physical weaknesses that can put stress on mental and learning states, the responses to different stressors that mitigate against proficient performance need to be studied while individuals are being assessed and while remedial interventions are being planned. Learning levels, learning styles, and learning load (amount), and mental load (difficulty level) corresponding to developmental performance levels need to be assessed in conjunction with physical and psychological stress assessments to arrive at adequate and appropriate methods and materials to be used for treatment and for remedial education.

Because of the significant individual differences in intercorrelated patterns of responses to achievable challenges and detrimental stress conditions, the study of individual cases must precede the statistical study of subgroups. For this reason, only individual case studies are now being accumulated to arrive at a better understanding of the dynamics of interaction of physical and mental conditions.

REFERENCES

1. CARMICHAEL, L. & M. D. DEARBORN. 1947. Reading and Visual Fatigue: 48. Riverside Press. Cambridge, Mass.
2. LINDSLEY, D. B. 1952. Psychological phenomena and the electroencephalogram. J. EEG Clin. Neurophysiol. **4:** 443–456 (see figs. 1, 2, and 4, and table 1).
3. KRIS, E. C. 1956. Use of eye-movements in the study of fixation shifts, with special reference to eye-dominance. J. EEG Clin. Neurophysiol. **8:** 343.
4. ———. 1959. Electrical measurement of eye movement during perception. Acta Psychologica, Proc. 15th Internatl. Congr. Psychology (Brussels, Belgium, 1957, pp. 247–249.
5. ———. 1960. Vision: Electro-oculography. *In* Medical Physics, Vol. III, O. Glasser, Ed.: 691–700. Yearbook Publ., Chicago.
6. ALEXANDER, L. & E. C. KRIS. 1958. Polygraphic studies of conditional reflexes in man: Diagnostic aspects of differentiation and generalization (see: Hypersynchronous alpha-like buildup in paradoxical response to stimulation in depressed patients). Acta Neurologica, Proc. 83rd Annu. Meet. of the American Neurological Association (Atlantic City, N.J.), Publ. 59.
7. ALEXANDER, L. & E. C. KRIS. 1960. Poligraphic measurement technique of conditioning sequences in mentally disturbed and normal control subjects. J. EEG Clin. Neurophysiol. **10:** 363–364.
8. KRIS, E. C. 1969. Developmental psychophysiological studies of binocular visuo-motor co-ordination, control and impairment. J. Psychophysiol. **5:** 587–588.
9. ———. 1969. Developmental and diagnostic EOG and EEG studies of binocular visual responsiveness and oculomotor control in children and adults with perceptual reading and learning difficulties. J. EEG Clin. Neurophysiol. **26:** 633–634.
10. ———. 1970. Simultaneous measurement of binocular EOG and bilateral EEG activation patterns in dyslexic children. J. EEG Clin. Neurophysiol. **29:** 413.
11. ———. 1972. Synchronized high voltage 5–7 cycle per second EEG, and EOG activation during open-eyed gaze, in dyslexic children. J. EEG Clin. Neurophysiol.
12. ———. 1973. Psychomotor activation through visuo-motor training in dyslexic children with intermittent "sleep-like states." *In* The Nature of Sleep: Proceedings of the Weitzburg International Symposium, V. J. Jovanich, Ed.: 115–116. Gustav Fischer Verlag. Stuttgart.
13. KRIS, E. C., S. B. REES & J. B. TAYLOR. 1971. Simultaneous EEG, ECG, and EOG recording before, during, and after hyperventilation: Studies of cardiac changes. J. EEG Clin. Neurophysiol. **31:** 413, 420.
14. KRIS, E. C. 1986. Psychophysiological EOG, EEG & ECG studies of binocular visuo-motor co-ordination and control-development during reading-readiness and graded reading tasks in perceptually handicapped and dyslexic children with special reference to differential diagnostic and training effects. Proc. 3rd Intl. Conf. of the International Organization of Psychophysiology (Vienna, Austria, July).
15. ———. 1990. Simultaneous binocular bidimensional EOG and bihemispheric bipolar EEC & ECG used in the differential diagnosis of vascular, oculomotor and hemispheric higher cortical perceptual dysfunctions and reading. Proc. 50th Anniversary Meet. of the Eastern Association of Electroencephalographers (J. EEG Clin. Neurophysiol. **76:** 80).

Auditory–Brainstem Synchronicity in Dyslexia Measured Using the REPs/ABR Protocol

JUDITH L. LAUTER AND SUZANNE B. WOOD

Department of Communication Disorders
University of Oklahoma Health Sciences Center
Oklahoma City, Oklahoma 73190

Eight individuals, five with a prior diagnosis of dyslexia, and three who were family members of one of the dyslexic patients, were tested using our Repeated Evoked Potentials[1-5] version of the Auditory Brainstem Response (REPs/ABR). The REPs method provides a way to quantify the *systematic variation* in EP waveforms, and yields *dramatically increased sensitivity to the characteristics of individual nervous systems, whether normal or disordered.*

The REPs scoring procedure compares an individual with a normal database to yield "positive" and "negative" neurological signs. Negative signs include latency *later* than normal, or absolute amplitude, amplitude stability, or latency stability *lower* than normal. These "late/low REP scores" are interpreted as signs of pathology affecting areas *in and around* the auditory pathways between cochlea and midbrain. Positive signs include latency *earlier* than normal, or absolute amplitude, amplitude stability, or latency stability *higher* than normal. These "early/high REP scores" are interpreted as "release signs," indicating a failure in top-down modulation of brainstem response, and thus localizing pathology to suprabrainstem regions.

Each of the eight adults in the current study was tested in a single one-hour REPs/ABR session, including an audiogram, vital statistics recording, consent form presentation, and ABR testing (Biologic Traveller). All procedures for ABR testing were based on standard clinical practice, with the single exception collection of 16 waveforms: four with left-ear, four with right-ear, and eight with binaural stimulation.

Analysis was based on calculation of mean, standard deviation, and coefficient of stability values (Cs = mean/s.d.) for latency and amplitude of peaks I–V tested under each ear condition. Only two of the dyslexics (AW and MG) were judged to have abnormal ABRs based on standard criteria[6] (both had normal behavioral hearing thresholds). This low rate of abnormal ABRs in dyslexia (2 of 5) is in agreement with previous reports.[7]

REP scores provide much more detail. FIGURE 1 summarizes the findings, plotting late/low versus early/high REP scores for each subject. The patterns of REP scores break subjects into four groups: nondyslexic sensorineural hearing loss; dyslexic with (predicted) brainstem involvement; dyslexic with mixed brainstem and suprabrainstem pathology; and dyslexic with predominantly suprabrainstem signs. (See figure legend for more detail.)

The predictions represented by these groupings will be tested with further examination of the same subjects using MRI and qEEG, as part of our Coordinated Noninvasive Studies (CNS) Project.[8,9] The CNS Project is designed to exploit the complementarity of several noninvasive brain-monitoring methods in order to generate CNS profiles of individual human subjects, linking neuroanatomy and neurophysiology to behavior. It is expected that further sophisticated application of non-

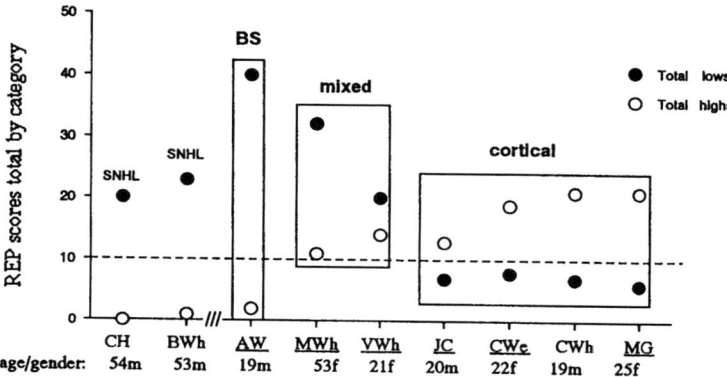

FIGURE 1. Summary data for nine subjects tested with REPs/ABR, arranged according to the number of late/low vs. early/high REP scores (see text for explanation). Subjects are identified on the abscissa by initials, age, and gender. *Underlined initials* indicates a prior diagnosis of dyslexia and/or anecdotal learning disability. Subjects are grouped according to the pattern of late/low vs. early/high REP scores, with a score of 10 selected as a tentative cutoff for grouping purposes. Groups including dyslexic individuals are indicated by *boxes*, with the interpretation of the localization of pathology (based on the REP-score pattern) indicated above. The neurological interpretations are based on previous findings in our laboratory using REPs/ABR in populations such as multiple sclerosis, learning disorder, stuttering, central auditory processing disorder (CAPD), and substance abuse (see references). Descriptions of the groups are as follows. **GROUP I (far left: "SNHL")**: Subjects CH and BWh. These are *nondyslexic* men in their early 50s, both with mild *sensorineural hearing losses (SNHL)*. BWh is the father of dyslexic subject VWh. **GROUP II ("BS")**: Subject AW. AW is a young adult *dyslexic* man. His very high number of late/low REP scores is interpreted as indicating that his learning and reading difficulties result from significant *brainstem* dysfunction. **GROUP III ("mixed")**: Subjects MWh and VWh. These are a *learning-disabled* mother and *dyslexic* daughter, respectively. Each has a *mixture* of "significant" (i.e., >10) late/low *and* early/high REP scores, taken to indicate a combination of brainstem and suprabrainstem involvement. **GROUP IV ("cortical")**: Subjects JC, CWe, CWh, and MG. All but CWh (the brother of dyslexic VWh) are *dyslexic;* their negligible late/low REP scores (<10) combined with >10 early/high REP scores are taken here to suggest that any neuropathology in these subjects involves primarily suprabrainstem levels of the CNS.

invasive methods, particularly exploring the range of individual differences in normal and disordered populations, will provide more insight into the neurological "signatures" of the subtypes of dyslexia.[10,11]

REFERENCES

1. LAUTER, J. L. & R. L. LOOMIS. 1986. Individual differences in auditory electric responses: Comparisons of between-subject and within-subject variability. I. Absolute latencies of brainstem vertex-positive peaks. Scand. Audiol. **15**: 167–172.
2. LAUTER, J. L. & R. G. KARZON. 1990. Individual differences in auditory electric responses: Comparisons of between-subject and within-subject variability. V. Amplitude-variability comparisons in early, middle, and late responses. Scand. Audiol. **19**: 201–206.

3. LAUTER, J. L. & J. M. LORD-MAES. 1991. Repeated-measures ABRs in multiple sclerosis: Demonstration of a new tool for individual neurological assessment. Paper presented to the Acoustical Society of America, San Diego, Calif. (Abstract: J. Acoust. Soc. Am. **88:** S18.)
4. LAUTER, J. L. & R. F. OYLER. 1992. Latency stability of auditory brainstem responses in children aged 10–12 years compared with younger children and adults. Brit. J. Aud. **26:** 245–253.
5. LAUTER, J. L. 1991. MacCAD and REP/ABRs: A new test battery for central auditory dysfunction. Paper presented to the Acoustical Society of America, Baltimore, Md. (Abstract: J. Acoust. Soc. Am. **89:** 1975.)
6. CHIAPPA, K., K. J. GLADSTONE & R. R. YOUNG. 1979. Brainstem auditory evoked responses: Studies of waveform variations in 50 normal human subjects. Arch. Neurol. **36:** 81–87.
7. GRONTVED, A., B. WALTER & A. GRONBORG. 1988. Normal ABRs in dyslexic children. Acta Otolaryngol. (Stockholm) **449:** 171–173.
8. LAUTER, J. L. & E. PLANTE. Human periSylvian cortex: Individual differences in electrophysiological correlates of anatomical asymmetries. Submitted for publication.
9. LAUTER, J. L. 1991. The Coordinated Noninvasive Studies (CNS) Project. Paper presented to the Third IBRO World Congress of Neuroscience, Montreal, Quebec, Canada; Society for Neuroscience, St. Louis, Mo.; American Association for the Advancement of Science, Washington, D.C.
10. DUFFY, F. H. & G. MCANULTY. 1990. Neurophysiological heterogeneity and the definition of dyslexia: Preliminary evidence for plasticity. Neuropsychologia **28**(6): 555–571.
11. GALABURDA, A. M., G. D. ROSEN & G. F. SHERMAN. 1992. Individual variability in cortical organization: Its relationship to brain laterality and implications to function. Neuropsychologia **28**(6): 529–546.

Assessing Reading Skills with a Computer-aided Set of Tests Based on the Dual-route Theory of Reading

H. LYYTINEN, S. HAVU, S. LEINONEN, E. HOLOPAINEN,
M. ARO & T. AHONEN
*Department of Psychology and Niilo Mäki Institute
University of Jyväskylä
40100 Jyväskylä, Finland*

INTRODUCTION

A battery of tests of elementary reading skills specified on the basis of a modification (FIG. 1) of the dual route theory of early reading[1] was constructed for diagnosing the deficient processes of developmental reading problems. Many of the tests were variants of those introduced by Seymour[2] and Höien and Lundberg.[3] The battery is a fully automatic computer version coded to the Amiga computer. The present study assesses the battery's ability to explain the variance associated with reading comprehension in two random samples of children.

METHOD

The subjects were 8–9 (SD 7.7 months) ($N = 100$) and 10–11-year-old children (SD 3.9 months) ($N = 114$). The criterion variable was reading comprehension (assessed using the Sentence Understanding test (SL60)—a Finnish translation of the test of Dansk Psykologisk Forlag). The older group was tested with a more extensive battery of comprehensive tests based on reading two expository text samples.

The following skills were assessed on the basis of accuracy and/or speed using the computer test: letter naming (1.2—the numbers refer to the location in the model in FIG. 1), letter matching (1.2.2), parsing (1.3), phonological decoding (2.1), phonological synthesis (2.3), reading pseudo- and nonwords (2.4), orthographic word recognition (3.1), and lexical decision.

Stepwise regression analyses were performed using the tests of the elementary skills as predictors and comprehension as the variable to be explained. Age and IQ (assessed using Raven Coloured Progressive Matrices) were forced to the model to examine the separate role of reading-specific skills in the explanation of reading comprehension. Only statistically significant ($p < 0.01$) contributions are mentioned in the present paper.

RESULTS

The rapid development of reading skills between the two age groups was accompanied by a decrease in the contribution of intelligence. The models were able

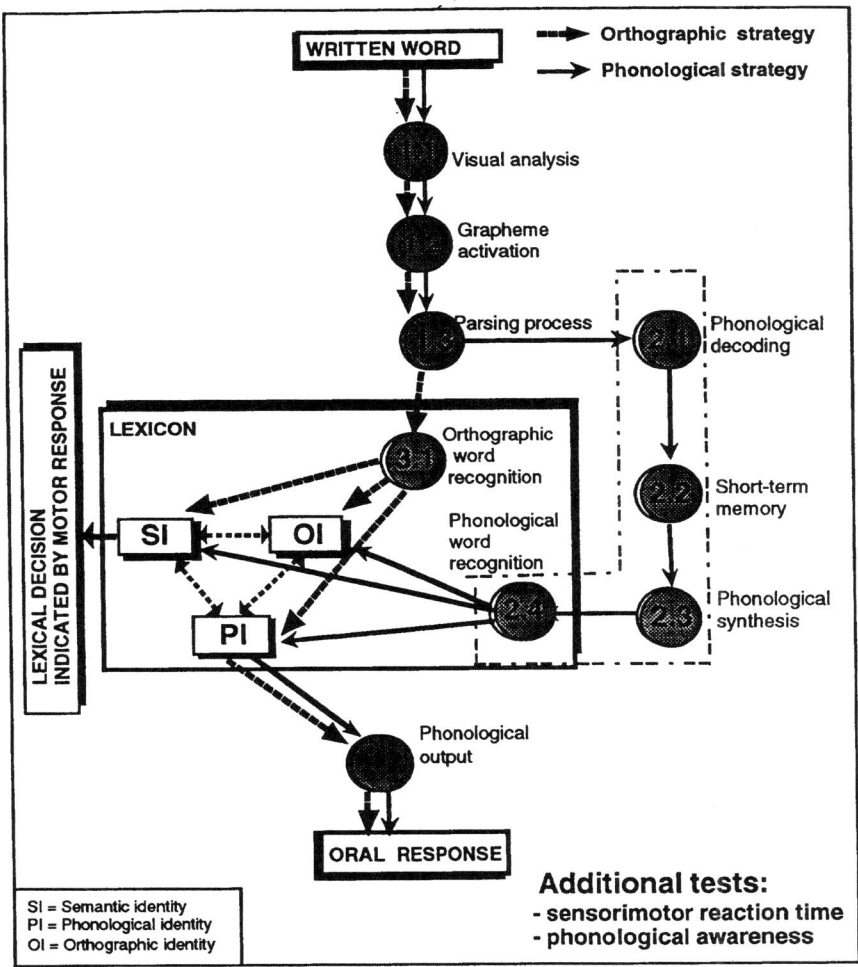

FIGURE 1. Our version of the dual-route model.

to explain almost 60 percent of the variance at ages 8–9 years, with the most significant single contribution coming from orthographic word recognition, as shown in TABLE 1. Phonological word recognition speed and letter naming accuracy (based only on the variation in the skill at naming the rarely used alphabets) added significantly to the explanation of variance based on word recognition, IQ, and age. At age 10–11 years, the total explanation was less (32 percent), but the contribution of basic reading skill variables was still substantial (30 percent in addition to IQ and age), as shown in TABLE 1. Again phonological word recognition speed and letter naming were significant predictors. On the other hand, at this age orthographic

TABLE 1. Regression Model: Elementary Reading Skills as Predictors of Reading Comprehension, IQ, and Age (within Group) Forced as First Variables

Predictor Variable	8–9-year-old Children			10–11-year-old Children		
	Correlation	Cumulative Explanation Multiple R	%	Correlation	Cumulative Explanation Multiple R	%
Intelligence	0.40	0.40	16	0.16	0.16	3
Age	0.24	0.44	19	−0.12	0.20	4
Orthographic word recognition—accuracy	0.68	0.70	50			
Phonological word recognition—reaction time	−0.13	0.75	55	−0.42	0.44	20
Letter naming—accuracy	0.43	0.77	59	0.41	0.54	29
Parsing process				0.27	0.56	32

processing made no contribution. Instead parsing rose to the model, explaining the equal proportion of the variance, as did IQ and age independently of all these variables.

CONCLUSIONS

Many single basic reading subskills, like orthographic and phonological recognition, parsing, and letter naming, still have a significant and cumulative ability to explain reading comprehension of 11-year-olds. Such skills explain a substantial portion of the variance of comprehension of the written text also after their variance common with IQ is excluded. Our experience from dyslexic children shows that the deficient processes may manifest in various locations in the separable routes/strategies of reading.

REFERENCES

1. MORTON, J. 1969. Interaction of information in word recognition. Psychol. Rev. **76:**165–178.
2. SEYMOUR, P. H. K. 1986. Cognitive Analysis of Dyslexia. Routledge & Kegan Paul. London.
3. HÖIEN, T. & L. LUNDBERG. 1989. A strategy for assessing problems in word recognition among dyslexics. Scand. J. Educ. **33:** 142–155.

Visible Persistence in Developmental Dyslexia

FRANCISCO J. MARTOS AND ANTONIO MARMOLEJO

*Departamento de Psicología Experimental y
Fisiología del Comportamiento
Campus de Cartuja
University of Granada
18071 Granada, Spain*

INTRODUCTION

The main aim of our study was to determine the existence of differences in the duration of visible persistence among dyslexic, retarded, and normal readers. Secondly, we wanted to find out whether the duration of visible persistence was related to the age of the subjects. Lastly, we wanted to know whether the longer visible persistence is a differential characteristic of the dyslexic readers, or whether, on the contrary, it is also present in other forms of reading disorders.

METHOD

Subjects-Design

A 3 × 3 × 2 factorial design was used, the first factor being *reading disability* at three levels (dyslexic, retarded, and normal readers), the second factor *age* at three levels (7–9, 10–11, and 12–14 years), and the third factor the two *methods* used to measure the visible persistence at two levels (*temporal* integration threshold and the *gap* detection threshold). The three reading groups of 30 subjects each (21 male and 9 female) were formed according to the following criteria:

- *Dyslexic Group:* Reading age two years behind chronological age; IQ > 95.
- *Retarded Reader Group:* Reading age two years behind chronological age; IQ between 75 and 90.
- *Normal Reader Group:* Reading age equal to or higher than chronological age; IQ > 95.

Experimental Tasks

Two different methods were used to measure visible persistence. In the determination of the temporal integration threshold, the researcher displayed, in a tachistoscope, two different stimuli (a vertical line followed by a horizontal line) in rapid succession, separated by an interstimuli interval (ISI) of variable duration. The display of both stimuli with a short ISI caused the observer to integrate them in a single image (a cross). The aim of the researcher was to establish the longest ISI at which the subjects were able to maintain an integrated perception of both stimuli.

TABLE 1. Means and Standard Deviations (in Brackets) of the ISIs (in ms) as a Function of Reading Disability and the Different Methods Used to Measure the Visible Persistence

	Reading Deficiency		
	Retarded	Dyslexic	Normal
Gap detection threshold	114.6 (40.7)	104.6 (40.4)	63.8 (24)
		*	
			*
Temporal integration threshold	85.3 (35.4)	79 (25.4)	56.1 (14.9)
		*	
			*

Note: Retarded = dyslexic > normal.
*Indicates significant differences between groups (Newman-Keuls Test). $p < 0.01$.

The second method was the determination of the gap detection threshold. In this case, the same stimulus (a horizontal line) was displayed twice in rapid succession with a blank ISI of variable duration inserted between each. The task was to determine the shortest ISI at which the subjects were able to distinguish the double flash from a single uninterrupted display. The main difference between the two methods is that in the temporal integration different retinal locations are stimulated, while in the gap detection threshold, the stimuli impinge on the same retinal receptors.

RESULTS

First Factor. Reading Disability

The results showed significant effects, $F(2,81) = 18.84$, $p < 0.001$. The analyses (Newman-Keuls Test) showed that the visible persistence of the normal readers was significantly shorter than that of dyslexic and retarded readers. However, there were no differences at all between dyslexic and retarded readers.

Second Factor. Age

Significant effects were also found, $F(2,81) = 4.76$, $p < 0.01$. The results indicated a linear decrease in the visible persistence of every subject as age increased. The decrease was greater in both groups of disabled readers and it was particularly remarkable in the dyslexic group.

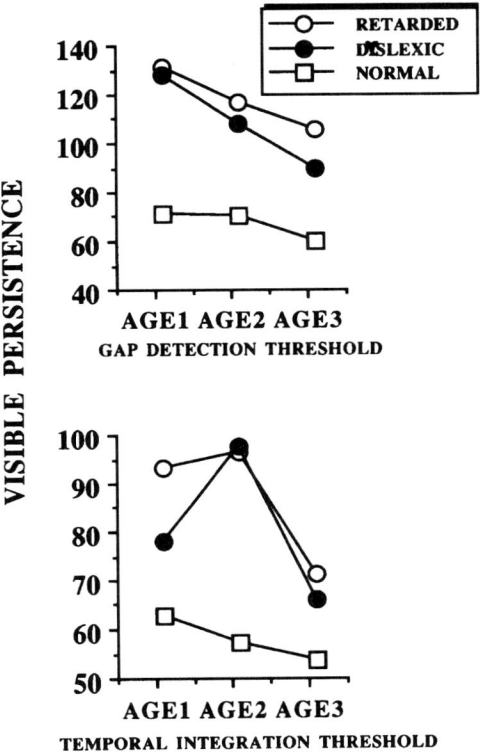

FIGURE 1. Mean values of the critical ISIs in the dyslexic, retarded, and normal groups as a function of age in the two methods used to determine the duration of visible persistence.

Third Factor. Method of Measure

The significant results ($F(1,81) = 21.05$, $p < 0.001$) showed that the method of determination of the gap-detection threshold produced a longer duration of visible persistence. However, the different method used did not produce differences in the general pattern of the results.

CONCLUSIONS

The results reflect that dyslexic and retarded readers maintain longer visible persistence than normal readers. These results confirm those obtained by Di Lollo, Hanson, and McIntire,[1] and Lovegrove, Martin, and Slaghuis.[2] These authors have explained that the longer duration of the persistence of the stimuli in the retina of dyslexic children could produce a stimulation overload in their visual system, causing an interruption or an integration in the processing of the stimuli.

With regard to age, the results show a general improvement in the visible persistence of every subject (see FIG. 1). This effect is particularly important in the dyslexic reader group. In this group, the critical ISI decrease progressively, and in such a way that in the last age level the differences between the dyslexic and the normal reader group has decreased considerably. Kail[3] has recently shown that the processing speed in normal subjects increases linearly in relation to age. In this sense, the results in the dyslexic group could reflect a maturative delay in their nervous system from which they recuperate progressively.

REFERENCES

1. DI LOLLO, V., D. HANSON & J. S. MCINTIRE. 1983. J. Exp. Psychol.: Hum. Percept. Perform. **9:** 923–935.
2. LOVEGROVE, W., F. MARTIN & W. SLAGHUIS. 1986. Cognitive Neuropsychol. **2:** 225–267.
3. KAIL, R. 1991. Psychol. Bull. **109**(3): 490–501.

Children with Dyslexia Classify Pure Tones Slowly

RODERICK I. NICOLSON AND ANGELA J. FAWCETT

Department of Psychology
Post Office Box 603
University of Sheffield
Sheffield S10 2 UR
United Kingdom

Developmental dyslexia is normally characterized by unexpected problems in learning to read for children of average or above average intelligence. Interestingly, however, slower speed of information processing appears to be a recurring symptom of dyslexia. There is a substantial literature on deficits in speed of access to the spoken word, initially discovered using the "rapid automatized naming" test.[1] This test involves the rapid sequential naming of a series of 50 familiar stimuli presented simultaneously on a card. The authors showed that dyslexic children were slower to name colors, pictures, digits, and letters than slow learners matched for reading age. Unfortunately, these and similar demonstrations of reduced speed of information processing have involved linguistic processing, and it is therefore not clear whether the deficit represents another correlate of the known linguistic abnormalities of dyslexic children or whether reduced speed of information processing reflects some deeper problem.

Five groups of children participated: 14 dyslexic children around 15 years old; 11 dyslexic children around 11 years old; 11 nondyslexic children matched to the other dyslexic children for age and full IQ; 12 nondyslexic children of similar IQ to the two dyslexic groups, matched for reading age with the older dyslexic children and for chronological age with the younger dyslexic children; and 9 nondyslexic children matched for full IQ and reading age with the younger dyslexic children. All the dyslexic children had been diagnosed between the ages of 7 and 10, based on discrepancies of at least 18 months between actual and reading age. Their IQ levels fell in the normal to superior range on the Wechsler Intelligence Scale for Children and they had no known neurological deficit or primary emotional difficulty.

In pilot studies we established that dyslexic children showed the expected speed deficit in complex linguistically based tasks. Consequently, in an attempt to find normal performance, we administered increasingly simple tasks—lexical decision, choice reaction, and finally simple reaction to a tone. In the lexical decision task, subjects were presented auditorily with a word (or, equally probably, a morphologically valid nonword) and had to say as quickly as possible Yes (if it was a word) or No (if it was a nonword). The dependent variable of interest was the response latency. In both reaction time experiments, subjects sat with a single button in their preferred hand, and their task was to press it as quickly as possible whenever they heard a low tone. In the simple reaction task (SRT), no other tone was ever presented, but in the selective choice reaction task (SCRT), there was an equal probability of a high tone being presented. If the high tone was presented, the subject had to do nothing. The SRT and SCRT experiments were controlled by a BBC microcomputer, using the sound generator to create the tones. The low tone used in both experiments was 350 Hz, and the high tone used in the SCRT experiment was 1400 Hz, a two-octave difference. In each task, subjects held a microswitched button in their preferred hand, and 100 trials were administered. Results were recorded automatically, and mean and median latencies, latency variance, and overall accuracy were calculated with a further program. For the lexical decision task, the stimuli used were 24 frequent single-syllable words, (e.g., *shop, king, meat*), matched with morphologically correct nonwords (e.g., *thop, hing, leat*), derived by altering the first consonant of each high-frequency real word. Subjects were instructed to say "yes" to a real word, or "no" to a nonsense word, as quickly as possible. Voice onset latency was recorded automatically.

For each experiment the mean latencies were calculated, as were the standard deviations. Furthermore, since reaction time distributions are skewed, it is important also to derive the median reaction times to avoid the danger of outliers biasing the means. The median results for the three tasks are shown in FIGURE 1, plotted on the same graph to facilitate comparison. To summarize the results: for the simple reaction task both groups of dyslexic children performed at the appropriate level for their age, and significantly faster than their reading age controls. However, for the SCRT and lexical decision conditions, the dyslexic children slipped back, to the extent that they were significantly slower than their chronological-age controls and equivalent to their reading-age controls. The same pattern of results applied for both mean and median latency. Furthermore, the dyslexic children were, if anything, less accurate than their age-matched controls, showing that the SCRT results cannot be attributed to some speed-accuracy trade-off effect. The "by item" analysis of the lexical decision data suggested that the dyslexic children showed a qualitative deficit in lexical access speed, performing even more slowly than their RA controls for access to words. Full details of the results and procedure are presented in reference 2.

Our original research strategy was to administer a series of less and less complex information processing tasks, with the hope of finding some task for which the speed impairment disappeared. As expected, the lexical decision data indicated a speed impairment, with the dyslexic groups responding significantly slower than their CA controls (and even slower than their RA controls). Rather more surprisingly, however, the SCRT data led to a similar pattern of impairment, with the dyslexic groups

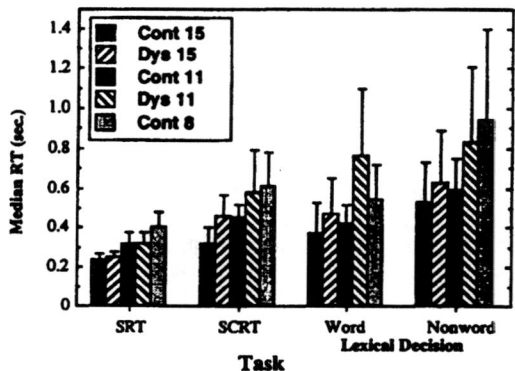

FIGURE 1. Median latencies for the three experiments. (*Key:* The *error bars* represent the within-group standard deviation of the medians. The *group labels* are as follows: "Cont 15"—15-year-old controls. "Dys 15"—15-year-old children with dyslexia. "Cont 11"—11-year-old controls; "Dys 11"—11-year-old children with dyslexia; "Cont 8"—8-year-old controls.

having significantly slower performance than their CA controls, though in this case the performance was equivalent to their RA controls. These results suggest that at least two processes are impaired, with an initial quantitative impairment on SCRT speed together with a further impairment on lexical access speed, which together result in an apparent qualitative deficit on the lexical decision task for words. Given the absence of phonological input or output in the SCRT task, these results suggest that, although differences in speed of lexical access may contribute to the overall problems in phonological processing, there is a further nonphonological deficit that is sufficient in itself to account for the quantitative impairment in SCRT.

In summary, the experiments reported here appear to be the first systematic, direct investigation of speed of information processing in dyslexic children. As the task complexity increased, the deficits shown by the dyslexic children became more marked. Both groups of dyslexic children performed normally on the simple reaction task. The two groups of dyslexic children showed an overall quantitative impairment on the selective choice reaction task. The two groups of dyslexic children showed an overall qualitative impairment on lexical decision time for words. It is likely that impairments of two processes combine to cause the lexical decision effect: namely, a phonological deficit in lexical access speed together with a nonphonological deficit in stimulus classification speed. The nonphonological deficit is consistent with speed impairments in either perceptual classification or central decision processes.

REFERENCES

1. DENCKLA, M. B. & R. G. RUDEL. 1976. Rapid 'Automatized naming (R.A.N.). Dyslexia differentiated from other learning disabilities. Neuropsychologia **14**: 471–479.
2. NICOLSON, R. I. & A. J. FAWCETT. 1992. Reaction times and dyslexia. Q. J. Exp. Psychol.: Hum. Exp. Psychol. In press.

Children with Dyslexia Automatize Temporal Skills More Slowly

RODERICK I. NICOLSON AND ANGELA J. FAWCETT

Department of Psychology
Post Office Box 603
University of Sheffield
Sheffield S10 2 UR
United Kingdom

Developmental dyslexia is normally characterized by unexpected problems in learning to read for children of average or above average intelligence. In recent research, however, we have established that dyslexic children also show problems in the gross motor skill of balance[1,2] and in speed of choice reaction to pure tones, even though their simple reaction speed is normal.[3] We interpreted the motor skill deficits as symptoms of incomplete automatization of skill, in that the deficits were apparent only when the children were prevented from consciously monitoring their performance, either through use of a dual task or by cutting out visual cues. The well-established reading and phonological deficits of dyslexic children are fully consistent with this "dyslexic automatization deficit" (DAD) hypothesis, since phonological skills evolve through long exposure to, and use of, speech, and of course, reading requires the fluent interplay of a number of subskills.[4] Unfortunately, the evidence for the DAD hypothesis is indirect, and therefore we undertook a further study testing the long-term learning of a temporal skill. Since we had established the deficit in choice reaction but not in simple reaction speed, the natural experimental design was to investigate the time course of the blending of two separate reactions into a choice reaction. Initially, children were tested on two separate simple reaction tasks: a finger press to an auditory tone and a foot press to a visual flash. Then a choice reaction task was constructed, using both modalities of stimulus, and the child had to make a finger press to the tone or a foot press to the flash as appropriate. Naturally, initial performance on this choice reaction task is much slower than the simple reactions, but through extended practice one would expect the latencies to diminish to near those for simple reactions, but through extended practice one would expect the latencies to diminish to near those for simple reactions.[5] The critical prediction, therefore, for DAD was that dyslexic children would improve their performance more slowly than nondyslexic children.

Two groups of children participated: 11 dyslexic children around 15 years old and 11 nondyslexic children matched for age and full IQ. All the dyslexic children had been diagnosed between the ages of 7 and 10, based on discrepancies of at least 18 months between actual and reading age. Their IQ levels fell in the normal to superior range on the Wechsler Intelligence Scale for Children and they had no known neurological deficit or primary emotional difficulty.

All reaction time tasks were computer administered and scored. The tone was 350 Hz and the flash duration was 100 ms. Initially, simple reaction performance was measured to each stimulus independently. Following this baseline testing, both stimuli were combined into a choice reaction task. One hundred trials were presented per run with stimuli presented pseudorandomly with equal probability. Three runs were carried out per session. Subjects returned for further testing as often as practicable, with up to 36 runs being completed per subject. Both speed and accuracy were monitored. Testing was discontinued if a subject appeared to have reached asymptote in their response speed and accuracy.

The median results for latency are shown in FIGURE 1, plotted on the same graph to facilitate comparison. It may be seen that baseline performance for both groups was similar, and that both groups showed the expected impairment following the change to choice reactions, and the expected improvement with practice over the subsequent sessions. Two factor analyses of variance indicated that the initial simple reactions were not significantly different between groups in latency; that the initial choice reaction performance was significantly slower for the dyslexic children ($p > 0.01$) for both hand and foot, and that the choice reaction performance was slower after training ($p > 0.01$) for both hand and foot. There were no significant differences in accuracy in the baseline condition, but the dyslexic children were significantly less accurate ($p > 0.001$) at asymptote. The critical issue, however, is whether the dyslexic children improved as fast as the controls. It is not appropriate merely to subtract posttraining latencies from pretraining latencies, because in general the control children had reached asymptote in less than 36 runs, whereas several of the dyslexic children were still improving even after 36 runs. Consequently, the mean data of latency per run (as in FIG. 1) was fit using a power law function of the form $CRT = Bt^{-\alpha}$, where the constant B represents the initial performance level, and the parameter α represents the rate of learning.[6] The best fit curves for hand responses were $CRT = 53.9t^{-0.073}$ for the dyslexic children and $CRT = 39.4t^{-0.141}$ for the controls. For the foot responses the corresponding best fit curves were $CRT = 62.3t^{-0.086}$, $CRT = 50.4t^{-0.116}$, respectively. The parameter α is the critical issue here, and it may be seen that α is twice as large for the controls than the dyslexic children for manual responses (0.141 vs. 0.073) and one-third larger for the foot responses (0.116 vs. 0.086). These are huge differences. Bearing in mind that the learning varies as a function of the time to the power α, if a skill takes a normal child 100 hours to master, it would, taking an average ratio of the learning rates as say 1.5, take a dyslexic child $100^{1.5}$, that is, 1000 hours (10 times as long) to learn the skill to the same criterion. Note that the longer the time taken for a normal child to acquire a skill, the greater the predicted decrement—for a skill taking a normal child say 400

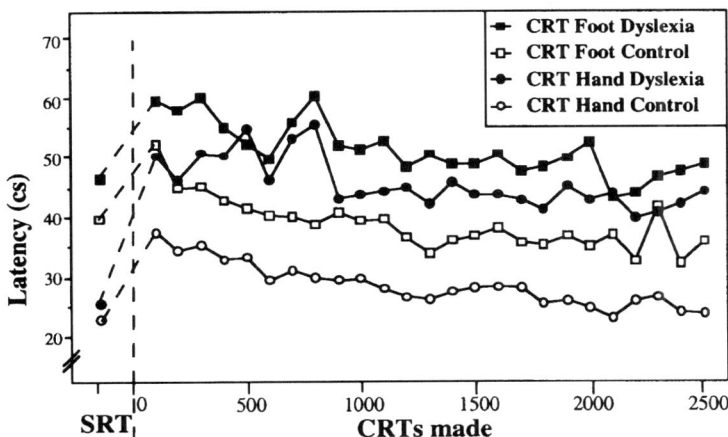

FIGURE 1. Median latencies over the period of training.

hours, it would take a dyslexic child 20 times as long, and so on. If these data are representative of long-term skill training, they raise important theoretical and applied issues regarding the teaching of dyslexic children.

In summary, the experiments reported here are the first systematic, direct investigations of long-term learning of a temporal processing skill in dyslexic children. Although performance on the two component subskills of the skill was initially equal, the dyslexic children had more difficulty combining the two skills at first and showed significantly less learning over the course of the training period, with final performance being both slower and less accurate. Furthermore, the theoretical learning rate estimated from the training data was around 50 percent slower for the dyslexic children, leading to the prediction that the proportionate slowing in acquisition time would increase as the square root of the normal acquisition time. These findings provide direct support for the DAD hypothesis, and occurring as they do for a combined visual–auditory skill with no linguistic component, they are very difficult to accommodate under any less broad theoretical framework.

REFERENCES

1. NICOLSON, R. I. & A. J. FAWCETT. 1990. Automaticity: A new framework for dyslexia research. Cognition **35:** 159–182.
2. FAWCETT, A. J. & R. I. NICOLSON. 1992. Automatisation deficits in balance for dyslexic children. Percept. Mot. Skills **75:** 507–529.
3. NICOLSON, R. I. & A. J. FAWCETT. 1992. Reaction times and dyslexia. Q. J. Exp. Psychol.: Hum. Exp. Pschol. In press.
4. LABERGE, D. & S. J. SAMUELS. 1974. Toward a theory of automatic information processing in reading. Cognitive Psychol. **6:** 293–323.
5. SPELKE, E., W. HIRST & U. NEISSER. 1976. Skills of divided attention. Cognition **4:** 215–230.
6. NEWELL, A. & P. S. ROSENBLOOM. 1981. Mechanisms of skill acquisition and the law of practice. *In* Cognitive Skills and Their Acquisition, J. R. Anderson, Ed. Erlbaum. Hillsdale, N.J.

Innovative Visual–Spatial Powers in Dyslexics: A New Perspective?

S. E. PARKINSON[a] AND J. H. EDWARDS[b]

[a]Lodge Cottage
Brabourne Lees
Ashford, Kent, TN25 6QZ
United Kingdom

[b]132 New Winchelsea Road
Rye, Sussex TN31 7TB
United Kingdom

INTRODUCTION

In our word-dominated society dyslexia is an obvious disability. Therefore expert research in this field has rightly concentrated on remediation. In this poster we concentrate on the *positive* aspects of dyslexia, the good visual–spatial faculties as observed in many instances and recorded in WISC (R) Subtests in psychologists' reports. Greater understanding of these faculties is urgently needed, and of the way in which they are used by professional artists/designers and innovative scientists. Further research is also required into the historical context of these skills, and their potential value to future generations. First steps toward a theoretical framework are proposed here that could support answers to some of the controversial questions still outstanding.

In formulating these proposals consideration has been given to:

(a) Current biological opinion on structure and function localization of the brain, starting from the documentation of important hemispherical differences by Sperry, Geschwind, and colleagues[1–4] in the 1960s and 1970s, and more recently advanced by Galaburda;[5]
(b) The development of lateralization theory by Gazzaniga,[6] for instance;
(c) The notion of connectionism, parallel distributed processing, neural networks, for example, Gazzaniga,[6] Dubai;[7]
(d) The results of research based on modern technology such as MRI and PET; Tallal and Katz,[8] and the apparent consensus regarding modularity of cerebral function and architecture;
(e) The work of artificial intelligence (AI) and computer scientists in attempting to model human vision and learning ability (Marr,[9] Rumelhart, McClelland, and the PDP Research Group[10]).
(f) The continuing debate on visual/neurological defects (Gordon; Ellis; Stein; Whyte[11]); here we present a new perspective by consideration of the viewpoint of artists/designers who are professionally reliant on their understanding and management of visual–spatial factors.

VISUAL–SPATIAL COGNITIVE SKILL

There is an extensive literature on the subject of language, and many penetrating studies of the way in which we order our thoughts in terms of words/numbers/logic.[12–14] There have also been many thorough studies of the deficient functioning of this mode in dyslexics. There is far less known and written on the visual–spatial mode of thought. In the first place, an adequate definition of "visual–spatial" is required.

We propose that visual–spatial skill should be defined as the understanding/awareness/management of one or more of ten factors (listed).

These categories are clearly distinguishable and well known to anyone who has worked in a college of art and design. They are less familiar, it would seem, to cognitive scientists, as there is a surprising lack of research results analyzed in these terms in the scientific literature. This is a pity, because we want to know in which of these categories the dyslexic strength shows itself most prominently. From our own observations we suggest that the visual–spatial categories in which dyslexics show greatest strength are:

(1) The understanding/awareness/management of three-dimensional form and space[a] (FIG. 1 shows an important aspect of this factor, the ability to move viewpoints);
(2) The understanding/awareness/management of innovative composition.

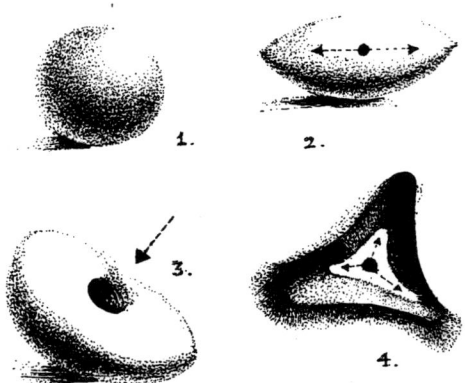

FIGURE 1. Movement in three-dimensional form observed from within. (1) Place yourself in the center of a sphere and you will see why it is called the only *static* form; force holding the peripheral skin out is no greater in one direction than another; this does not, of course, prevent mobility being given to a sphere from *outside* by cricket bat/golfclub/etc., but movement from *within* is still static so long as the sphere stays spherical. (2) Movement/pressure is required in the direction *arrowed* to change a sphere into this form. (3) A force (often called *negative*) exerted from *outside* that alters the shape of the original sphere, while positive movement *within* the form remains the same as in (2). (4) Movement can similarly be viewed from the center of a three-dimensional *space*.

---

[a]The usual appending of "spatial" to "visual" or "visuo," though undefined, can be taken to imply some general acceptance of this factor.

PARKINSON & EDWARDS: INNOVATIVE VISUAL–SPATIAL POWERS 395

Discussion of these points[15-20] forms the heart of our poster. FIGURE 2 illustrates one example of the visual–spatial ways of organizing/reorganizing information, which is condusive to innovative thought.

CONCLUSION

The hypothesis we put forward for discussion and testing is based on the difference between the *cognitive* processes concerned with making sense out of the *one*-dimensional aspects of language and the *three*-dimensional aspects of vision, as we have outlined very briefly. Our contention is that the nature of this difference may be responsible for *both* the dyslexic weakness (in language) and the dyslexic strength (in vision).

Finally, it is proposed that the extent of the success of language in helping to empower the dominance of the human race may have detrimentally masked another crucial survival factor: the brain's capacity to invent new response patterns—to *create*.

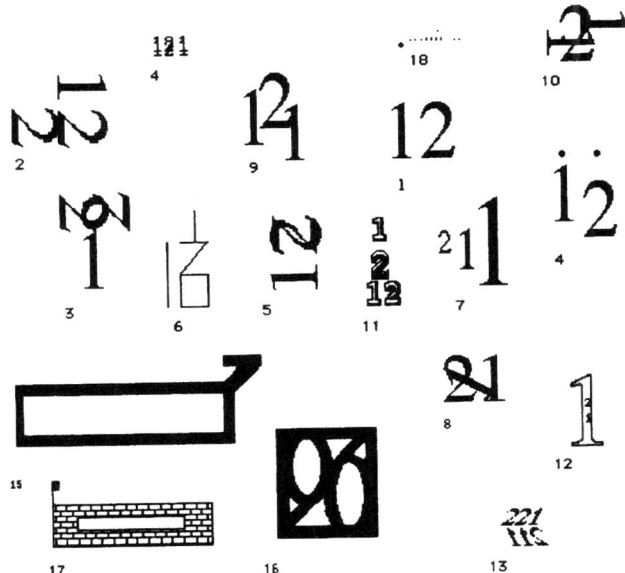

FIGURE 2. Two-dimensional 12 + 12 (processed one dimensionally) = 24. Three-dimensionally many answers are possible; here are some from dyslexic artists/designers. From (**1**) to (**16**), each version introduces or changes one new visual–spatial element: stacking (one 12 put on top of the other); orientation; overlapping; scale; inversion; typeface; perspective; until (**14**), (**15**), and (**16**), in which the two 12s are barely discernible.

REFERENCES

1. SPERRY, R. W. & M. GAZZANIGA. 1967. Language following disconnection of the hemispheres. *In* Brain Mechanism Underlying Speech and Language, H. M. Clark and H. M. Darley, Eds.: 108–115. Grune & Stratton. New York.
2. GESCHWIND, N. & A. M. GALABURDA, Eds. 1984. Cerebral Dominance: The Biological Foundations. Harvard Univ. Press. Cambridge, Mass.
3. GESCHWIND, N. 1974. Specializations of the human brain. Sci. Am. **241**(3).
4. ———. 1972. Language and the brain. Sci. Am. **226**(4):340.
5. GALABURDA, A. M. 1983. Developmental dyslexia: Current anatomical research, Ann. Dyslexia **33**: 41–53.
6. GAZZANIGA, M. 1985. The Social Brain. Basic Books. New York.
7. DUBAI, Y. 1990. The Neurobiology of Memory. Oxford Univ. Press. Oxford.
8. TALLAI, P. & W. KATZ. 1989. Neuropschychological and neuroanatomical studies of developmental language/reading disorders: Recent advances. *In* Brain and Reading, C. Von Euler, I. Lundberg, and G. Lennerstrand, Eds. Macmillan. London.
9. MARR, D. 1982. Vision. Freeman. New York.
10. RUMELHART, D. E., J. L. MCCLELLAND & THE PDP RESEARCH GROUP. 1986. Parallel Distributive Processing. MIT Press. Cambridge, Mass.
11. WHYTE, J., Ed. 1989. Dyslexia current research issues. Irish J. Psychol. **10**(4).
12. JOHNSON-LAIRD, P. N. 1983. Mental Models: Towards a Cognitive Science of Language, Inference, and Consciousness. Cambridge Univ. Press. Cambridge, England.
13. SIMON H. E. & A. K. CRAIG. 1989. *In* Foundations of Cognitive Science. M. I. Posner, Ed. MIT Press. Cambridge, Mass.
14. CHOMSKY, N. 1980. Rules and Representations. Columbia Univ. Press. New York.
15. HUNT, M. 1982. The Universe Within. Simon & Schuster. New York.
16. GARDNER, H. 1983. Frames of Mind: The Theory of Multiple Intelligences. Basic Books. New York.
17. ———. 1984. The Minds New Science: A History of the Cognitive Revolution, 2nd ed. Basic Books. New York.
18. ROOT-BERNSTEIN, R. S. 1989. Discovering: Inventing and Solving Problems at the Frontiers of Scientific Knowledge. Harvard Univ. Press. Cambridge, Mass.
19. KOESTLER, A. 1964. The Act of Creation. Hutchinson. London.
20. WEST, T. 1991. In the Mind's Eye. Prometheus. New York.

Ophthalmologic Aspects of Dyslexia: The Influence of Full Prismatic Correction of Heterophoria on Dyslexic Symptoms

D. PESTALOZZI

Ophthalmologist FMH
Solothumerstrasse 19
CH-4600 Olten
Switzerland

INTRODUCTION

This poster shows the result of the author's 10 years' experience with 367 dyslexic patients. They all had an *heterophoria* (H). By definition this is a squint compensated for by *motor and sensory fusion*. Both kinds of compensation need, however, nervous energy in order to maintain binocular single vision and stereopsis. Under stress an H may decompensate and cause asthenopic troubles. Headache, glare, burning, and chronically irritated eyes are then the most frequent complaints. We presume that *dyslexic symptoms are also part of an asthenopia*. The sensory compensation is called *fixation disparity* (FD). This condition is a shift of the sense of "straight ahead" in binocular vision from the very center of the retina to a slightly eccentric spot. Conventional methods of measuring H may miss it partly or altogether; this includes conventional tests as Ogle's or Mallet's. So far only the Zeiss-Polatest®[a] with its three different kinds of test charts (conventional, FD charts, stereo charts) permits us to detect the full amount of an FD in addition to the motor deviation, and hence to correct it with prisms. The device and the theory were developed by H.-J. Hasse,[1] former lecturer at the "SFOF, Berlin," during the 1980s and earlier. The *point of our binocular correction* is to save the patients' nervous energy, allowing them effortless comfortable seeing. The corrections are done by prismatic spectacles. Only full prismatic correction of an H allows effortless bicentral fixation, comparable to the condition orthophoric subjects find themselves in. Conventional methods, however, and incomplete examination by Polatest, not using the stereo test charts, may give an incomplete correction (FIG. 1[2]).

RESULTS

Samples of handwriting (FIG. 2) show a considerable improvement after full prismatic correction. Six graphs display a *case study* of all the dyslexics seen so far by the author: altogether 367 cases, whereof 278 were selected; distribution of age and sex (2/3 males); time until improvement (70 percent within the first half year; 12 percent in the next six months; the rest in up to 3 years); results concerning

---

[a]The author has no proprietary interest in the Zeiss-Polatest®.

398   ANNALS NEW YORK ACADEMY OF SCIENCES

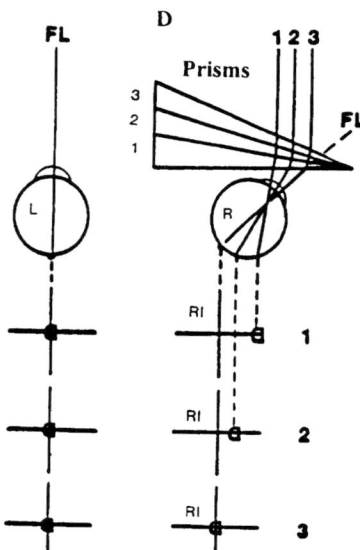

FIGURE 1. Under- and full correction of a heterophoria with FD-II. The fixation line (FL) of the *left eye* (L) points to a far distant fixation object (D). This D is represented in the left eye's retinal center (symbolized by a *cross*). The *right eye's* (R) FL is deviated outside. By correction with **Prism 1**, found by *conventional* examining techniques, the retinal image (RI) lies outside the center of the retina. By **prism 2**, which restores the *fixation-disparity charts* of the Polatest, the retinal image lies closer to the center. By **prism 3**, found by the *stereo charts* of the Polatest, central position of the retinal image is achieved and bicentral fixation restored. (After Goersch.[2] Used by permission.)

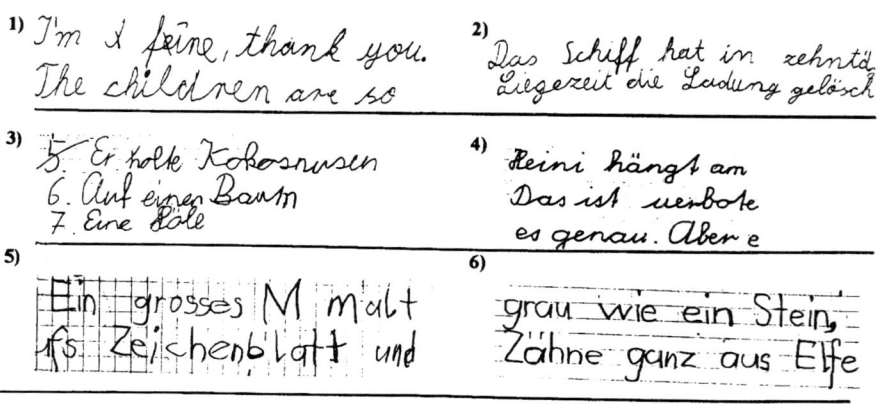

FIGURE 2. Samples of handwriting before and after prismatic correction. **(1)** Boy (10) before. **(2)** Ten weeks after correction. **(3)** Girl (10) before. **(4)** Three months after correction. **(5)** Boy (9) before. **(6)** Two months after correction.

dyslexia (11 percent very good, 60 percent good results, 17 percent at least relief of asthenopic complaints, and 12 percent no improvement); improvement of reduced visual acuity in 175 eyes; development of sensory state: after full correction 60 percent with ideal binocular vision (initially 2 percent), while the number of FD cases dropped from 70 to 22 percent. This stresses the fact that FD, in contrast to anomalous retinal correspondence (ARC), is reversible. Nevertheless, the number of cases with pathologic binocular vision dropped from over 20 percent to 10 percent (last column in the graph), showing that binocular correction by Polatest may be helpful even with ARC.

CONCLUSIONS

We concur with Stein's[3] hypothesis that dyslexia may be caused by disorders in the *left and right hemispheres.* We thus think that prismatic corrections would probably not help in dyslexia caused mainly by the left hemisphere, but would improve it in those caused by right hemisphere disorders. In mixed cases some improvement might be expected.

By full prismatic correction of the motor and sensory parts of a heterophoria, patients get better visual input, thus saving nervous energy; asthenopic symptoms and dyslexia may improve, but *dyslexia will not be cured by prismatic corrections alone.* So far only the Zeiss-Polatest® allows us to find and correct completely an H with FD. It is now used by an increasing number of ophthalmologists and many optometrists in the German-speaking and some other countries of Europe, but is virtually unknown in the United States. The author does not know why FD is not considered important for the correction of H in the United States.

REFERENCES

1. HAASE, H.-J. Zur Fixationsdisparation. Deutsche Optikerzeitung. Heidelberg. In press.
2. GOERSCH, H. 1987. Die drei notwendigen Testarten zur vollständigen Heterophoriebestimmung: 14, Fig. 14. Deutsche Optikerzeitung. Heidelberg.
3. STEIN, J. 1989. Visuospatial perception and reading problems. Ir. J. Psychol. **10**(4): 521–533.

Dyslexia, Schizotypy, and Visual Direction Sense

A. J. RICHARDSON[a] AND J. F. STEIN

University Laboratory of Physiology
Parks Road
Oxford OX1 3PT, England

We have previously shown that adult dyslexics score highly on a scale measuring schizotypal personality traits in the normal population.[1] These traits in normals have also been linked with unusual hemispheric specialization (particularly with unusual right-hemisphere performance), and with abnormal functioning of the transient visual system. Dyslexic children show poor visual direction sense on a nonverbal "dot localization" task,[2] and make significantly more errors on the left. This pattern of results has also been interpreted as suggesting disordered visual transient and right-hemisphere function. We therefore proposed that (1) adult dyslexics would show poor visual direction sense, with an excess of errors on leftward judgments, and (2) high scores on the schizotypal personality scale (STA) would be associated with poor visual direction sense, with a similar pattern of errors.

Twenty-two adult dyslexics and 28 controls matched for age, sex, and educational/occupational status were assessed for personality and handedness. The latter did not differ between groups, and only on the schizotypal personality scale[3] did dyslexics differ from controls ($p < 0.04$), as previously found. Visual direction sense was tested using a paradigm in which the subject had to indicate by keypress whether a test spot (0.25 degrees, duration 200 ms) was presented to the right or to the left of a previously presented "priming" spot (0.25 degrees, duration 2 s). A mask of visual noise was presented for 500 ms between priming spot and test spot. One hundred and sixty trials were given (40 at each of 4 displacement distances, with equal numbers of left and right trials).

FIGURE 1 shows the percentage of errors across all distances for left and right trials by dyslexic and control groups split by STA. Errors were subjected to multiple correlation analysis, with independent variables DISTANCE (1,2,3,4), DYSLEXIC STATUS (D,N), SCHIZOTYPY (High, Low), and DIRECTION (Left, Right). Highly significant independent main effects were found for DISTANCE ($p < 0.0001$), DYSLEXIC STATUS ($p < 0.0001$), STA ($p < 0.0001$), and DIRECTION ($p < 0.0001$). Dyslexics made more errors than controls, as did high schizotypes, independent of their dyslexic status. There was a significant interaction of DYSLEXIC STATUS*DIRECTION ($p < 0.026$); dyslexics made more errors on the left, replicating our previous finding. There was no interaction between STA and dyslexic status, nor between STA and direction, though within the control group, high schizotypes produced the "dyslexic pattern" of more total errors and more errors on the left, giving rise to a three-way interaction in the whole sample of DYSLEXIC STATUS*DIRECTION*STA ($p < 0.022$). No significant effects were found for age, sex, handedness, or any of the other personality scales used.

We have confirmed our previous findings that dyslexia is associated with poor visual direction sense, particularly when a leftward judgment is required. Schizotypy

---

[a]To whom correspondence should be addressed.

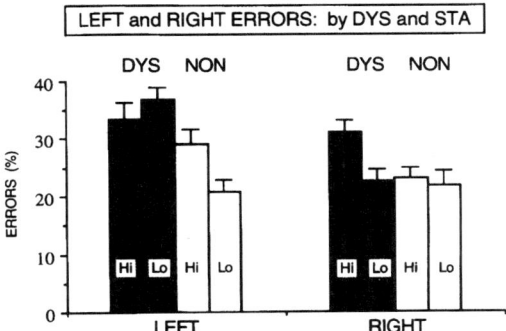

FIGURE 1. Left and right errors on the dot localization task for dyslexic and control groups, split by median STA scores.

was also associated with poor task performance (independent of the association we again found between dyslexia and STA); and in the control group, high STA scorers showed increased errors on the left. These results support the view that both dyslexia and schizotypal personality traits may be associated with impairment of visual transient and right-hemisphere function.

REFERENCES

1. RICHARDSON, A. J. & J. F. STEIN. 1993. Personality characteristics of adult dyslexics. *In* Studies in Visual Information Processing, R. Groner and S. Wright, Eds. Elsevier/North-Holland. In press.
2. RIDDELL, P., M. S. FOWLER & J. F. STEIN. 1990. Inaccurate visual localisation in dyslexic children. Percept. Mot. Skills **70:** 707–718.
3. CLARIDGE, G. & P. BROKS. 1984. Schizotypy and hemisphere function—I: Theoretical considerations and the measurement of schizotypy. Pers. Individ. Differ. **5:** 633–648.

Associations of Dyslexia with Epilepsy, Handedness, and Gender

STEVEN C. SCHACHTER,[a] ALBERT M. GALABURDA,[a]
AND BERNARD J. RANSIL[b]

[a]Department of Neurology
Beth Israel Hospital and Harvard Medical School
330 Brookline Avenue
Boston, Massachusetts 02215

[b]Harvard-Thorndike Laboratory of Beth Israel Hospital
Department of Medicine
Beth Israel Hospital and Harvard Medical School
Boston, Massachusetts 02215

Based on the observations of developmental cortical abnormalities in the brains of some dyslexic[1] and epileptic[2] patients, we tested for an association between epilepsy and a history of dyslexia in 200 adult epileptic patients and 130 age-matched controls. We also evaluated the interrelationships of handedness scores,[3,4] gender, and dyslexia in epileptics given the literature on dyslexia, male gender, and left-handedness.[5]

A history of dyslexia was significantly increased in patients with epilepsy compared with controls (9 vs. 2.3 percent; odds ratio = 4.19; 95 percent confidence interval = 1.21 to 15). Further, dyslexic epileptic males had significantly younger age of seizure onset than nondyslexic males, consistent with other epileptic syndromes associated with cortical anomalies.[6-10] Left-handed epileptic females were also at greater risk for dyslexia—among epileptic dyslexic patients, 15 percent of males versus 45 percent of females wrote with the left hand, possibly the first demonstration of elevated left-handedness in females compared to males.

The possible explanations for an association between dyslexia and epilepsy are (1) the cortical lesions seen in dyslexic brains may be epileptogenic and/or the structural abnormalities associated with epilepsy may also include neural networks involved in reading, (2) subclinical electrical discharges of the cortex may cause reading impairment, (3) epilepsy and dyslexia may be genetically linked, (4) reading impairment may result from anticonvulsant toxicity.

Adult patients referred to an epilepsy center may be at increased risk for dyslexia compared to controls, especially left-handed women and males with seizure onset by age 12. These findings supplement previous studies of reading achievement in epileptics and suggest that maintaining a high index of suspicion for dyslexia in these subgroups of epileptic patients may facilitate earlier recognition and intervention.

REFERENCES

1. GALABURDA, A. M., G. F. SHERMAN, G. D. ROSEN, F. ABOITIZ & N. GESCHWIND. 1985. Developmental dyslexia: Four consecutive patients with cortical anomalies. Ann. Neurol. **18**(2): 222–233.
2. ARMSTRONG, D. D. & C. J. BRUTON. 1987. Postscript: What terminology is appropriate for tissue pathology? How does it predict outcome? *In* Surgical Treatment of the Epilepsies, J. Engle, Ed.: 541–552. Raven Press. New York.

3. OLDFIELD, R. C. 1971. The assessment and analysis of handedness: The Edinburgh inventory. Neuropsychologia **9**(1): 97–113.
4. SCHACHTER, S. C., B. J. RANSIL & N. GESCHWIND. 1987. Associations of handedness with hair color and learning difficulties. Neuropsychologia **25**(1B): 269–276.
5. SCHACHTER, S. C. Studies of handedness and anomalous dominance: Problems and progress. *In* The Extraordinary Brain, A. M. Galaburda, Ed. Harvard Univ. Press. Cambridge, Mass. In press.
6. MEENCKE, H. & J. D. JANZ. 1984. Neuropathological findings in primary generalized epilepsy: A study of eight cases. Epilepsia **25**(1): 8–21.
7. BARKOVICH, A. J., D. J. JACKSON & R. S. BOYER. 1989. Band heterotopias: A newly recognized neuronal migration anomaly. Radiology **171**(2): 455–458.
8. KAZEE, A. M., L. W. LAPHAM, C. F. TORRES & D. D. WANG. 1991. Generalized cortical dysplasia. Clinical and pathologic aspects. Arch. Neurol. **48**(8): 850–853.
9. KUZNIECKY, R., J. H. GARCIA, E. FAUGHT & R. B. MORAWETZ. 1991. Cortical dysplasia in temporal lobe epilepsy: Magnetic resonance imaging correlations. Ann. Neurol. **29**(3): 293–298.
10. PALMINI, A., F. ANDERMANN, A. OLIVIER, D. TAMPIERI, Y. ROBITAILLE, E. ANDERMANN & G. WRIGHT. 1991. Focal neuronal migration disorders and intractable partial epilepsy: A study of 30 patients. Ann. Neurol. **30**(6): 741–749.

Correlation of Ocular Motor Reading Strategies to the Status of Adaptation in Patients with Hemianopic Visual Field Defects

DIETER SCHOEPF AND WOLFGANG H. ZANGEMEISTER[a]

Department of Neurology
University of Hamburg
Martinistrasse 52
D-2000 Hamburg 20
Germany

INTRODUCTION

To compensate for hemianopia it is necessary to have appropriate ocular motor strategies for efficient use of the remaining half of the visual field.[1] In reference 2 we demonstrated that patients with pure hemianopia and foveal sparing optimally learn to compensate their visual handicap in reading by active and motivated visual training. The purpose of the present study is to analyze in detail the different ocular motor reading strategies that hemianopic patients develop to compensate their visual handicap corresponding to their "relative" status of ocular motor adaptation in reading. Therefore, the eye and head reading path of ten well-selected patients with hemianopic visual field defects due to different aetiology was completely analyzed under this aspect. The "relative" status of ocular motor adaptation was marked according to the *mean reading rate,* the *frequency of acoustical reading errors,* and the most frequently applied *ocular motor reading strategies.* The apparatus and methods used were the same as previously described.[2] All patients had to read two groups of four different texts with distinct content. In a low-letter density mode the texts had 28 letters per line, and in high-letter density mode each text had 46 letters per line. The task was performed under two varying conditions: a head-fixed condition and a head-free-to-move condition. The patients were asked to read the texts as accurately and as quickly as possible.

RESULTS

The aetiology of the hemianopia, the visual field defect, and the reading efficiency of eight hemianopic patients of the experimental group are represented in TABLE 1, and the different reading strategies are shown in FIGURE 1. The upper two strategies were demonstrated by left hemianopic patients, the lower four by right hemianopic patients.

Patients with additional signs of visual hemi-inattention did not develop any adaptive ocular motor reading strategies. A normal "stop and go" reading pattern was

---

[a]To whom correspondence should be addressed.

TABLE 1. Description of Visual Field Defects, Aetiology, and Reading Efficiency of Eight Patients with Homonymous Hemianopia

RHH Patients	Age	Visual Field Defect	Aetiology	Neuro-psychological Testing	Male Reading Rate in Eye and Head Reading Path	Frequency of Acoustical Reading Error	Mostly Used Reading Strategies	Relative Status of Adaptation
D.H.	24	—Complete *right* hemifield loss without macular sparing —Slowly developing over 4 years	—Stenosis of Basilar At. —No CCT/MRI correlation —Psychogenic ätiology in question	No signs of visual hemi-inattention	11.5 L/S	—No acoustical reading error	—B. hemifield oversh. strategy —Increased error of line lex. during strategy	+ 9
E.S.	56	—Complete dense *right* lower hemifield loss reaching far over the horizontal meridian into the right upper quadrant	—Infarction left lower ocular lobe —CCT correlation —Acute event [3 months]	No signs of visual hemi-inattention	7.1 L/S	—No acoustical reading error	—End of line detection strategy —Sacc. resolution strategy —B. hemifield oversh. strategy	+ 5
A.S.	36	—*Right* wedgeshaped defect reaching from the papilla into the periphery —Additional right paracentral sco. —*Left eye patched*	—Isolated neuritis of the optic nerve (R.E.) —No other neurological diseases	No signs of visual hemi-inattention	7.5 L/S	—<1 error/text	—End of line detection strategy —Sacc. resolution strategy —(B. hemifield oversh. strategy)	+ 4
Z.Z.	46	—Incomplete *right* hemifield loss with determination of the upper quadrant —Macular sparing [3–5°] (left quadrant)	—Infarction left P.C.A. —Temporal contusion —CCT correlation —Acute event [11 months]	No signs of visual hemi-inattention	6.6 L/S	—>1 error/text	—End of line detection strategy —Sacc. resolution strategy	− 2
R.K.	48	—Incomplete *right* hemifield loss with determination of the upper quadrant —Macular sparing [3–5°] CCT (+)	—Recurrent cerebral embolism with transient dysphasia and hemiparesis	—*Poor test* with additional signs of visual neglect	< 4 L/S	—>4 error/text	—Disorganized reading pattern	− 8

(continued)

TABLE 1. (Continued)

LHH Patients	Age	Visual Field Defect	Aetiology	Neuro-psychological Testing	Male Reading Rate in Eye and Head Reading Path	Frequency of Acoustical Reading Error	Mostly Used Reading Strategies	Relative Status of Adaptation
G.S.	56	—Irregular *left* hemifield loss reaching into the right upper quadrant —Macular sparing [2°]	—Vascular embolism —Infarction P.C.A. —CCT correlation —Acute event [22 days]	No signs of visual hemi-inattention	8.3 L/S	—<1 error/text	—General oversh./reg. strategy	+5
K.U.	73	—Incomplete *left* hemifield loss —Macular sparing [5°]	—Vascular embolism —Infarction P.C.A. —CCT correlation —Acute event [31 days]	No signs of visual hemi-inattention	7.9 L/S	—No acoustical reading error	—Beginning of line detection strategy	+4
J.S.	59	—Complete dense *left* upper quadrantic loss —Visus right eye 0.1 —Visus left eye 1.0	—Cerebral embolism —CCT correlation —Acute event [12 days]	No signs of visual hemi-inattention	6.7 L/S	—>2 error/text	—Beginning of line detection strategy	−5

Note: Left [LHH] and right hemianopic patients [RHH] are ordered according to their "relative" status of ocular motor adaptation. The highest status of ocular motor adaptation in reading is reflected by plus ten; minus ten reflects the lowest status of adaptation.

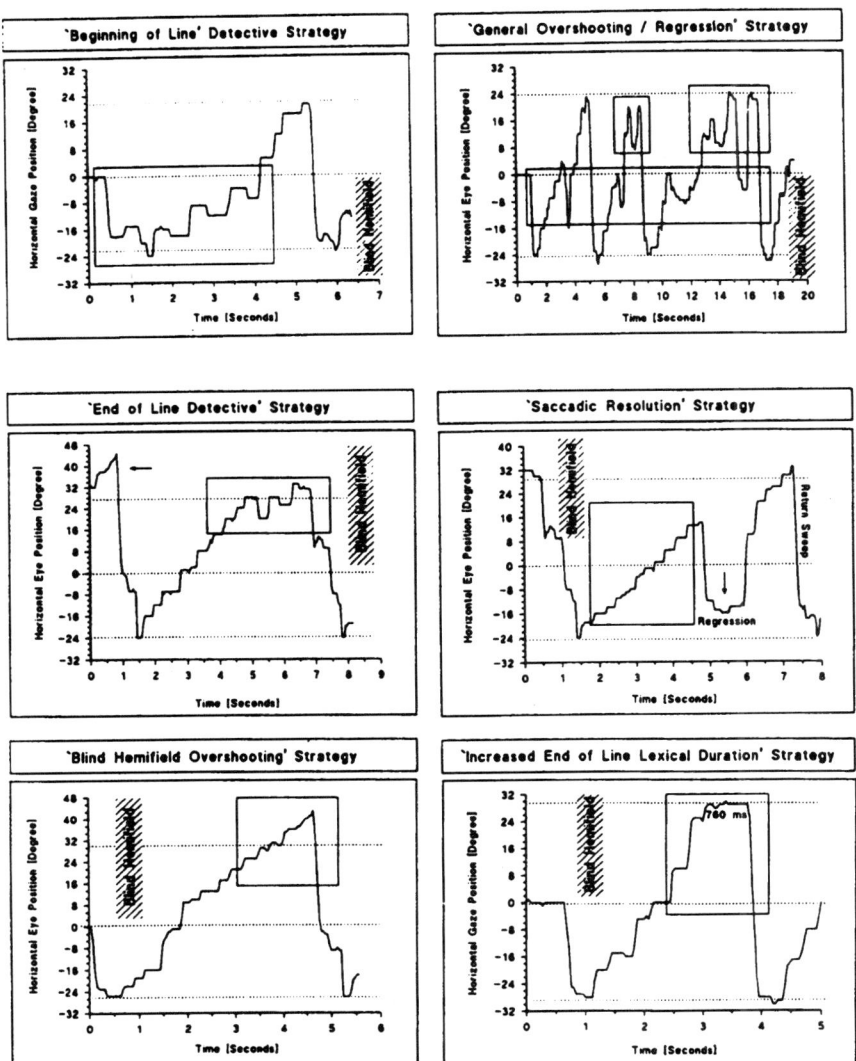

FIGURE 1. Ocular motor reading strategies that hemianopic patients demonstrated in the "eye and head reading path." *Often applied strategies* were the "beginning of line detective" strategy, the "end of line detective" strategy, and the "saccadic resolution" strategy. *Rarely used strategies* were the "general overshooting/regression" strategy, the "blind hemifield overshooting" strategy, and the "increased end of line lexical duration" strategy.

diminished, and the reading saccades appeared as strongly "disorganized." The mean reading rate was greatly decreased. Because of the disturbed ocular motor reading behavior, an increased number of acoustical reading errors resulted.

Simple adaptive reading strategies used by "poorly adapted" patients were as follows: the "beginning of line detective" strategy, the "end of line detective" strategy, and the "saccadic resolution" strategy. Higher adaptive reading strategies used by "better adapted" patients included the "general overshooting/regression" strategy, the "blind hemifield overshooting" strategy, and the "increased end of line lexical duration" strategy.

Delimitation of the Term "Subcortical Reading Ability"

In our experimental setup, with special respect to the patient D.H., who demonstrated clinically a maximal statokinetical dissociation,[3] a mean reading rate faster than nine letters per second, in combination with the "increased end of line lexical duration" strategy, was directed either to a "simulated," that is, hysterically, hemianopia, or to subcortical reading abilities.

CONCLUSION

The mean reading rate and the number of acoustical reading errors of the hemianopic patients were directly correlated with the "relative" status of ocular motor adaptation and to the aetiology of the visual field defect.

REFERENCES

1. ZANGEMEISTER, W. H., O. MEIENBERG, L. STARK & W. F. HOYT. 1982. Eye head coordination in homonymous hemianopia. J. Neurol. **226:** 243–254.
2. SCHOEPF, D. & W. H. ZANGEMEISTER. 1992. Eye and head reading path in hemianopic patients. *In* Studies in Visual Information Processing, R. Groner, Ed.: 267–290. North-Holland/Elsevier. Amsterdam.
3. RIDDOCH, G. 1917. Dissociation in visual perception due to occipital injuries, with special reference to appreciation of movement. Brain **40:** 15–57.

The Performance of Good and Poor Readers on Simultaneous and Temporal–Sequential Memory Tasks

ANN M. STAUNTON[a]

Department of Psychology
University College Dublin
Dublin, Ireland

INTRODUCTION

The theoretical framework of Working Memory incorporates the Articulatory Loop (AL) and The Visuospatial Sketch Pad (VSSP). The AL is used for recycling speech-based material in order to refresh the memory trace. The AL system makes an important contribution to serial order recall, and visual stimuli must be labeled if the stimuli are to avail of it.[1] The labeling of visual stimuli is a skill that is absolutely essential for learning to read. The VSSP is utilized for the maintenance of spatial stimuli and for storing images, but it is not equipped for storing temporal sequences of visual items.[1] A simultaneous visual presentation along with the prevention of auditory recoding and labeling of the stimuli is necessary to elicit the use of the VSSP.[2] The present study investigated the performance of good reading students (GRS) and students with reading difficulties (SRD) on Simultaneous and Temporal–Sequential visual memory tasks.

In Experiment 1 a simultaneous two-dimensional presentation of stimuli was employed to elicit the involvement of the VSSP[1] and to investigate the parallel processing powers of the subjects.[3] Twenty male SRD were matched with 20 male GRS according to chronological age and nonverbal IQ. Seven sets of stimuli "concrete words," "shapes," "household objects," "stones," "digits," "tones of pink," and "function words" were presented. Each stimulus set consisted of nine individual items. Access to imagery and to verbalization were manipulated by varying the concreteness of the stimuli and also the possibility of labeling them. Stimuli were presented in a predetermined order on a square chart containing 3 × 3 individual boxes. Viewing time of 3 seconds per item was allowed, and the responses were recorded on individual Response Forms. FIGURE 1 gives a comparison of the level of performance achieved by the SRD and the GRS for the various types of stimuli presented. Performance was comparable for both groups on all of the stimulus sets with the exception of the Function Words ($p < 0.05*$). Both groups performed well on items that were easily labeled, for example, "words," "objects," "digits," and less well on nonverbal stimuli, for example, "stones" and "tones of pink."

In Experiment 2 a Temporal–Sequential method of stimulus presentation was used. This type of presentation was expected to involve the use of the AL, and S's were expected to rely more heavily on verbalization. The same subjects and stimuli were again employed in this experiment. The items were presented in a Temporal–Sequential order, allowing 3 seconds of viewing time per item. The Response Form

---

[a]Current address: 4 Clyde Court, Clyde Road, Ballsbridge, Dublin 4, Ireland.

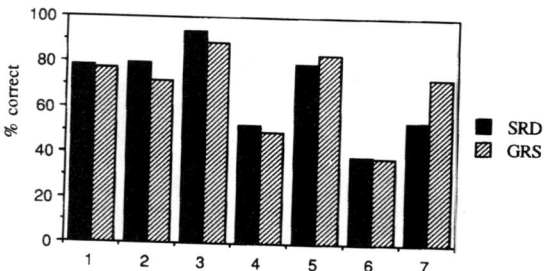

FIGURE 1. Overall performance achieved by the SRD and the GRS for the various sets of stimuli presented in Experiment 1, i.e., the Simultaneous Memory Tasks. Stimuli: 1 = words; 2 = shapes; 3 = objects; 4 = stones; 5 = digits; 6 = pinks, 7 = function words.

and the Display Chart were changed to take account of the sequential presentation order of the stimuli. The S's gave their responses by reconstructing the correct serial order of the stimuli on a rectangular display chart that contained 9 × 1 individual boxes. An outline of the overall performance is shown in FIGURE 2. Significant intergroup differences were found in relation to the following items: "Words" ($p < 0.01^{**}$), "Shapes" ($p < 0.001^{***}$), "Pinks" ($p < 0.01^{**}$). "Function Words" ($p < 0.001^{***}$). No difference in performance was observed for the highly familiar "Objects" and "Digits," nor was there any intergroup difference on the highly unfamiliar nonverbal "Stones."

In Experiment 3 the same sets of stimuli were presented in one- and two-dimensional arrays to a new but similar group of SRD. The same procedure was followed, that is, a simultaneous presentation of the stimuli, and the same S's tested for both presentations. Any observed differences in performance for this group of S's could be attributed directly to the type of presentation used. High scores were achieved by this group of SRD for both presentation methods. Scores obtained for the two-dimensional presentations were significantly better for "words" ($p < 0.01^{**}$) and "objects" ($p < 0.05^{*}$).

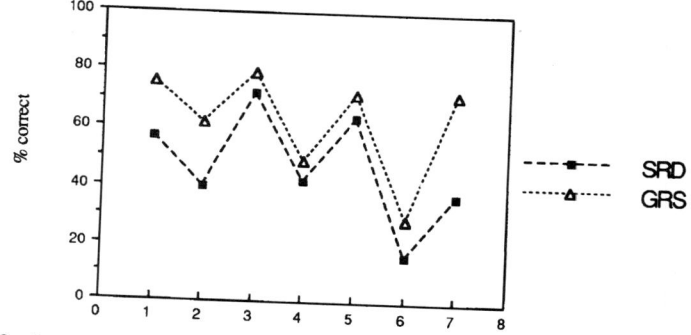

FIGURE 2. Overall performance achieved by the SRD and the GRS for the various sets of stimuli presented in Experiment 2, i.e., the Temporal–Sequential Memory Tasks. Stimuli: 1 = words; 2 = shapes; 3 = objects; 4 = stones; 5 = digits; 6 = pinks; 7 = function words.

DISCUSSION AND CONCLUSIONS

When the SRD performance on Simultaneous tasks was compared with their performance on the Temporal–Sequential tasks, I found that they had scored significantly better in the simultaneous presentation method on all of the stimulus sets with the exception of "stones." No such differences were observed for the GRS. It has been suggested that simultaneous and successive information processing are available to an individual for use in accordance with the demands of a task and the habitual method of problem solving that he or she uses.[4] The high level of performance (FIG. 1) by the SRD in Experiment 1 may be attributed to a tendency to rely on the VSSP. The poor performance of the SRD on the nonverbal "shapes" and "pinks" in Experiment 2 could be the result of some form of interitem interference among the consecutively presented visual items.[5] The use of control processes such as chunking may have facilitated better performance for familiar items in the two-dimensional presentations. Observed differences in performance on simultaneous presentations were related to difficulties at the central positions in the one-dimensional presentations. The SRD aptitude for simultaneous presentations was confirmed in Experiment 3, and they performed best when a two-dimensional array of the stimuli was employed.[6]

REFERENCES

1. BADDELEY, A. D. 1986. Working Memory. Clarendon Press. Oxford.
2. FRICK, R. W. 1988. Br. J. Psychol. **79:** 289–308.
3. PAVIO, A. & K. CSAPO. 1969. J. Exp. Psychol. **80:** 279–285.
4. DAS, J. P. 1973. J. Educational Psychol. **65**(1): 103–108.
5. NAIRNE, J. S. 1988. Mem. Cognition **6**(4): 342–352.
6. STAUNTON, A. M. 1991. The aetiology and remediation of reading difficulties. Unpublished Ph. D. Thesis. Submitted to the National University of Ireland, Dublin.

Frequency Modulation Analysis in Children with Landau-Kleffner Syndrome

GERRY A. STEFANATOS

Department of Psychiatry
Medical College of Pennsylvania
3200 Henry Avenue
Philadelphia, Pennsylvania 19129

Landau-Kleffner syndrome (LKS) is a progressive aphasic disturbance in children that is often characterized by a significant impairment of auditory language comprehension considered to involve disordered phonological decoding of speech. The specific nature of the phonological disorder has not been established, but is potentially related to (1) an *apperceptive* disturbance in which there is primary impairment of processes subserving the auditory analysis of acoustical features [amplitude modulation (AM) or frequency modulation (FM)] necessary for speech perception, or (2) an *associative* disturbance that may impede the intact acoustical representation from being mapped to an appropriate referent in the phonological system. In order to address this issue we examined neurophysiological processes subserving FM analysis in children with LKS. Given that formant frequency modulations serve as fundamental cues to distinguish speech sounds and may serve a cohesive function in binding speech sounds together, we reasoned that a disturbance involving FM analysis could result in the substantial comprehension difficulties characteristic of the syndrome. We employed a steady-state evoked-response methodology to obtain cortical responses to tones whose frequency was modulated at rates relevant to the phonetic analysis of speech, and compared responses of LKS children to those obtained from children with expressive developmental dysphasia and normal language controls.

The stimuli consisted of a continuous 1-kHz pure tone carrier frequency modulated at rates of 10, 20, and 40 Hz (see FIG. 1). The neurophysiological responses to these stimuli, recorded differentially over the left and right cerebral hemispheres (F3 and F4, referred to the ipsilateral mastoid), approximate sinusoids with a frequency of 4 Hz.[1] For comparison purposes we routinely also record responses to pure tone to serve as a "no response" control condition. As shown in FIGURE 1, responses to the FM tones in the normal ($n = 6$) and expressive developmental dysphasic group ($n = 6$) are well-formed potentials with a substantial 4-Hz frequency component and consistent phase characteristics. By contrast, the responses of the LKS group ($n = 6$) did not have a prominent 4-Hz component, nor regular phase characteristics. Indeed, their responses to frequency-modulated tones were similar to their responses to pure tones. This suggests that in many instances the frequency modulations present in the experimental stimuli evoked little if any time-locked neural activity. This was confirmed by analysis of the fast Fourier transform of these responses (FIG. 2). In two LKS cases, small but evident responses were identified by Fourier analysis at the 20-Hz modulation rate with no response at 10 Hz or 40 Hz. No overall hemispheric differences were noted.

These findings suggest that LKS is associated with aberrations in the neural mechanisms that respond to FM in sound and support an apperceptive basis to their

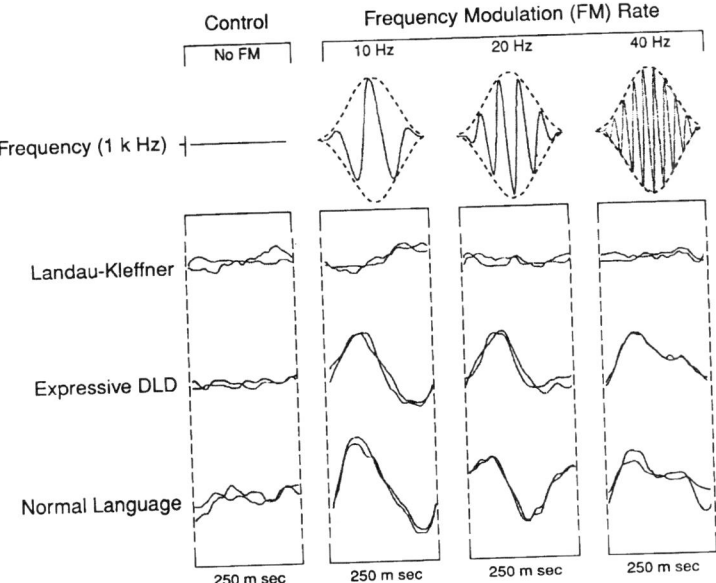

FIGURE 1. The stimuli consisted of a continuous 1-kHz pure tone carrier frequency modulated at rates of 10, 20, and 40 Hz. The depth of FM was modulated 100 percent by a 4-Hz sinusoid such that the carrier varied from a pure tone to a fully frequency modulated one, four times per second. Responses are time locked to the envelope imposed by the depth modulation (4 Hz) and occur at the same frequency. The two responses depicted for each condition represent potentials derived from the left and right hemisphere of representative cases.

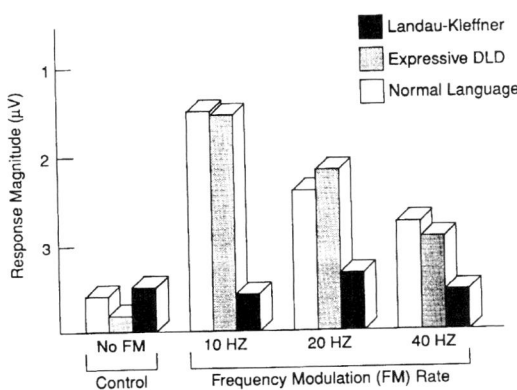

FIGURE 2. Histograms represent mean response magnitude derived from the fast Fourier transform for each group in each condition. The magnitude in the control pure tone condition represents a measure of the baseline activity present at 4 Hz.

difficulties with auditory language comprehension. The pathophysiological basis for this finding may involve neural mechanisms known to exist in the auditory system that are specifically concerned with FM analysis, particularly in processing the temporal attributes of frequency change in sound.[2] These mechanisms comprise parallel, physiologically distinguishable, rate-sensitive channels that are also attuned to such instantaneous temporal characteristics as the shape and direction of frequency modulation. The response profiles in LKS children to various rates of modulation presented here suggest that there may be some selectivity in their FM processing deficits, with relative sparing of particular rate-sensitive FM channels in some cases. The bilateral depression of responses to the FM tones is compatible with collateral clinical evidence in this population that bitemporal pathophysiology plays a critical role in the development of the syndrome. These findings add to a growing number of studies suggesting that anomalies of FM analysis contribute to some neurologically based problems with speech perception.[1,3]

REFERENCES

1. STEFANATOS, G. A., G. G. R. GREEN & G. G. RATCLIFF. 1989. Neurophysiological evidence of auditory channel anomalies in developmental dysphasia. Arch. Neurol. **46:** 871–875.
2. KAY, R. H. 1982. Hearing of modulation in sounds. Physiol. Rev. **63**(3): 894–975.
3. QUINE, D. B., D. REGAN, K. I. BEVERLY & T. J. MURRAY. 1984. Multiple sclerosis patients experience hearing loss specifically for shifts of tone frequency. Arch. Neurol. **41:** 506–508.

Temporal Encoding of Phonetic Features in Auditory Cortex[a]

M. STEINSCHNEIDER,[b] C. E. SCHROEDER,
J. C. AREZZO, AND H. G. VAUGHAN, JR.

[b]*Departments of Neurology and Neuroscience*
Rose F. Kennedy Center
Albert Einstein College of Medicine
Bronx, New York 10461

Neural encoding of temporal features of speech is a key component of language perception. This process is exemplified clinically by the selective deficits in processing rapidly changing sounds seen in dysphasic children,[1] and physiologically by the temporally precise pattern of activity evoked by speech in the auditory nerve.[2] Despite the crucial role of auditory cortex in language processing,[3] little is known about the temporal encoding of speech within primary auditory cortex (A1).

We investigated the temporal encoding of speech in A1 by examining laminar profiles of auditory evoked potentials (AEP), current source density (CSD), and multiple unit activity (MUA) in 7 awake monkeys to the synthetic syllables /da/, /ta/, and /ba/. These syllables differ in the phonetic parameters of voice onset time (VOT) and place of articulation, and are discriminated by monkeys in a manner similar to that seen in humans.[4] The recording procedures yield measures of net postsynaptic-potential (CSD) and action potential (MUA) activity in neuronal ensembles, and are directly applicable to AEP scalp recordings in humans. Click-evoked potentials were used to differentiate cortical responses from activity in thalamocortical (TC) afferents, and to define physiologically the laminar locations of the recording sites.[5]

Multiple phonetic features are encoded in short-latency and temporally precise response patterns within A1 and its TC afferents.[6,7] Syllable fundamental frequency (f_0) is encoded by phase-locked responses of equal frequency. Place of articulation (/da/ versus /ba/) is reflected by discriminative "on" and phase-locked responses occurring to the formant transition regions of the syllables. VOT (/da/ versus /ta/) is encoded by "on" responses time-locked to constant release and voicing onset, and phase-locked to the syllables' f_0- (FIG. 1). The phase-locked response pattern reflecting VOT occurs more commonly in TC afferents, while the "on" responses time-locked to consonant release and voicing onset are more prominent in cortical responses. This latter cortical response pattern correlates with the perceptual VOT boundary for /da/ and /ta/ (FIG. 2).

We conclude that important features of speech, including syllable f_0, VOT, and place of articulation, are rapidly encoded by temporally precise responses within A1. Subtle abnormalities in these temporal encoding mechanisms may underlie the perceptual deficits in certain dysphasic populations.

---

[a]This work was supported in part by grant DC00657, in part by grant MH06723, and in part by the McDonnell-Pew Program in Cognitive Neuroscience.
[b]To whom correspondence should be addressed.

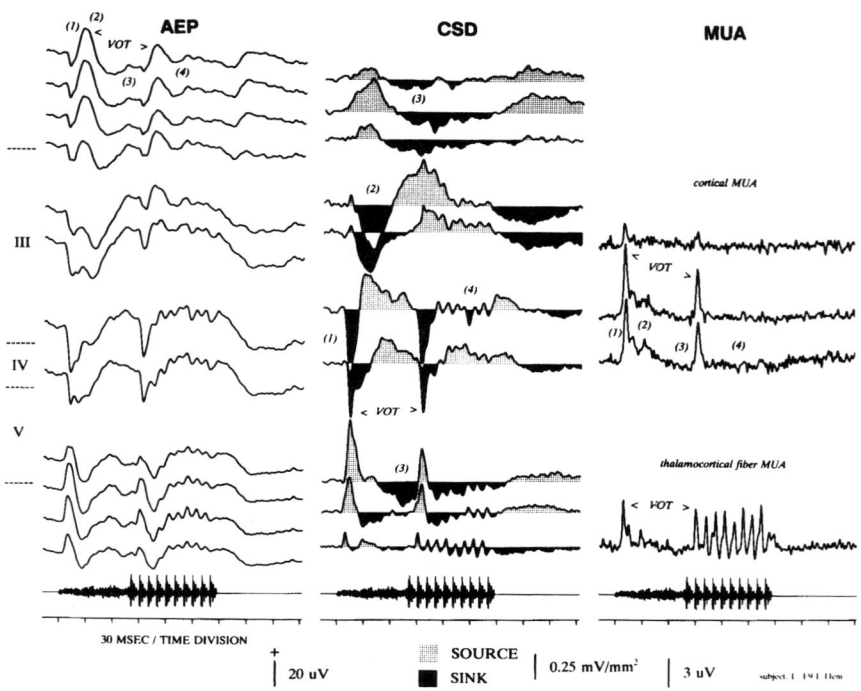

FIGURE 1. Laminar profiles of the AEP, CSD, and MUA to /ta/ recorded at 200-μm intervals through A1. Approximate laminar boundaries are shown at the left. Prominent cortical "on" responses in the AEP, CSD, and MUA are evoked by the onsets of the aperiodic and periodic stimulus segments and reflect syllable VOT. In contrast, the TC fiber MUA contains an "on" response to consonant release followed by phase-locked responses to the f_0. Syllables initiate a characteristic laminar sequence of current sinks, labeled (1) to (4) in the CSD. The initial sink (1) is located in lamina 4 and lower lamina 3 and is followed by current sinks in more superficial regions of lamina 3 (2), very superficial and infragranular current sinks (3), and a subsequent lower lamina 3 sink (4). Activity reflecting voicing onset is superimposed upon these responses. Concurrent MUA increases and decreases, labeled (1)–(4), indicate that current sinks (1), (2), and (4) represent locations of net excitatory synaptic activity, while current sinks (3) at least partially represent passive current return for inhibitory synaptic activity and active current sources in lamina 3. The superficial AEP waveform is similarly labeled to indicate the timing of the current sinks. Comparisons with the CSD indicate that the AEP is a composite waveform generated by a sum of the multilaminar sources and sinks.

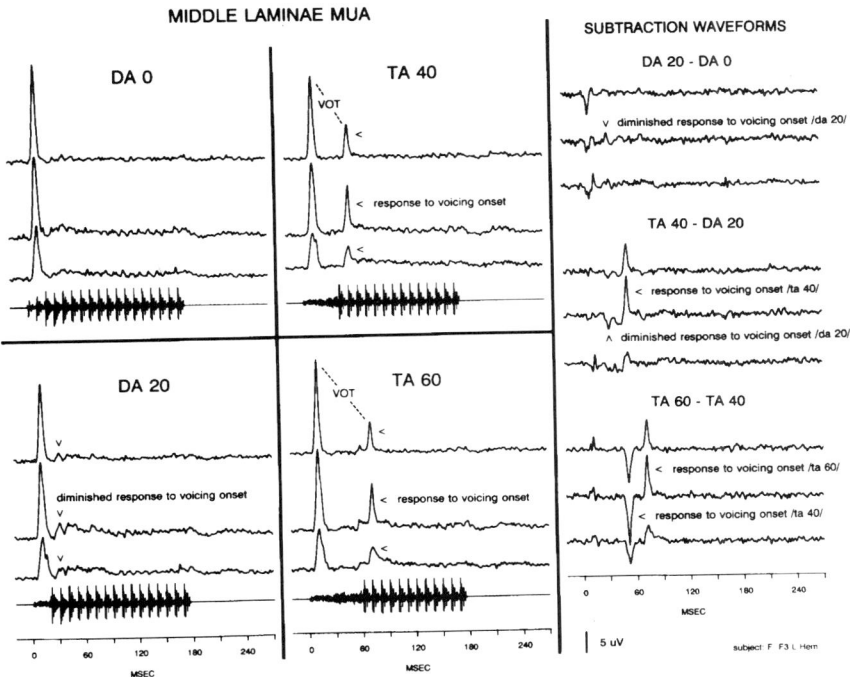

FIGURE 2. MUA recorded from 3 locations in laminae 3 and 4 separated by 150-μm intervals. Only /ta/ syllables (VOT = 40 and 60 ms) elicit 2 "on" responses, while /da/ syllables (VOT = 0 and 20 ms) elicit a single "on" response. This pattern reflects the psychoacoustic boundary for VOT.

REFERENCES

1. TALLAL, P. & R. E. STARK. 1981. J. Acoust. Soc. Am. **69:** 568–574.
2. DELGUTTE, B. 1980. J. Acoust. Soc. Am. **68:** 843–857.
3. WISE, R., et al. 1991. Brain **114:** 1803–1817.
4. KUHL, P. K. 1986. Exp. Biol. **45:** 233–265.
5. STEINSCHNEIDER, M., et al. 1992. Electroenceph. Clin. Neurophysiol. **84:** 196–200.
6. STEINSCHNEIDER, M., J. C. AREZZO & H. G. VAUGHAN, JR. 1982. Brain Res. **252:** 353–365.
7. ———. 1990. Brain Res. **519:** 158–168.

Auditory Temporal Processing in Relation to Reading and Math Disabilities

BETTY U. WATSON AND CHARLES S. WATSON

Department of Speech and Hearing Sciences
Indiana University
Bloomington, Indiana 47405

Previous studies have demonstrated degraded auditory temporal processing by reading-disabled students, compared to students with normal reading skills. This study examined the auditory temporal processing skills of reading-disabled, math-disabled, and normally achieving students. The math-disabled group was included to control for the possibility that poor temporal processing is a "marker" variable for learning disabilities rather than being related specifically to reading disability.

Twenty reading-disabled and ten math-disabled college students who met the federal discrepancy and exclusionary guidelines[1] for diagnosis of learning disability served as subjects. Twenty-five college students with normal reading and math skills composed the normal group. All subjects passed bilateral audiometric screenings.

The Test of Basic Auditory Capabilities (TBAC)[2] was used to assess temporal abilities. This test battery includes eight subtests, five of which measure aspects of temporal processing. The five temporal subtests include: Single-Tone Duration (DT), Pulse/Train Discrimination (PT), Embedded Test-Tone Loudness (ET)—in which the subject must detect the presence of an extra tone in a word-length, nine-tone sequence—Temporal Order for Tones (TO), and Syllable Sequence (SS). The remaining subtests are: Pitch Discrimination (DF), Loudness Discrimination (DL), and Syllable Identification (SI), in which the subject identifies nonsense syllables in noise. With the exception of the Syllable Identification subtest, all tasks are conducted using a modified two-alternative forced-choice psychophysical procedure. This battery yields large and reliable differences among adult listeners.[3]

FIGURE 1 shows the means and standard errors of the mean for the three groups on the TBAC. A composite score on the five temporal tasks was calculated for each subject, and an analysis of variance of this score showed the mean of the reading-disabled group to fall significantly below the mean of the normal group. The means of the math-disabled and normal groups were not significantly different.

FIGURE 2 shows the performance of the individual subjects on each subtest. This figure reveals considerable overlap in the range of performance by the three groups on all of the tasks in spite of the finding of a significant difference between the reading-disabled and normal subjects on the mean composite score for the temporal tasks.

These results confirm an association between reading disability and auditory temporal processing that is specific to reading disability, as the math-disabled group performed similarly to the normal subjects on the temporal tasks. However, the overlap in performance of the three groups suggests that impaired temporal processing is neither a sufficient nor necessary cause of specific reading disability.

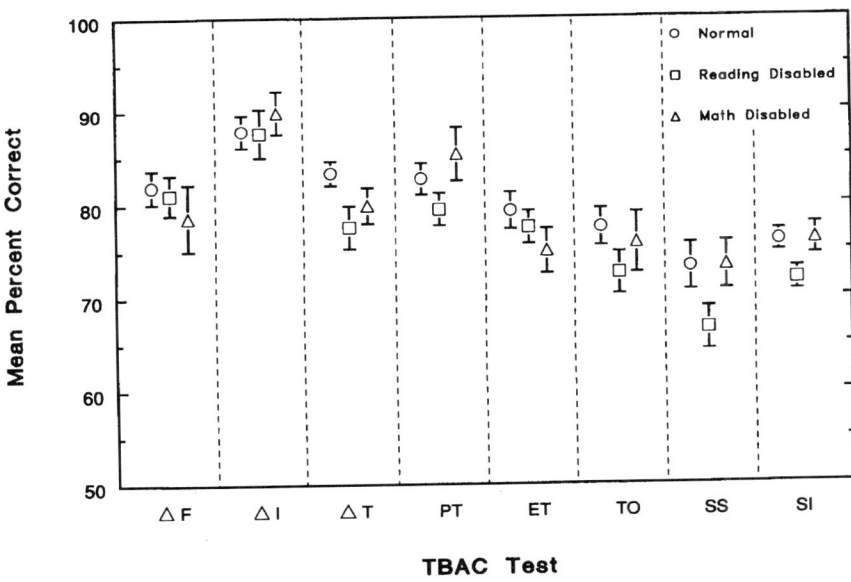

FIGURE 1. Mean percent correct and standard errors of the mean on the eight subtests of the Test of Basic Auditory Capabilities for the reading-disabled, math-disabled, and normal subjects. (*Key:* DF—pitch discrimination; DL—loudness discrimination; DT—single-tone loudness; PT—pulse/train discrimination; ET—embedded test-tone loudness; TO—temporal order for tones; SS—syllable sequence; SI—syllable identification.)

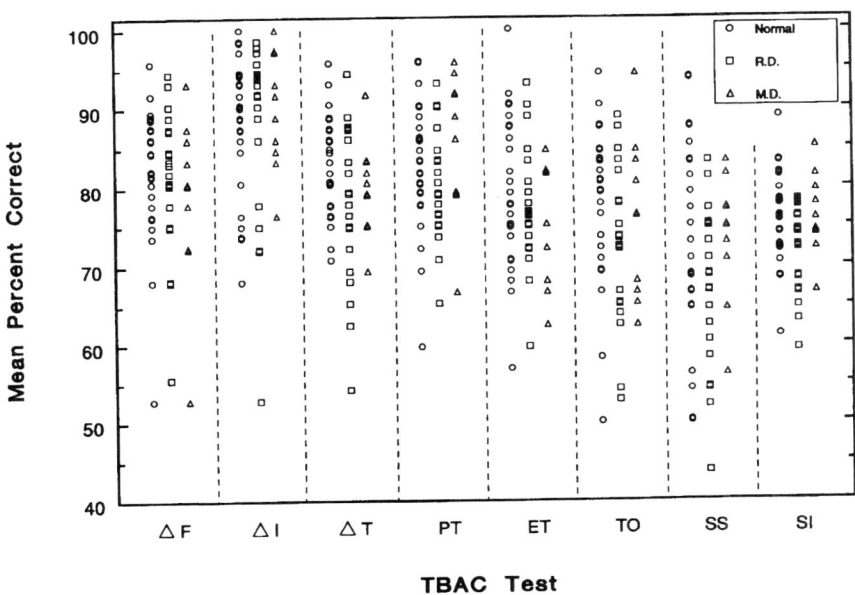

FIGURE 2. Performance of all subjects on the eight subtests of the Test of Basic Auditory Capabilities.

REFERENCES

1. UNITED STATES OFFICE OF EDUCATION. 1977. Rules and regulations implementing Public Law 94-142 (The Education for All Handicapped Children Act of 1975). Fed. Regist. **42.**
2. WATSON, C. S., D. M. JOHNSON, J. R. LEHMAN, W. J. KELLY & J. K. JENSEN. 1982. An auditory discrimination test battery. J. Acoust. Soc. Am. Suppl. **71:** S73.
3. CHRISTOPHERSON, L. A. & L. E. HUMES. 1992. Some psychometric properties of the Test of Basic Capabilities (TBAC). J. Speech Hear. Res. **35:** 929–935.

Auditory Perception, Phonological Processing, and Reading Ability/Disability

BETTY U. WATSON AND CHARLES S. WATSON

Department of Speech and Hearing Sciences
Indiana University
Bloomington, Indiana 47405

Auditory perception, including temporal processing, has been proposed as one source of individual differences in the phonological abilities that play a major role in skilled reading as well as in reading disability. It has been suggested that subtle perceptual deficits may lead to the development of degraded representations of verbal information in memory and also to problems in segmenting words into phonemes.[1,2] Although a number of previous investigations have demonstrated differences between good and poor readers on a variety of auditory perceptual tasks, only a few studies have directly examined relationships between the auditory and phonological domains. This study investigated the relationship between the two domains.

The subjects for this study were 94 undergraduate students. Twenty-four of the subjects had been previously identified as reading-disabled using the discrepancy and exclusionary criteria of the federal guidelines.[3] The remaining subjects volunteered for the study and demonstrated a wide range of reading proficiency. All subjects passed bilateral audiometric screenings.

A battery of experimental and standardized tests was administered to each subject to assess reading, phonological, and auditory abilities. The auditory tasks included tests of speech perception, nonverbal auditory temporal processing, and simple auditory discrimination.

The test results were first analyzed using confirmatory factor analysis[4] to identify factors or latent variables. TABLE 1 shows the latent variables and the measures contributing to each variable.

Relationships among the latent variables were then assessed using a latent variable model approach,[4] or path analysis. FIGURE 1 shows the model that proved to be the best fit. The insignificant paths, or those with insufficient parameter estimates, have been removed. The original form of this model hypothesized that *both* nonverbal temporal processing and speech perception affected phonological processing. However, none of the relationships between nonverbal temporal processing and the various phonological latent variables were significant, and those paths have therefore been deleted from the final version of the model.

These findings indicate a strong relationship between speech perception, which included a measure of temporal processing, and several of the phonological processes involved in reading. Nonverbal temporal processing, however, was not related to the phonological abilities independently of intelligence and speech perception.

TABLE 1. Latent Variables and Component Measures

Latent Variables	Component Measures
Auditory Perception	
Simple discrimination	Pitch discrimination
	Loudness discrimination
	Duration discrimination
Nonverbal temporal processing	Rhythm discrimination
	Discrimination of patterns with an embedded tone
	Discrimination of temporal order of tones
Speech perception	Syllable sequence test
	Syllable identification test
	Staggered spondaic word test
	Sound mimicry test
Phonological Processing	
Short-term auditory memory	Digit span
	Letter span
Long-term auditory memory	Paired associates task—Real words
	Paired associates task—Artificial words
Phoneme segmentation	Word reversal tasks
	Sound analysis task
Reading	
Word identification (reading words)	Woodcock-Johnson Word Identification
	Woodcock Reading Mastery Word Identification
Word attack	Woodcock-Johnson Word Attack
	Woodcock Reading Mastery Word Attack
Passage comprehension	Woodcock-Johnson Passage Comprehension
	Woodcock Reading Mastery Passage Comprehension

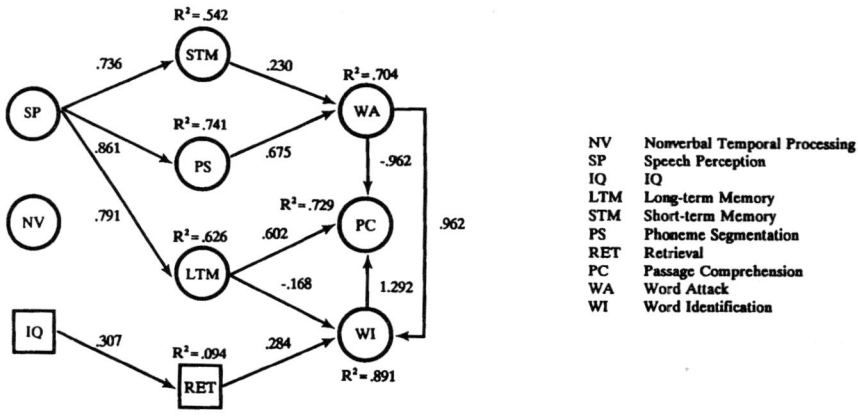

FIGURE 1. Path diagram showing the significant relationships between auditory perception, phonological processing, and reading. Squared multiple correlation coefficients are given for each of the dependent variables, and standardized path coefficients are also presented.

REFERENCES

1. TALLAL, P. 1980. Auditory perception, phonics, and reading disabilities in children. Brain Lang. **9:** 182–198.
2. TORGESEN, J. K. 1985. Memory processes in reading disabled children. J. Learn. Disabilities **18:** 350–357.
3. UNITED STATES OFFICE OF EDUCATION. 1977. Rules and regulations implementing Public Law 94-142 (The Education for All Handicapped Children Act of 1975). Fed. Regist. **42.**
4. JÖRESKOG, K. G. & D. SÖRBOM. 1990. LISREL 7: Estimation of Linear Structural Equation Systems. Program Version 7.16. Scientific Software. Mooresville, Ind.

Temporal Information Processing in Adults with Reading Difficulties

JEAN WHYTE

Clinical Speech and Language Studies
Trinity College
Dublin 2, Ireland

DISCUSSION

Research into neuropsychological correlates of reading disability in adults has been very sparse.[1,2] If the deficiencies in language subskills and in the integration of subskills found to be associated with reading difficulties in children subsist in adults, there would be support for the notion of a deficiency in an underlying mechanism affecting both language and reading skills, and for the interrelationship of the skills involved. Adults with reading difficulties would perform at a lower level than normally reading peers on tasks using nonverbal cognitive skills and language skills, but more basic mechanisms such as temporal processing might be ultimately responsible.

Cognitive and linguistic correlates of reading disability were investigated in a sample of 20 adult males (C.A. 25–45) in Belfast, Northern Ireland.[3] They were in employment, of average nonverbal IQ, had attended normal schools, and had estimated reading ages < 9. They were compared with matched normal readers ($N = 22$) on the time taken:

(a) To process nonlinguistic material;[4,5]
(b) To transform immediate linguistic input;[6]
(c) To recall and reorganize linguistic input;[7]
(d) To generate linguistic output independent of input (giving instructions to an unseen listener with and without a stimulus present).

RESULTS

Both groups scored within the normal range on the nonlinguistic material (WAIS Performance IQ of 96.6 for poor readers, 106.96 for controls; $P < 0.01$), but poor readers scored significantly lower on all subtests. The Associative Grouping Task demanded that input be matched to previously acquired linguistic knowledge and then transformed. Subjects were presented with two sets of nine sequentially presented nouns, first spoken aloud and then laid out on cards, and asked to state how the first two were alike, how the third differed from the first two, how it was like them, and so on. Poor readers were significantly slower and scored significantly lower on the first list. They were not slower, but still scored significantly lower on the second list, suggesting that more than processing time is involved.

But poor readers did not differ significantly from normal readers in time or in results when they were required to recall ideas from immediate linguistic input (3 × 100 word passages). They were not significantly slower in giving titles, but scored significantly lower for title 1 ($P < 0.01$) and title 2 ($P < 0.05$), and similarly to the normal readers for title 3. The progressive improvement suggested that their problem with transforming and integrating material could be overcome.

There were no significant differences in time or scores between the groups on the two tasks requiring generation of linguistic output without presented input to an unseen listener [instructions on changing a plug (stimulus present) and an automobile wheel (stimulus absent)].

It was concluded that adult poor readers have failed to develop certain cognitive skills that enable normal readers to transform language at a complex level. These deficiencies may have prevented them from forming particular concepts in the past and are now associated with slower processing time for these tasks. But the finding that poor readers performed equally with normal readers in language tasks demanding less complex processing suggests that any underlying deficiency, such as a weakness in temporal processing, does not operate at all levels of functioning in adult subjects.

REFERENCES

1. SPREEN, O. 1989. *In* Learning Disabilities: Neurological correlates and treatment, Vol. 1, D. J. Bakker and H. van der Vlugt, Eds.: 55–71. Swets & Zeitlinger. Amsterdam.
2. KINSBOURNE, M., D. T. RUFO, E. GAMZU, R. L. PALMER & A. K. BERLINER. 1991. Dev. Med. Child Neurol. **33**(9): 763–776.
3. WHYTE, J. 1979. Cognitive and linguistic correlates of reading disability in adults. Unpublished Ph.D. Thesis, Queen's University, Belfast.
4. RAVEN, J. C. 1956. Progressive Matrices, rev. ed. H. K. Lewis. London.
5. WECHSLER, D. 1955. Wechsler Adult Intelligence Scale. Psychological Corporation. New York.
6. BRUNER, J. S. & R. OLVER. 1962. The development of equivalence transformations in children. *In* Cognitive Development in Children: 5 Monographs. Society for Research in Child Development. Univ. of Chicago Press. Chicago.
7. BATE, S. M. 1970. Reading Test EH1-3. Test 2, Comprehension. National Foundation for Educational Research. Slough, Bucks., England.

Long-term Effects of Rehabilitative Interventions for Dyslexic Children

EVELIN WITRUK[a]

Martin Luther University
Halle-Wittenberg, Germany

For 3–5 percent of children in the eastern part of Germany, dyslexia represents a substantial learning and developmental handicap. Although these children have the opportunity of learning in special rehabilitative classes in grades 2 and 3, in grade 4 they go back to their normal classes.

We looked at the long-term effects of these special classes in regard to compensation of partial perceptive, cognitive, and memory deficits and with reference to the development of the whole personality in these dyslexic children.

The developmental analysis of cognitive, motivational, and emotional traits on the basis of longitudinal and cross-sectional comparisons performed from grade 2 to grade 8 showed an increase in interindividual differences [see FIG. 1(a) and (b)]. Two divergent types of personality development of dyslexic children were statistically verified. After reintegration into grade 4, a large number of dyslexic children require continued care and support. Boys predominate in the negative developmental cluster, where we found underachievement still in grade 8. These clusters include about 60 percent of our dyslexic children, and is characterized by lower and lower school performances. We therefore suggest that further rehabilitation is urgently needed after grade 3 [see FIG. 1(a)].

The smaller positive developmental cluster, which includes about 40 percent of the dyslexics, with girls predominating, shows very good school performance development. They are obviously able to compensate better for the partial deficits. Until grade 8 these students have developed so well that underachievement cannot be seen anymore.

Personality characteristics distinguish these two developmental clusters [see FIG. 1(b)]. We note an increasing differentiation, even in motivational and emotional traits, from grade 4 to grade 8. Thus we have to assume that there are clear compensations—for example, high learning motivation, better learning behavior, higher self-esteem, but also greater fear of failure—within the positive developmental group. The high degree of fear of failure is an especially important characteristic of this group of dyslexic children (see FIG. 2). In comparison with the normal, nonselected, and nondiscrepancy student group it seems to be an overcompensation. Interestingly enough, however, even the negative developmental cluster of dyslexic students differs from the normal control group only in the learning behavior, not in their whole personality structure.

---

[a]Current address. Universität Leipzig, Fachbereich Psychologie "Wilhelm Wundt," Tieckstrasse 2, Leipzig 0-7030.

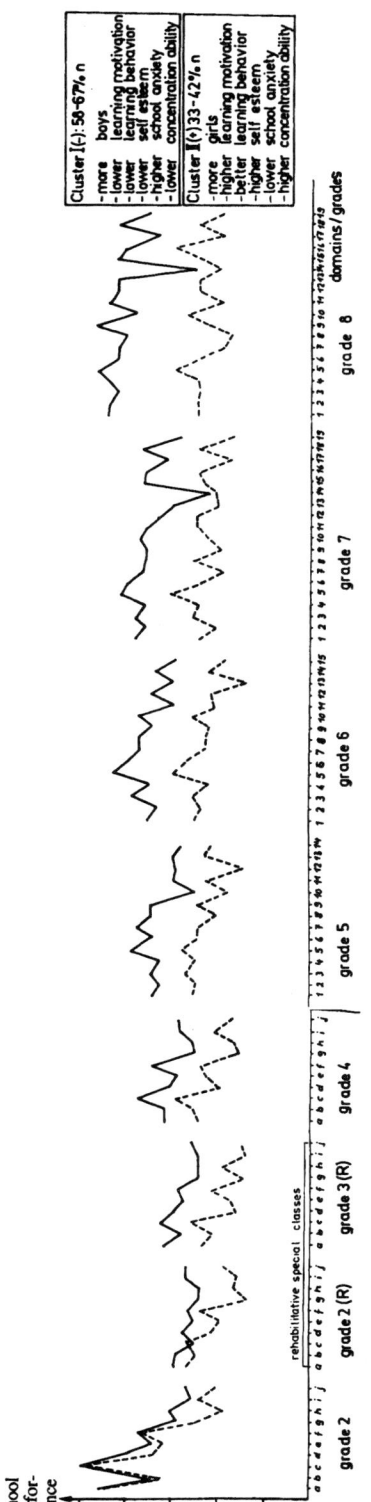

FIGURE 1. Developmental analysis of dyslexic children from grade 2 to grade 8 on the basis of profile-time-series-cluster analysis with longitudinal and cross-sectional dates. (From Witruk.[1] Reproduced by permission.) Two divergent types of personality development! (a) School performance development of the two types of dyslexic children.

428   ANNALS NEW YORK ACADEMY OF SCIENCES

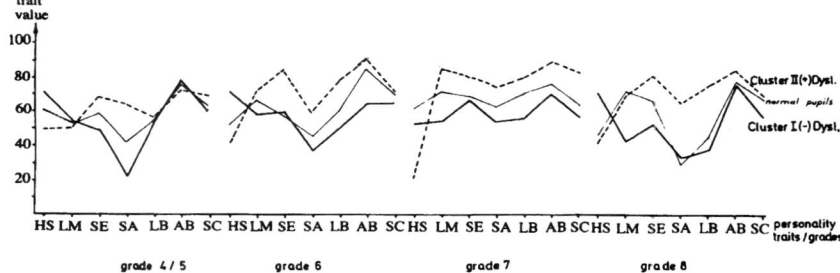

FIGURE 1. (b) Development of emotional, motivational, and behavioral traits on the two types of dyslexic children in comparison with a normal pupil group. (*Key:* HS—hope for success–fear for failure; LM—learning motivation; SE—self-esteem; SA—school anxiety; LB—learning behavior; AB—abnormal deviant behavior; SC—self-concept.)

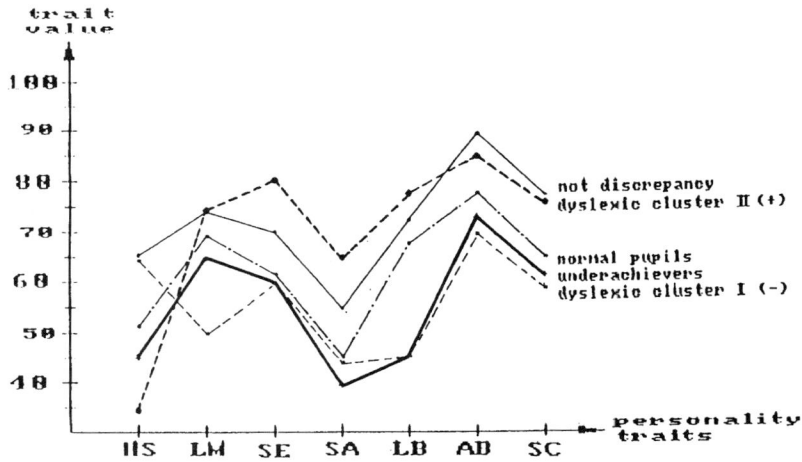

FIGURE 2. Emotional and motivational traits of pupils in grades 6–9 (Ronstanz Questionnaire: HS—hope for success–fear for failure; LM—learning motivation; SE—self-esteem; SA—school anxiety; LB—learning behavior; AB—abnormal behavior; SC—self-concept) (Reiss, Janicke 1989; Thiele, Dixie 1989). Do dyslexic children stay underachievers?

On the basis of our results we can estimate and compare the differential, long-term effects of the special rehabilitative intervention in our country. We can conclude that additional support or psychotherapy is necessary.

REFERENCES

1. WITRUK, E. 1990. Learning and developmental problems of dyslexic children. Paper presented at the IVth European Conference for Developmental Psychology, Stirling, Scotland.

Memory Deficits of Dyslexic Children

EVELIN WITRUK[a]
Martin Luther University
Halle-Wittenberg, Germany

We assume that dyslexia is represented by a complex of syndromes consisting of various combinations of partial disabilities on the basis of minimal cerebral dysfunctions. For 3–5 percent of our children, dyslexia exhibits a substantial learning and developmental handicap, and they have the opportunity of taking special rehabilitative classes in grades 2 and 3.

The question of the existence and the specifics of memory deficits and their chances for compensation are important points in our dyslexia research program. In our studies we examined the internal representation and the use of various complex levels of the language system in the acts of reading and writing in regard to acute primary symptoms and secondary reasons and with reference to the degree of compensation in later years. The acquisition of literacy is based on learning processes which lead to an internal representation of the various complex levels of the language system. The generation of reading and writing acts occurs by the interaction of working and long-term memory components.

We present for discussion some selected examples and results that agree with our plan of purpose and methods.

The acute primary status (primary symptoms and secondary reasons) was checked in regard to deficits of working memory in the processing of visual, phonological, and intermodal sequences (Witruk, Weber, Fuchs 1991). The rehabilitative effects were checked against cross-sectional and longitudinal comparisons from first to second grade (see FIG. 1). We found no significant differences in the demands on the memory of visual sequences between normal and dyslexic children. The longitudinal analysis shows a significant compensation effect. In accordance with other results (see FIG. 3 and compare with Siegel 1992) it seems to be an overcompensation in the direction of the visual analysis with a high perceptive effort. The opposite relations we found on the memory demands of phonological sequences. Here exist significant differences between normal and dyslexic children, and we cannot see a compensation tendency. We assume here a high resistance to therapy. Normal reading and writing acts suppose intermodal sequential memory performances. Here we can see a high deficit in comparison with normal children, but also a high, significant compensation effect in the longitudinal and cross-sectional analysis.

In regard to deficits in long-term memory parameters within the acute primary status of dyslexia, we examined the recognition of semantic relations under the demands of analogies, associations, and omission texts. We compared the intelligence of homogeneous groups of normal, dyslexic, and speech disturbed children in grade 2 (Witruk, Born 1987, Witruk, Weber 1991) (see FIG. 2). We did not find any

---

[a]Current address. Universität Leipzig, Fachbereich Psychologie "Wilhelm Wundt," Tieckstrasse 2, Leipzig 0-7030.

FIGURE 1. Working memory deficits and their compensation of dyslexic children. (Cross-sectional comparison by Rosendahl (1986) and longitudinal comparison by Witruk *et al.* (1991). Reproduced by permission.)

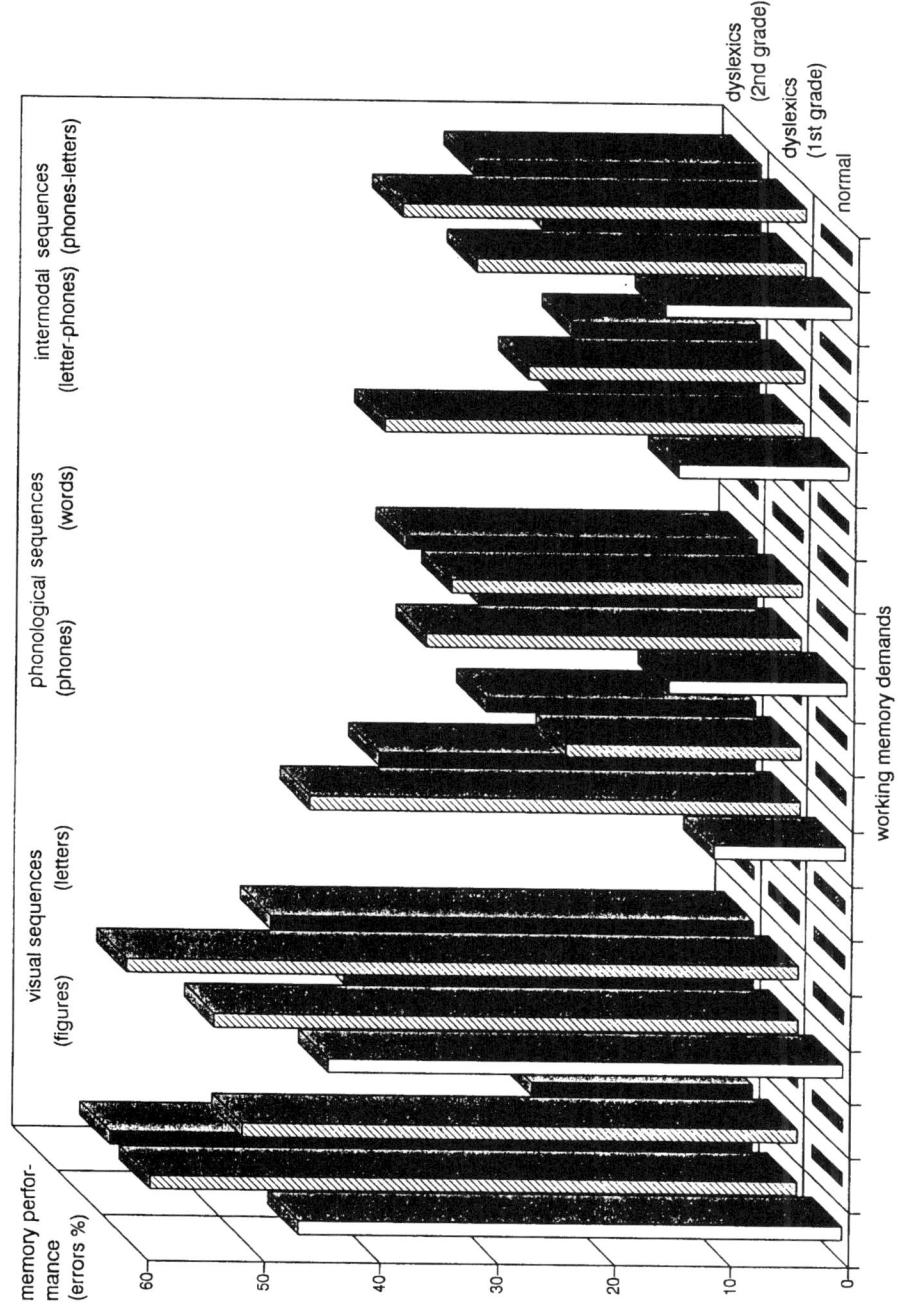

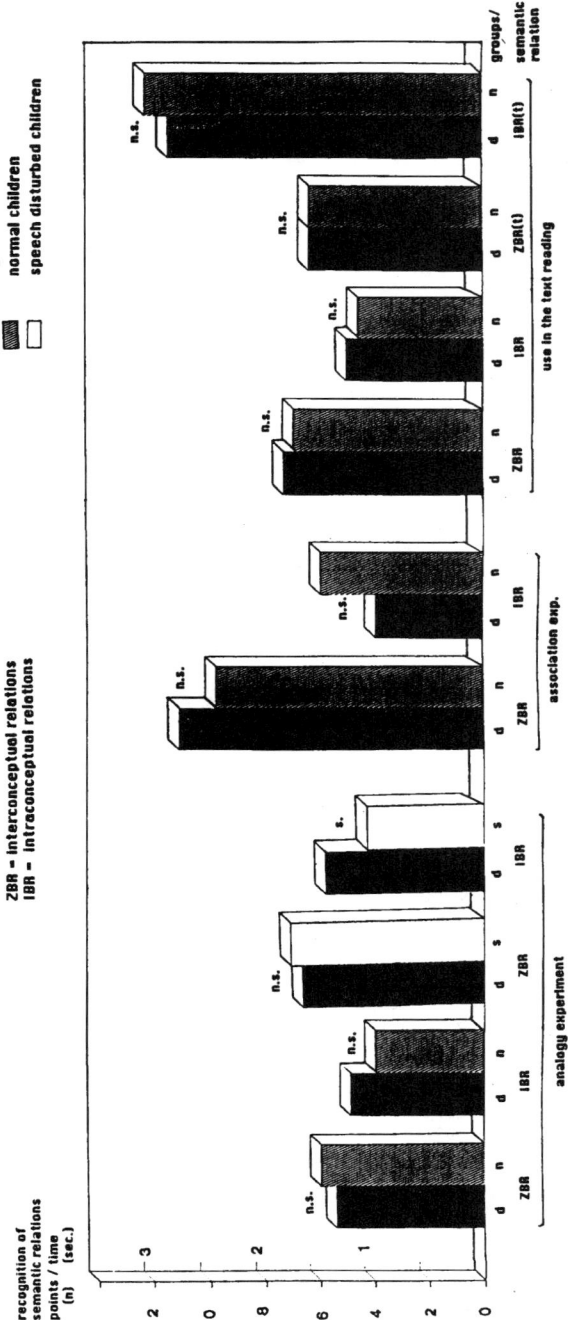

FIGURE 2. Recognition of semantic relations of dyslexic, normal, and speech-disturbed children in second grade. (From Witruk et al. (1991). Reproduced by permission.) No significant differences between normal and dyslexic children!

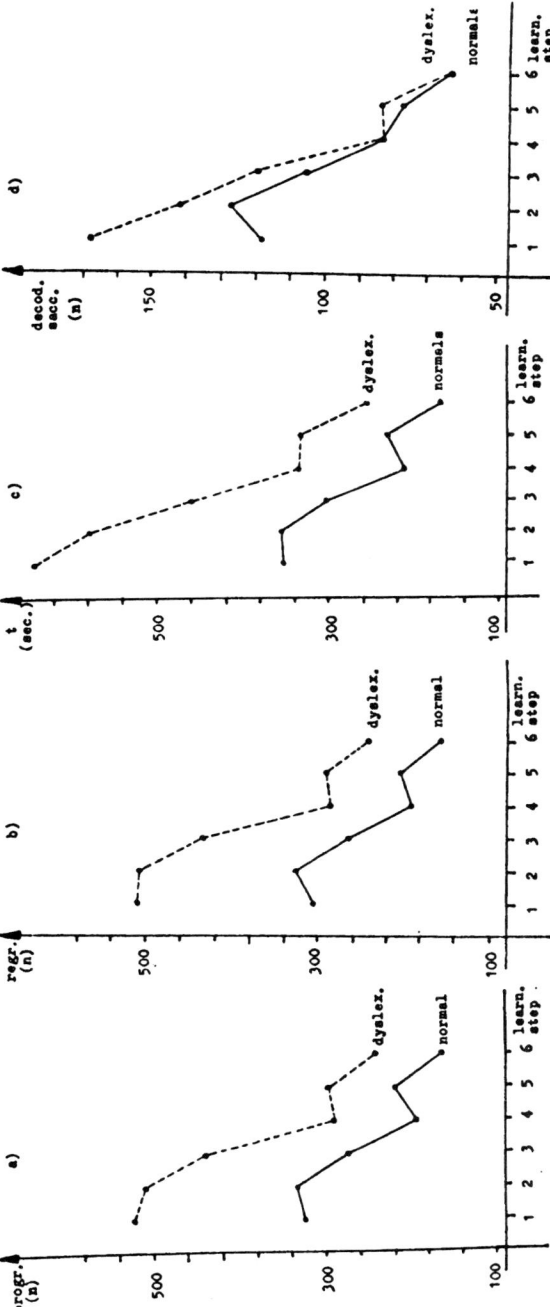

FIGURE 3. Efficiency of working memory in the course of second reading learning with normal and dyslexic children in seventh grade. (From Witruk and Staats (1983). Reproduced by permission.) (a) Differential learning course analysis in terms of working memory parameters progressions a), regressions b), reading time c), and decoding saccades d).

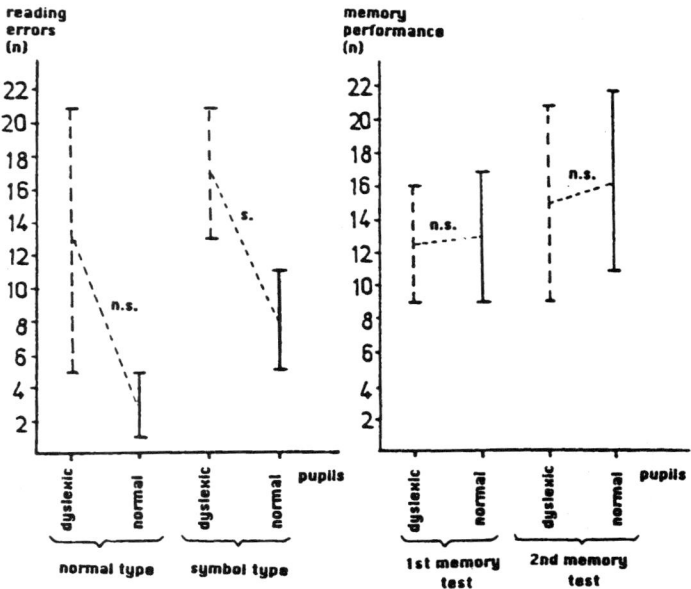

FIGURE 3. (b) Differential comparisons of learning effects on the basis of second reading learning with a new graphical code.

indications of a dyslexia-specific deficit in regard to semantic representation. All differences with the normal group are not significant, and in comparison to the speech-disturbed children, dyslexic children have a significantly higher value in the recognition of intraconceptual relations.

The second part of our research program is directed at the *long-term effects* of the rehabilitative classes in regard to compensation of partial perceptive, cognitive, and memory deficits, and with reference to the development of the whole personality of dyslexic children. We studied children in the seventh grade, using the memory of a new graphemic code and its learning-contingent retrieval when reading. The second reading learning on the basis of graphemic–phonetic recoding involved six learning steps and two memory tests. The learning course and the efficiency of the working memory are represented in eye movement and time parameters. The two groups are intelligence homogeneous (see FIG. 3). No group differences were found in the two recall tests of the new graphemic code [see FIG. 3(b)]. This does not mean, however, that for the dyslexics the visual code stored was as readily retrievable and usable during the reading act as it was for the normals. Dyslexic children show a significantly higher number of reading errors. The learning patterns of the two groups became similar, but level differences remained clear-cut, especially in regard to eye movement and time parameters. The two groups have the same recall capacity, but differ in retrieval when processing units sequentially [see FIG. 3(a)]. These results also refer to a dyslexia-specific deficit in working memory, and it seems to be highly therapy-resistant (Witruk, Staats 1983).

The question of long-term effects in regard to compensation or to therapy resistance of deficits in long-term memory parameters is especially connected with the orthography performances of dyslexic children. We investigated the inner repre-

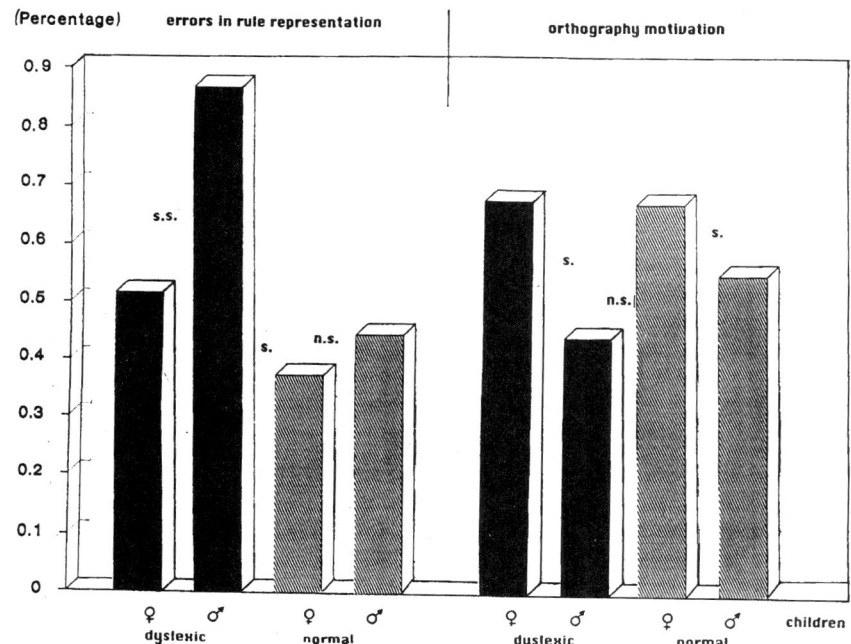

FIGURE 4. Differential analysis of representation of a hierarchical orthographical rule system and orthographical motivation of pupils in eighth grade. (From Witruk *et al.* (1990). Reproduced by permission.)

sentation and the use of a hierarchic orthographic rule system (capitalization of verbs) in eighth grade pupils at normal secondary schools and in pupils in the same grade, who learned in special classes for dyslexics in grades 2 and 3 (Witruk, Knotek, Altenkirch 1990) (see FIG. 4). On the basis of a gap-text investigation, we found that dyslexic children, according to gender and motivation, have significant deficits in using orthographical rules. Girls seems to be more able to compensate for partial performance disturbances. We have to consider these results as therapy-resistant deficits in using procedural orthographical knowledge.

To sum up, our results show memory deficits as acute primary symptoms, and in later years as therapy-resistant symptoms, especially in regard to restrictions in working memory in sequential processing demands. We have not found long-term deficits in regard to semantic representations, but some indications for therapy-resistant deficits in procedural orthographical knowledge.

REFERENCES

1. WITRUK, E., H. J. MUSIOL & F. PIONTEK. 1991. Underachievement and dyslexia—Conditions and specific problems of development. Paper presented at the 11th Biennial Meeting of ISSBD, Minneapolis, Minn.
2. WITRUK, E. 1992. The specific of memory deficits on dyslexic children. Paper presented at the 25th International Conference on Psychology, Brussels.

The Directional Motor Link in Reading Disabilities[a]

ROWE A. YOUNG AND BENSON E. GINSBURG

Biobehavioral Sciences Graduate Degree Program/Psychology
The University of Connecticut
Storrs, Connecticut 06269-4154

INTRODUCTION

Where reading disabilities occur in persons of average-to-superior intelligence, these are often associated with a lack of motor directionality and a mixed constellation of motor and perceptual patterns. We have been working to develop an instrument to assess these patterns. During the past several years, we have been interested in observing and measuring various rotational and lateral behavior patterns in normal and learning-disabled (LD) subjects. In our past work with several hundred such subjects[1,2] we reported that inconsistency in fine motor bimanual behavior was associated with male academic underachievement. We also found that this profile applied to female subjects only when other characteristics, such as inverted left handedness for writing, was included in the profile. During the process of testing these past samples, we began to notice interesting differences from the norm in some subjects showing inconsistent patterns. One such difference was a preference for using the bottom hand to perform a bimanual, three-dimensional rotation task. This preference was associated with a history of learning disability. Curiously, some of our subjects were found to have an unusual arm characteristic that we have never seen reported in the literature on this subject. This characteristic is the ability to rotate the arm so it faces outward without a corresponding movement in the hand region when hyperextending the arm. A few of the subjects stated that the arm felt that it was "backwards" in a directional sense.

The subjects also reported reading and writing difficulties. These observations led us to suspect that what we had previously labeled as inconsistency in performing a rotational motor task was actually a manifestation of an inverted spatial motor feedback that contributed to expressive and receptive written language disabilities. In the present analysis, we present our results based on the newly designed subtests used to help identify these additional characteristics.

POPULATION

The sample population was derived from a private suburban Connecticut day school with a good mix of male and females, both LD diagnosed and reportedly non-LD. We used a middle school population consisting of 47 females and 49 males ($n = 96$). Twenty-four percent of the males were considered "normal" learners and

---

[a]This research was supported in part by grants from The University of Connecticut Research Foundation.

27 percent were diagnosed as LD; 37 percent of the females were considered "normal" learners and 13 percent were diagnosed as LD.

METHODS

Portions of our test battery (Young-Ginsburg Lateral Direction Assessment) were administered to this population to whose diagnoses we, the testers, were blind. The tests were administered in a classroom setting. The procedures described are only for the tasks we used for this report.

Bimanual, Three-dimensional Rotation Task

A bimanual, three-dimensional rotation task was executed by first presenting a small container (one-inch-diameter cap) to each student. The students were then asked to try each possible pattern for unscrewing the lid. These patterns were first demonstrated and then described on the answer sheets they were furnished. They were then instructed to mark each answer that felt both comfortable and familiar.

Arm Hyperrotation Identification

The students were asked to stretch their arms down at their sides as stiffly as possible. As each student tried this, we looked for a turning motion in the elbow region. The hand and wrist will not turn as this motion occurs. In a relaxed position, the arms appear to be alike. In the stiffened position, they are unquestionably dissimilar in appearance. Every student who was found to have arm hyperrotation was noted.

We then divided our total sample by, first, gender and then by the bimanual, three-dimensional rotation categories of (1) consistently performing the task with the left hand on top; (2) inverting the performing hand (this group could also contain any other answer along with "inverted"); (3) consistently performing the task with the right hand on top; (4) either right hand or left hand on top. [Four males and three females were classified as either left or right (ambilateral) without being "inverted." Because these groups were statistically insignificant, they are not included in this report.] After the testing sessions were completed, the school provided information describing the subjects either as "normal" learners or certified learning disableds. The students were also given a battery of aptitude and achievement tests (ERB, 1982).[3] For our analysis, we used the mean of each of the ERB aptitude–achievement subtests for each of the three groups analyzed according to gender and LD status [see FIG. 1(a) and (b)].

RESULTS

The higher achieving LD male group ($n = 12$) was characterized by both display and self-description of preference for using an inverted hand position when unscrewing the lid. No non-LD male subjects were found to use this schema comfortably. Only five of the twelve LD females in the sample preferred an inverted hand

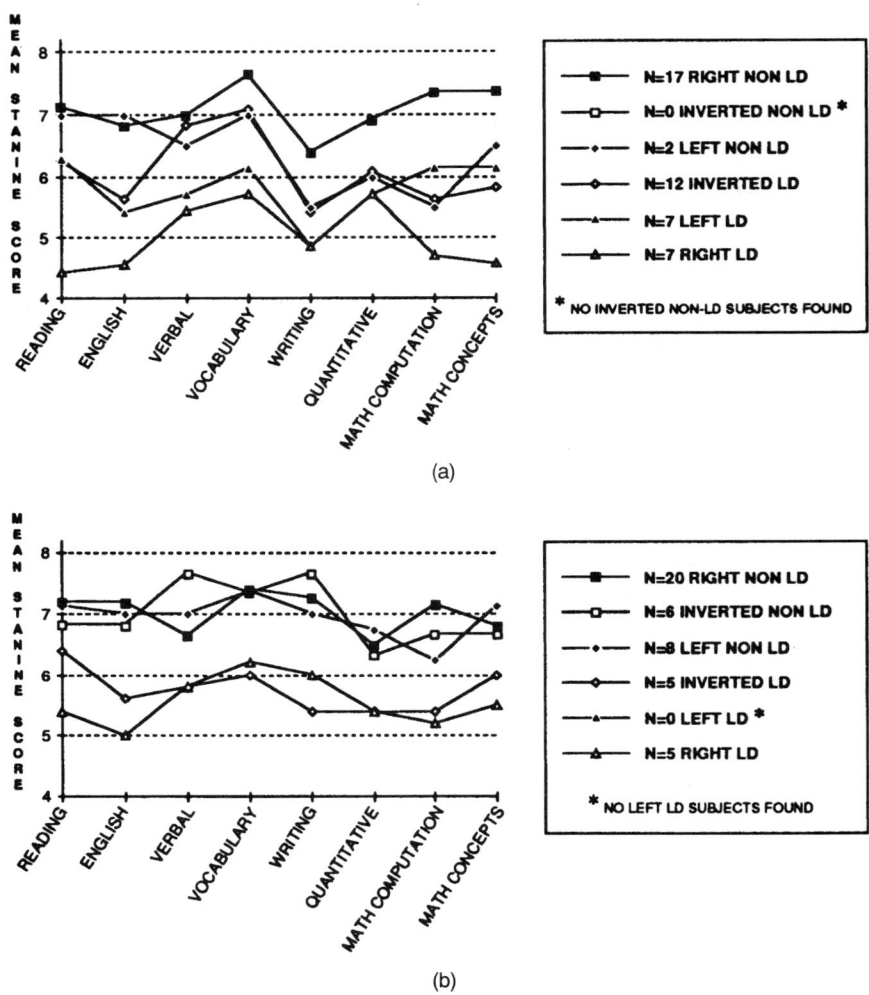

FIGURE 1. ERB Aptitude and Achievement Tests compared to bimanual rotation task. (a) Males. (b) Females.

position when performing this task and, unlike the male population, non-LD identified females ($n = 6$) were also found with this characteristic. Seven of the nine males who consistently used the left hand in the top position were found to be LD. None of the females using this pattern ($n = 8$) were diagnosed as LD. Right top-hand consistent rotators are both the highest and the lowest achieving populations in the male groups, while males with left and inverted rotational preference patterns fluctuate irregularly in between. Six of the seven students with hyperrotated arms were also diagnosed as LD.

DISCUSSION

Using the bimanual, three-dimensional rotation task, we have managed to separate the diagnosed LD male students with a higher mean level of standardized academic achievement from the lower achieving LD males. That there were no non-LD males who demonstrated use or reported preference for an inverted hand position out of forty-nine males tested is highly significant. That both the highest and the lowest achieving groups in the male population are "right-consistent" argues that another factor is involved in the overall achievement problems for the right-consistent LD groups. Male LD students in the "inverted" and "left" groups were characterized by problems in the written language aspects of achievement. This argues that their problem may be primarily the result of a maladaptive motor pattern involving aberrant feedback. Based upon this one subtest, there are marked differences in the association between the bimanual, three-dimensional rotation patterns and learning disability between the sexes. As mentioned, five of the twelve females in our sample were LD with the inverted rotation characteristic. Unlike the non-LD inverted rotation female group, they, like our previous samples, demonstrated the other unusual hand use characteristics, such as mixed handedness. In viewing the figures, the similarly shaped (unlike the males), relatively flat female LD profiles seem to argue for a different neurological motor organization affecting language between the sexes. The female groups also cluster into only two aggregates, LD and non-LD, by contrast with the males, who fall into three patterns. We also present evidence from a five-generation pedigree of a genetic etiology involving this directional motor link as well as a physical marker (hyperrotation of the arm) for this link.

REFERENCES

1. YOUNG, R. A. & B. E. GINSBURG. 1987. Genetic variations in motor and cognitive patterns associated with reading disabilities—Diagnosis and remediation (Abstract). Behav. Genet. **17:** 644.
2. ———. 1989. Motor directionality as a tool for diagnosis and remediation in reading disabilities. Paper presented at the Second National Scientific Conference on Jewish Children and Young Adults with Learning Disabilities, New York, March.
3. EDUCATIONAL RECORDS BUREAU. 1982. The Educational Records Bureau Aptitude and Achievement Tests; Level 4-Form C. Educational Testing Service, Princeton, N.J.

Index of Contributors

Ahonen, T., 380–382
Altmann, G., 272–282
Arezzo, J. C., 415–417
Aro, M., 380–382
Ashe, J., 179–191

Benasich, A. A., 312–314
Bennett, H. W., 315–317
Bowers, P. G., 318–320
Breznitz, Z., 321–322
Broman, M., 323–325
Brown, C. P., 346–347
Bruck, M., 351–353

Cavanagh, P., 351–353
Chase, C., 326–329
Chattopadhyay, A. K., 342–345
Christophe, A., 272–282
Cornelissen, P., 330–332
Curtiss, S., 359–362

Denckla, M. B., 23–26
Duane, D. D., 333–334
Dudley, J. G., 348–350
Dupoux, E., 272–282

Eden, G. F., 335–338
Edwards, J. H., 393–396

Farmer, M. E., 339–341
Fawcett, A. J., 342–345, 387–389, 390–392
Fitch, R. H., 27–46, 346–347
Fortin, J., 348–350
Fowler, S., 330–332

Galaburda, A., 70–82, 402–403
Georgopoulos, A. P., 179–191
Ginsburg, B. E., 436–439
Goswami, U., 296–311

Havu, S., 380–382

Hayduk, S., 351–353
Hodgson, J. M., 354–356
Holopainen, E., 380–382
Hutchens, T. A., 357–358

Ingvar, D. H., 240–247
Ivry, R., 214–230

Jacobsson, C., 231–239
Jarratt, J. A., 342–345
Jenkins, W., 1–22
Jenner, A. R., 326–329
Joanette, Y., 348–350
Johnson, G., 354–356

Kandler, R. H., 342–345
Katz, W. F., 359–362
Kegl, J., 192–213
Kemp, S. L., 363–365
Kennedy, A., 318–320
Kirk, U., 363–365
Klein, R., 339–341
Kraft, R. H., 366–368
Kris, E. C., 369–376
Kuhl, P. K., 248–263

Lauter, J. L, 377–379
Leinonen, S., 380–382
Lennerstrand, G., 231–239
Levelt, W. J. M., 283–295
Liberman, A. M., 264–271
Livingstone, M., 70–82
Llinás, R., 48–56
Lovegrove, W., 57–69
Lyytinen, H., 380–382

Marmolejo, A., 383–386
Martos, F. J., 383–386
Mason, A., 330–332
Mehler, J., 272–282
Merzenich, M. M., 1–22
Miller, S., 27–46
Moore, B. C. J., 119–136
Mountcastle, V. B., 150–170

Nicolson, R. I., 342–345, 387–389, 390–392

Pallier, C., 272–282
Parkinson, S. E., 393–396
Pestalozzi, D., 397–399
Phillips, D. P., 104–118
Poizner, H., 192–213
Proctor, M., 342–345

Ransil, B. J., 402–403
Read, H. L., 171–178
Richardson, A. J., 400–401

Schachter, S. C., 402–403
Schoepf, D., 404–408
Schreiner, C., 1–22
Schroeder, C. E., 415–417
Sebastian, N., 272–282
Siegel, R. M., 171–178
Staunton, A. M., 409–411
Sefanatos, G. A., 412–414
Stein, J. F., 83–86, 330–332, 335–338, 400–401

Steinschneider, M., 415–417

Tallal, P., ix, 27–46, 312–314, 346–347, 359–362
Trehub, S. E., 137–149

Vaughan, H. G., Jr., 415–417

Wang, X., 1–22
Watson, B. U., 418–420, 421–423
Watson, C. S., 418–420, 421–423
Whyte, J., 424–425
Witruk, E., 426–429, 430–435
Wolff, P. H., 87–103
Wood, F. B., 335–338
Wood, M. H., 335–338
Wood, S. B., 377–379

Ygge, J., 231–239
Young, R. A., 436–439

Zangemeister, W. H., 404–408